AF598422

Methods in Neurosciences

Volume 21

Providing Pharmacological Access to the Brain: Alternate Approaches

Methods in Neurosciences

Editor-in-Chief

P. Michael Conn

Methods in Neurosciences

Volume 21

Providing Pharmacological Access to the Brain: Alternate Approaches

Edited by

Thomas R. Flanagan
Chatham Associates
Barrington, Rhode Island

Dwaine F. Emerich
Shelley R. Winn
CytoTherapeutics
Providence, Rhode Island

ACADEMIC PRESS
San Diego New York Boston London Sydney Tokyo Toronto

Front cover photograph: Fluorescent photomicrograph of galactocerebroside-positive oligodendrocytes (green) double labeled with the nuclear stain Hoechst 33258 (blue). Cells were derived from a continuous line of epidermal growth factor-stimulated neuroepithelial cells. Courtesy of Dr. Malcolm Schinstine, CytoTherapeutics, Inc., Providence, Rhode Island.

This book is printed on acid-free paper. ♾

Academic Press, Inc.
A Division of Harcourt Brace & Company
525 B Street, Suite 1900, San Diego, California 92101-4495

United Kingdom Edition published by
Academic Press Limited
24-28 Oval Road, London NW1 7DX

International Standard Serial Number: 1043-9471

International Standard Book Number: 0-12-185291-1

PRINTED IN THE UNITED STATES OF AMERICA
94 95 96 97 98 99 EB 9 8 7 6 5 4 3 2 1

Table of Contents

Contributors to Volume 21 ix

Preface xv

Volumes in Series xvii

Section I Characterizing the Blood–Brain Barrier

1. Cellular Response of Central Nervous System Tissue to Invasive Therapeutic Measures 3
Ann Logan and Martin Berry

2. Models of Angiogenesis and the Blood–Brain Barrier 20
Jeffrey M. Rosenstein and Janette M. Krum

Section II Transiently Removing the Blood–Brain Barrier

3. Osmotic Opening of the Blood–Brain Barrier and Brain Tumor Chemotherapy 35
Peter J. Robinson

4. Osmotic Blood–Brain Barrier Modification: Increasing Delivery of Diagnostic and Therapeutic Agents to the Brain 52
Edward A. Neuwelt and Robert A. Kroll

Section III Facilitated Transport through the Blood–Brain Barrier

5. Peripheral Administration of Nerve Growth Factor Conjugated to an Anti-transferrin Receptor Antibody Increases Cholinergic Neuron Survival in Intraocular Forebrain Transplants 71
Ann-Charlotte Granholm, Paul T. Biddle, Cristina Bäckman, Ted Ebendal, Greg Gerhardt, Barry Hoffer, Ludmila Mackerlova, Lars Olson, Stine Söderström, Lee Walus, and Phillip Friden

6. Ferrotransferrin and Antibody against the Transferrin Receptor as Potential Vehicles for Drug Delivery across the Mammalian Blood–Brain Barrier into the Central Nervous System 93
Richard D. Broadwell, Belinda J. Baker, William A. Banks, Phillip Friden, Majorie Moran, Constance Oliver, and Juan C. Villegas

7. Depofoam-Mediated Drug Delivery into Cerebrospinal Fluid 118
Sinil Kim

Section IV Polymeric Release Systems for the Central Nervous System

8. Interstitial Drug Delivery to the Central Nervous System Using Controlled Release Polymers: Chemotherapy for Brain Tumors 135
Rafael J. Tamargo, Robert Langer, and Henry Brem

9. Sustained Intracerebral Delivery of Nerve Growth Factor with Biodegradable Polymer Microspheres 150
Alejandro Mendez, Paul J. Camarata, Raj Suryanarayanan, and Timothy J. Ebner

10. Polymeric Drug Carrier Systems in the Brain 169
Abraham J. Domb and Israel Ringel

Section V Using Pump Delivery Devices within the Brain

11. Using Osmotic Minipumps for Intracranial Delivery of Amino Acids and Peptides 187
Jeffrey D. White and Michael W. Schwartz

12. Continuous Central Nervous System Infusion with Alzet Osmotic Pumps 201
Theo Hagg

13. Injection of Biologically Active Substances into the Brain 214
Paul M. Carvey, Terrence J. Maag, and Donghui Lin

Section VI Using Implanted Living Tissues within the Brain

14. Factors Important in the Survival of Dopamine Neurons in Intracerebral Grafts of Embryonic Substantia Nigra 237
Roger Barker, Rosemary Fricker, and Steven B. Dunnett

15. Techniques in Adrenal Medullary Transplantation for Experimental Nonhuman Primate Parkinsonism 253
Massimo S. Fiandaca and Jeffrey H. Kordower

16. Technical Aspects of Transplantation of the Adrenal Medulla to the Caudate Nucleus as a Treatment for Parkinson's Disease 272
Stephen W. Carmichael, Susan L. Stoddard, and Patrick J. Kelly

Section VII Creating Cell Lines for Transplant Therapies

17. Transplantation of Epidermal Growth Factor-Responsive Neural Stem Cell Progeny into the Murine Central Nervous System 281
Joseph P. Hammang, Brent A. Reynolds, Samuel Weiss, Albee Messing, and Ian D. Duncan

18. Application of Astrocyte Transplants as a Therapeutic Intervention 294
J. Patrick Kesslak and Richard J. Bridges

19. Development of Immortalized Cell Lines for Transplantation in Central Nervous System Injury and Degeneration Models 308
M. Giordano, H. Takashima, M. Poltorak, H. M. Geller, and W. J. Freed

Section VIII Using Implanted Living Cells within the Central Nervous System

20. Use of Genetically Modified Cells to Deliver Neurotrophic Factors and Neurotransmitters to the Brain 329
Lisa J. Fisher, Gordon R. Chalmers, and Fred H. Gage

21. Neuropeptide and Catecholamine Delivery to the Central Nervous System by Implanted Chromaffin Cells 348
Jacqueline Sagen, John D. Ortega, and George D. Pappas

Section IX Using Implanted Encapsulated Cells within the Brain

22. Microencapsulation of Cells in Thermoplastic Copolymer (Hydroxyethyl Methacrylate-Methyl Methacrylate) 371
M. V. Sefton, H. Uludag, J. Babensee, T. Roberts, V. Horvath, and U. De Boni

23. Hydrogel Applications for Encapsulated Cellular Transplants 387
Shelley R. Winn and Patrick A. Tresco

24. Test for Validating the Safety of Encapsulated Xenografts 403
T. R. Flanagan, B. Frydel, B. Tente, M. Lavoie, E. Doherty, D. Rein, D. F. Emerich, and S. R. Winn

Section X Induced Gene Expression in Intrinsic Central Nervous System Cells with DNA Injected into the Brain

25. Particle Bombardment for Gene Transfer into Nerve Cell Systems 427
Ning-Sun Yang, Shoushu Jiao, and Carolyn De Luna

Section XI Viral Transfection of Intrinsic Cells within the Brain

26. A Defective Herpes Simplex Virus Vector System for Genetic Intervention in the Adult Brain: Applications to Gene Therapy and Neuronal Physiology 443
Alfred I. Geller, Mathew J. During, and Rachael Neve

27. Expression of Neurotropic Factor Genes from Herpes Simplex Virus Type 1 Vectors: Modifying Neuronal Phenotype 462
Michael D. Geschwind, Bing Lu, and Howard Federoff

Section XII Predicting the Future of Central Nervous System Delivery System Technologies

28. Assessing the Commercial Potential of Central Nervous System Delivery Approaches 485
John S. Swen, Thomas R. Flanagan, and Thomas G. Wiggans

Index 499

Contributors to Volume 21

Article numbers are in parentheses following the names of contributors. Affiliations listed are current.

J. BABENSEE (22), Departments of Chemical Engineering and Applied Chemistry, Center for Biomaterials, University of Toronto, Toronto, Ontario, Canada M5S 1A4

CRISTINA BÄCKMAN (5), Department of Basic Science, University of Colorado Health Sciences Center, Denver, Colorado 80262

BELINDA J. BAKER (6), Laboratory of Molecular Medicine and Neuroscience, National Institute of Neurological Diseases and Stroke, National Institutes of Health, Bethesda, Maryland 20892

WILLIAM BANKS (6), Section of Medicine, Veterans Affairs Medical Center, New Orleans, Lousiana 70146, and Department of Medicine, Tulane University, School of Medicine, New Orleans, Louisiana 70118

ROGER BARKER (14), MRC Cambridge Centre for Brain Repair, and Department of Experimental Psychology, University of Cambridge, Cambridge CB2 3EB, United Kingdom

MARTIN BERRY (1), Department of Anatomy and Cell Biology, United Medical and Dental Schools, London SE1 9RT, United Kingdom

PAUL T. BIDDLE (5), Department of Basic Science, University of Colorado Health Sciences Center, Denver, Colorado 80262

HENRY BREM (8), Department of Neurosurgery, The Johns Hopkins University School of Medicine, Baltimore, Maryland 21287

RICHARD J. BRIDGES (18), Department of Pharmaceutical Science, School of Pharmacy, University of Montana, Missoula, Montana 59812

RICHARD D. BROADWELL (6), Office of Research Integrity, U.S. Public Health Service, Rockville, Maryland 20852

PAUL J. CAMARATA (9), Department of Neurosurgery, University of Minnesota, Minneapolis, Minnesota 55455

STEPHEN W. CARMICHAEL (16), Department of Anatomy, Mayo Clinic/ Mayo Foundation, Rochester, Minnesota 55905

PAUL M. CARVEY (13), Department of Neurological Sciences, Neuropharmacology Research Laboratories, Rush-Presbyterian-St. Luke's Medical Center, Chicago, Illinois 60612

GORDON R. CHALMERS (20), Department of Neurosciences, University of California, San Diego, La Jolla, California 92093

U. DE BONI (22), Department of Physiology, University of Toronto, Toronto, Ontario, Canada M5S 1A4

E. DOHERTY (24), CytoTherapeutics, Inc., Providence, Rhode Island 02906

ABRAHAM J. DOMB (10), Department of Pharmaceutical Chemistry and the Department of Pharmacology, School of Pharmacy, Faculty of Medicine, The Hebrew University of Jerusalem, Jerusalem, Israel 91120

IAN D. DUNCAN (17), School of Veterinary Medicine, University of Wisconsin—Madison, Madison, Wisconsin 53706

STEPHEN B. DUNNETT (14), MRC Cambridge Centre for Brain Repair, and Department of Experimental Psychology, University of Cambridge, Cambridge CB2 3EB, United Kingdom

MATHEW J. DURING (26), Neuroendocrine Program, Yale University School of Medicine, New Haven, Connecticut 06510

TED EBENDAL (5), Department of Developmental Biology, Uppsala University, S-751 23 Uppsala, Sweden

TIMOTHY J. EBNER (9), Department of Neurosurgery, University of Minnesota, Minneapolis, Minnesota 55455

D. F. EMERICH (24), CytoTherapeutics, Inc., Providence, Rhode Island 02906

HOWARD FEDEROFF (27), Departments of Medicine and Neuroscience, Albert Einstein College of Medicine, Bronx, New York 10461

MASSIMO S. FIANDACA (15), Department of Neurosurgery, The Johns Hopkins Medical Center, Baltimore, Maryland 21287

LISA J. FISHER (20), Department of Neurosciences, University of California, San Diego, La Jolla, California 92093

THOMAS R. FLANAGAN (24, 28), Chatham Associates, Barrington, Rhode Island 02806

W. J. FREED (19), National Institute of Mental Health, National Institute of Health, Neuroscience Center at St. Elizabeths, Washington, D. C. 20032

ROSEMARY FRICKER (14), MRC Cambridge Centre for Brain Repair, and Department of Experimental Psychology, University of Cambridge, Cambridge CB2 3EB, United Kingdom

PHILLIP FRIDEN (5, 6), Alkermes, Inc., Cambridge, Massachusetts 02139

B. FRYDEL (24), CytoTherapeutics, Inc., Providence, Rhode Island 02906

FRED H. GAGE (20), Department of Neurosciences, University of California, San Diego, La Jolla, California 92093

ALFRED I. GELLER (26), Division of Endocrinology, Children's Hospital, Boston, Massachusetts 02115

H. M. GELLER (19), Department of Pharmacology, University of Medicine and Dentistry at New Jersey, Robert Wool Johnson Medical School, Piscataway, New Jersey 08854

GREG GERHARDT (5), Departments of Pharmacology and Psychiatry, University of Colorado Health Sciences Center, Denver, Colorado 80262

MICHAEL D. GESCHWIND (27), Departments of Medicine and Neuroscience, Albert Einstein College of Medicine, Bronx, New York 10461

M. GIORDANO (19), National Institute of Mental Health, National Institute of Health, Neuroscience Center at St. Elizabeths, Washington, D. C. 20032

ANN-CHARLOTTE GRANHOLM (5), Department of Basic Science, University of Colorado Health Sciences Center, Denver, Colorado 80262

THEO HAGG (12), Department of Anatomy and Neurobiology, Dalhousie University, Halifax, Nova Scotia, Canada B3H 4H7

JOSEPH P. HAMMANG (17), Cell and Molecular Neurobiology, CytoTherapeutics, Inc., Providence, Rhode Island 02906

BARRY HOFFER (5), Departments of Pharmacology and Psychiatry, University of Colorado Health Sciences Center, Denver, Colorado 80262

V. HORVATH (22), Departments of Chemical Engineering and Applied Chemistry, Center for Biomaterials, University of Toronto, Toronto, Ontario, Canada M5S 1A4

SHOUSHU JIAO (25), Department of Pediatrics and Medical Genetics, Waisman Center, University of Wisconsin–Madison, Wisconsin 53705

PATRICK J. KELLY (16), Department of Neurologic Surgery, Mayo Clinic/Mayo Foundation, Rochester, Minnesota 55905

J. PATRICK KESSLAK (18), Department of Neurology, I.R.U. in Brain Aging, University of California, Irvine, Irvine, California 92717

SINIL KIM (7), DepoTech, La Jolla, California 92037

JEFFREY H. KORDOWER (15), Department of Neurological Sciences, Rush-Presbyterian-St. Luke's Medical Center, Chicago, Illinois 60612

ROBERT A. KROLL (4), Department of Neurology, School of Medicine, Oregon Health Sciences University, Portland, Oregon 97201

JANETTE M. KRUM (2), Departments of Anatomy and Neurosurgery, The George Washington University Medical Center, Washington, D. C. 20037

ROBERT LANGER (8), Department of Chemical Engineering, The Massachusetts Institute of Technology, Boston, Massachusetts 02139

M. LAVOIE (24), CytoTherapeutics, Inc., Providence, Rhode Island 02906

DONGHUI LIN (13), Department of Neurological Sciences, Neuropharmacology Research Laboratories, Rush-Presbyterian-St. Luke's Medical Center, Chicago, Illinois 60612

ANN LOGAN (1), Department of Clinical Chemistry, University of Birmingham, Birmingham B15 2TT, United Kingdom

BING LU (27), Departments of Medicine and Neuroscience, Albert Einstein College of Medicine, Bronx, New York 10461

CAROLYN DE LUNA (25), Mammalian Genetics, Agracetus, Inc., Middleton, Wisconsin 53562

TERRENCE J. MAAG (13), Department of Neurological Sciences, Neuropharmacology Research Laboratories, Rush-Presbyterian-St. Luke's Medical Center, Chicago, Illinois 60612

LUDMILA MACKERLOVA (5), Department of Cell Biology, University of Linkoping, Faculty of Health Sciences, S-581 85 Linkoping, Sweden

ALEJANDRO MENDEZ (9), Department of Neurosurgery, University of Minnesota, Minneapolis, Minnesota 55455

ALBEE MESSING (17), School of Veterinary Medicine, University of Wisconsin—Madison, Madison, Wisconsin 53706

MARJORIE MORAN (6), Alkermes, Inc., Cambridge, Massachusetts 02139

EDWARD A. NEUWELT (4), Departments of Neurology, Surgery, and Biochemistry and Molecular Biology, Division of Neurosurgery, School of Medicine, Oregon Health Sciences University, Portland, Oregon 97201

RACHAEL NEVE (26), Molecular Neurogenetics Laboratory, McLean Hospital, Belmont, Massachusetts 02178

CONSTANCE OLIVER (6), National Institute for Dental Research, National Institutes of Health, Bethesda, Maryland 20892

LARS OLSON (5), Department of Histology and Neurobiology, Karolinska Institute, S-104 01 Stockholm, Sweden

JOHN D. ORTEGA (21), Department of Anatomy and Cell Biology, University of Illinois, Chicago, Chicago, Illinois 60612

GEORGE D. PAPPAS (21), Department of Anatomy and Cell Biology, University of Illinois, Chicago, Chicago, Illinois 60612

M. POLTORAK (19), National Institute of Mental Health, National Institute of Health, Neuroscience Center at St. Elizabeths, Washington, D. C. 20032

D. REIN (24), CytoTherapeutics, Inc., Providence, Rhode Island 02906

BRENT A. REYNOLDS (17), NeuroSpheres Ltd., Calgary, Alberta, Canada T2N 4N1

ISRAEL RINGEL (10), Department of Pharmaceutical Chemistry and the Department of Pharmacology, School of Pharmacy, Faculty of Medicine, The Hebrew University of Jerusalem, Jerusalem, Israel 91120

T. ROBERTS (22), Departments of Chemical Engineering and Applied Chemistry, Center for Biomaterials, University of Toronto, Toronto, Ontario, Canada M5S 1A4

PETER J. ROBINSON (3), Miami Valley Laboratories, The Procter & Gamble Company, Cincinnati, Ohio 45239

JEFFREY M. ROSENSTEIN (2), Departments of Anatomy and Neurosurgery, The George Washington University Medical Center, Washington, D. C. 20037

JACQUELINE SAGEN (21), Department of Anatomy and Cell Biology, University of Illinois, Chicago, Chicago, Illinois 60612

MICHAEL W. SCHWARTZ (11), Division of Endocrinology and Metabolism, Department of Medicine, University of Washington and Veterans Administration Medical Center, Seattle, Washington 98108

M. V. SEFTON (22), Departments of Chemical Engineering and Applied Chemistry, Center for Biomaterials, University of Toronto, Toronto, Ontario, Canada M5S 1A4

STINE SÖDERSTRÖM (5), Department of Developmental Biology, Uppsala University, S751 23 Uppsala, Sweden

SUSAN L. STODDARD (16), Department of Anatomy, Indiana University School of Medicine, Fort Wayne, Illinois 46805

RAJ SURYANARAYANAN (9), Department of Pharmaceutics, University of Minnesota, Minneapolis, Minnesota 55455

JOHN S. SWEN (28), CytoTherapeutics, Inc., Providence, Rhode Island 02906

H. TAKASHIMA (19), Kawatana National Hospital, Nagasaki 859-36, Japan

RAFAEL TAMARGO (8), Department of Neurosurgery, The Johns Hopkins University School of Medicine, Baltimore, Maryland 21287

B. TENTE (24), CytoTherapeutics, Inc., Providence, Rhode Island 02906

PATRICK A. TRESCO (23), Department of Bioengineering, University of Utah, Salt Lake City, Utah 84112

H. ULUDAG (22), Departments of Chemical Engineering and Applied Chemistry, Center for Biomaterials, University of Toronto, Toronto, Ontario, Canada M5S 1A4

JUAN VILLEGAS (6), Department of Cell Biology, Faculty of Medicine, University of Cantaberia, 39005 Santander, Spain

LEE WALUS (5), Alkermes, Inc., Cambridge, Massachusetts 02139

SAMUEL WEISS (17), Neuroscience Research Group, Faculty of Medicine, University of Calgary, Calgary, Alberta, Canada T2N 4N1

JEFFREY D. WHITE (11), Department of Cell Biology and Biochemistry, Trophix Pharmaceuticals, Inc., South Plainfield, New Jersey 07080

THOMAS G. WIGGANS (28), CytoTherapeutics, Inc., Providence, Rhode Island 02906

SHELLEY R. WINN (24, 23), CytoTherapeutics, Inc., Providence, Rhode Island 02906

NING-SUN YANG (25), Mammalian Genetics, Agracetus, Inc., Middleton, Wisconsin 53562, and Department of Pathology and Laboratory of Medicine, University of Wisconsin—Madison, Madison, Wisconsin 58705

Preface

This volume focuses on contemporary approaches for delivering experimental and therapeutic agents into the brain. Its unifying theme is appropriately reflected by its title: *Providing Pharmacological Access to the Brain: Alternate Approaches*.

Throughout the history of pharmacological research, the brain has presented a unique spectrum of problems for therapeutic manipulation. Given the large number of researchers currently active in this field together with the myriad of approaches being evaluated, it would be inappropriate to suggest that the scopes of activity across this field were fully reflected in this one volume. Rather, nontraditional experimental approaches have been chosen to illustrate rapidly developing therapeutic themes. To provide the reader with the best understanding of these approaches, we have included comparisons of similar experimental approaches taken by different groups. In instances where an alternate drug delivery theme seems particularly close to entering traditional practice, an appropriate overview has been included. In keeping with the spirit of this series, reviews are included only where they provide the reader with valuable insights into the evolution of the central nervous system drug delivery process. The contributions provide methodological details that are typically not available in the literature. Subtleties and shortcuts critical to each procedure are included to facilitate their use by both experienced researchers and students.

The volume is organized into twelve sections. Experimental characterization of the blood–brain barrier includes consideration of wound responses and vascularization. Two sections discuss means of circumventing the blood–brain barrier: one approach through transiently removing the barrier and a second by employing facilitated transfer through the barrier. Another is devoted to now broadly used infusion and pump strategies. Four sections describe drug delivery from cells implanted into the brain; one describes tissue transplants, another cell lines created for transplants, a third cell line transplants, and the fourth encapsulated cell transplants. Two sections consider approaches that promote therapeutic gene expression from intrinsic cells within the brain; one describes direct gene transfer and the second virus-mediated gene transfer into intrinsic cells. A final section discusses methods of identifying economic factors that can promote successful academic and corporate partnerships for funding central nervous system drug delivery programs.

All groups working on developing methods for delivering pharmacological agents to the brain share the same ultimate goal: improving the quality of life of individuals with neurological disorders. Some approaches are currently being evaluated in clinical trials, while others are still experimental and at the level of basic research. Within the brain, where drug delivery requirements may call for trace level dosing to precisely defined target sites, alternate delivery strategies will require the emergence of new validation philosophies. Means of conducting pharmacokinetic studies, dosimetry controls, and chronic delivery quantitation present special problems. With some classes of therapeutic agents (e.g., native hormones and transmitter substances), therapeutic windows are likely to be much wider than they are for conventional pharmaceuticals. Natural hormone-inactivating systems may lessen the demand for stringent dosage control within the central nervous system. Clearly, the use of natural products and their precursors as therapeutic agents delivered into the central nervous system represents a significant frontier in biomedical research. The methods included in this volume will doubtless play a key role in the growth of this field.

Thomas R. Flanagan
Dwaine F. Emerich
Shelley R. Winn

Methods in Neurosciences

Volume 1 Gene Probes
Edited by P. Michael Conn

Volume 2 Cell Culture
Edited by P. Michael Conn

Volume 3 Quantitative and Qualitative Microscopy
Edited by P. Michael Conn

Volume 4 Electrophysiology and Microinjection
Edited by P. Michael Conn

Volume 5 Neuropeptide Technology: Gene Expression and Neuropeptide Receptors
Edited by P. Michael Conn

Volume 6 Neuropeptide Technology: Synthesis, Assay, Purification, and Processing
Edited by P. Michael Conn

Volume 7 Lesions and Transplantation
Edited by P. Michael Conn

Volume 8 Neurotoxins
Edited by P. Michael Conn

Volume 9 Gene Expression in Neural Tissues
Edited by P. Michael Conn

Volume 10 Computers and Computations in the Neurosciences
Edited by P. Michael Conn

Volume 11 Receptors: Model Systems and Specific Receptors
Edited by P. Michael Conn

Volume 12 Receptors: Molecular Biology, Receptor Subclasses, Localization, and Ligand Design
Edited by P. Michael Conn

Volume 13 Neuropeptide Analogs, Conjugates, and Fragments
Edited by P. Michael Conn

Volume 14 Paradigms for the Study of Behavior
Edited by P. Michael Conn

Volume 15 Photoreceptor Cells
Edited by Paul A. Hargrave

Volume 16 Neurobiology of Cytokines (Part A)
Edited by Errol B. De Souza

Volume 17 Neurobiology of Cytokines (Part B)
Edited by Errol B. De Souza

Volume 18 Lipid Metabolism in Signaling Systems
Edited by John N. Fain

Volume 19 Ion Channels of Excitable Membranes
Edited by Toshio Narahashi

Volume 20 Pulsatility in Neuroendocrine Systems
Edited by Jon E. Levine

Volume 21 Providing Pharmacological Access to the Brain: Alternate Approaches
Edited by Thomas R. Flanagan, Dwaine F. Emerich, and Shelley R. Winn

Volume 22 Neurobiology of Steroids (in preparation)
Edited by E. Ronald deKloet and Win Sutanto

Volume 23 Peptidases and Neuropeptide Processing (in preparation)
Edited by A. Ian Smith

Volume 24 Neuroimmunology (in preparation)
Edited by M. Ian Phillips and Dwight E. Evans

Volume 25 Receptor Molecular Biology (in preparation)
Edited by Stuart C. Sealfen

Volume 26 PCR in Neuroscience (in preparation)
Edited by Gobinda Sarhar

Volume 27 G Proteins (in preparation)
Edited by Patrick C. Roche

Section I

Characterizing the Blood–Brain Barrier

[1] Cellular Response of Central Nervous System Tissue to Invasive Therapeutic Measures

Ann Logan and Martin Berry

Introduction

After injuries that penetrate either the mature brain or spinal cord, damaged neurons begin initially to regrow, but this regeneration is aborted as a permanent fibrotic scar is laid down that effectively reforms the glia limitans externa in the lesion area. Functional recovery from such injuries is poor and morbidity severe, particularly for those patients with spinal cord damage. Clinically, no long-term therapeutic treatments are available to inhibit scarring and promote nerve growth and reconnection of compromised nerve pathways. Consequently, the prevalence of patients permanently disabled from head and spinal cord injury is high, estimated at more than 1 : 1000 of the population of North America (Office of Technology Assessment USA, 1990). The lack of available treatment provides the impetus for further definition of the cellular and trophic mechanisms underlying nerve regeneration in laboratory models of neural injury.

Definition of Cellular Response to Injury

Mature Central Nervous System

The response to injury of the adult central nervous system (CNS) is characterized by two sequential and overlapping stages: one of acute hemorrhage and inflammation, the other of glial/collagen scar organization (1, 2). We have analyzed and defined the reaction of glial, mesodermal, and neural elements within cerebral lesions using immunohistochemical procedures.

Briefly, animals with lesions are anesthetized and perfused through their left ventricle at atmospheric pressure with the descending aorta clamped and both external jugular veins incised. Perfusion with physiological saline for 1 min is followed by fixative for 5 min. The fixative is 4% (w/v) glutaraldehyde in 0.1 *M* phosphate buffer, pH 7.2. The brain is removed from the cranium, and immersed in the same fixative for 1 hr at 4°C before washing in phosphate-

Methods in Neurosciences, Volume 21

buffered saline (PBS) overnight at 4°C. On the next day, brains are dehydrated in graded alcohols, embedded in a low melting point polyester wax (3, 4), and stored at 4°C. Sections, 7 μm thick, are cut through the lesion site on a microtome fitted with a cooled chuck and floated onto a gelatin solution (10 g/liter) on subbed slides and air dried.

The antibodies used to detect and identify cellular elements within lesions are commercially available and include rabbit anti-bovine glial fibrillary acidic protein (GFAP) to detect activated astrocytes; rabbit anti-carbonic anhydrase II (CAII) to identify oligodendrocytes; rabbit antibodies to antigens ED1 and OX42, which mark cells of the monocyte/macrophage/microglial lineage; and rabbit anti-mouse sarcoma laminin, rabbit anti-fibronectin, rabbit anti-collagen I, II, and IV, and monoclonal anti-chondroitin-6-sulfate proteoglycan, to detect matrix molecules. Regeneration is assessed using specific axonal markers, including a polyclonal antibody raised against the 200-kDa phosphorylated component of the neurofilament triplet (RT97), anti-growth-associated protein 43 (GAP-43), and anti-protein product PGP 9.5, an antibody to ubiquitin carboxy-terminal hydrolase. All dilutions are made in PBS containing 1% (w/v) bovine serum albumin (BSA).

Sections are dewaxed, rehydrated before soaking (or immersion) in PBS containing 0.1% (v/v) Tween 20 for 15 min, and then incubated in the specific primary antibody for 1–12 hr at room temperature. Slides are washed in three changes of PBS before incubation in the labeled secondary antibody for 1 hr; this antibody is goat anti-rabbit or anti-mouse IgG conjugated to fluorescein isothiocyanate (FITC) or tetramethylrhodamine isothiocyanate (TRITC). Sections are then washed in three changes of PBS and mounted in a nonquenching mountant. For controls, either the first or second antibody is omitted. Finally, sections are examined on a microscope with a fluorescent attachment and photomicrographs taken on Ilford HP5 film, rated 400 ISO.

By using such techniques we have identified the cellular changes that occur in the immediate postinjury response period. At first the lesion is hemorrhagic and extravasated platelets play a major role in initiating both clotting in the lesion lumen and vasoconstriction in the wound edges associated with edema and necrosis. Polymorphs, monocytes, and later macrophages appear in large numbers. Their concentration in the wound is probably controlled by a homing response organized both by platelet factors and also by the expression of addressins on the endothelium of the brain vasculature and counterreceptors on leukocytes, as elsewhere in the body (reviewed in Refs. 5–8), although little is known of the details of this process in the damaged CNS. By 3–5 days, most of the extravasated erythrocytes have disappeared. The wound and its margins are filled with macrophages, monocytes, and a few polymorphs. Fibroblasts and collagen fibers first appear at this stage to form a mesenchymal core in which extracellular matrix molecules, such as laminin and fibronectin, are deposited. The necrotic neuropil at the mesenchyme–CNS parenchymal interface is also absorbed over the 3- to 5-day period and large numbers of reactive astrocytes, with upregulated GFAP expression, appear in the CNS surrounding the wound. Microglia, which become reactive at about 2 days, also accumulate in the same perilesion neuropil. Scar tissue is laid down between 5 and 8 days postinjury. The cytoplasmic processes of astrocytes become concentrated at the CNS–mesenchymal boundary, form a continuous multilayered sheet, and become locked together by tight junctions. Between those astrocytic processes and the mesenchymal core, a basal lamina is deposited, probably by the astrocytes under the influence of fibroblasts. Macrophages are lost from the mesenchymal core but much fibrous collagen and fibronectin is deposited by fibroblasts (see Fig. 1).

Central nervous system scarring essentially establishes a glia limitans in the wound (identical to and continuous with that of the external limiting membrane), composed of the mesenchymal elements of the leptomeninges externally, a basal lamina, and astrocytic end feet bound together by tight junctions internally. Fibroblasts in the central core of the lesion migrate in from the meninges. Thus, the scar matures sequentially from pial surface to the depths of the lesion. By 8–14 days, the scar is fully formed, the central mesenchymal core contracted, and the palisades of astrocyte processes compacted at the lesion margins. The GFAP activity in astrocytes declines, except at the wound margins. A small number of macrophages remain in the core but none are seen in the surrounding CNS tissue.

Embryonic/Neonatal Central Nervous System

The mature response to injury described above is acquired neonatally, in the rat for example, between 8 and 12 days postpartum (dpp) (1, 9). Before 8 dpp, no mesenchymal elements accumulate in the wound and, although some astrocytes become reactive, a glia limitans is not formed and the neuropil grows together, obliterating all signs of the original lesion. Typical scarring first appears at 8 dpp subpially and, over the next 4 days, invades the depths of the wound. Although the microglial response is qualitatively mature in the neonate, macrophage and fibroblast invasion from the pia into the wound is minimal. Curiously, however, the glia limitans externa is repaired after injury, even before 8 dpp. Clearly, understanding the biology of scar acquisition in the perinatal CNS could lead to a pharmacological strategy aimed at replicating the neonatal response to injury in the adult.

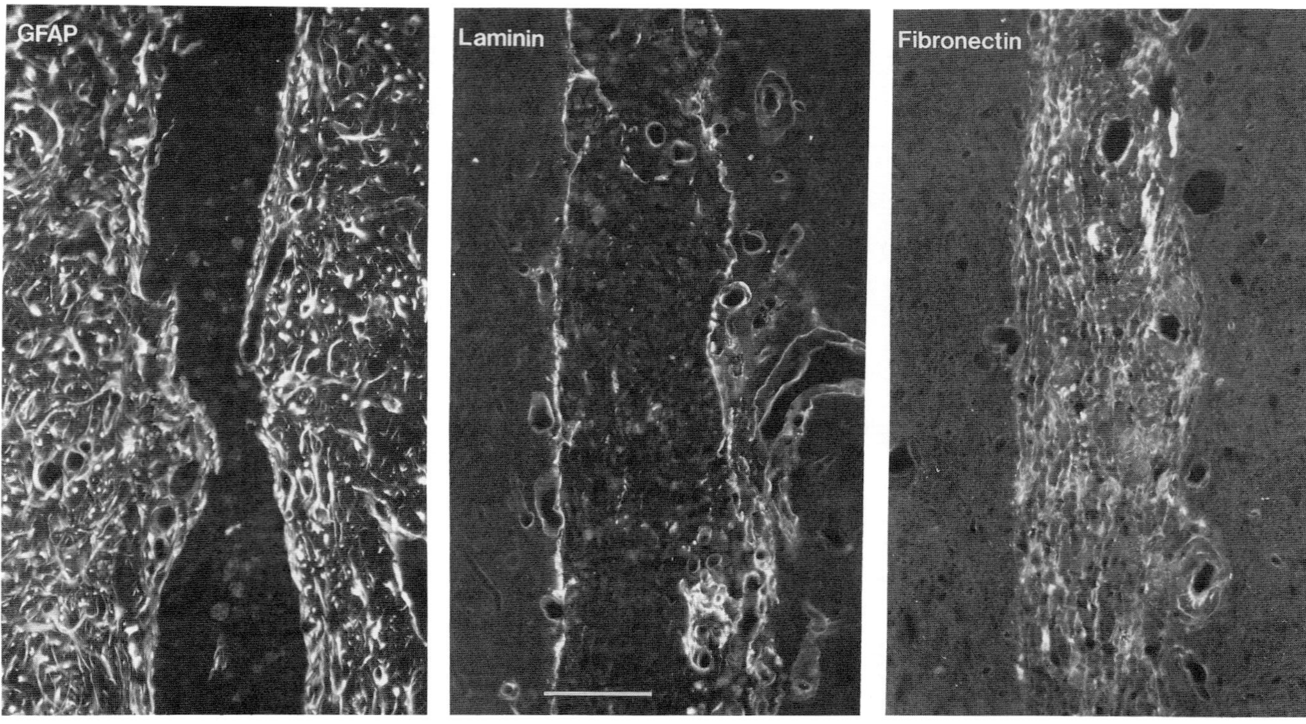

FIG. 1 Fourteen-day-old stereotactic lesion in the midcortical region of the cerebral cortex of an adult rat showing the astrocytic (GFAP) and matrix (laminin/fibronectin) responses. By 14 days, astrocytic processes have walled off the lesion site and their end feet have secreted a basal lamina (laminin), which lines the wound and is continuous with the glia limitans externa. The central core is filled with fibroblasts that secrete collagen and fibronectin. Bar: 300 μm.

Degeneration/Regeneration of Neurons and Their Processes

The classic response of mature neurons to injury is an initial sprouting reaction from the terminals of cut axons, followed by degeneration. By 16 days after injury, all newly grown processes have died back to their original parent axons, a large number of which remain *in situ* in perpetuity, making no further attempt to grow (10). It is not known if this abortive growth response of axons is also exhibited by dendrites. It is also not known why axons fail to sustain growth after injury. An early explanation was that growth arrest is scar related, because the cicatrix constitutes a physical barrier through which axons are unable to pass. But neuromata never form around a scar and, accordingly, this idea has received little support. Nonetheless, it is clear that if regeneration becomes a possibility, concomitant inhibition of scarring is essential if axons are to restore disconnected functional pathways.

A contemporary explanation for the failure of regeneration in the CNS is that glia, probably both astrocytes and oligodendrocytes (1), have surface membrane ligands that, when engaged by specific axonal membrane receptors, trigger the inhibition of growth by a Ca^{2+}-dependent intracellular signals (reviewed in Refs. 11 and 12). This hypothesis predicts successful regeneration in sites where either axonal receptors, glia ligands, or both are not expressed. For example, the florid regeneration of the axons from fetal brain grafts implanted into adult brain (13, 14) is probably explained if embryonic neurons do not express the receptor for the ligand on mature host glia about the transplant site in the adult brain.

It is generally held that neurons have an absolute dependency on trophic molecules for growth and survival. It is possible that, in the adult CNS, viability of neurons is maintained by a continuous flow of neurotrophic molecules derived from the target and retrogradely transported along the axon to the perikaryon. Some neuronal cell death always follows axonal damage. In neonates, the parent cell bodies are particularly sensitive to axotomy. In embryonic and neonatal retina, for example, almost all retinal ganglion cells die after transection of the optic nerve, whereas in adults 20–30% survive. Separating perikaryon from target might cause cell death if the neuron is thereby deprived of essential target-derived trophic factors. Differential viability of neural centers in the adult may be explained by differences in the degree of multiple-target innervation by collaterals.

Neural degeneration is probably augmented by the release of proteases from microglia amassing in the wound and surrounding neuropil in the acute postinjury period (15). Cell death may also be enhanced by activation of proteases by Ca^{2+} flooding into the wound area from the blood as the blood–brain barrier is breached. The *N*-methyl-D-aspartate (NMDA) receptor-mediated cytotoxicity associated with excitatory amino acid release immediately after trauma also contributes to neuronal cell death.

Definition of Trophic Mechanisms of Injury Response

The spatiotemporal trophic cascade that results from invasive injuries of the CNS and that regulates the subsequent cellular responses involves multiple paracrine regulatory factors. By using molecular hybridization and immunochemical techniques to analyze histological sections and extracts of damaged neural tissue, the individual elements of this cascade are beginning to be defined. If DNA probes and antibodies are available, methods such as Northern blotting, ribonuclease protection assays, and radioimmunoassays can quantify gross changes in specific populations of mRNA and protein. *In situ* hybridization and immunocytochemistry can localize the mRNA and protein at the cellular level.

Ribonuclease Protection Assay

Total RNA is extracted from snap-frozen CNS tissue using the RNAzol B method (protocol supplied in kit form by Cinna/Biotecx Laboratories, Inc., Houston, TX). For analysis, 10 μg of vacuum-dried, extracted total RNA is dissolved in 30 μl of hybridization solution [80% (v/v) formamide, 40 m*M* piperazine-*N*,*N'*-bis(2-ethanesulfonic acid) (PIPES), pH 6.4, 400 m*M* sodium chloride, and 1 m*M* ethylenediaminetetraacetic acid (EDTA)] containing 10^5 cpm of ^{32}P-labeled cRNA probes. After being heated to 85°C for 4 min, the cRNA probe is allowed to anneal to the endogenous RNA at 55°C overnight. At the end of hybridization, the solution is diluted with 350 μl of RNase digestion buffer [300 m*M* sodium chloride, 10 m*M* Tris (pH 7.4), and EDTA (pH 7.5)], containing RNase A (40 μg/ml) with RNase T_1 (500 U/ml), and incubated for 30 min at 37°C. Proteinase K [100 μg in 10% (w/v) sodium dodecyl sulfate (SDS)] is added to the sample and the mixture incubated at 37°C for an additional 20 min. Following a phenol–chloroform extraction and ethanol precipitation, the pellet containing the RNA : RNA hybrid is briefly dried and resuspended in loading buffer [80% (v/v) formamide, 0.1% (v/v) xylene cyanol, 0.1% (v/v) bromophenol blue, and 2 m*M* EDTA]. The samples are boiled at 85°C for 4 min and separated on a 4% (w/v) polyacrylamide–8 *M* urea gel. ^{32}P-end-labeled (DNA polymerase I), *Hind*I-digested pBR322 fragments are used as molecular markers. The protected mRNA fragments are visualized by autoradiography against Amersham (Arlington Heights, IL) Hyperfilm at −70°C.

In Situ Hybridization

Polyester wax sections are prepared as previously described from lesioned CNS tissue. Sections are mounted on poly-L-lysine-coated slides, digested with proteinase K (10 μg/ml, 37°C, 30 min), acetylated for 10 min, rinsed in 2× SSPE [1× SSPE is 0.18 *M* NaCl, 10 m*M* $NaPO_4$, and 1 m*M* EDTA (pH 7.7)], dehydrated through a graded series of ethanol washes, and then air dried for 2 hr before hybridization. Hybridization with specific radiolabeled cRNA probes is performed at 55°C overnight in 10 m*M* Tris (pH 8.0) containing 50% (v/v) formamide, 0.3 *M* NaCl, 1 m*M* EDTA, 0.05% (v/v) tRNA, 10 m*M* dithiothreitol (DTT), 1× Denhardt's solution, and 10% (w/v) dextran sulfate. After hybridization, sections are treated with ribonuclease A (25 mg/ml, 37°C, 30 min) and washed in 0.1× SSPE, 1 m*M* DTT at 65°C. Dehydrated slides are exposed to β_{max} film for 5 days. For microscopic analysis, slides are coated with Kodak (Rochester, NY) NTB-2 liquid autoradiographic emulsion, and exposed at 4°C for 2 weeks. They are developed in Kodak D-19 for 3.5 min, rinsed, and fixed. After washing in distilled water, the sections are counterstained with hematoxylin.

Peroxidase Immunohistochemistry

Immunostaining for trophic factors within CNS tissue is performed on the polyester wax sections previously described, using the ABC Vectastain Elite kit (Vector Laboratories, Inc., Burlingame, CA). The avidin–biotin complex (ABC) technique requires the endogenous peroxidase to be quenched by treating the sections (7 μm thick) in 0.5% (v/v) hydrogen peroxide in PBS for 30 min. Sections are rinsed and incubated in 1.5% (v/v) normal goat serum and then incubated at 4°C overnight with primary antibodies diluted in PBS containing 1% (w/v) BSA. The tissue sections are incubated in goat biotinylated anti-rabbit followed by ABC. Finally, the sections are treated with 0.5% (w/v) diaminobenzidine (DAB) in PBS containing 0.01% (v/v) hydrogen peroxide. The DAB-treated sections are rinsed, dehydrated, and protected with coverslips. For control experiments, sections are incubated with the primary antibody preabsorbed with the immunogenic peptide or with the eluate from a peptide affinity column. Sections are examined under Normaski illumination with a Zeiss (Thornwood, NY) Axioscope microscope and photomicrographs taken on Kodak Gold II film, rated 100 ASA.

All of these methods are now being used to define the trophic components of CNS wounding responses (16, 17). Penetrating wounds rupture the blood–cerebrospinal fluid (CSF)–brain barrier, directly damaging blood vessels in the meninges and the microvasculature of the neuronal parenchyma.

In the acute phase, damage is accompanied by extravasation of plasma proteins, such as endocrine insulin-like growth factor 1 (IGF-I), together with activated platelets into the CNS tissues and recruitment of monocytic cells into the site of injury. These constitute some of the earliest trophic events, because these elements bring multiple cytokines into the wound. Platelet lysis releases factors such as platelet-derived growth factor (PDGF) and transforming growth factors (TGFs), and recruited macrophages synthesize and release interleukins, TGFs, fibroblast growth factors (FGFs), and tumor necrosis factors (TNFs), all of which may themselves be trophic and also stimulate the production of trophic substances from target cells. The accompanying gliosis contributes another tier of regulatory molecules. Reactive astrocytes and microglia are thought to be a primary source of many growth factors and cytokines, including basic FGF, TGF-βs, and IGF-I. Damaged neurons release a number of trophins into wounds, such as TGF-β_1 and acidic and basic FGF. Finally, the CSF is also a source of active molecules, such as TGF-β_1 and IGF-II, which may influence neuronal and glial responses.

Despite the application of new and sensitive techniques for this analysis, definition of the relative contribution of individual factors *in vivo* is difficult, particularly because cooperativity and redundancy of trophic molecules in effecting cellular responses seems to be the rule. Nevertheless, *in vivo* and *in vitro* evidence is implicating a role for many of these factors in the CNS injury response.

Models for Therapeutic Manipulation

Cerebral Lesion

Several techniques have been used to injure the cerebral cortex: these include dropping weights onto the exposed brain to produce a contusion and the application of cold instruments to the brain surface. Surgical penetration of the pia mater and underlying neuropil has the advantage that both dendrites and axons are severed, and that scarring is studied with minimal ischemic necrosis. Thus, unilateral incisional lesions of the cerebral cortex provide a good model for analysis of the overall cellular and trophic responses to penetrating CNS injuries (2). The cellular changes seen within such wounds are representative of those seen throughout the CNS and are relatively simple to analyze, because the resultant cicatrization is well organized. Furthermore, any resultant sensory or motor impairment is minimal, ensuring rapid, uncomplicated recovery and easy postsurgery management of the lesioned animals. Owing to the relative complexity of the neural network at this location, this model is probably not the method of choice for studying regenerative responses in isolation.

Adult rats (200–250 g) are anesthetized and the cranium of each is shaved. They are placed into a stereotactic apparatus and, using aseptic technique, a longitudinal skin incision is made to expose the surface of the skull. Overlying connective tissue is cleared from the operative area and a strip of calvarium over the hemisphere to be lesioned is removed with a dental drill. A unilateral vertical incisional lesion is then made with a disposable, sterile scalpel blade along the stereotactic coordinates [taken from Paxinos and Watson (18)] 1.5 mm lateral of the midline, running from −1.3 mm posterior through +2.5 mm anterior of bregma, to a depth of 5 mm, thus penetrating the lateral ventricle (see Fig. 2).

Infusion of this lesion site with test reagents is achieved through a stainless steel cannula introduced into the lateral ventricle posteriorly (19) at the same time as placement of the lesion. The cannula is made from a modified flow moderator (supplied by Alza Corporation, Palo Alto, CA), positioned in the lateral ventricle ipsilateral to the lesion 1.5 mm lateral to the midline, −1.3 mm posterior to bregma, and 3.5 mm below the cranial surface (see Fig. 3). The cannula is cemented to the cranium by a dental acrylic platform, stabilized with three stainless steel screws driven into the cranium distal to the

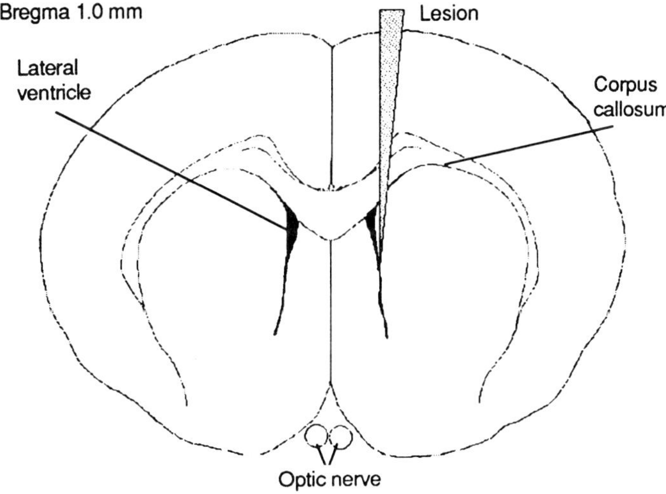

FIG. 2 Diagram to show the position of the incisional cortical lesion in coronal section, illustrating the structures incised after surgery. The lesion extends from the superior pial surface, through the cortex and corpus callosum, to penetrate the lateral ventricle.

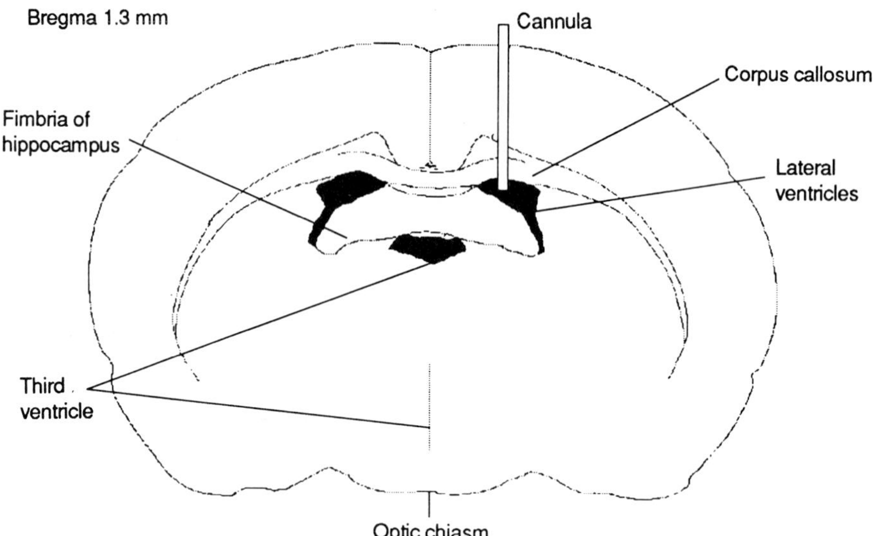

FIG. 3 Diagram to show the site of cannulation of the lateral ventricle. The vertical stainless steel cannula is lowered to a depth of 3.5 mm through the cortex until its tip penetrates the lateral ventricle.

site of cannulation and lesion. The proximal end of the cannula can be joined by tubing to a subcutaneously embedded miniosmotic pump to deliver reagents continuously into the cerebrospinal fluid of the lateral ventricle, or exteriorized through the skin and sealed with a removable cap, allowing access for daily injections of a 10-μl maximum volume with a Hamilton syringe through the cannula.

The brains of treated animals are perfusion fixed at specific postlesion times and processed to generate polyester wax sections as previously described. Immunocytochemical staining of tissue sections documents matrix deposition in the wound (antibodies to laminin, fibronectin, tenascin, and collagen I, II, and IV) and the cellular reactions of macrophages and microglia (ED1 and OX 42 antibodies), astrocytes (GFAP antibodies), and axons (antibodies to GAP-43 and RT97). If required, the dimensions and trophic/tropic characteristics of the wound can be quantified in a standard coronal plane at the same depth below the pial surface in each animal, using image analysis methods described elsewhere (19).

Optic Nerve

The visual system is an excellent model for regenerative research. All axons in the optic nerve are unequivocally severed surgically under direct vision, and regeneration measured in the nerve by immunocytochemistry, using both the specific axonal markers already indicated (Fig. 4) and by anterograde/retrograde tracing techniques (20–22). Retrograde tracing fills the parent ganglion cells and thus the regenerative response of axons in the optic nerve can be quantified by counting filled ganglion cells in retinal whole mounts (Fig. 5). Moreover, functional restitution in the visual system can be accurately assessed electrophysiologically and behaviorally.

Practically, the optic nerve is accessible through the orbit under the upper lid under anesthesia and, after opening the dural sheath, it may be completely severed or crushed without damaging the central retinal artery. Pharmacological agents may be applied directly to the lesion by a cannula cemented to the frontal bone or by implanting cells transfected with the cDNA of specific trophic proteins. Agents can also be introduced directly to the ganglion cells to promote survival by intravitreal injection. At intervals postlesion animals are perfusion fixed and their optic nerves dissected and processed for histochemistry as described. Changes in individual cell populations and the endogenous expression of trophic factors and their receptors can be determined by the immunocytochemical and *in situ* hybridization techniques previously described.

Spinal Cord

Hemisection of the dorsal column avoids the animal morbidity associated with paralysis, anesthesia, and bladder and bowel dysfunction that occurs after complete cord lesions. Contained in rat dorsal columns are two major projection systems: descending corticospinal tract fibers with cell bodies in the contralateral sensorimotor cortex, and ascending first-order sensory fibers of ipsilateral dorsal root ganglion cells. At the T12 level both tracts are easily lesioned in the dorsal funiculi without disturbing the L4/L5 root entry zone. Thus, the ipsilateral L4/L5 dorsal root ganglia and pyramidal neurons in layers V and VI of the contralateral sensorimotor cortex can be retrogradely labeled by applying rhodamine dextran to the T12 lesion site. The numbers of labeled dorsal root ganglia in the ipsilateral L4/L5 ganglia and also pyramidal cells in the contralateral cortex can be counted 36–48 hr after lesion by histological examination of perfusion-fixed tissues. The reaction of gracile tract axons can be monitored histologically by either the fluorescent carbocyanine lipophylic dye, DiI, or horseradish peroxidase transganglionic labeling after sciatic nerve injection, because 99% of the L4/L5 dorsal root ganglia project into the sciatic nerve.

The response to injury of the cord is modifiable by application of reagents through an indwelling catheter cemented to the vertebral spine adjacent to the lesioned segment, with the tip of the cannula sited at the base of the

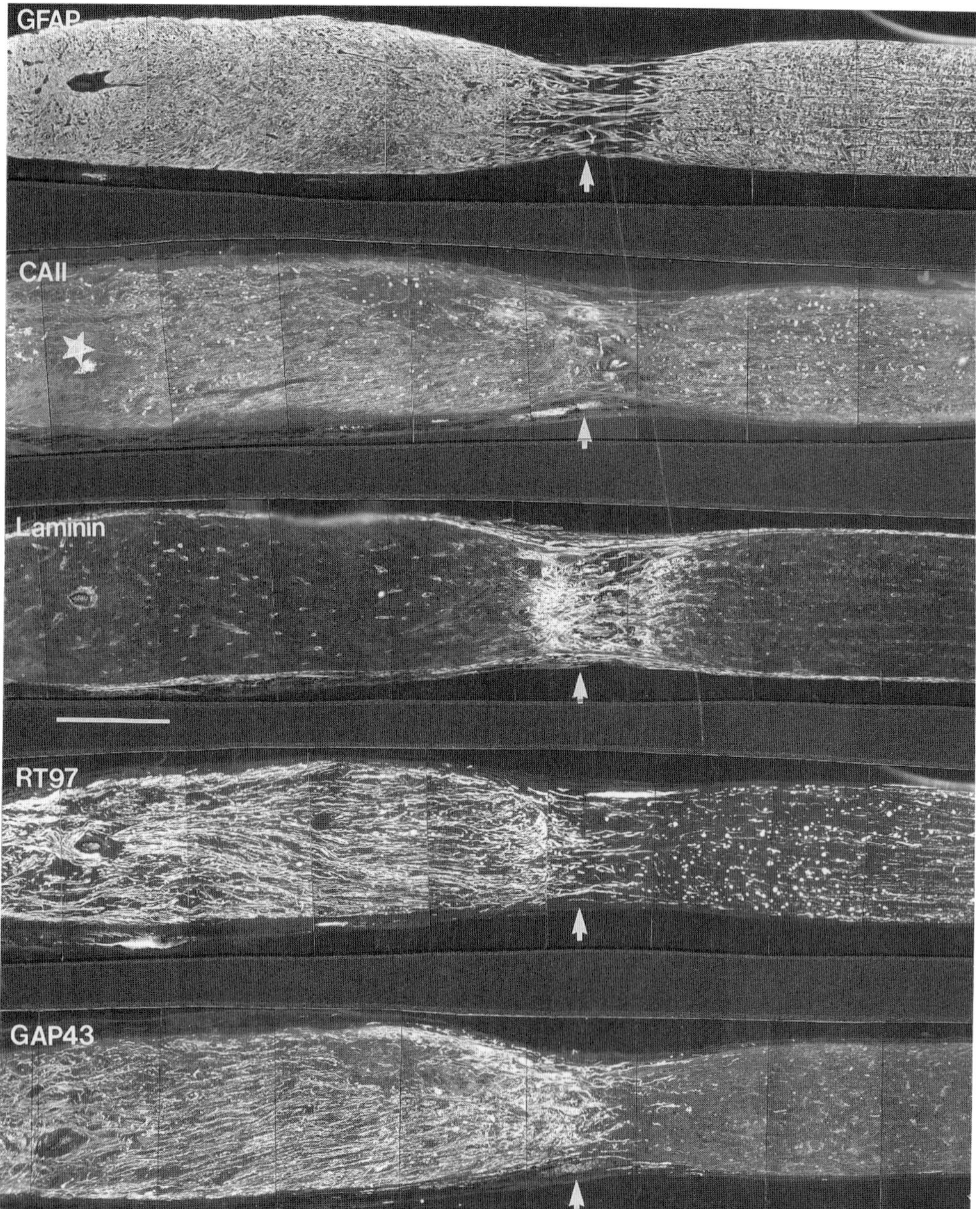

FIG. 4 Rat optic nerve 20 days after a crush injury, showing astrocyte (GFAP), oligodendrocyte/CNS myelin (CAII), and laminin and axon (RT97/GAP-43) immunostaining of serial sections through the same nerve. The retina is to the left of the

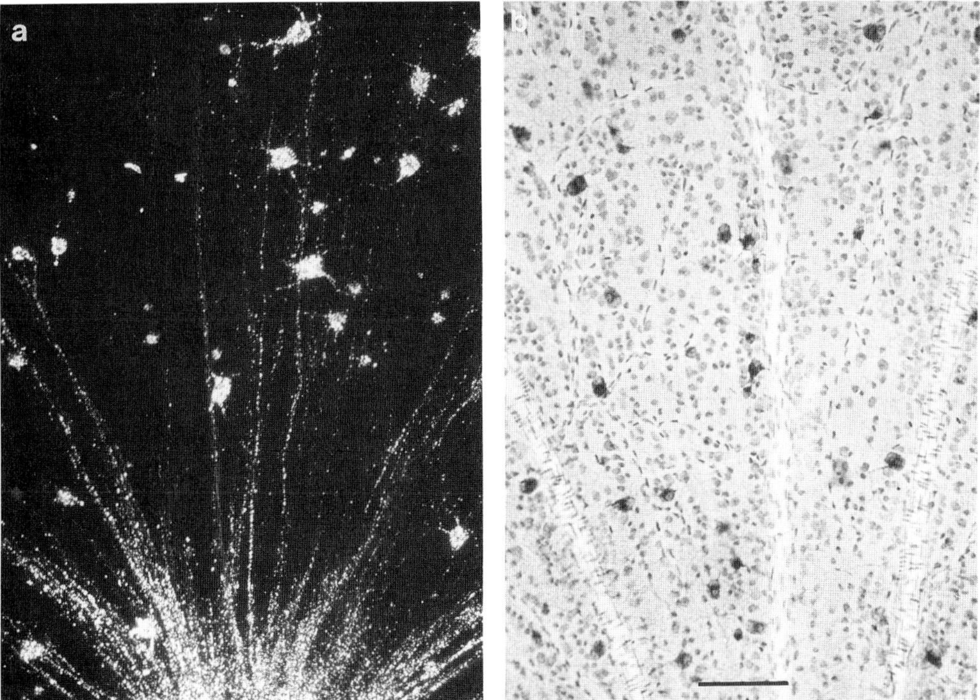

FIG. 5 Two whole mounts of different rat retinas, showing ganglion cells and their axons retrogradely filled with horseradish peroxidase applied to the cut end of the optic nerve 12 hr previously in (a) dark-field and (b) bright-field view. In (a) the axons of retinal ganglion cells converge on the optic disk before leaving the retina in the optic nerve. Horseradish peroxidase-filled ganglion cells are seen among other unlabeled cells in the retina in (b). Bar: 250 μm.

---

lesion (proximal, arrowed), the chiasma to the right (distal). At the site of the lesion, laminin-rich matrix material is deposited through which astrocyte processes run (GFAP). The myelin (CAII) of intact fibers is normal proximal to the lesion [myelin is absent at the lamina cribrosa (star)], but fragmented beyond. Large numbers of axons (RT97, GAP-43) survive in the proximal optic nerve segment after injury, but none regenerate into the distal segment, although a few fibers ramify within the lesion. There is much RT97-positive axonal debris in the nerve distal to the lesion. Monoclonal mouse anti-RT97 and polyclonal rabbit anti-GFAP antibodies have been applied to the same section. Bar: 300 μm.

dorsal funiculus, or by introducing into the lesion site cells transfected with the cDNAs of trophic molecules.

Efficacy of Therapeutic Measures

Scarring

The fibrotic scar that is laid down within CNS wounds presents a formidable mechanochemical barrier for regenerating axons. Any neuronotrophic strategy must also include a regime for scar reduction. We have used classic endocrinological strategies to investigate novel methods for manipulation of CNS scarring. By delivering specific protein agonists and antagonists into CNS wounds, via cannulation and injection or transfected cell implantation, we are able to add and subtract individual growth factor activities *in vivo*. Following such treatments, we can examine the consequences for different components of the cellular wounding response, using established immunohistological techniques already described.

For example, we have demonstrated that TGF-β_1 is a primary regulator of glial scarring in the CNS and have shown that modulation of this factor alone can determine the extent of matrix deposition within wounds (19). Injection or infusion of TGF-β_1 antagonists locally into the cerebrospinal fluid inhibits fibrogenesis at lesion sites. A number of proteoglycan-related molecules (such as decorin) are able to replicate the effects of immunoneutralizing anti-TGF-β_1 antibodies to prevent scar formation in wounds in disease and after injury, and these may prove to be clinically significant (23). However, to what extent this treatment might enhance neuronal repair or affects the restoration of homeostasis within the damaged CNS awaits investigation.

Regeneration

Although a regenerative response is easily detected in some areas of the CNS, in others false-positive results are possible. One means of detecting unequivocal regeneration is by the use of the double-labeling technique. The first tracer is introduced into the lesion site at the time of injury to label all the parent cell bodies of severed axons—easily done in the optic nerve and spinal cord, for example, but difficult in the cerebrum and brainstem. The criterion for definitive regeneration is the labeling, with a second tracer, of neurons already filled with the first label, after infusion of the second dye into neuropil distal to the lesion into which axons are expected to regenerate. Regeneration can be quantified by counting all double-labeled neurons.

Central nervous system axons will regenerate into segments of peripheral nerve implanted into the brain/spinal cord. However, if all Schwann cells are killed in the peripheral nerve graft, no growth is seen. The acellular peripheral grafting technique is a useful method for studying the role of trophic molecules in CNS regeneration. Thus, if acellular peripheral nerve grafts are soaked in solutions of neurotrophins and sutured into a CNS tract of interest, the trophic requirements of the axons can be discerned (24). Regeneration can be measured in terms of the number of axons entering the graft and the number of parent neurons back-labeled after applying different tracers, first to the fresh-cut surface of the tract and then by injecting the graft after a delay period sufficient to allow regenerating fibers to penetrate deep into the grafts. The marker anti-GAP-43 is particularly useful in regenerative studies because GAP-43 is expressed only in growing (*de novo*) and regenerating CNS axons. It is, however, a wise precaution to double label axons with GAP-43 and another axonal marker (e.g., for neurofilaments), because GAP-43 is not specific and may label other elements in the nervous system.

Neuronal Death

Cell death is measured by determining the decrement in number of neurons, labeled at the time of injury, at different times after wounding. Cell death may be prevented pharmacologically by the application of trophic molecules either to the lesion site or in the nucleus containing the parent cell bodies, as described. At this latter site, protease inhibitors may be administered to counteract the enzyme-induced degeneration initiated by microglia (15). Protease inhibitors are delivered as a 5-μl injection cocktail containing pepstatin (0.03 μg), leupeptin (0.05 μg), aprotinin (0.015 μg), *N*-neuraminidase inhibitor (2 μg), and E-64 (0.01 μg). Furthermore, Thanos and co-workers have demonstrated that treatment of CNS wounds with a macrophage inhibitor factor (MIF), which suppresses macrophage and microglia activity, retards neuronal degradation and enhances axonal regeneration (25). Other experiments (26) have demonstrated that treatment of damaged CNS tissue with interleukin 1 receptor antagonists and lipocortin 1 (an endogenous phospholipid) can significantly reduce the neuronal degeneration resulting from the release of cytotoxic excitatory amino acids, thus implicating these two factors as neuroprotective agents.

Conclusions

It is now clear that the development of effective therapies for patients with compromised CNS pathways is within grasp. Because the wounding response is complex and multifactorial, a thorough understanding of its biological regulation is an important first step toward this goal. The cellular changes occurring in damaged tissues are well characterized, using established techniques, and we are now also identifying key trophic molecules that regulate these responses. However, it seems that changing the CNS environment into one conducive to sustained regeneration will ultimately involve the manipulation of multiple trophic and tropic components.

References

1. M. Berry, W. L. Maxwell, A. Logan, A. Mathewson, P. McConnell, D. Ashhurst, and G. Thomas, *Acta Neurochir., Suppl.* **32,** 31 (1983).
2. W. L. Maxwell, R. Follows, D. E. Ashhurst, and M. Berry, *Philos. Trans. R. Soc. London, B* **328,** 479 (1990).
3. A. P. Kent, *Microsc. Anal.* **24,** 39 (1991).
4. H. F. Steedman, *Nature (London)* **179,** 1345 (1957).
5. G. J. Roth, *Immunol. Today* **13,** 100 (1992).
6. Y. Shimizu, W. Newman, Y. Tanaka, and S. Shaw, *Immunol. Today* **13,** 106 (1992).
7. T. A. Springer, *Nature (London)* **346,** 425 (1990).
8. G. A. Zimmerman, S. M. Prescott, and T. M. McIntyre, *Immunol. Today* **13,** 93 (1992).
9. W. L. Maxwell, R. Follows, D. E. Ashhurst, and M. Berry, *Philos. Trans. R. Soc. London, Ser. B* **328,** 501 (1990).
10. S. R. Y. Cajal, "Degeneration and Regeneration in the Nervous System." Oxford Univ. Press, London, 1928.
11. J. W. Fawcett, *Trends Neurosci.* **16,** 164 (1993).
12. M. Berry, S. Hall, D. Shewan, and J. Cohen, *Eye* **8** (1994) (In press).
13. S. J. A. Davies, P. M. Fidd, and G. Raisman, *Eur. J. Neurosci.* **5,** 95 (1993).
14. K. Wictorin, P. Brundin, H. Sauer, O. Lindvall, and A. Bjorklund, *J. Comp. Neurol.* **323,** 475 (1992).
15. S. Thanos, *Eur. J. Neurosci.* **3,** 1189 (1991).
16. A. Logan, S. A. Frautschy, A. M. Gonzalez, and A. Baird, *J. Neurosci.* **12**(10), 3828 (1992).
17. A. Logan, S. A. Frautschy, A. M. Gonzalez, A. Baird, and M. B. Sporn, *Brain Res.* **587,** 216 (1992).
18. G. Paxinos and C. Watson, "The Rat Brain in Stereotactic Coordinates." Academic Press, San Diego, 1986.
19. A. Logan, M. Berry, A. M. Gonzalez, S. A. Frautschy, M. B. Sporn, and A. Baird, *Eur. J. Neurosci.* **6,** 355 (1994).
20. M. Berry, L. Rees, S. Hall, P. Yui, and J. Sievers, *Brain Res. Bull.* **20,** 223 (1988).
21. M. Berry, S. Hall, R. Follows, L. Rees, N. Gregson, and J. Sievers, *J. Neurocytol.* **17,** 727 (1988).

22. M. Berry, S. Hall, L. Rees, J. Carlile, and J. P. H. Wyse, *J. Neurocytol.* **21,** 426 (1992).
23. W. A. Border, N. A. Noble, T. Yamamoto, J. R. Harper, Y. Yamaguchi, M. D. Pierschbacher, and E. Ruoslahti, *Nature* (*London*) **360,** 361 (1992).
24. T. Hagg, A. K. Gulati, M. A. Behzadian, H. L. Vahlsing, S. Varon, and M. Manthorpe, *Exp. Neurol.* **112,** 79 (1991).
25. S. Thanos, J. Mey, and M. Wild, *J. Neurosci.* **13,** 455–466 (1993).
26. J. K. Relton and N. Rothwell, *Brain Res. Bull.* **29,** 243 (1992).

[2] Models of Angiogenesis and the Blood–Brain Barrier

Jeffrey M. Rosenstein and Janette M. Krum

Introduction

Angiogenesis, the formation of new blood vessels, is a requisite developmental event in organ and tissue formation. In the embryonic brain, endothelial cells that comprise the vasculature proliferate at a moderate pace and essentially cease division by day 20–25 in the rat. In the mature brain, the cerebral endothelia are stable and their turnover rate is extremely low. It follows that angiogenesis in adult brain is an event that occurs only under conditions of an injury or pathological event. Concurrent with new endothelial growth and vessel formation following a pathological occurrence is a breakdown of the blood–brain barrier (BBB). There are many different conditions, both clinical and experimental, in which BBB breakdown occurs. In certain neurobiological disorders such as multiple sclerosis and encephalitis it has long been known that there are focal and global barrier changes, and reports have appeared of possible BBB dysfunction in acquired immunodeficiency syndrome (AIDS)-related dementia. The significant permeability found in many brain tumors after vascular administration of contrast medium, as seen in computerized tomography (CT) or magnetic resonance imaging (MRI), is a major determinant that directs the course of surgical intervention. Although, as in all tumors, angiogenesis in and around brain tumors is evident, the permeability observed is almost exclusively confined to the tumor tissue itself. Thus, in cerebral tumors, the blood–tumor barrier is highly compromised whereas the BBB in the adjacent brain is largely unaffected.

In several experimental paradigms, endothelial cell division can be documented in mature rat brain. The experiments that are described in this chapter involve the implantation of tissues and cells into the brain and the subsequent examination of vascular growth and changes in the BBB. The surgical placement of any material into the brain causes both direct mechanical damage to blood vessels and incipient BBB breakdown. Normally, this permeability resolves in 10–14 days and it is important to separate or distinguish between acute, traumatic leakage and that which may occur over time in the experimental system.

Methods in Neurosciences, Volume 21

Techniques for Localization of Proliferating Vasculature (Angiogenesis)

[³H]-Thymidine Autoradiography

[^{3}H]Thymidine autoradiography, although time intensive, remains an excellent technique for the visualization of growing blood vessels. The procedure may be easily combined with immunocytochemical labeling appropriate (1, 2). Following systemic injection into laboratory animals, the exogenous [^{3}H]thymidine is incorporated into the replicating DNA of cells that are about to divide, that is, in the S phase of the cell cycle. Most of the [^{3}H]thymidine is taken up by the cells within 1 hr (3). After autoradiographic processing, the endothelial cells and pericytes that would have undergone mitotic division exhibit radioactive foci (in the form of silver grains) over their nuclei. In counterstained sections, both labeled and unlabeled cells may be counted within a designated area. The labeling index (percentage of labeled nuclei) is determined as follows:

$$\text{Labeling index (\%)} = \frac{\text{number of labeled endothelial cells}}{\text{total number of endothelial cells}} = \frac{X}{100}$$

To circumvent the problem of background silver grains, which may occasionally be present over nuclei, endothelial cells are considered to be labeled when five or more silver grains lie over the nucleus (Fig. 1).

Experimental animals, in our case neonatal or adult Wistar rats, are injected intraperitoneally with [^{3}H]thymidine (5 μCi/g body weight; specific activity, 78 Ci/mmol; New England Nuclear, Boston, MA) mixed with Earle's balanced salt solution. After 1 hr, the animals are deeply anesthetized with 35% chloral hydrate (0.1 ml/100 g body weight) and intracardially perfused with 3% (v/v) glutaraldehyde in an aqueous solution of 0.1 *M* sodium cacodylate and 3% (w/v) sucrose. The desired central nervous system (CNS) regions are removed and placed in the same fixative overnight at 4°C. Tissues are postfixed in 1% (v/v) osmium tetroxide for 2 hr at room temperature. After dehydration in a graded series of ethanols, tissues are embedded in Polybed 812 (Polysciences, Warrington, PA).

The autoradiographic technique used is a modification of the method of Kornhauser *et al.* (4) that has been developed in our laboratory. For light microscopic autoradiography, 1-μm sections are cut on an ultramicrotome, placed on precleaned glass slides, and stained with toluidine blue on a hot plate for 15–30 sec. The slides are then coated with Parlodion film. The film is prepared by placing one pyroxylin-purified strip (Fisher, Pittsburgh, PA)

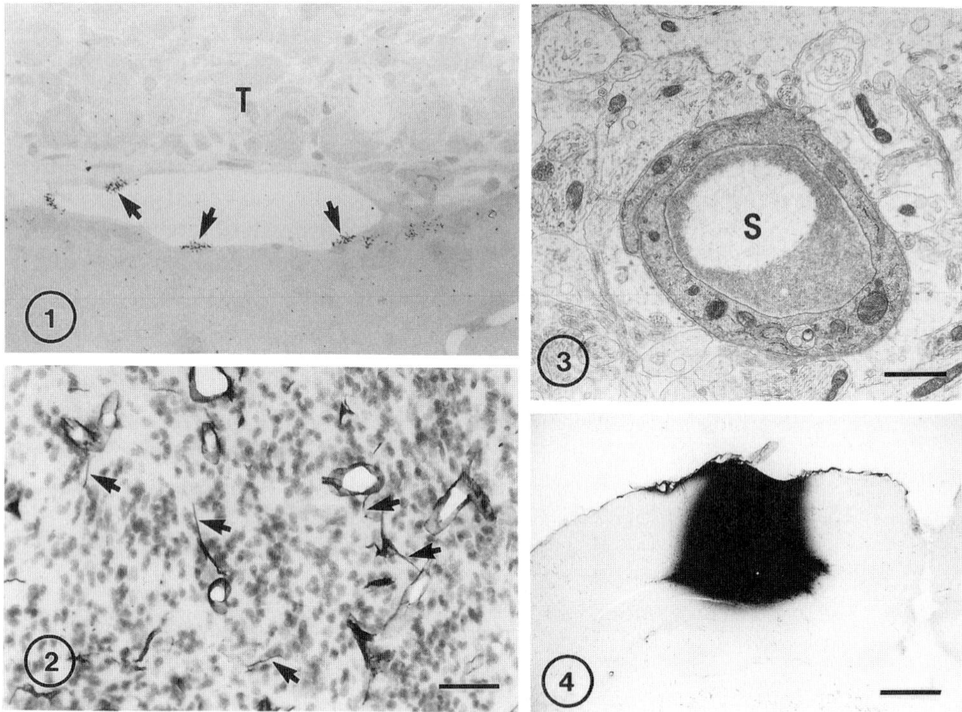

Fig. 1 Autoradiograph showing labeled endothelial cells (arrows) adjacent to a ganglion transplant (T). Bar: 35 μm.

Fig. 2 Vascular sprouts (arrows) within an experimental glioma are depicted with anti-laminin immunostaining. Bar: 40 μm.

Fig. 3 Electron micrograph of a capillary sprout (S) in a neural transplant. Bar: 1 μm.

Fig. 4 A large focal leakage of administered HRP is produced by an adrenal medulla transplant, which is not visible in the center of the permeable (dark) region. Bar: 400 μm.

in 50 ml of isoamyl acetate (anhydrous; Sigma, St. Louis, MO) for 1 week or until completely dissolved. Three milliliters of this solution is added to 45 ml of isoamyl acetate. The film is then cast on glass slides and floated in a large trough filled with double-distilled water. The film should have a light gray-to-clear interference color indicative of an approximate thickness of 30 nm. The film is then slowly and carefully picked up from underneath with the slide, so as to cover the 1-μm sections, taking care not to trap air bubbles between the sections and the film. The coated slides are then left to dry in a dust-free area overnight.

The slides are coated with undiluted Kodak (Rochester, NY) NTB-2 emulsion melted at 40°C in an entirely lightproof darkroom containing a safelight with a Wratten series No. 2 filter (Kodak, Rochester, NY). The backs of the slides are wiped clean of emulsion and they are allowed to dry for 1 hr. The slides are then boxed in lightproof black boxes containing a small bag of desiccant (Drierite). The boxes are sealed with black adhesive tape, labeled, and stored on edge at 4°C with the slides in the horizontal position, emulsion side up, with the desiccant bag on the bottom of the box.

After 3 weeks of exposure, the slides are developed in D-19 developer diluted 1 : 1 with distilled water for 4 min and fixed in Kodak Ectaflo fixer (1 : 7 dilution), followed by rinsing in five changes of distilled water. The temperature of all solutions is maintained at 20°C.

If a particular immunocytochemical reaction is desired in conjunction with autoradiography, the changes in the above protocol are as follows: the perfusion fixative may be whatever is appropriate for optimal preservation of the antigen to be examined; usually 4% (v/v) paraformaldehyde is used. The osmium postfixation is eliminated, and the tissue is processed for paraffin embedment. Sections 6 μm in thickness are cut and placed on clean glass slides. Standard immunocytochemical procedures appropriate for the particular antibody are then performed on the tissue sections, which may then be counterstained if desired and processed for autoradiography as described above.

When electron microscopic visualization is desired, silver to pale gold sections are cut with a diamond knife and placed directly in the center of 200/300-mesh copper grids, on the shiny side. Care is taken to keep the grids completely flat. A narrow strip of adhesive tape is placed on slides that have been cleaned with chromic acid. A long groove (having a width slightly less than the grid diameter) is cut in the tape with a clean razor blade. The grids are placed over the groove, touching the edges of the tape, with sections facing up. There is a free space between the glass slide and the grid. The slides bearing the grids are then coated with Parlodion film as described above. The slides are next coated with 1% Ilford L-4 (0.14 mm) emulsion with a semiautomatic coating instrument (5), according to the method established by Kopriwa (6). The coated slides are stored in light-proof boxes at 4°C. After 8–9 weeks of exposure, the slides are developed for 3 min in D-19 developer diluted 1 : 1 with distilled water. They are rinsed in a distilled water stop bath for 30 sec and fixed for 4 min in 24% sodium thiosulfate, then rinsed in five changes of distilled water. All solutions are kept at 20°C; slides are left overnight to dry. The grids are carefully loosened from the adhesive tape, using fine forceps and the edge of a clean razor blade. The grids are routinely stained with lead citrate and uranyl acetate.

Anti-Bromodeoxyuridine Immunocytochemistry

Bromodeoxyuridine (BrdU) is a thymidine analog to which monoclonal antibodies have been developed. This methodology allows detection of endothelial cells in the S phase at the light microscopic level but, unlike autoradiography, there is no 3- to 4-week exposure period. Labeling indices can be calculated immediately after the immunocytochemical reaction is complete. Data obtained from BrdU studies have been shown to be as reliable as those obtained using [^{3}H]thymidine (7, 8).

Experimental animals are injected intraperitoneally with BrdU (50 mg/kg body weight) in Earle's balanced salt solution and allowed to survive for 1–2 hr. After intracardial perfusion with 4% (v/v) paraformaldehyde in 0.1 *M* sodium cacodylate and 4% (w/v) sucrose, the appropriate brain regions are removed and processed for routine paraffin embedment. Sections cut at 4–5 μm are deparaffinized and pretreated with 2 *M* HCl for 30 min, followed by neutralization with 0.1 *M* $Na_2B_4O_7$, 0.3% (v/v) H_2O_2–methanol for 30 min, and 0.1% (w/v) trypsin for 10 min at 37°C. The sections are then incubated successively with anti-BrdU monoclonal antibody (Becton Dickinson, Paramus, NJ) diluted 1 : 100 overnight at 4°C, goat anti-mouse IgG (1 : 100) for 1 hr, and mouse peroxidase–anti-peroxidase (1 : 100) for 30 min at room temperature. The standard diaminobenzidine (DAB) reaction is used to visualize the immunocytochemical reaction product, which is localized over the nuclei of mitotically active cells. All reactants are diluted in Tris-buffered saline (TBS).

Anti-Laminin Immunocytochemistry

Laminin is one of the component glycoprotein molecules of the vascular basement membrane. Newly formed vessels in brain typically demonstrate enhanced expression of laminin (9–11). Immunocytochemical localization of perivascular laminin in free-floating cryostat (9, 10) or vibratome (Teo Pella, Tustin, CA) sections (11) is a rapid method for detecting proliferating vasculature in the CNS.

Experimental animals are anesthetized and perfused with 4% (v/v) paraformaldehyde as described above. The desired brain areas are removed and placed in the same fixative overnight. After blocking the tissue to a suitable size, sections 40 μm thick are cut on a vibratome. The free-floating sections are then washed in TBS and endogenous peroxidatic activity is blocked with a solution of 10% (v/v) methanol and 3% (v/v) H_2O_2 in TBS for 20 min. The sections are next incubated in TBS plus 10% (v/v) normal goat serum (NGS) for 30 min, followed by an overnight incubation at 4°C in anti-laminin polyclonal antibody (GIBCO, Grand Island, NY) diluted 1 : 500 in TBS with 0.03%

(v/v) Nonidet P-40 (NP-40) and 2% (v/v) NGS added. Further processing is done according to the peroxidase–antiperoxidase method of Sternberger *et al.* (12).

Although the vasculature of the circumventricular organs always appears strongly immunoreactive, only newly formed vessels and vascular sprouts such as those in a growing brain tumor (Fig. 2) in the CNS are immunostained with anti-laminin in the adult rat. The quiescent vasculature remains completely free of reaction product.

Electron Microscopic Analysis: Vascular Sprouts

Ultrastructural observations of newly formed vessels within the neural transplants can provide information about whether or not normal endothelial/astrocytic relationships are developing, which may have implications for the function of the blood–brain barrier (13).

A new capillary arises when endothelial cells migrate through the fragmented basement membrane of the parent vessel wall to form a sprout. Endothelial cell proliferation is observed only proximal to the migrating tip of the sprout; eventually, the sprout becomes canalized and filled with blood (14). Ultrastructurally, vascular sprouts in the CNS are characterized as having a diameter of 5–6 μm, with the endothelial cells resting on a thin basal lamina (Fig. 3). Often, only one endothelial cell will form the sprout profile and junctional complexes are not evident. Sprouts usually have an incomplete complement of astroglial foot processes. The lumen may vary from appearing slitlike to being completely patent. The endothelial cells have become activated; that is, they are thickened, contain abundant rough endoplasmic reticulum and many free ribosomes, and they have irregular ablumenal surface. Pericytes are usually not present.

Strategies for Determining Temporal Sequence and Source of Neovascularization in Neural Transplants

The formation of new blood vessels is requisite for neural transplant survival and must occur rapidly to prevent ischemic insult to grafted neurons. We have focused on the temporal sequence of angiogenic events in peripheral nervous system (PNS) (15) or CNS (16) tissues grafted to the rat brain, as well as on the source of the newly formed vessels. Host CNS vessels might directly anastomose with the surviving transplant vasculature, or host vessels could replace those in the graft either partially or completely. Because the time course and mechanism of transplant revascularization could vary with the type of graft tissue used and the transplantation site, we have used two sources of graft tissue: autonomic tissue, either superior cervical ganglion or adrenal medulla, and CNS tissue, generally fetal neocortex. We have also utilized two different sites for grafted tissues, the fourth ventricle and parietal neocortex.

The superior cervical ganglion was removed from outbred stains of young Wistar rats, decapsulated, and cut into 1.0-mm^3 pieces as previously described (17, 18). The pieces were bathed briefly in Earle's balanced salt solution, followed by immersion in biologically inert Pelikan ink (Gunther Wagner, Hannover, Germany) to delineate its borders after fixation. For neocortical transplants, timed-pregnant Wistar rats (17–21 days postcoitus) were anesthetized with ether and the fetuses removed under aseptic conditions. Pieces of parietal cortex (1.0 mm^3) with meninges removed were excised and placed in ice-cold balanced salt solution.

Recipient animals were deeply anesthetized with chloral hydrate (35%, 0.1 ml/g body weight). For intraventricular transplants, the cisterna magna was opened and the transplant tissue gently pushed through with a fire-polished glass rod and carefully prodded into the fourth ventricle. Great care was taken not to injure the brain surface; in most attempts no bleeding was visible. The surgical wound was sutured in layers and the recipients returned to their cages. A 2-mm burr hole was drilled into the parietal bone of intraparenchymal transplant recipients, followed by excision of the underlying dura. For ganglion or adrenal medulla grafts, a stab wound was created with sharp forceps to a depth slightly above the corpus callosum. The graft was placed in the wound with forceps and the host neocortex allowed to recoil to its original configuration. For fetal neocortical transplants, an injection device consisting of a polypropylene tube fitted to a plunger from a Hamilton syringe was used. Graft tissue was aspirated into the tube, which was then inserted at a 45° angle into the recipient's parietal cortex. The fetal tissue was injected at a depth of 2 mm, where it usually came to rest just above the corpus callosum. The skull defects were sealed with bone wax and the skin was sutured and bathed with iodine scrub.

To determine the temporal sequence of graft revascularization, recipient animals were injected with [^{3}H]thymidine, as described above, at postgrafting survival times ranging from 4 hr to 4 weeks. The endothelial labeling index was determined by counting labeled and unlabeled cells both within the transplant and in the adjacent host vasculature, and statistical determinations were carried out using Student's t test for unpaired data.

To determine the source of graft vasculature in fetal neocortical transplants, the strategy of prelabeling either the host animal or the transplant tissue was used. Pregnant rats were injected with 10 μCi of [^{3}H]thymidine 24 hr prior to removal of the fetuses. This enabled the developing vasculature within the fetal brain tissue to take up the radioactive label. The recipient animals were killed without further [^{3}H]thymidine administration between 1 and 7 days following the operation. After two or more cell divisions, the radioactive label becomes diluted, and therefore analysis of labeled endothelial cells was slightly more difficult. A cell was considered labeled if it had two or three grains over the nucleus that were also present in sequential 1-μm sections. The presence of labeled endothelial cells in healthy, patent graft vessels indicated that the transplant vasculature survived and proliferated. To determine if host vessels also invaded the transplants, transplant recipients ranged in age from 8 to 12 days old, an age in which vascular endothelial cells are actively proliferating within the growing CNS (19). Recipients were injected with [^{3}H]thymidine (5 μCi/g body weight) twice daily for 3 days prior to surgery. The grafted fetal tissue was therefore not exposed directly to the radiolabel. The recipients survived for 1–7 days without further administration of [^{3}H]thymidine. The presence of labeled vessels within the transplants indicated that host vessels grew in to anastomose with the nascent transplant vessels.

Techniques to Determine Blood–Brain Barrier Permeability

We have used immunocytochemical, histochemical, and autoradiographic methods to visualize the presence of the BBB following experimentation. The two most reliable methods, the histochemical detection of horseradish peroxidase (HRP; an enzyme with a molecular weight of 40,000) and the immunoexpression of serum albumin (SA), are complementary to one another. Horseradish peroxidase is injected in an aqueous solution directly into the vasculature and permitted to circulate for allotted times. In this manner, a temporal sequence of potential permeability can be deduced. Normally, because of its large size, charge, and lack of any significant transporting mechanism through the endothelia, this exogenous protein will never be exhibited in the extracellular space within the neuropil. In the experimental situation, if only a small amount of reaction product appears after a few minutes of circulation, it is likely but not necessarily universal that more product will be found after a much longer period, that is, 1 hr.

Similarly, endogenous SA (M_r 69,000) should not be present in the extracellular space. In examining the immunocytochemical expression of SA, we are not looking for a temporal sequence but for the extent of serum protein extravasation over the life of the graft or tumor (see below), up until the time that the experimental animal was perfused. The physical extent of the sensitive SA immunostaining should represent the furthest extent of protein dissemination under normalized physiological conditions. In contrast, the elevated blood volume produced by the HRP injectant followed by perfusion could, in a small rodent, affect some vessels and produce a spurious appearance of protein leakage (20, 21).

A third method to visualize permeability is the vascular administration of a radiolabeled neurotransmitter. Because large proteins may leak in the system, it does not necessarily follow that a smaller molecule will also leak. The neurotransmitter should not only have competent biological activity, but there must be knowledge beforehand that transmitter-specific neurons are present in the region of potential leakiness. For instance, only γ-aminobutyric acid (GABA) neurons will take up [^{3}H]GABA if it is available in the extracellular space. Another transmitter, even if the region is highly permeable, will be washed out of the neuropil, although nonspecific binding is often found in the circumventricular organs. This method can produce interesting results but the autoradiographic methods must be carefully controlled to avoid overexposure and overinterpretation of the results.

In addition to the above methods, which have a physiological context, there are other, more indirect methods that mark specific aspects of cerebral endothelia. These immunocytochemical methods do not directly show protein extravasation in the brain extracellular space. Instead, these antibodies depict vessels that have BBB characteristics; lack of staining indicates that barrier properties are missing in the endothelium. The first such antibody we have used is the endothelial barrier antigen (EBA) first described by Sternberger and Sternberger (22). The EBA is a triplet protein identified with molecular weights of 25,000–35,000. The monoclonal antibody stains only cerebral vessels in rat brain after postnatal day 3 but does not stain vessels of the circumventricular organs, which lack a barrier. Under conditions in which brain tissue is known to be lacking a BBB such as experimental allergic encephalomyelitis (EAE), stab wounds, or in some CNS transplants, the antibody is not expressed on vessels at these sites (23). Similarly, the glucose transporter antibody that labels the facilitative glucose transporter in human erythrocytes and cerebral microvessels (GLUT 1) will mark only known barrier tissues in particular cerebral endothelia (24). Unlike the EBA, however, GLUT 1, a rabbit antiserum to a synthetic peptide homologous to the C terminal of rat brain glucose transporter, is expressed in the embryonic state in cells that have a barrier, such as those of the choroid plexus epithelium. In this case a lack of label would suggest a loss of facilitative transport that may or may not be correlated with protein leakage.

Determining Blood–Brain Barrier Changes in Neural Transplants and Experimental Glioma

The methods to deliver neural transplants in our system has already been described. Barring unforseen anesthesia problems the success rate for ganglia and fetal neocortical grafts is greater than 95%. Adrenal medullary grafts between rats, however, have a much lower rate of success, below 50%. This inconsistency has lead to their virtual abandonment in primate and clinical trials but they are still useful to study permeability changes in the host brain.

An additional method that is routinely used in our laboratories involves the implantation of C_6 glioma cells into the brain. The subsequent prolific tumor growth is ideal for the study of angiogenesis and protein permeability. For this procedure C_6 cells were cultured in Dulbecco's modified Eagle's medium (DMEM) containing 10% (v/v) fetal bovine serum and 10% (v/v) glutamine. The T150 flasks were seeded with 10^4 cells and were confluent (over 1×10^7) within 3 days. The cells were trypsinized, washed in phosphate-buffered saline (PBS), and centrifuged to a loose pellet. A small portion of the pellet was aspirated in just 0.5 μl of medium (cell counts have determined as 2×10^5 cells) and implanted through a burr hole in the skull of an anesthetized rat into the cortex and striatum.

To determine HRP permeability, an aqueous solution consisting of 1 mg of type VI HRP (10,000 U; Sigma) per 7 g body weight dissolved in 0.6 ml of balanced salt solution is injected into the femoral vein over a period of 20 sec. For young rats, as little as 0.1–0.3 ml is used and injected into external jugular veins. With circulation times of 30 min or more, the furthest extent of protein exudation is realized. In a leaky structure such as an adrenal medulla graft the marker spills well past the graft boundaries and inundates the surrounding host brain in a relatively uniform manner (Fig. 4). On the other hand, short circulation times can depict the location of leaky vessels. This is particularly important when using the tetramethylbenzidine (TMB) (25) method to visualize the reaction product in CNS grafts (Fig. 5), because

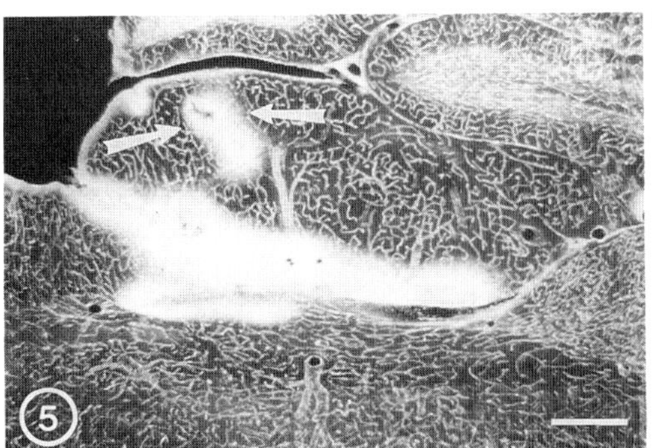

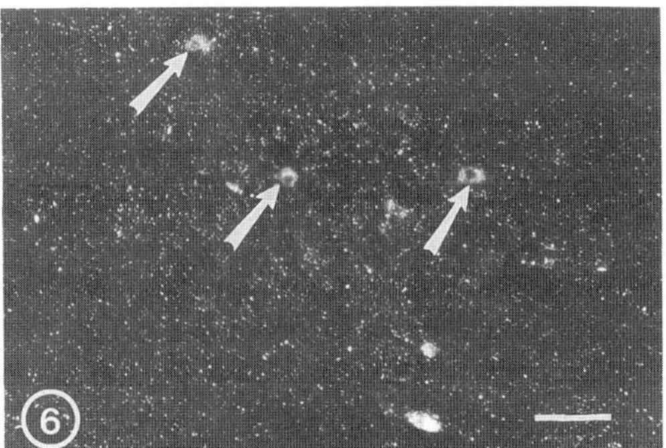

FIG. 5 Small leakage of administered HRP (arrows) is visible after a short circulation time, using TMB methodology. Bar: 200 μm.

FIG. 6 Autoradiograph showing several neurons (arrows) in a fetal neocortical transplant that have taken up vascularly administered [^{3}H]GABA. Bar: 50 μm.

it shows that not all vessels are permeable; if HRP circulation were allowed to continue the leak would obscure the vascular source.

In determining the penetration of the neurotransmitter GABA into CNS grafts the same injection and circulation procedures are used, with an adult rat receiving 200 μCi of [^{3}H]GABA (specific activity, 32 Ci/mmol; New England Nuclear). In this case the maximum uptake of the radiolabeled compound is desired. Using our standard autoradiographic development this method shows that many GABA-ergic neurons can be visualized in the graft (Fig. 6), but more importantly it indicates the neurotransmitters can bypass the BBB in the graft model.

To depict immunocytochemical expression of SA the animals must be perfused with 4% (v/v) paraformaldehyde in 0.1 *M* cacodylate or phosphate buffer, because glutaraldehyde in the fixative will eliminate most of the protein staining. The GLUT 1 antibody can tolerate glutaraldehyde fixation but this often results in higher background staining. With paraformaldehyde

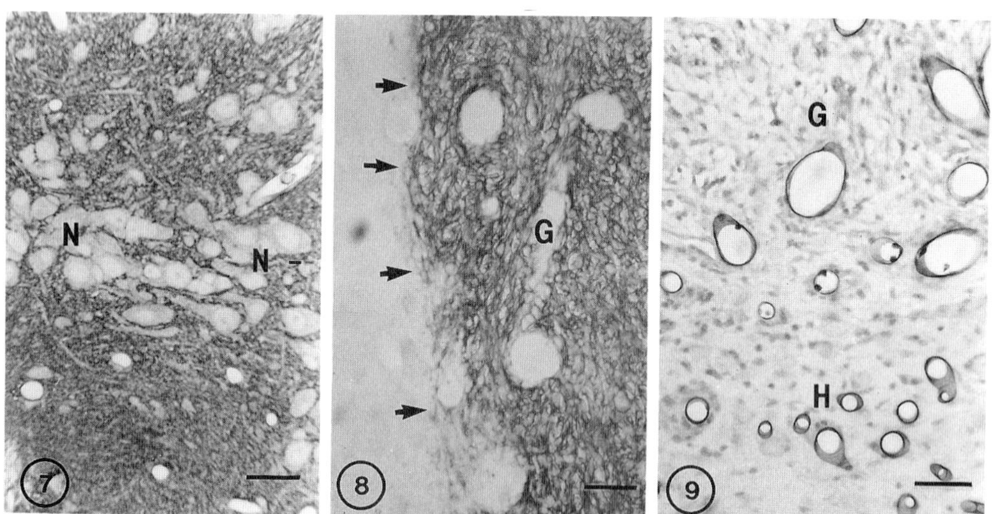

FIG. 7 Immunostaining for anti-serum albumin reaction product filling the extracellular spaces and outlining clusters of neurons (N) in a fetal neocortical transplant. Bar: 30 μm.

FIG. 8 Immunostaining for anti-serum albumin shows extensive reaction in an experimental glioma (G) that stops abruptly at the interface with host brain (arrows). Bar: 50 μm.

FIG. 9 Immunostaining for anti-GLUT 1 shows intense expression both in glioma (G) vessels and in host brain (H). Bar: 50 μm.

fixation anti-SA, a direct peroxidase-labeled polyclonal antibody, can be seen in paraffin sections (dilution, 1 : 1000) outlining grafted neurons (Fig. 7) or in 40-μm vibratome sections (dilution, 1 : 2000), showing that protein permeability always ends at the tumor–brain interface (Fig. 8). Examination of Fig. 8 might suggest that the vessels in the tumor are completed leaky and those in the adjacent brain are not. However, when we examine this region for the GLUT 1 antibody we see that all vessels in this region are positive for this cerebrovascular barrier marker (Fig. 9). These findings confound the issue of brain tumor permeability because these tumor vessels, presumably leaky, have the barrier marker. Moreover, the immunocytochemical labeling of SA reveals the significant finding of an as yet unknown barrier at the interface; in contrast to the tumor situation, HRP, the artificial marker for (serum) protein in a permeable transplant model, can have free access through the brain neuropil. From a normal physiological perspective, a barrier should not exist to prevent the movement of a solute, particularly from a tumor with a great degree of physical extracellular space, into the brain. These methods have detected a region with restrictive permeability characteristics and a vasculature with unusual molecular characteristics.

Acknowledgments

We wish to thank Gilda Kornhauser and Newton More for excellent technical assistance on these projects and Uma Gupta for expert secretarial assistance. This work is supported by Jacob Javits Neuroscience Investigation Award NS-17468.

References

1. N. Latov, G. Nilaver, E. A. Zimmerman, W. G. Johnson, A.-J. Silverman, R. Defendini, and L. Cote, *Dev. Biol.* **72,** 381–384 (1979).
2. K. Janeczko, *Brain Res.* **485,** 236–243 (1989).
3. B. Messier and C. P. Leblond, *Am. J. Anat.* **106,** 247–265 (1960).
4. G. V. Kornhauser, J. M. Krum, and J. M. Rosenstein, *J. Histochem. Cytochem.* **40,** 879–882 (1992).
5. B. M. Kopriwa, *J. Histochem. Cytochem.* **14,** 923–928 (1967).
6. B. M. Kopriwa, *Histochemistry* **37,** 1–17 (1973).
7. A. H. Cawood and J. R. K. Savage, *Cell Tissue Kinet.* **16,** 51–57 (1983).
8. H. Sugihara, T. Hattori, and M. Fukuda, *Histochemistry* **85,** 193–195 (1986).
9. K. Shigematsu, H. Kamo, I. Akiguchi, M. Kameyama, and H. Kimura, *Neurosci. Lett.* **99,** 18–23 (1989).
10. K. Shigematsu, H. Kamo, I. Akiguchi, J. Kimura, M. Kameyama, and H. Kimura, *Brain Res.* **501,** 215–222 (1989).

11. J. M. Krum, N. S. More, and J. M. Rosenstein, *Exp. Neurol.* **111,** 152–165 (1991).
12. L. A. Sternberger, P. H. Hardy, J. J. Cuculis, and H. G. Meyer, *J. Histochem. Cytochem.* **18,** 315–333 (1970).
13. J. M. Krum and J. M. Rosenstein, *Exp. Neurol.* **103,** 203–212 (1989).
14. P. A. D'Amore and R. W. Thompson, *Annu. Rev. Physiol.* **49,** 453–464 (1987).
15. J. M. Krum and J. M. Rosenstein, *J. Comp. Neurol.* **258,** 420–434 (1987).
16. J. M. Krum and J. M. Rosenstein, *J. Comp. Neurol.* **271,** 331–345 (1988).
17. J. M. Rosenstein and M. W. Brightman, *Nature (London)* **275,** 83–85 (1978).
18. J. M. Rosenstein and M. W. Brightman, *J. Neurocytol.* **8,** 359–379 (1979).
19. P. L. Robertson, M. DuBois, P. D. Bowman, and G. D. Goldstein, *Dev. Brain Res.* **23,** 219–223 (1985).
20. B. Balin, R. Broadwell, M. Salcman, and M. El-Kalliny, *J. Comp. Neurol.* **251,** 260 (1986).
21. J. M. Rosenstein, *J. Comp. Neurol.* **305,** 676 (1991).
22. N. H. Sternberger and L. A. Sternberger, *Proc. Natl. Acad. Sci. U.S.A.* **84,** 8169 (1987).
23. J. M. Rosenstein, J. M. Krum, L. A. Sternberger, M. T. Pulley, and N. H. Sternberger, *Dev. Brain Res.* **66,** 47 (1992).
24. S. I. Harik, R. N. Kalaria, L. Anderson, P. Lungdahl, and G. Perry, *J. Neurosci.* **10,** 3862 (1990).
25. M. M. Mesulan, *J. Histochem. Cytochem.* **26,** 106 (1978).

Section II

Transiently Removing the Blood–Brain Barrier

[3] Osmotic Opening of the Blood–Brain Barrier and Brain Tumor Chemotherapy

Peter J. Robinson

The permeability characteristics of the blood–brain barrier can be modified in a number of ways, including arterial hypertension, hypercapnia, some drugs, and by the administration of hyperosmotic solutions. The latter method has been the most extensively studied and characterized, and has been used as the basis for enhancing the entry of water-soluble drugs or high molecular weight compounds into the brain for the treatment of some brain tumors and in enzyme replacement therapies. Transient increases in barrier permeability are followed by restoration of normal permeability within 30 min to a few hours, providing a therapeutic window for treatment. It is likely that such reversible opening of the blood–brain barrier to water-soluble materials is mediated by osmotically induced shrinkage of cerebrovascular capillary endothelial cells and consequent widening of tight junctions. Movement of compounds across the blood–brain barrier during this time can be characterized in terms of the molecular size and charge of the compound, pore size and number, and bulk fluid flow from blood to brain. Although some brain tumors may have an ineffective blood–brain barrier, it is likely that the barrier is completely or partially intact at the proliferating edge of the tumor. Access of chemotherapeutic agents to brain tumor and surrounding brain regions following osmotic opening can be modeled quantitatively, and the osmotic method for enhancing blood–brain barrier permeability has been shown to have therapeutic effectiveness in the treatment of primary lymphomas and glioblastomas in humans.

Introduction

The blood–brain barrier (BBB) in mammals separates the blood from the two major compartments of the central nervous system: the brain and the cerebrospinal fluid (CSF). The sites of the barrier are the choroid plexus, the subarachnoid membrane that overlies the subarachnoid space, and, most importantly for the present discussion, the blood vessels of the brain and the subarachnoid space (see Fig. 1).

All barrier sites are composed of cells connected by tight junctions that restrict intercellular diffusion, so that they act like a continuous cell layer,

Methods in Neurosciences, Volume 21

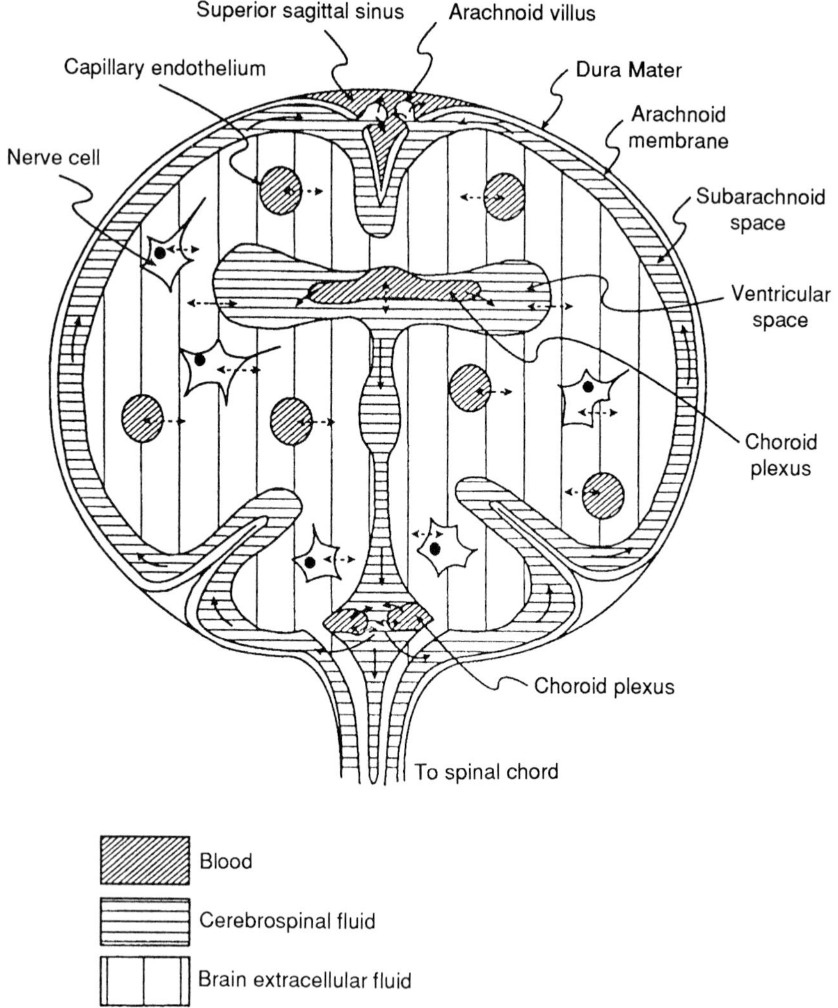

FIG. 1 The major fluid compartments of the central nervous system. Dashed arrows show major pathways for solute exchange; solid arrows show bulk circulation of fluid. [From Robinson and Rapoport (33).]

effectively preventing significant entry into the brain of lipid-insoluble substances and proteins, and substances bound to proteins (see Fig. 2). The brain is thus protected by the BBB from potentially disruptive fluctuations of such substances in the blood stream, and from exogenous substances of this type that may reach significant levels in the blood.

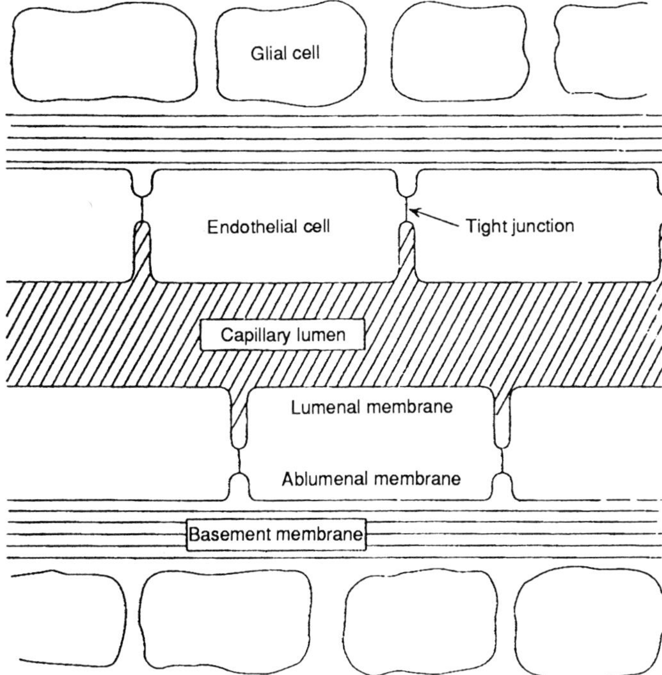

FIG. 2 Schematic representation of cerebral capillary defined by endothelial cells connected by continuous belts of tight junctions. [From Robinson and Rapoport (33).]

On the other hand, lipophilic substances easily penetrate the plasma membranes of the cells and enter the brain at rates determined in large part by their ability to partition into lipids; hence the relationship between cerebrovascular permeability and octanol–water partition coefficients (a measure of lipid solubility) for a wide range of compounds illustrated in Fig. 3.

In addition to lipid-soluble compounds, substances that are essential for brain metabolism, for synthesis of brain proteins and neurotransmitters, and some exogenous compounds chemically similar to these (as well as some inorganic ions) can make use of specific transport systems that facilitate their entry into the brain. Thus the role of the BBB in regulating the internal chemical environment of the brain is achieved by combining low passive permeability with highly selective transport between blood and brain.

In such a situation, it is likely that any particular chemical substance, such as an anticancer agent, may, unless it happens to be particularly lipophilic (and not significantly bound to plasma proteins) or sufficiently similar to particular endogenous compounds as to be able to take advantage of specific

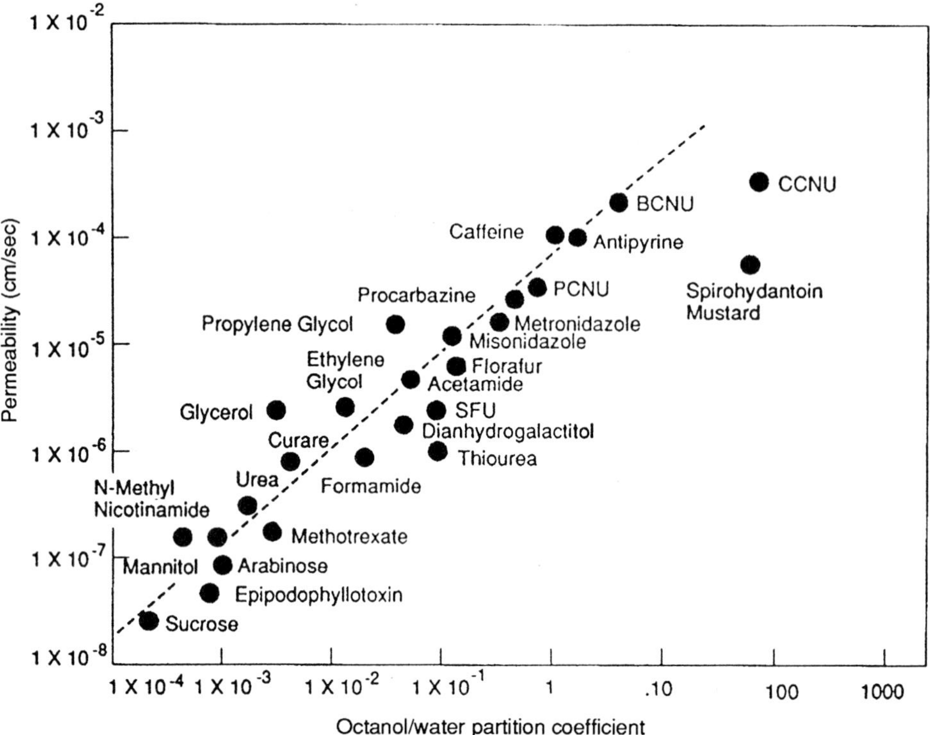

FIG. 3 Relationship between cerebrovascular permeability and octanol–water partition coefficients for a variety of drugs and other compounds. [From Robinson and Rapoport (33).]

transport processes, be effectively prevented from entering the brain to any significant extent. However, three major approaches suggest themselves for overcoming the particularly effective isolation of the brain from the blood and enhancing the entry of compounds into the brain from the blood for therapeutic purposes: (a) chemical modification to enhance lipophilicity, (b) chemical modification to allow a compound to take advantage of existing transport mechanisms across the BBB, and (c) modification of the BBB itself to facilitate entry of the compound.

Of these approches, the first two are chemical specific. This is clearly an advantage in that brain homeostasis is only minimally disrupted. The third approach appears more draconian, but is useful when other approaches may not be feasible or effective. Techniques of chemical modification are discussed elsewhere in this book (see, for example, Sections II and IV). The focus of the present chapter is a particularly effective technique for modifying

BBB permeability by exposing the blood vessels of the brain to hyperosmotic solutions; this technique has proved useful in a clinical context, particularly in the treatment of certain types of brain tumors.

Osmotic Opening of Blood–Brain Barrier

Hypertonic solutions can disrupt the BBB, both when applied topically to the pia–arachnoid surface of the cortex (18), or when infused to the blood side of the BBB (24). Thompson (43), using a perfused rat head preparation, showed that brain uptake of [^{14}C]sucrose and [^{14}C]urea was enhanced by perfusion of hyperosmolar solutions of mannitol, urea, thiourea, and glycerol. Similar results were found when hyperosmolar solutiolns were infused into the external carotid artery of intact animals and the opening of the blood–brain barrier was assessed with Evans blue-labeled albumin (19, 24) or with ^{22}Na (42). Intracarotid infusion of lactamide, mannitol, urea, or arabinose opened the blood–brain barrier reversibly, whereas solutions of lipid-soluble solutes such as propylene glycol or ethanol acted irreversibly (24, 25, 40). Electron microscopy has confirmed that reversible opening is mediated by increased permeability of interendothelial tight junctions to tracers such as horseradish peroxidase and $La(OH)_3$ (3, 5, 14). It is likely that reversible BBB opening to water-soluble materials is mediated by osmotically induced shrinkage of cerebrovascular endothelial cells, and consequent reversible widening of interendothelial tight junctions, through which the tracers pass in an aqueous phase (18, 25); see Fig. 4.

Radiotracer experiments have been used to quantify the degree and time course of BBB opening, the critical parameters that determine such opening, and the reversibility of opening. Blood–brain barrier opening (as quantified by the regional cerebrovascular permeability-surface area product, or PA), was found to be critically dependent on the osmolality of the solution infused into the carotid circulation. For example, regional [^{14}C]sucrose PA between 5 and 15 min following osmotic treatment was found to be 7- to 10-fold higher than control PA values for 30-sec infusions of 1.6 and 1.8 *M* arabinose, but showed little increase following a 1.4 *M* arabinose infusion in awake rats (25). There was a threshold arabinose concentration of 1.6 *M* for barrier opening. A similar threshold for infusion duration, for a fixed infusate concentration, suggested a more general threshold of concentration times duration to produce BBB opening (25).

The time course of PA following hypertonic arabinose infusion shows that measured PA values tend to return to control values by 1 hr following osmotic treatment (25), and lack of histological evidence for brain cell damage or

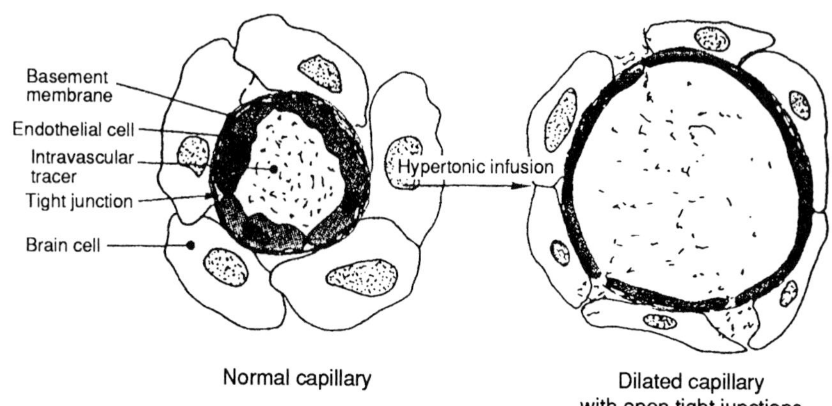

FIG. 4 Postulated mechanism for osmotic opening of the BBB at the cerebral capillary. Hypertonic perfusate in the cerebral capillaries absorbs water from the endothelial cells, inducing cell shrinkage, stretching of cell membranes, and widening of intercellular tight junctions. [From Rapoport and Robinson (21).]

long-term neurological sequelae following osmotic opening (16, 23, 38) further demonstrates the reversible nature of the phenomenon.

Size Dependence of Blood–Brain Barrier Permeability

Blood–brain barrier permeability following hypertonic infusion has been most extensively characterized by means of double-tracer experiments, with (neutral) tracers of different molecular sizes (such as sucrose and dextran) injected simultaneously (1, 45, 46). If the opened BBB did not discriminate at all on the basis of molecular size, the ratio of the PA values for two such substances would equal 1. This would be the case if both molecules crossed the BBB by unrestricted bulk flow. On the other hand, if each molecule passed through the opened BBB by simple (unrestricted) diffusion in an aqueous phase, then the PA ratio would equal the ratio of their respective free aqueous diffusion coefficients. If, however, larger molecules were further hindered to a greater extent than smaller molecules (e.g., by passage through relatively small, diffusion-limiting pores), the PA ratio would be greater than the ratio of the free diffusion coefficients by a factor which depends on the molecular radii, and the pore radius or half slit width (31). This factor takes into account both the steric hindrance and the frictional resistance of the molecule in the pore, relative to free solute (6). Its functional form depends on the particular pore geometry (4).

Table I gives PA ratios for sucrose to dextran for 14 brain regions following carotid infusion of 1.6 *M* arabinose in the rat (46). These data are representative of other pairs of compounds studied in a similar way. Because the PA ratios generally are less than the ratio of the free diffusion coefficients for sucrose to detran [5.3; Lanman *et al.* (12)] for the 6-min experiment, there must, at early times after osmotic infusion, be an additional mechanism apart from diffusion that reduces discrimination on the basis of molecular size. It has been proposed that this process is bulk water flow from blood to brain (31, 46). Such an interpretation is consistent with the independent observation of a transient increase in brain water content by 1–1.5% of wet weight within the first 10 min following a hypertonic arabinose injection (25), and evidence that the brain shrinks during the infusion procedure itself (7, 8).

A quantitative model describing BBB permeability following osmotic opening in terms of restricted diffusion through cylindrical pores (or narrow slits), together with bulk fluid flow and solute drag, has been developed and applied to data on the size dependence of BBB permeability (28, 31, 46). Assuming a bulk flow value consistent with observed changes in brain water content, such a model suggests an effective open pore radius of about 200 Å, or an

TABLE I Ratio of PA Products for [^{14}C]Sucrose and [^{3}H]Dextran (M_r 79,000) after Hypertonic Arabinose Infusion[a]

Brain region	PA ratio ([^{14}C]sucrose/[^{3}H]dextran) 6-min exp.	35-min exp.	55-min exp.
Olfactory bulb	2.7 ± 0.5	13.0 ± 3.6	7.9 ± 1.2
Caudate nucleus	3.8 ± 0.7	12.3 ± 2.5	10.7 ± 1.5
Hippocampus	4.5 ± 0.7	11.4 ± 1.7	13.8 ± 3.0
Frontal lobe	3.6 ± 0.6	11.4 ± 1.5	8.1 ± 0.6
Occipital lobe	3.7 ± 0.9	16.0 ± 1.2	12.7 ± 1.5
Thalamus and hypothalamus	3.3 ± 0.6	11.7 ± 2.1	9.4 ± 0.9
Superior colliculus	2.5 ± 0.4	10.9 ± 2.0	10.4 ± 1.1
Inferior colliculus	3.1 ± 0.9	8.1 ± 1.2	9.4 ± 1.1
Cerebellum	4.2 ± 0.9	9.2 ± 1.3	9.1 ± 1.5
Pons	3.2 ± 0.4	10.1 ± 1.5	8.9 ± 2.0
Medulla	4.3 ± 0.8	14.9 ± 1.7	13.0 ± 3.5
Midbrain	3.0 ± 0.3	11.0 ± 1.5	8.5 ± 0.7
Parietal lobe	3.3 ± 0.9	9.9 ± 1.2	9.5 ± 1.2
White matter (corpus callosum)	3.5 ± 0.4	30.3 ± 9.0	15.8 ± 1.5

[a] Values are means ± SE; n = 10 rats. In all regions 35- and 55-min PA ratios are significantly higher ($p < 0.05$) than 6-min values. Values for 35 and 55 min are not significantly different ($p > 0.05$) from each other.

[b] From Ziylan *et al.* (48).

effective slit width of about 220 Å (31). Changes in PA values for sucrose and dextran can be explained on the basis of this model in terms of reductions in bulk water flow from blood to brain, by a factor of about 10, from 6 to 35 min as the barrier recloses, without any changes in the effective pore size (31). The pore density also seems to remain fairly constant, changing from about 1 pore/200 μm^2 of membrane surface area at 6 and 35 min after osmotic opening, to about 1 pore/300 μm^2 at 55 min (31).

Once the effective pore size, pore density, and time course for bulk water flow have been estimated, such a model can be used to predict the entry of other neutral, water-soluble drugs into the brain following osmotic BBB opening (28). Figure 5A summarizes the results of such an analysis. The ordinate gives the effective PA value for a neutral, water-soluble, and roughly spherical drug as a function of its molecular size at various times after BBB opening (28). As the BBB recloses, the effective permeability decreases with time, reaching a particular permeability threshold (horizontal broken lines) much sooner for a larger molecule. Larger molecules therefore have a shorter "window" following osmotic opening, during which time appreciable quantities of drug can enter the brain for therapeutic effect; see Fig. 5B.

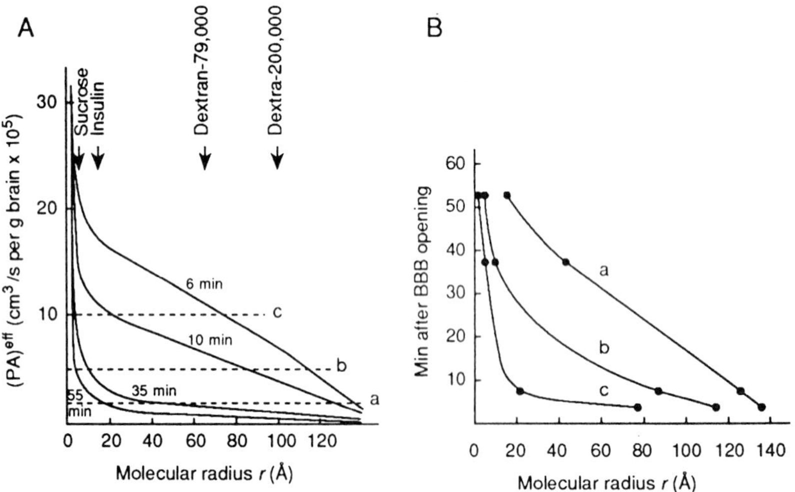

FIG. 5 Predicted variation (A) of effective cerebrovascular permeability-surface area product $(PA)^{eff}$ (equivalent to brain clearance from plasma) at four time points after osmotic opening of the BBB in rat, as a function of molecular radius. Broken lines represent three arbitrary threshold permeability values for therapeutic effectiveness of a drug. (B) The "therapeutic window" in terms of time after osmotic BBB opening as a function of molecular radius for the three threshold permeability values in (A).

In addition to molecular size, molecular charge may also play an important role in the entry of drugs into the brain following osmotic opening. A negative surface charge associated with interendothelial pores should restrict the passage of negatively charged molecules to a greater extent than their neutral or positively charged counterparts. A number of models have been developed to describe the interaction of charged molecules with charged pores. For example, Smith and Deen (41) solved the Poisson–Boltzmann equation for a sphere on the axis of a cylindrical pore to evaluate the interaction potential between the sphere and the pore wall. Deen *et al.* (4a) developed a pore model that describes exclusion and diffusion of solutes in the presence of a uniformly distributed space charge in the pore. There have also been a number of experimental studies in this area (4). Furthermore, Armstrong *et al.* (1) observed possible charge effects on BBB permeability to polysaccharides following osmotic BBB opening in rats. Charge modification, in conjunction with osmotic BBB opening, may be a potential technique for further enhancing drug entry into the brain.

An important class of drugs that may be significantly hindered from entering the brain by an intact BBB are those that are highly and tightly bound to circulatig plasma proteins (29, 34). These substances would clearly benefit from the temporary increases in BBB permeability resulting from osmotic treatment by allowing some bound, as well as free, drug to enter the brain. Total drug entry would in this case be made up of two components: both the bound and the free components would follow a time course for entry into the brain determined by the relevant physicochemical properties of the complex and the free drug, respectively, as well as the time-dependent characteristics of the BBB (28). It is important to note also that a drug entering the brain, if attached to a plasma protein, would have to dissociate from that protein before producing its therapeutic effect. A similar process has been proposed as a model for kernicterus in infants (13, 30): hypoxic damage to brain lets in protein-bound bilirubin, which dissociates from protein in the brain and, among other things, inhibits the coupling between oxidation and phosphorylation.

Osmotic Opening and Brain Tumor Chemotherapy

Although the BBB in brain tumors may be partially disrupted, it still is a major factor limiting the efficacy of chemotherapy with water-soluble drugs. The degree of BBB disruption depends critically on the type of tumor. For example, transfer constants for α-aminoisobutyric acid (AIB) in a number of brain tumor models in rat range from 1.5 times that of normal cortex for ethylnitrosourea-induced brain tumors to 29 times that of normal cortex for

H-54 transplanted human gliomas (2). As a result, the effect of osmotic treatment in enhancing drug delivery to brain tumors may be more moderate than to normal cortex (11), especially for those tumors with normally high brain–tumor barrier (BTB) permeabilities.

In addition, some chemotherapeutic agents are toxic to normal brain cells (17, 20), as well as to other cells in the body, and therefore it is desirable to limit exposure of these cells while at the same time maximizing exposure of the tumor cells. Although it is possible by the osmotic method to expose tumor cells to the same amount of drug at a lower total dose, allowing less exposure of cells in the rest of the body, this advantage may be outweighed by exposing surrounding normal brain to even higher levels of drug. Thus, in assessing the efficacy of the osmotic method, the relative toxicities of the drug to tumor cells, normal brain cells, and cells in the rest of the body need to be taken into account. Neuwelt *et al.* (17) established a drug-screening procedure in animals and concluded that Adriamycin (doxorubicin), cisplatin, bleomycin, 5-fluorouracil, and mitomycin C are too neurotoxic to be used clinically in conjunction with the osmotic method, whereas cyclophosphamide and methotrexate were found suitable.

The relative exposure of tumor and normal brain to a drug also depends on the infusion schedule of the drug combined with the time course for barrier opening and reclosure both within the tumor and surrounding brain, because the permeability of the BBB and BTB influences not only the time course for brain and tumor uptake of the drug, but also its rate of return to the blood stream once the bolus has passed. This leads to complex uptake characteristics in both brain and tumor.

This complexity is further enhanced because of possibly large spatial permeability inhomogeneities in a brain with a brain tumor, which set up concentration gradients of drug along which the drug may diffuse. In the untreated brain, a higher concentration of the drug in the tumor than in the surrounding brain establishes a concentration gradient from tumor to brain along which the drug may diffuse ("sink effect") (20, 44), as well as possible bulk fluid flow between tumor and brain asociated with peritumoral edema (26). The net result of these processes is to reduce the concentration of a drug at the proliferataing edge of a tumor to levels considerably lower than at its center.

Indeed, it is likely that it is particularly important to deliver drug, not to the center of a tumor, but rather to this proliferating edge, where barrier properties may be more akin to normal brain than tumor and drug delivery may benefit particularly from barrier disruption. Not only will osmotic treatment presumably enhance entry of drug from blood, but it will also prevent loss of drug from tumor to surrounding brain by the sink effect and bulk flow. To assess the relative effects of each of these processes on the exposure of a particular tumor (as well as brain surrounding tumor and normal brain) to a particular drug both with and without osmotic treatment, Robinson and Rapoport (32) developed a mathematical model of a spherically symmetric brain tumor that provides a quantitative framework essential for discussing the therapeutic effectiveness of the osmotic method in any particular case.

Figure 6 shows the effect of osmotic treatment on the calculated relative 1-hr exposures to a representative compound [in this case α-aminoisobutyric acid (AIB)] as a function of the distance from the center of (Fig. 6A) a Walker 256 carcinoma and (Fig. 6B) a C6 glioma following the onset of (a) a continuous infusion and (b) a bolus injection. The effect of osmotic treatment on exposure of a particular brain region can be expressed in terms of an enhancement factor γ, defined as the ratio of exposure to a drug following osmotic opening to exposure without osmotic treatment. Enhancement factors for AIB in Walker 256 carcinomas and C6 gliomas are given in Table II.

For normal brain, the enhancement factors range from 16 to 37, whereas for the tumor centers, enhancement factors are about 5 for the Walker 256 carcinoma, and only about 1.3–1.4 for the relatively leaky C6 glioma. Such relatively large enhancement factors for normal brain relative to tumor have led to some concern over the effectiveness of the osmotic method for enhancing drug entry into the brain for chemotherapeutic purposes (9, 10, 36, 37). It has also been suggested that it may be an advantage to allow the BBB to remain intact to optimize its protective capacity for normal brain, while the tumors that have only partially intact barriers would be exposed to the drug to a relatively greater extent. However, a number of other factors need to be taken into account in order to assess the efficacy of the osmotic method for brain tumor chemotherpay, including (32) the following.

1. There is considerable variability in vascular permeabilities among different types of tumors.
2. Diffusion from surrounding brain into tumor following osmotic treatment (rather than in the reverse direction, as in untreated brain: "sink effect") should be taken into account.
3. Localized drug concentration at the proliferating edge of the tumor, or in the brain tissue surrounding the tumor, is more relevant for efficacy than is concentration in the center of the tumor.
4. Osmotic treatment reduces the overall dose of drug necessary to achieve therapeutic effect against the tumor, reducing the potential for toxic effect on peripheral organs.
5. The time course of drug plasma concentration relative to that of BBB opening affects integrated exposure of brain and tumor to the drug. This depends both on the drug and its method of administration.
6. A rigorous program of drug toxicity testing should be employed in conjunction with the osmotic method, as has been done by Neuwelt and coworkers (14a, 17).

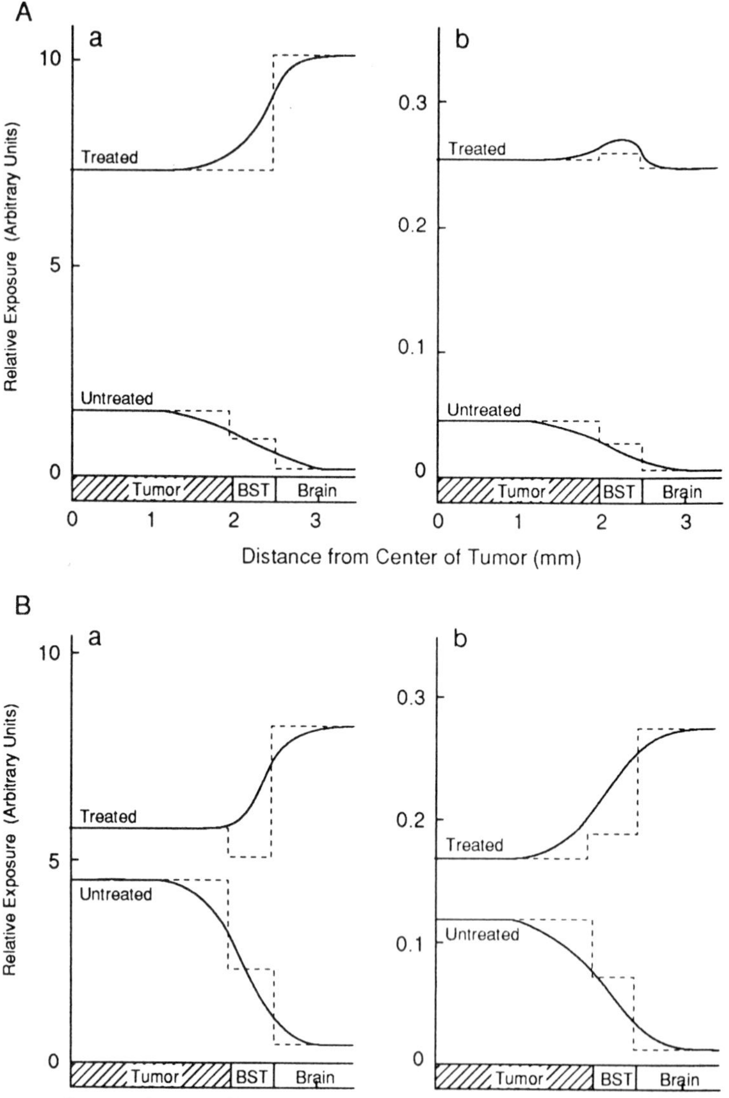

FIG. 6 Calculated relative 1-hr exposure to α-aminoisobutyric acid (AIB) as a function of the distance from center of (A) a Walker 256 carcinoma, and (B) a C6 glioma following the onset of (a) a continuous infusion and (b) a bolus injection. In all four graphs, the lower curves represent the untreated case, whereas the upper curves show the effect of osmotic treatment concurrent with the onset of the AIB injections. Broken lines represent exposure in the absence of diffusion within tissue. BST, Brain surrounding tumor.

TABLE II Calculated Enhancement Factors γ for Exposure to α-Aminoisobutyric Acid for Tumor, Tumor Edge, Brain Surrounding Tumor, and Normal Brain for 1 Hr following Osmotic Treatment[a]

		Enhancement factor γ[b]			
Tumor type	Input	Center of tumor	100 μm into tumor	BST	Brain
Walker 256 carcinoma	Continuous infusion	4.8	6.2	9.9	37
	Bolus	5.6	8.1	11.5	30
C6 glioma	Continuous infusion	1.3	1.7	2.9	16
	Bolus	1.4	2.4	3.8	17

[a] From Robinson and Rapoport (34).

[b] Defined as ratio of integrated exposure to drug following osmotic treatment to exposure without osmotic treatment.

A quantitative model of blood–brain barrier permeability changes following osmotic opening, both in normal brain and brain tumor, such as the one outlined here, is essential for assessing the relevance and importance of each of these factors for drug delivery to brain tumors in each case.

Conclusions

The main conclusions concerning the nature of the BBB, the effect of osmotic treatment, and implications for brain tumor chemotherapy, can be summarized as follows.

1. The BBB prevents entry of many drugs into the brain, particularly hydrophilic compounds, proteins, and protein-bound compounds.
2. Blood–brain barrier permeability can be increased reversibly by administration of hyperosmotic solutions.
3. There is a precise threshold (concentation times time) for osmotically induced opening of the BBB. In the evaluation of the clinical effectiveness of the osmotic method, it is essential that the brain be adequately perfused so that this threshold is reached.
4. Osmotic BBB opening is mediated by osmotically induced shrinkage of cerebrovascular endothelial cells, and consequent reversible widening of interendothelial tight junctions.

5. Size and charge dependence: Quantitative studies of BBB permeability following osmotic opening in rats suggest an induced pore size of about 200 Å, with a pore density of about 1 pore/200 μm^2 of membrane surface area, within 35 min of osmotic treatment.
6. Bulk fluid flow: Enhanced entry into brain following osmotic treatment is mediated by bulk fluid flow from blood to brain accompanied by solute drag, primarily within the first 10 min or so following osmotic treatment. Initial "reclosure" of the BBB is mediated primarily by reductions in bulk flow rather than reductions in pore size or density.
7. The osmotic method can increase vascular permeability in many brain tumors, and when it is combined with methotrexate, cyclophosphamide, and procarbazine administration the tumor regresses and survival is prolonged in patients with primary lymphomas and glioblastomas (11, 15, 27, 35, 41).
8. Blood–tumor barrier permeability is highly dependent on the type of tumor, and the osmotic method is most effective in the case of tumors with at least a partial BTB.
9. To assist in evaluating the efficacy of the osmotic method in brain tumor chemotherapy and in assessing the effect of factors such as tumor type and dosage regimen, drug entry into brain and tumor has been modeled in terms of time-dependent BBB and BTB permeabilities and bulk flow, as well as drug plasma profiles, concentration gradients, and diffusion of drug within the brain and brain tumor, to give quantitative estimates of the effect of osmotic treatment on exposure of tumor, brain surrounding tumor, and normal brain to the drug (32).

References

1. B. K. Armstrong, P. J. Robinson, and S. I. Rapoport, Size-dependent blood–brain barrier opening demonstrated with 14-C sucrose and a 200,000 dalton dextran. *Exp. Neurol.* **97,** 686–696 (1987).
2. R. G. Blasberg and D. R. Goothuis, Chemotherapy of brain tumors: Physiological and pharmacokinetic considerations. *Semin. Oncol.* **13,** 70–82 (1986).
3. M. W. Brightman, M. Hori, S. I. Rapoport, T. S. Reese and E. Westergaard, Osmotic opening of tight junctions in cerebral endothelium. *J. Comp. Neurol.* **152,** 317–326 (1973).
4. F. E. Curry, Mechanics and thermodynamics of transcapillary exchange. *In* "Handbook of Physiology" (E. M. Renkin and C. C. Michel, eds.), Sect. 2, Vol. IV, pp. 309–374. Am. Physiol. Soc., Bethesda, MD, 1984.

4a. W. M. Deen, B. Satvat, and J. M. Jamieson, Theoretical model for glomerular filtration of charged solutes. *Am. J. Physiol.* **238,** F126–F189 (1980).

5. K. Dorvini-Zis, M. Sato, G. Goping, S. I. Rapoport, and M. Brightman, Ionic lanthanum passage across cerebral endothelium exposed to hyperosmotic arabinose. *Acta Neuropathol.* **60,** 49–60 (1983).
6. H. Faxen, About T. Bohlin's paper: On the drag of rigid spheres moving in a viscous liquid inside cylindrical tubes. *Kolloid. Zh.* **167,** 146 (1959).
7. J. D. Fenstermacher and J. A. Johnson, Filtration and reflection coefficients of the rabbit blood–brain barrier. *Am. J. Physiol.* **211,** 341–346 (1966).
8. J. D. Fenstermacher and S. I. Rapoport, Blood–brain barrier. *In* "Handbook of Physiology" (E. M. Renkin and C. C. Michel, eds.), Sect. 2, Vol. IV, pp. 969–1000. Am. Physiol. Soc., Bethesda, MD, 1984.
9. R. A. Fishman, Editorial: Is there a therapeutic role for osmotic breaching of the blood–brain barrier? *Ann. Neurol.* **22,** 298–299 (1987).
9a. R. A. Fishman, Reply. *Ann. Neurol.* **24,** 680 (1988).
10. D. R. Groothuis and R. G. Blasberg, Reply. *Ann. Neurol.* **24,** 682–684 (1988).
11. E. M. Hiesiger, R. M. Voorhies, G. A. Basler, L. E. Lipschutz, J. B. Posner, and W. R. Shapiro, Opening the blood–brain and blood–tumor barriers in experimental rat brain tumors: The effet of intracarotid hyperosmolar mannitol on capillary permeability and blood flow. *Ann. Neurol.* **19,** 50–59 (1986).
12. R. C. Lanman, J. A. Burton, and L. S. Schanker, Diffusion coefficients of some 14-C labeled saccharides of biological interest. *Life Sci.* **10,** 803–811 (1971).
13. R. Levine, W. Fredericks, and S. I. Rapoport, Entry of bilirubin into the brain due to opening of the blood–brain barrier. *Pediatrics* **69,** 255–259 (1982).
14. Z. Nagy, H. M. Pappius, G. Mathieson, and I. Huttner, Opening of tight junctions in cerebral endothelium. I. Effect of hyperosmolar mannitol infused through the internal carotid artery. *J. Comp. Neurol.* **185,** 569–578 (1979).
14a. E. A. Neuwelt and P. A. Barnett, Blood–brain barrier disruption in the treatment of brain tumors. Animal studies. *In* "Implications of the Blood–Brain Barrier and Its Manipulation," Vol. 2, pp. 107–193. Plenum, New York, 1989.
15. E. A. Neuwelt and S. I. Rapoport, Modification of the blood–brain barrier in the chemotherapy of malignant brain tumors. *Fed. Proc., Fed. Am. Soc. Exp. Biol.* **43,** 214–219 (1984).
16. E. A. Neuwelt, E. P. Frenkel, J. Diehl, L. H. Vu, S. I. Rapoport, and S. Hill, Reversible osmotic blood–brain barrier disruption in humans: Implications for the chemotherapy of malignant brain tumors. *Neurosurgery* **7,** 44–52 (1980).
17. E. A. Neuwelt, M. Glasberg, E. Frenlel, and P. Barnett, Neurotoxicity of chemotherapeutic agents after blood–brain barrier modification: Neuropathological studies. *Ann. Neurol.* **14,** 316–324 (1983).
18. S. I. Rapoport, Effect of concentrated solutions on blood–brain barrier. *Am. J. Physiol.* **219,** 270–274 (1970).
19. S. I. Rapoport, "Blood–Brain Barrier in Physiology and Medicine." Raven Press, New York, 1976.
20. S. I. Rapoport, Osmotic opening of the blood–brain barrier. *Ann. Neurol.* **24,** 677–679 (1988).
21. S. I. Rapoport and P. J. Robinson, Tight junctional modification as the basis of osmotic opening of the blood–brain barrier. *Ann. N.Y. Acad. Sci.* **481,** 250–267 (1986).

22. S. I. Rapoport and P. J. Robinson, Response to letter to the editor by R. G. Blasberg and D. G. Groothuis. *J. Cereb. Blood Flow Metab.* (1990).
23. S. I. Rapoport and H. K. Thompson, Osmotic opening of the blood–brain barrier in the monkey without associated neurological deficits. *Science* **180,** 971 (abstr.) (1973).
24. S. I. Rapoport, and I. Klatzo, Testing of a hypothesis for osmotic opening of the blood–brain barrier. *Am. J. Physiol.* **223,** 323–331 (1972).
25. S. I. Rapoport, W. R. Fredericks, K. Ohno, and K. D. Pettigrew, Quantitative aspects of reversible osmotic opening of the blood–brain barrier. *Am. J. Physiol.* **238,** R421–R431 (1980).
26. H. J. Reulen, S. Graber, P. Huber, and U. Ito, Factors affecting the extension of peritumoral brain oedema. A CT study. *Acta Neurochir.* **95,** 19–24 (1988).
27. C. G. Rhodes, R. J. S. Wise, and J. M. Gibbs, In vivo disturbance of the oxidative metabolism of glucose in human cerebral gliomas. *Ann. Neurol.* **14,** 614–626 (1983).
28. P. J. Robinson, Facilitation of drug entry into brain by osmotic opening of the blood–brain barrier. *Clin. Exp. Pharmacol. Physiol.* **14,** 887–901 (1987).
29. P. J. Robinson and S. I. Rapoport, Kinetics of protein binding determine rates of uptake of drugs by brain. *Am. J. Physiol.* **251,** R1212–R1220 (1986).
30. P. J. Robinson and S. I. Rapoport, Effect of binding to albumin on uptake of bilirubin by brain. *Pediatrics* **79,** 553–557 (1987).
31. P. J. Robinson and S. I. Rapoport, Size-selectivity of blood–brain barrier permeability after osmotic opening. *Am. J. Physiol.* **253,** R458–R466 (1987).
32. P. J. Robinson and S. I. Rapoport, Model for drug uptake by brain tumors: effects of osmotic treatment and diffusion in brain. *J. Cereb. Blood Flow Metab.* **10,** 153–161 (1990).
33. P. J. Robinson and S. I. Rapoport, Blood–brain barrier. *In* "Encyclopedia of Human Biology" (R. Dulbecco, ed.), Vol. 1, pp. 715–727. Academic Press, San Diego, 1991.
34. P. J. Robinson and S. I. Rapoport, Transport of drugs. *In* "Handbook of Experimental Pharmacology" (G. V. R. Born, P. Cuatrecasas, H. Herken, and A. Schwartz, eds.), Vol. 103, Chapter 11, pp. 279–300. Springer-Verlag, Berlin, 1992.
35. S. C. Saris, D. C. Wright, E. H. Oldfield, and R. G. Blasberg, Intravascular streaming and variable delivery to brain following carotid artery infusions in the Sprague-Dawley rat. *J. Cereb. Blood Flow Metab.* **8,** 116–1120 (1988).
36. W. R. Shapiro, Reply. *Ann. Neurol.* **24,** 680–682 (1988).
37. W. R. Shapiro, R. M. Voorhies, E. M. Hiesiger, P. B. Sher, G. A. Basler, and L. E. Lipschutz, Pharmacokinetics of tumor cell exposure to [14-C]methotrexate after intracarotid administration without and with hyperosmotic opening of the blood–brain and blood–tumor barriers in rat brain tumors: A quantitative autoradiographic study. *Cancer Res.* **48,** 694–701 (1988).
38. N. Simionescu, M. Simionescu, and G. E. Palade, Permeability of muscle capillaries to small heme peptides. Evidence for the existence of patent transendothelial channels. *J. Cell Biol.* **64,** 586–607 (1975).

39. F. G. Smith and W.M. Deen, Electrostatic double-layer interactions for spherical colloids in cylindrical pores. *J. Colloid Interface Sci.* **78,** 444–465 (1980).
40. M. Spatz, S. Z. Rap, S. I. Rapoport, and I. Klatzo, Effects of hypertonic solutions of mercuric chloride on the uptake of 14-C glucose analogues by rabbit brain. *Neuropathol. Appl. Neurobiol.* **2,** 53–61 (1976).
41. P. A. Stewart, K. Hayakawa, C. L. Farrell, and R. F. Del Maestro, Quantitative study of microvessel ultrastructure in human peritumoral brain tissue. Evidence for a blood–brain barrier defect. *J. Neurosurg.* **67,** 697–705 (1987).
42. R. K. Studer, D. M. Welch, and B. A. Siegel, Transient alteration of the blood–brain barrier: Effect of hypertonic solutions administered via carotid artery injection. *Exp. Neurol.* **44,** 266–263 (1974).
43. A. M. Thompson, Hyperosmotic effects on brain uptake of non-electrolytes. *In* "Capillary Permeability" (C. Crone and N. Lassen, eds.), pp. 459–467. Munksgaard, Copenhagen, 1970.
44. M. D. Walker and H. Weiss, Chemotherapy in the treatment of malignant brain tumors. *Adv. Neurol.* **13,** 149–191 (1975).
45. Y. Z. Ziylan, P. J. Robinson, and S. I. Rapoport, Differential blood–brain barrier permeabilities to 14-C sucrose and 3-H inulin after osmotic opening in the rat. *Exp. Neurol.* **79,** 845–857 (1983).
46. Y. Z. Ziylan, P. J. Robinson, and S. I. Rapoport, Blood–brain barrier permeability to sucrose and dextran after osmotic opening. *Am. J. Physiol.* **247,** R634–R638 (1984).

[4] Osmotic Blood–Brain Barrier Modification: Increasing Delivery of Diagnostic and Therapeutic Agents to the Brain

Edward A. Neuwelt and Robert A. Kroll

Introduction

The demonstration that dopamine deficiency of the basal ganglia, resulting in Parkinson disease, could be improved by the administration not of dopamine itself (a substance that does not cross the blood–brain barrier) but of its precursor (which does cross) was a major breakthrough in the treatment of this neurological disease. Furthermore, it highlights the importance of the blood–brain barrier (BBB) in clinical medicine. More recently, significant advances have been made in the treatment of central nervous system (CNS) infection and brain tumors through the delivery of drugs across the BBB. Evidence is also accruing that manipulation of the BBB will be important in the treatment of CNS genetic disorders. Certainly, animal studies have played a fundamental role in advancing our understanding of the BBB and will continue to serve an integral function in our continuing efforts to improve the diagnosis and treatment of a number of neurological disorders, based primarily on manipulation of the BBB.

Blood–Brain Barrier

When compared to other body systems, the CNS has a unique function in the exchange of metabolites. Many metabolic products are not freely exchanged between the blood and brain tissue (7). This aspect of the CNS has led to the notion of the BBB. Not only does this awareness of the BBB help explain questions of metabolite exchange, but it is important in understanding the permeability of the CNS to antibodies, toxins, and infectious agents, and the ability of many drugs to penetrate the CNS (7, 46).

Endothelium of the CNS vasculature demonstrates a number of structural differences, when compared with that of other organs. Fenestrations between the vascular endothelial cells within some organs (i.e., kidney, intestine, and endocrine, salivary, and lacrimal glands) that contribute to water and metabolite exchange are not seen within normal mammalian brain (27). This

Methods in Neurosciences, Volume 21

is true except for certain areas of the brain, such as the area postrema and adenohypophysis, that correspond to areas lacking a BBB. In many other organs, such as striated muscle, pinocytotic vesicles provide a transport function across the endothelial cell. In contrast, endothelium of the brain microvasculature has few vesicles (6). Cerebral endothelial cells also differ from those of other organs with regard to their intercellular attachments. Adjacent outer layers of cytoplasmic membranes are fused together to form a continuous belt around the vessel (1, 7). These unique attachments are called tight junctions or zonula occludens, and are yet another morphological feature of the BBB. The ionic conditions around the endothelium have been emphasized. The net negative charge of the lumenal surface of CNS endothelium influences the BBB function (19). The sialic acid residues of glycocalyx account for this net negative charge (29). Extracellular Ca^{2+} plays a significant role in maintaining structural integrity of the tight junctions as well (30).

Blood–Brain Barrier Disruption

Blood–brain barrier disruption must be reversible to have any role in the delivery of therapeutic or diagnostic agents. Several methods to modify the BBB have been described. Greig and Cavanagh have demonstrated that pentylenetetrazol, a CNS stimulant, provided reversible disruption of the BBB (16). Johansson has shown breakdown of the BBB in acute hypertension; however, there is associated structural damage (25). Clemedson *et al.* (8) and Cutler and Barlow (9) have shown increased cerebrovascular permeability in the face of hypercapnia, with the degree of opening related to the CO_2 concentration and duration of exposure. It has been reported that dimethyl sulfoxide (DMSO) safely and reversibly opens the BBB (3, 4); however, others have not been able to demonstrate any increased BBB permeability with DMSO (15, 33). Spigelman and others have achieved reversible disruption of the BBB with the intracarotid infusion of etoposide (54, 55). The alteration in barrier integrity associated with etoposide lasts for 4 days or more (54), however, making clinical usefulness unlikely.

Intracarotid infusion of a hypertonic solution is the most carefully evaluated and proven method available for reversible disruption (32). Hypertonic solutions used to disrupt the BBB include mannitol, arabinose, lactamide, saline, urea, glycerol, and several radiographic contrast agents (32). Osmotic disruption of the BBB appears to cause endothelial cell shrinkage, associated with the hypertonic environment, opening the endothelial tight junctions that constitute the anatomical basis of the barrier (2, 49).

Blood–brain barrier modification is currently being utilized clinically to increase the delivery of chemotherapeutic agents for the treatment of brain tumors in humans. In a report of 30 patients with primary CNS lymphoma, unrelated to immune system compromise, 17 patients had a statistically significant increase in median survival (44.5 months) following initial BBB disruption chemotherapy (methotrexate and cyclophosphamide regimen), compared to 13 patients who had received standard radiation therapy prior to chemotherapy (median survival, 17.8 months) (39). Questions raised in the clinical setting continue to guide the direction of preclinical research and results of preclinical studies in animal models continue to find direct application in the treatment of patients.

Development of Animal Models

Osmotic BBB disruption has been reported for several animal models. The technique for the rat has been studied extensively and used in many BBB experiments (21, 34).

Blood–Brain Barrier Modification in Rat

The technique requires retrograde cathether placement in the external carotid artery for cephalad infusion into the internal carotid artery. Catheter placement is greatly aided by the use of a dissecting or operating microscope. The surgical instruments and supplies that we use are listed in Table I.

For acute studies, the rat is anesthetized with intraperitoneal pentobarbital sodium at a dose of 50 mg/kg and a tracheostomy tube [an ~3-cm length of polyethylene tubing (PE-240)] is placed for airway management and later ventilatory assistance. For chronic studies, because of the rapid recovery from anesthesia as well as the consistency of successful disruption, the rat

TABLE I Instruments and Supplies Useful in Performing Blood–Brain Barrier Disruption in Rat

Dissecting microscope	Biemer clip and applicating forceps
Umbilical tape	3 or 4 Needle retractors
Cellophane tape	4-0 silk thread
Scalpel	PE-50 tubing (~10 in.)
Metzenbaum scissors	Three-way stopcock
Iris scissors	Luer stub adapter (Intramedic, Becton Dickinson and Co., Franklin Lakes, NJ)
2 Microthumb forceps	
2 Microneedle holders	3-cc syringe with heparinized saline

is anesthetized with and maintained on isoflurane (AErrane, Anaquest, Inc., Liberty Corner, NJ). Following anesthetic induction (5% isoflurane) in a small chamber, an endotracheal tube (fashioned from a 14-gauge intravenous catheter with the needle stylet removed) is placed and the rat is maintained on a ventilator with 2% isoflurane. For both acute and chronic studies, the rat is placed in dorsal recumbancy, with its limbs and head tied in slight distraction. Umbilical tape ($\frac{1}{8}$-in. wide) works well as restraining ties, with cellophane tape used to secure it to the work surface. A ventral midline skin incision (~4 cm) is made from between the angles of the mandible to the manubrium sternum. If a tracheostomy is needed, the trachea is exposed, a small nick incision is made between tracheal rings, and a tracheostomy tube is inserted. Blunt dissection is used to expose the carotid artery at the level of the bifurcation of internal and external branches. Hooked needles with thread attached can be used as effective muscle retractors. Branches from the external carotid artery, the occipital and superior thyroid arteries, must be ligated or cauterized prior to infusion. It is not necessary to occlude the pterygopalatine branch of the internal carotid. The external carotid artery is freed from fascial attachments from rostral to the superior thyroid artery to just caudal to the carotid bifurcation. The external carotid artery is ligated as far rostral as possible and a fine Biemer clip is placed on the external carotid, just rostral to the bifurcation. Iris scissors are used to make a small nick incision in the external carotid, approximately 2 mm caudal to the rostral ligature. A few drops of lidocaine (2%) applied to the arteriotomy will cause vasodilation and permit easier introduction of the catheter. A cannula of polyethylene tubing (PE-50) with a bevel at the end and filled with heparinized saline is introduced retrograde through the arteriotomy and advanced to the Biemer clip. The cannula is then secured in place with a ligature rostral to the bifurcation, the Biemer clip is carefully removed, and, after aspirating to clear the cannula of any air bubbles, heparinized saline is flushed through. If the cannula is correctly placed, blood from the common carotid artery should flow through the internal carotid and the saline should flow cephalad through the internal carotid artery. Correct placement of the carotid cannula in the rat is illustrated in Fig. 1. In adult rats, the osmotic agent is infused at a constant rate (0.9–1.2 ml/sec) for 30 sec. Because the animals become apneic during administration of the osmotic agent, they must be mechanically ventilated during the infusion. The agent of study can then be administered through the carotid catheter. The procedure is finished by reapplying the Biemer clip, withdrawing the cannula, and tying off the external carotid artery caudal to the arteriotomy site, as it is already ligated rostrally. The wound can be closed in a single layer by apposing the skin edges with skin staples or sutures. It is important to remember that this is a one-time procedure in the rat, because the external carotid artery is sacrificed.

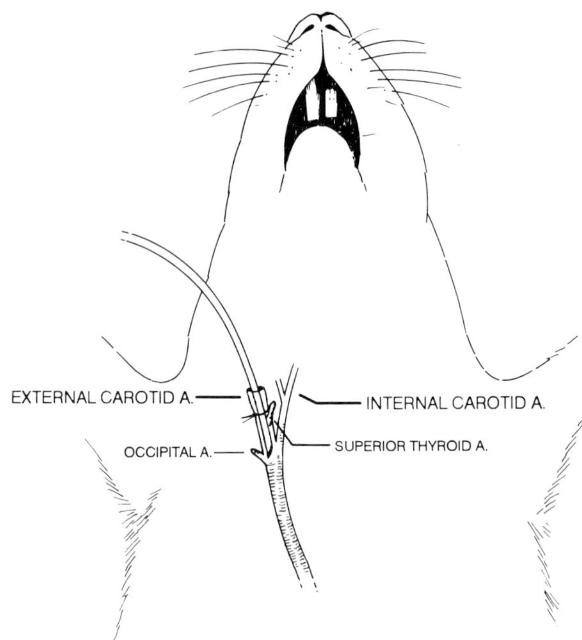

FIG. 1 Illustration of the surgical placement of a cannula into the carotid artery of the rat. For osmotic blood–brain barrier modification, the carotid artery is isolated at the level of the bifurcation of internal and external branches, the superior thyroid and occipital arteries are ligated, and a cannula is inserted retrograde in the external carotid artery. The tip of the cannula is placed so as to provide blood pressure-dependent cephalad infusion into the internal carotid artery.

Blood–Brain Barrier Modification in Dog

A canine model for reversible, osmotic disruption of the cerebral BBB has also been developed. Because a dog is larger, it provides sufficient cerebrospinal fluid (CSF) for serial evaluation and may be more accurately evaluated from a behavioral and imaging standpoint (32). Initial canine studies in which hypertonic mannitol was infused into the common carotid artery, after fluoroscopic cathether placement via the femoral artery, resulted in variable disruption (37, 40). Cannulation of the internal carotid artery, a relatively small vessel in dogs as compared to humans, can be readily accomplished by surgical exposure of the common carotid artery. Cephalad infusion of mannitol through this cannula has resulted in consistent disruptions (37).

It is important to be aware of the presence of external-to-internal carotid artery anastomoses (23). We have found that blood flow in the external carotid must be maintained to prevent diversion of internal carotid flow via these anastomoses and resultant suboptimal delivery of mannitol. With the availability of Tracker catheter systems (Target Therapeutics; Fremont, CA), BBB disruption through a fluoroscopically guided internal carotid catheter may now be more consistent. However, direct surgical cannulation has been routinely used.

The surgical technique is as follows: an angled, ventrolateral skin incision is made from the ramus of the mandible caudoventrally to a point lateral to the rostral end of the trachea. The platysma muscle is incised along this line and fascia is bluntly dissected to expose the jugular vein and parotid and mandibular salivary glands. The capsule of the mandibular salivary gland is incised so that the gland can be retracted ventrally while the jugular vein is retracted caudodorsally. Gentle, blunt dissection is used to expose and free the bifurcation of the carotid artery. A length of umbilical tape is passed once around the common carotid artery and then secured loosely with a hemostat. A Rummel clamp (length of 0 suture passed around the vessel and then both ends passed through a piece of soft tubing) is placed around the proximal end of the internal carotid artery and then loosely secured with a hemostat. While retracting the common carotid artery caudally and laterally with the umbilical tape, with just enough tension to occlude blood flow, a 14-gauge, over-the-needle indwelling catheter is inserted into the common carotid artery just caudal to the bifurcation and on the side opposite the internal carotid artery. It is imperative that the needle tip not perforate the opposite side of the artery. Once the catheter tip is within the arterial lumen, the catheter is advanced over the needle (without advancing the needle) and directed and advanced into and through the carotid sinus, the bulbous enlargement at the origin of the internal carotid artery (approximately 1 cm). Once this is accomplished, the needle is withdrawn, a three-way stopcock is attached to the catheter hub to stop the backflow of blood, and the catheter is held in place by snugging down the Rummel clamp and securing it with the hemostat. The catheter is then flushed with heparinized saline. Correct placement of the catheter for cerebral BBB disruption in the dog is illustrated in Fig. 2. In adult dogs, the osmotic agent is infused at a constant rate of 1.5 ml/sec for 30 sec. As in rats, the dog must be mechanically ventilated during the infusion. The agent of study can then be administered through the carotid catheter. Atraumatic vascular clamps are applied just above and below the site of arterial puncture when the catheter is removed. The arterial wound can then be sutured (6-0 Prolene; Ethicon, Inc.; Somersville, NJ) to maintain patency in the artery. The surgical wound should be closed in 3 layers—deep tissue, superficial fascia and subcutaneous tissue, and skin—to prevent a pocket of serum from accumulating.

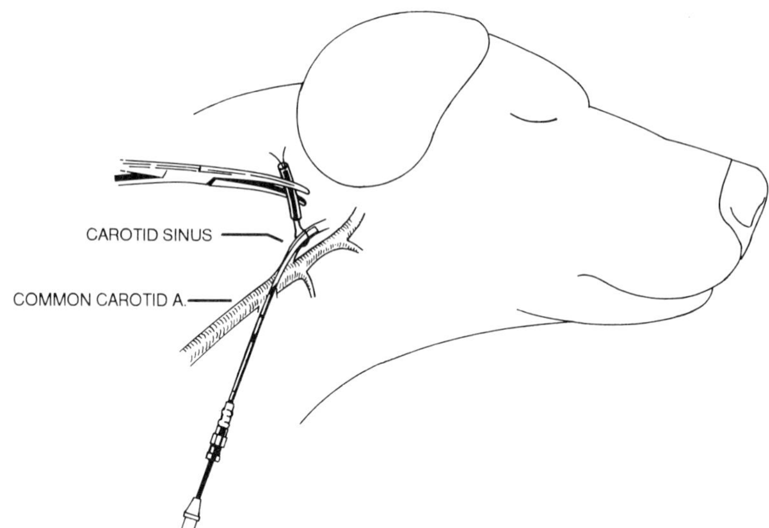

FIG. 2 Illustration of the surgical placement of a catheter into the internal carotid artery of the dog. Following isolation of the carotid bifurcation, a 14-gauge, over-the-needle indwelling catheter is inserted into the common carotid artery just caudal to the bifurcation and advanced 1 cm, through the carotid sinus, into the internal carotid artery. A Rummel clamp is utilized to secure the catheter in place temporarily.

Blood–brain barrier disruption of the posterior fossa (cerebellum and brainstem) can also be performed in dogs (38). Under fluoroscopic guidance, a percutaneous transfemoral catheter system can be placed in the vertebral artery for infusion of the osmotic agent, providing the potential for repeated barrier disruptions. The catheter is advanced to the level of the third cervical vertebra. The rate of mannitol infusion into the vertebral artery was found to be critical. An infusion rate of 2.47 ml/sec resulted in frequent neuropathological abnormalities, predominantly hemorrhagic infarction. An infusion rate of 2.08 ml/sec resulted in a reduced occurrence of successful barrier disruption (63%), but neurological complications were markedly reduced.

Blood–Brain Barrier Modification in Other Animal Models

Blood–brain barrier disruption has also been performed successfully in rabbits and primates (5, 47, 50, 56, 57). Attempts to disrupt the BBB reversibly in the cat have been frustrating. The cat lacks a continuous, patent internal carotid artery, but rather has a rete mirabile just proximal to the circle of Willis (14). This anatomical difference appears to result in infusate dilution.

With the availability of steerable Tracker catheter systems, which allow fluoroscopically guided transfemoral catheter placement to vessels with an inside diameter as small as 0.6 mm, current efforts are aimed at posterior fossa disruption in the cat (Fig. 3).

Confirming Blood–Brain Barrier Disruption

The agent most commonly used for acute studies of osmotic barrier opening, to assess BBB integrity, is Evans blue–albumin. Evans blue dye binds tightly but reversibly to albumin *in vivo* (48), resulting in an M_r 68,500 marker that does not cross an intact BBB, but that will stain brain parenchyma following disruption (Fig. 4) and will provide a semiquantitative visual measure of osmotic BBB modification. A 2% solution of Evans blue is administered intravenously (iv) (2 ml/kg) and staining of brain is graded on a scale of 0 to 3+ (Table II). As a matter of practicality, if surgical placement of a carotid cannula is being performed, Evans blue should not be administered until the cannula is placed, because the artery will be difficult to distinguish from adjacent tissues if they are all the same deep blue color. Fluorescein dye (10% solution, 0.6 ml/kg iv) can be used as a low molecular weight marker (M_r 376) of barrier opening.

The success of BBB disruption can be assessed antemortem via nuclear scintigraphy, computerized tomography (CT), or magnetic resonance imaging (MRI). The agents that have been used include technetium (^{99m}Tc)-labeled glucoheptonate for scintigraphy, iodinated contrast agents such as meglumine iothalamate and iopamidol for CT, and gadopentetate dimeglumine and microcrystalline iron oxide for MRI (Fig. 5) (40, 42, 43, 52, 53). Imaging BBB disruption in the dog, utilizing nuclear scintigraphy, is difficult because of the large temporal muscle mass in the dog and the associated high background activity of the ^{99m}Tc. Ionized iodinated contrast agents, as well as gadopentetate dimeglumine, have been found to be associated with an increased frequency of seizures when given across a disrupted BBB (53). Nonionic, iodinated agents have not been associated with increased seizure frequency.

Factors Influencing Successful Blood–Brain Barrier Disruption and Agent Delivery

Osmotic disruption of the BBB is a threshold event, requiring a minimum osmolality of the hypertonic solute as well as a minimum duration of infusion. Assuring an appropriate rate of solute infusion into the selected artery is critical (31, 36, 37). An insufficient infusion rate will result in a subthreshold

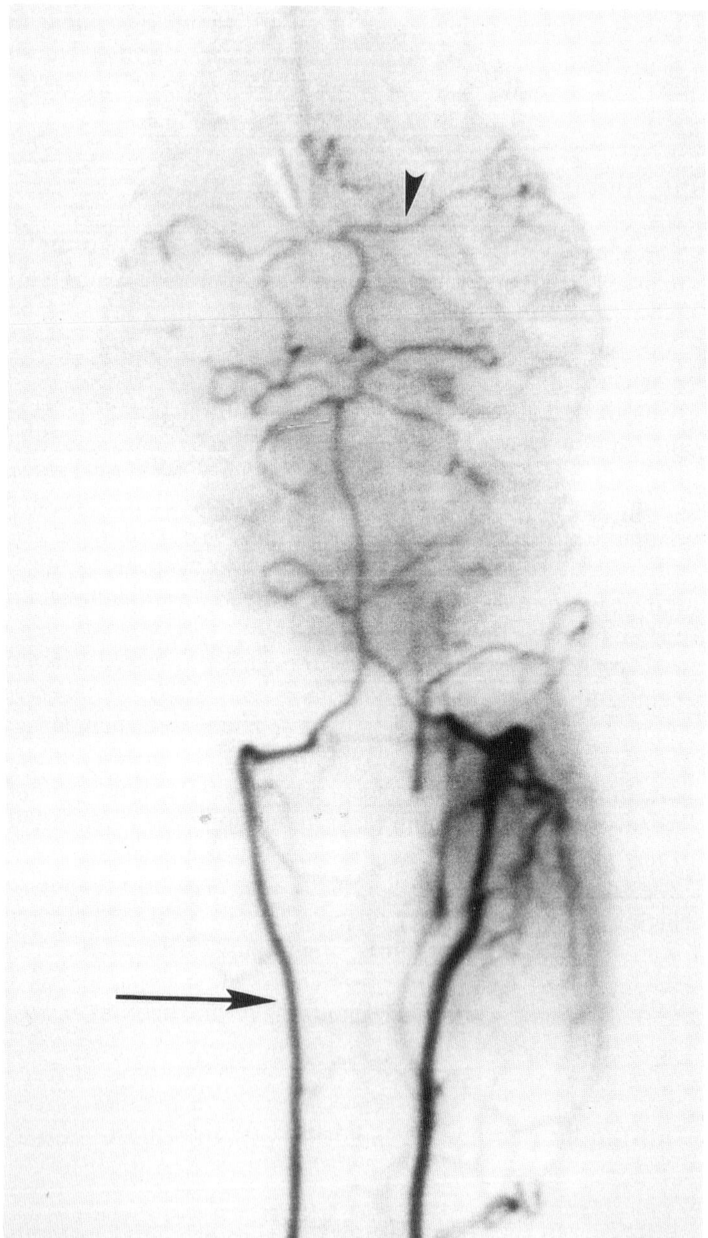

FIG. 3 Cerebral angiogram of a cat. A Tracker-18 catheter was inserted into the femoral artery and fluoroscopically guided into the left vertebral artery. Iodinated

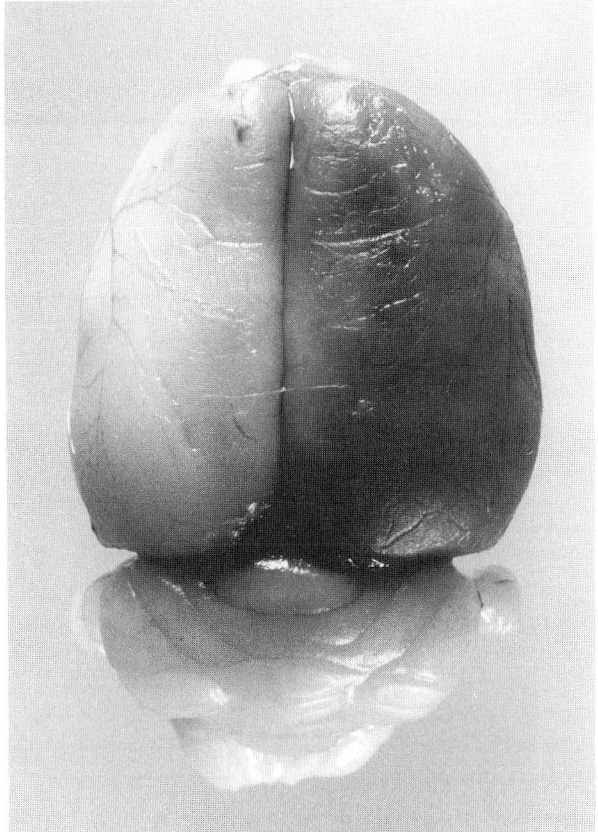

FIG. 4 Formalin-fixed rat brain 2 days after osmotic BBB disruption with mannitol infusion into the right internal carotid artery. The dark areas represent penetration of Evans blue–albumin (M_r 68,500) across the BBB.

event associated with dilution of the infusate by blood from the ipsilateral carotid artery or from collateral flow via the circle of Willis. Excessive infusion rates, on the other hand, may lead to intravascular hypertension and irreversible damage (25). A rare complication of cerebral BBB disruption has been observed in the dog, even with the previously described infusion

---

contrast was injected at a rate of 2 ml/sec to produce this image. Immediately thereafter, mannitol was infused at a similar rate to effect osmotic blood–brain barrier disruption. The right vertebral artery (arrow) and left middle cerebral artery (arrowhead) are identified.

TABLE II Scale of Brain Staining by Evans Blue–Albumin following Osmotic Blood–Brain Barrier Modification

Degree of tissue staining	Grading scale
No apparent staining	0
Just noticeable	1+
Moderate staining	2+
Excellent staining	3+

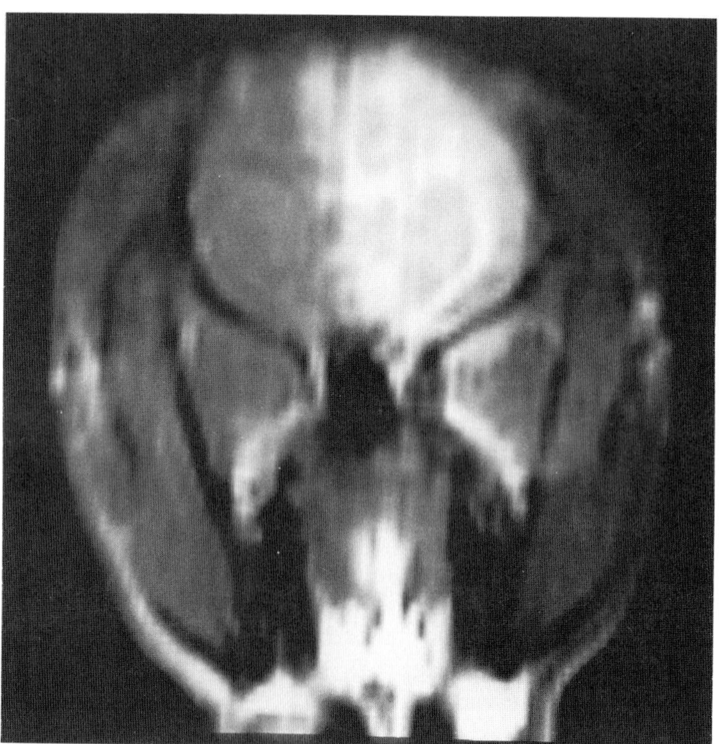

FIG. 5 Transaxial, T1-weighted magnetic resonance image of a rat following intravenous administration of monocrystalline iron oxide particles (iron dose, 10 mg/kg) and blood–brain barrier disruption of the right cerebral hemisphere. Note the signal enhancement (white) of the right hemisphere.

rate of 1.5 ml/sec for 30 sec. Overdisruption, resulting in malignant cerebral edema with increases in intracranial pressure as high as 140 mmHg, has been observed in about 5% of canine subjects (32). Rarely, similar severe disruptions occur in rats.

Measuring cerebrovascular permeability times capillary surface area (*PS*) to sucrose in rats, Ohno and colleagues found that the threshold for BBB disruption with arabinose is 1.6 *M* infused for a minimum of 20 sec (45). Higher arabinose concentrations or longer infusions did not increase the *PS* value. When methotrexate was administered following BBB disruption with 1.4 *M* mannitol for 30 sec, the increase in drug delivery to the disrupted hemisphere was similar to that when 1.6–2.0 *M* arabinose was used. Drug concentration was not significantly increased with increasing osmolalities of mannitol above 1.4–1.6 *M* (36).

Additional factors that affect successful BBB modification and subsequent agent delivery include anesthetics used, $PaCO_2$ level, steroid administration, and route and duration of agent administration.

The effects of various anesthetic agents on osmotic BBB disruption were evaluated in Sprague-Dawley rats, comparing pentobarbital, ketamine–xylazine, isoflurane, methoxyflurane, and fentanyl–droperidol (17). With pentobarbital, ketamine–xylazine, or isoflurane, excellent disruption (3+, Evans blue staining) of the mannitol-infused cerebral hemisphere was observed. Fentanyl–droperidol anesthesia was associated with tachycardia and methoxyflurane with hypotension. Both resulted in poor Evans blue staining. Following pharmacological manipulation to normalize the cardiac index (ml of blood/min/kg), excellent disruption was achieved with both drugs, suggesting that the cardiovascular changes associated with these anesthetic agents are important in obtaining optimal BBB disruption. Quantitative evaluation of ^{99m}Tc-labeled glucoheptonate (M_r 226) and ^{125}I-labeled albumin (M_r 68,000) delivery was also assessed in this study, with results that paralleled Evans blue staining.

Johansson, Neuwelt, and co-workers (24, 26, 37) have studied the effects of $PaCO_2$ on BBB opening. Hypercapnia has been shown to increase brain permeability to protein (9) and, in the acute hypertension model of BBB disruption, protein extravasation may correlate directly with $PaCO_2$ (24). Neuwelt *et al.* evaluated the effect of $PaCO_2$ on methotrexate delivery with osmotic BBB disruption and found a nonlinear relationship between $PaCO_2$ and drug delivery (37). However, cardiovascular parameters were not monitored and it has been suggested that the differences observed may have been due to changes in the cardiac index (17).

Adrenocortical steroids are commonly used in brain tumor patients because they rapidly decrease vasogenic edema around CNS tumors (18, 51) and, therefore, have a dramatic effect on clinical signs. Steroid administration leads to decreased contrast enhancement on CT scans and decreased uptake of radionuclide agents on brain scans (28) and positron emission tomography (PET) scans (22). Also, in an intracerebral C6 rat glioma tumor model, Reichman *et al.* reported decreased extravasation of Evans blue–albumin in tumor, brain adjacent to tumor, and contralateral brain when the rats were pretreated with dexamethasone, methylprednisolone, or indomethacin (51). These effects suggest steroids decrease vascular permeability. They may also result in decreased delivery of drugs or other agents given in conjunction with BBB disruption.

In a study of Neuwelt *et al.*, when dexamethasone (96 $mg/m^2/day$ for 3 days) was administered to normal (non-tumor-bearing) rats prior to BBB disruption and methotrexate administration, there was a slight but not significant decrease in methotrexate concentration in the disrupted hemisphere as compared to non-dexamethasone-pretreated controls (34). However, in rats with an intracerebral avian sarcoma virus-induced glioma, dexamethasone pretreatment prior to BBB disruption resulted in a dramatic reduction of methotrexate delivery to tumor, brain adjacent to tumor, and ipsilateral brain distant to tumor. Compared to animals that did not receive steroids prior to BBB disruption, there was a 40–60% decrease of methotrexate concentration in the tumor, and to a lesser degree in brain adjacent to tumor and brain distant to tumor.

Intrinsically related are dose, method of administration (bolus, slow infusion, or continuous), and route of administration [iv versus intraarterial (ia)] of an agent when given with BBB modification. Fenstermacher and Gazendam found a distinct advantage to ia administration for target tissues with a low blood flow in the infused artery or associated capillary bed or when drug biotransformation or excretion is high (11). Methotrexate has a rapid plasma clearance (35, 44). Intracarotid administration of methotrexate (4 mg/kg) following BBB disruption resulted in a 7- to 10-fold increase in delivery as compared to iv administration after BBB disruption (20, 37, 44). When a higher dose of methotrexate (14 mg/kg) was administered as an iv bolus (1 min) or iv drip (40 min) after intracarotid saline, the concentration in brain ranged from 1500 to 2500 ng/g (41). Methotrexate administered in the same manner after BBB disruption resulted in an 8- to 18-fold increase in drug levels in the ipsilateral hemisphere when compared to saline-infused control animals. However, the difference in drug levels between the iv bolus and iv drip groups was not significant. When methotrexate was administered ia (over 15 min) after intracarotid infusion of saline, the concentration in brain was 500–2000 ng/g; after BBB opening, the concentration increased to 50,000 ng/g in the ipsilateral hemisphere. This increase was significantly higher ($p < 0.025$) than the increases associated with other routes.

Conclusion

Thus far, osmotic modification of the blood–brain barrier has been studied most commonly as a method of improving brain tumor therapy. The chemotherapeutic dose–response curve for responsive tumors is known to be quite steep, therefore any factor that decreases drug delivery can significantly diminish therapeutic efficacy (10, 12, 13). Vascular permeability to small molecules (e.g., aminoisobutyric acid), large biomolecules (e.g., antibodies), and even virus-sized iron oxide particles is increased transiently following infusion of hypertonic mannitol, after which it decreases rapidly, returning to preinfusion levels within 2 hr (32, 43). Although this is an invasive procedure, this method has been shown in human patients to be a safe and effective means of treating certain types of malignant brain tumors while maintaining cognitive function (39). One limitation of this technique is that increased agent delivery to spinal cord is not achieved, although delivery to cerebrospinal fluid is increased (37).

Current directions of BBB disruption research include delivery of monoclonal antibodies conjugated to iron particles for tumor-specific magnetic resonance imaging, monoclonal antibodies conjugated to drugs and toxins for tumor-specific therapy, and delivery of viral vectors for global therapy of genetic disorders. We anticipate that osmotic blood–brain barrier modification will continue to have a role in increasing delivery of diagnostic and therapeutic agents to the brain.

References

1. M. W. Brightman and T. S. Reese, *J. Cell. Biol.* **40,** 647 (1969).
2. M. W. Brightman, M. Hori, S. I. Rapoport, T. S. Reese, and E. Westergaard, *J. Comp. Neurol.* **152,** 317 (1973).
3. R. Broadwell, R. Kaplan, and M. Salcman, *Soc. Neurosci.* **7,** 244 (1981).
4. R. Broadwell, M. Salcman, and R. Kaplan, *Science* **217,** 164 (1982).
5. T. Broman and O. Olsson, *Acta Radiol.* (*Stockholm*) **30,** 326 (1948).
6. J. Cervós-Navarro, *Arch. Psychiat. Nervenkr.* **204,** 484 (1963).
7. J. Cervós-Navarro, S. Kannuki, and Y. Nakagawa, *Histol. Histopathol.* **3,** 203 (1988).
8. C. Clemedson, H. Hartelius, and A. Holmberg, *Acta Pathol. Microbiol. Scand.* **42,** 137 (1958).
9. R. Cutler and C. Barlow, *Arch. Neurol.* **14,** 54 (1966).
10. V. T. DeVita, *J. Clin. Oncol.* **4,** 1157 (1986).
11. J. D. Fenstermacher and J. Gazendam, *Cancer Treat. Rep.* **65,** 27 (1981).
12. E. Frei and G. P. Canellos, *Am. J. Med.* **69,** 585 (1980).
13. E. A. Gehan, *Cancer* **54,** 1204 (1984).

14. N. G. Ghosal and B. S. Nanda, *in*: "Sisson and Grossman's The Anatomy of the Domestic Animals" (R. Getty, ed.), 5th ed., p. 1594. Saunders, Philadelphia, 1975.
15. N. Greig, D. Sweeney, and S. Rapoport, *Cancer Treat. Rep.* **69,** 305 (1985).
16. N. Greig and J. Cavanagh, *J. Neuropathol. Appl. Neurobiol.* **8,** 245 (1982).
17. M. K. Gumerlock and E. A. Neuwelt, *Neurosurgery* **26,** 268 (1990).
18. P. H. Gutin, *Semin. Oncol.* **2,** 49 (1975).
19. M. N. Hart, L. F. VanDyk, S. A. Moore, D. M. Shasby, and P. A. Cancilla, *J. Neuropathol. Exp. Neurol.* **46,** 141 (1987).
20. H. Hasegawa, J. E. Allen, B. M. Mehta, W. R. Shapiro, and J. B. Posner, *Neurology (N.Y.)* **29,** 1280 (1979).
21. E. M. Hiesiger, R. M. Voorhies, G. A. Basler, L. E. Lipschultz, J. B. Posner, and W. B. Shapiro, *Ann. Neurol.* **19,** 50 (1986).
22. J. O. Jarden, V. Dhawan, A. Poltorak, J. B. Posner, and D. A. Rottenberg, *Ann. Neurol.* **18,** 636 (1985).
23. P. A. Jewell, *J. Anat.* **86,** 83 (1952).
24. B. B. Johansson, *Stroke* **9,** 588 (1978).
25. B. B. Johansson, *in:* "Implications of the Blood–Brain Barrier and Its Manipulation" (E. A. Neuwelt, ed.), Vol. 2, p. 389. Plenum, New York, 1989.
26. B. B. Johansson and L. E. Linder, *Acta Anaesthesiol. Scand.* **24,** 65 (1980).
27. J. C. Lee, *in:* "Progress in Neuropathology" (H. M. Zimmermann, ed.), Vol. 1, p. 84. Grune & Stratton, New York, 1971.
28. R. Marty and M. L. Cain, *Radiology* **107,** 117 (1973).
29. S. Nag, *Acta Neuropathol. (Berlin)* **70,** 38 (1986).
30. Z. Nagy, U. G. Goehlert, L. S. Wolfe, and I. Hüttner, *Acta Neuropathol. (Berlin)* **68,** 48 (1985).
31. H. Nakagawa, D. Groothuis, and R. G. Blasberg, *Neurology (N.Y.)* **34,** 1571 (1984).
32. E. A. Neuwelt and P. A. Barnett, *in:* "Implications of the Blood–Brain Barrier and Its Manipulation" (E. A. Neuwelt, ed.), Vol. 2, p. 107. Plenum, New York, 1989.
33. E. A. Neuwelt, P. Barnett, and J. Barranger, *Neurosurgery* **12,** 29 (1983).
34. E. A. Neuwelt, P. A. Barnett, D. Bigner, and E. P. Frenkel, *Proc. Natl. Acad. Sci. U.S.A.* **79,** 4420 (1982).
35. E. A. Neuwelt, P. A. Barnett, and E. P. Frenkel, *Neurosurgery* **14,** 145 (1984).
36. E. A. Neuwelt, P. A. Barnett, C. I. McCormick, and E. P. Frenkel, *in:* "Developmental Neurosciences: Physiological, Pharmacological, and Clinical Aspects" (F. Caciagli, E. Giacobini, and R. Paoletti, eds.), p. 173. Elsevier Science Publishers, New York, 1984.
37. E. A. Neuwelt, E. P. Frenkel, S. Rapoport, and P. Barnett, *Neurosurgery* **7,** 36 (1980).
38. E. A. Neuwelt, M. Glasberg, J. Diehl, E. P. Frenkel, and P. Barnett, *J. Neurosurg.* **55,** 742 (1981).
39. E. A. Neuwelt, D. L. Goldman, S. A. Dahlborg, J. Crossen, F. Ramsey, S. Roman-Goldstein, R. Braziel, and B. Dana, *J. Clin. Oncol.* **9,** 1580 (1991).

40. E. A. Neuwelt, K. R. Maravilla, E. P. Frenkel, P. Barnett, S. Hill, and R. J. Moore, *Neurosurgery* **6,** 49 (1980).
41. E. A. Neuwelt, M. Pagel, P. Barnett, M. Glasberg, and E. P. Frenkel, *Cancer Res.* **41,** 4466 (1981).
42. E. A. Neuwelt, H. D. Specht, J. Howieson, J. E. Haines, M. J. Bennett, S. A. Hill, and E. P. Frenkel, *Am. J. Neuroradiol.* **4,** 829 (1983).
43. E. A. Neuwelt, R. Weissleder, G. Nilaver, R. A. Kroll, S. Roman-Goldstein, J. Szumowski, M. A. Pagel, R. S. Jones, L. G. Remsen, C. I. McCormick, E. M. Shannon, and L. L. Muldoon, *Neurosurgery* **34,** 777 (1994).
44. K. Ohno, W. R. Fredericks, and S. I. Rapoport, *Surg. Neurol.* **12,** 323 (1979).
45. K. Ohno, K. D. Pettigrew, and S. I. Rapoport, *Am. J. Physiol.* **253,** H299 (1978).
46. I. F. Pollack and R. D. Lund, *Exp. Neurol.* **108,** 114 (1990).
47. S. I. Rapoport, "Blood–Brain Barrier in Physiology and Medicine." Raven, New York, 1976.
48. S. I. Rapoport, W. R. Fredericks, K. Ohno, and K. D. Pettigrew, *Am. J. Physiol.* **238,** R421 (1980).
49. S. I. Rapoport, *Am. J. Physiol.* **219,** 270 (1970).
50. S. I. Rapoport and H. K. Thompson, *Science* **180,** 971 (1973).
51. H. R. Reichman, C. L. Farrell, and R. F. Del Maestro, *J. Neurosurg.* **65,** 233 (1986).
52. W. D. Rhine, D. A. Benaron, D. R. Enzmann, C. Chung, R. Gonzales-Mendez, J. R. Sayre, and D. K. Stevenson, *J. Comput. Assist. Tomogr.* **17,** 563 (1993).
53. S. M. Roman-Goldstein, P. A. Barnett, C. I. McCormick, M. J. Ball, F. Ramsey, and E. A. Neuwelt, *Am. J. Neuroradiol.* **12,** 885 (1991).
54. M. Spigelman, R. Zappulla, J. Holland, L. I. Malis, and L. Norton, *Proc. Am. Assoc. Cancer Res.* **25,** 383 (1984).
55. M. K. Spigelman, R. Zappulla, J. Johnson, S. J. Goldsmith, L. I. Malis, and J. F. Holland, *J. Neurosurg.* **61,** 674 (1984).
56. I. J. Strausbaugh and G. S. Brinker, *Antimicrob. Agents Chemother.* **24,** 147 (1983).
57. J. Wilcox, C. A. Evill, and M. R. Sage, *Neuroradiology* **28,** 271 (1986).

Section III

Facilitated Transport through the Blood–Brain Barrier

[5] Peripheral Administration of Nerve Growth Factor Conjugated to an Anti-transferrin Receptor Antibody Increases Cholinergic Neuron Survival in Intraocular Forebrain Transplants

Ann-Charlotte Granholm, Paul T. Biddle, Cristina Bäckman, Ted Ebendal, Greg Gerhardt, Barry Hoffer, Ludmila Mackerlova, Lars Olson, Stine Söderström, Lee Walus, and Phillip Friden

Introduction

Selective death of specific neuronal populations in the brain is characteristic of certain neurological disorders such as senile dementia of the Alzheimer type (SDAT). Memory impairment in patients with Alzheimer's disease has been linked to the degeneration of forebrain cholinergic neurons (1). It is now established that neurotrophic molecules play a role in the survival and maintenance of some adult central neurons (2). Nerve growth factor (NGF) was the first trophic factor to be characterized and sequenced (3). Cholinergic neurons of the basal forebrain, which degenerate in the brains of patients with SDAT, are sensitive to NGF, which is delivered to the cell body through retrograde axonal transport from their synaptic target areas in the hippocampal formation and the cerebral cortex (4). The midline of the basal forebrain contains the largest cholinergic nucleus in the brain (5). Antibodies directed against the enzyme choline acetyltransferase (ChAT) have been utilized frequently to visualize cholinergic neurons (6). In addition, there is a high correlation between the distribution of cholinergic afferents in the adult rat hippocampal formation and the distribution of NGF mRNA, NGF-like biological activity, and NGF-like immunoreactivity (7–12).

If the clinical symptoms of Alzheimer's disease are a function of the loss of cholinergic neurons, then therapy to limit their loss would be of great benefit. The observations discussed above, that medial septal cholinergic neurons respond to NGF as a neurotrophic factor, combined with the findings that NGF can significantly prevent lesion-induced loss of both developing and mature cholinergic neurons in the basal forebrain (13), suggest that NGF

Methods in Neurosciences, Volume 21

may have a role in the treatment of patients with SDAT. The blood–brain barrier (BBB) presents one of the primary obstacles to clinical testing of NGF for neurodegenerative disorders. The BBB is composed primarily of specialized capillary endothelial cells joined by highly restrictive tight junctions. This barrier functions to maintain homeostasis of the brain. The entry into the brain of nonlipophilic substances, including large proteins that might be used for therapeutic treatments, is hindered by the BBB (14). Currently, there is no efficient, noninvasive delivery system for the NGF peptide across the BBB to target cells. Attempts to circumvent this barrier such as intraventricular injection utilizing an implanted cannula (15, 16), although effective, present possible side effects such as infections or changes in blood flow and intracerebral pressure. Therefore, a noninvasive transport system for NGF would significantly improve its therapeutic utility.

The most efficient means to transport substances into the brain would be to access a preexisting mechanism. Iron, which must gain access to the brain from the periphery, plays an integral role in the function of the central nervous system (CNS) in, for example, the synthesis of neurotransmitters such as serotonin (17) and γ-aminobutyric acid (GABA) (18). Transferrin, a plasma glycoprotein, binds iron in the blood and functions as the primary iron transport protein. Iron is delivered to cells through the interaction of the iron–transferrin complex with specific transferrin receptors located on the cell surface (19, 20) and is internalized through receptor-mediated endocytosis. Iron is released from transferrin in a pH-dependent manner into the interior of the cell as an ATP-dependent proton pump drives the pH of the endosome toward 5.5. In the brain, there is evidence suggesting both that the iron–transferrin complex undergoes direct transcytosis across the capillary endothelial cells and that iron is released from transferrin within the endothelial cells and then transported into the brain. Figure 1 depicts simplified schematics of the transferrin receptor-mediated pathway for the transport of iron–transferrin across the endothelial cell membrane. On the basis of the hypothesis that the transferrin transport mechanism could be used as a drug delivery system across the BBB, antibodies against the transferrin receptor were tested for their ability to penetrate the BBB (14, 19). Monoclonal antibodies against rat and human transferrin receptors were found to label blood capillaries in the brain, but not the blood vessels in other tissues. Furthermore, the binding of the antibody to brain capillary endothelial cells after intravenous injection was dose dependent (14, 18). Drugs conjugated to these antibodies have been found to accumulate in the brain (14). This penetration across the BBB suggests a possible role for transferrin receptor antibodies in the delivery of brain-targeted agents.

On the basis of the initial studies of BBB penetration by the transferrin

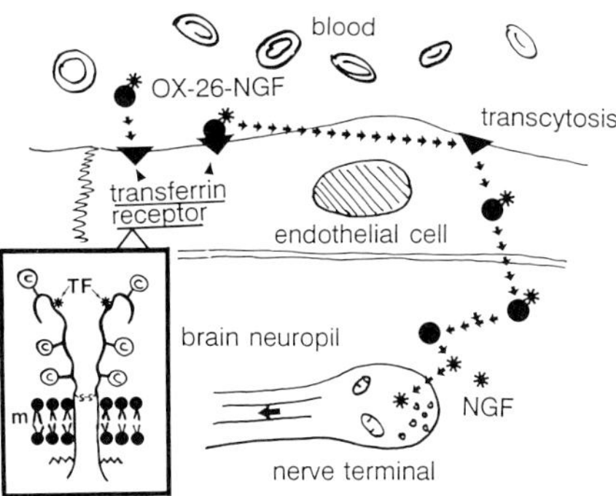

FIG. 1 Schematic illustration of the hypothesized binding and transfer of the OX-26–NGF conjugate on brain capillary endothelial cells. The conjugate is thought to bind to the transferrin receptor on the surface of the endothelial cell, and then to be transferred by transcytosis into the brain parenchyma. *Inset:* Demonstrates the transferrin receptor location in the cell membrane (m) and the two sites for transferrin (TF) binding on the extracellular portion of the receptor.

receptor antibodies, we have shown that NGF can be covalently linked to the OX-26 antibody while retaining biological activity (21). It was also shown that this OX-26–NGF conjugate can be delivered across the BBB and exert physiological effects earlier observed with direct administration of NGF into the brain (21). Presumably, the conjugate-delivered NGF is able to interact with its receptor on the target neurons and elicit a biological response. In this chapter we present evidence that peripheral administration of the antibody–drug conjugate OX-26–NGF delivers biologically active NGF by means of transferrin receptor transcytosis to stimulate the survival and growth of cholinergic forebrain neurons in brain tissue transplants. To enable studies of region-specific effects of this trophic factor conjugate in a controlled environment, transplantation techniques were employed.

The intraocular transplantation technique has been utilized for many years to investigate the effects of different factors on development and differentiation of discrete areas of the peripheral and central nervous systems (22, 23). Previous studies have shown that intraocular brain tissue grafts become well vascularized within approximately 1 week after transplantation (22), and develop barrier mechanisms consistent with a functional BBB (24, 25). When fetal medial forebrain tissue is grafted to the anterior chamber of the eye, cholinergic neurons will survive and develop a network of neurites within the grafted brain tissue (21, 26). The neurons will manifest many morphological characteristics resembling those of cholinergic neurons *in situ* (26). Medial forebrain tissue grafts *in oculo* have been shown to be stimulated by local application of NGF into the anterior eye chamber, in terms of overall growth and cholinergic neuron survival (26). In the present studies, intraocular grafting of fetal septal tissue was utilized for comparative studies using intravenous (iv) injections of free NGF, OX-26–NGF, OX-26, or saline. Overall growth of septal tissue, as well as cholinergic neuron survival, was utilized to evaluate the effects of systemic administration of NGF conjugated to a transferrin receptor antibody.

Methods and Results

Dissection and Transplantation Procedures

The recipients of intraocular transplants are young, adult, female Fischer 344 rats (150 g; Harlan Laboratories, Indianapolis, IN). Embryonic day 18 rat fetuses are donors of fetal forebrain tissue. The dams are sacrificed using an overdose of metophane; the entire uterus is placed on ice after dissection. The septal region is removed from the dissected fetal brain (23, 26). Tissue pieces are placed in ice-cold Ringer solution until transplantation. Recipient rats are anesthetized with chloral hydrate (300 mg/kg, i.p.) and pretreated with eye drops containing 1% atropine to retract the iris. A small incision is made in the cornea (this corneal incision heals extremely rapidly); one fetal brain tissue piece is subsequently injected in each eye, using a modified syringe. The grafts are placed in the lateral corner of the eye, to avoid interference with the pupil. The transplants quickly undergo vascularization from the host iris and have survival rates greater than 95% (23). Transplants are monitored twice weekly through the cornea until cessation of growth, and thereafter once a month, using microscopic observation in lightly metophane-anesthetized recipients (see Fig. 2); growth curves were generated as previously described (23).

Antibody–Nerve Growth Factor Conjugation

The OX-26–NGF conjugate is produced by introducing a protected sulfhydryl group onto the anti-transferrin receptor antibody OX-26 through lysine ε-amines and a heterobifunctional cross-linker that contains a thiol-reactive group onto NGF through carboxyl groups (Fig. 3A; see also Ref. 21). This approach avoids homoprotein polymer formation in that the coupling is performed in a stepwise fashion (21).

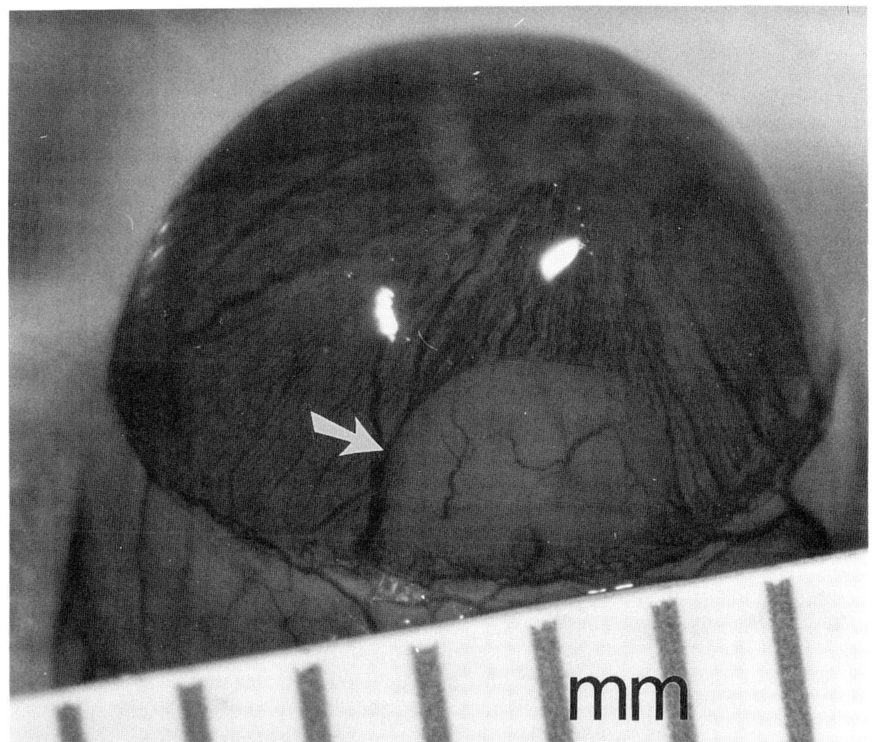

FIG. 2 Septal transplant *in oculo* (arrow). Note the numerous blood vessels located on the transplant surface. A reticule is used to measure the surface area of each transplant to demonstrate growth.

Nerve Growth Factor Biological Activity

One obvious concern in the conjugation process is maintenance of biological activity of the trophic factor. To determine what, if any, effect the modification of the NGF carboxyl group has on the biological activity of the trophic factor, the PC-12 cell neurite outgrowth assay was used. These cells adopt a neuronal phenotype and extend neurites after undergoing a reversible differentiation in response to NGF stimulation (21). This assay can be used as a semiquantitative test for the biological activity of NGF (27). The results shown in Fig. 3B clearly demonstrate the retention of specific biological activity of conjugated OX-26–NGF versus unmodified NGF in the PC-12 cell neurite outgrowth (21).

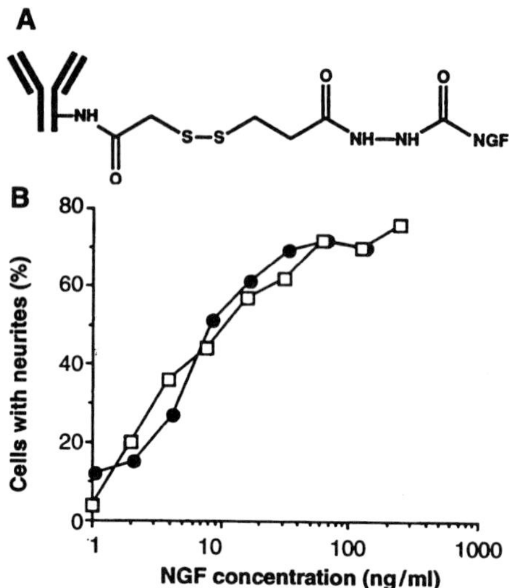

FIG. 3 Conjugation of biologically active NGF to the transferrin receptor antibody OX-26 (A) PDP-hydrazide was used to attach a reactive thiol group to NGF by means of carboxyl groups that had been activated with EDC. SATA was reacted with lysine amines on the antibody to introduce a protected sulfhydryl group. The sulfhydryl group on the antibody exchanged with the 2-pyridyl-sulfide group on NGF, forming a cleavable disulfide bond between the two proteins. (B) The neurite outgrowth response of PC-12 cells treated with either unmodified NGF (open squares) or OX-26–NGF (closed circles) was examined over a range of doses. Response is expressed as the percentage of cells extending neurites as a function of NGF dose. [Reproduced from Friden *et al.*, *Science* **259,** 373–377 (1993). Copyright 1993 by the AAAS.]

Furthermore, we used chick embryo sympathetic trunk ganglia to assay NGF bioactivity. Sympathetic ganglia from 9-day White Leghorn chick embryos are embedded in a collagen gel matrix (28–31). Serial dilutions of NGF or OX-26–NGF are added over the collagen gels and the cultures are incubated at 37°C, 5% CO_2, and 92% relative humidity. An inverted dark-field microscope is used at low magnification to examine the coded cultures after 2 days. The fiber outgrowth response is scored on a scale where 0 biological units (BU) indicates total absence of outgrowth, and 1 indicates a dense, circular fiber halo. Each analysis is repeated several times and the mean ± SEM is calculated. Figure 4 shows examples of chick embryo sympathetic ganglia used to assay NGF bioactivity. In the absence of NGF, there was no fiber outgrowth (Fig. 4A). Maximal response was observed with the OX-26–NGF conjugate in concentrations corresponding to an NGF dose of 10 ng/ml (Fig. 4B). A similar response was observed with the nonconjugated NGF at an equal concentration (10 ng/ml; Fig. 4C).

Delivery of OX-26–NGF Conjugate to Brain Vasculature

In addition to the biological activity of the NGF, it is also critical to determine that the conjugation process has not altered the ability of the antibody to target the brain vasculature. Immunohistochemical procedures were used to visualize both components of the OX-26–NGF conjugate in the brain vasculature 1 hr after intravenous injection (20). There was no difference between localization of the antibody–NGF conjugate in the brain vasculature and the antibody OX-26 alone (Fig. 5A). This indicates that, following NGF conjugation, the OX-26 antibody retains the ability to target brain vasculature. Furthermore, NGF was localized in the vasculature of the brain after intravenous OX-26–NGF injection, as evidenced with an NGF probe (Fig. 5B and C; see also Ref. 25). No immunoreactivity was observed in the brain

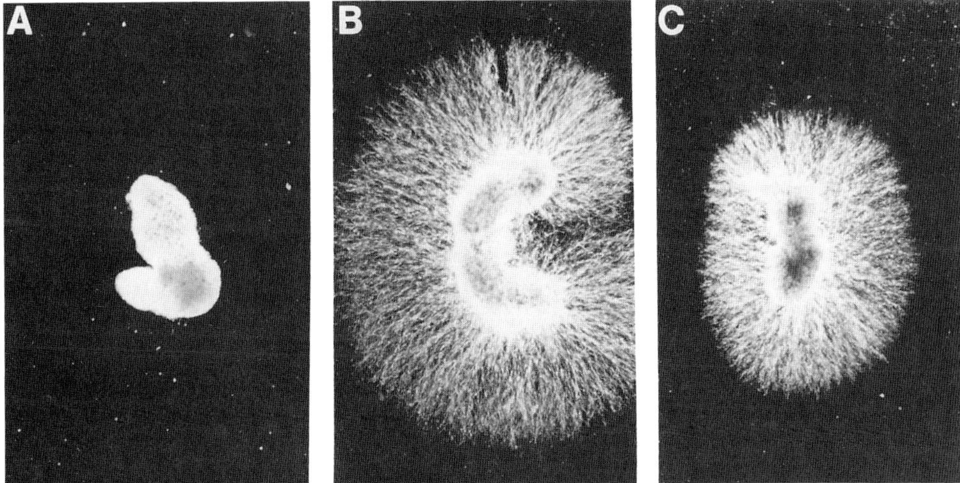

FIG. 4 Chick embryo sympathetic trunk ganglia used to assay NGF bioactivity. Ganglia were cultured for 2 days, and the fiber outgrowth was estimated. In the absence of NGF (A) there was no fiber outgrowth, whereas OX-26–NGF at a β-NGF dose of 10 ng/ml elicited a maximal response (B), and the same dose of unconjugated β-NGF likewise elicited a maximal fiber growth response (C). [Reproduced from Granholm *et al.* (25).] Copyright William & Wilkins, 1993.

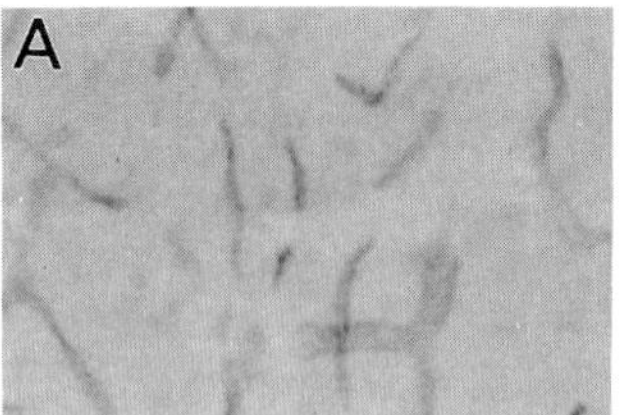

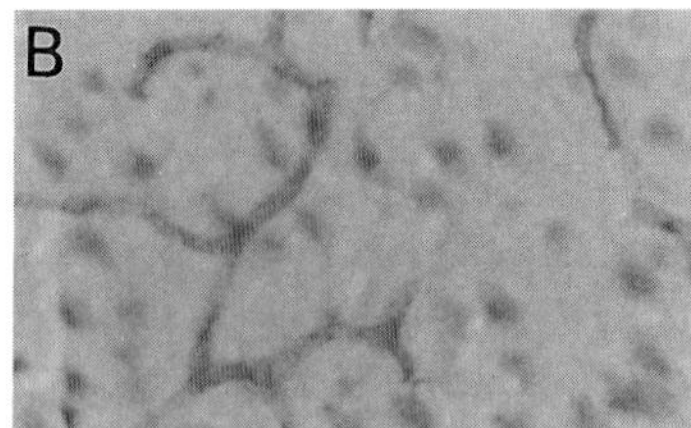

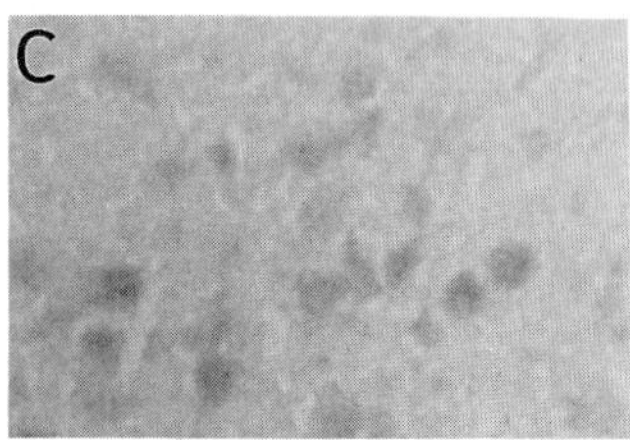

FIG. 5 Targeting of OX-26–NGF conjugate to brain vasculature. (A) Distribution of OX-26-like immunoreactivity in host brain after OX-26–NGF injection intravenously. (B) Distribution of NGF-like immunoreactivity in the host hippocampus after iv injection of OX-26–NGF, (C) NGF-like immunoreactivity in a control brain injected intravenously with NGF alone. Note that no immunoreactivity to NGF is observed in the brain vessels in the NGF-injected animal, whereas the OX-26–NGF-injected animal has abundant NGF immunoreactivity in the blood vessels. Magnification: ×40. [Reproduced from Granholm *et al.* (25).] Copyright William & Wilkins, 1993.

parenchyma after intravenous injection of NGF alone (Fig. 5C). Thus, NGF reached the blood vessel wall only after intravenous injection with the OX-26–NGF conjugate.

OX-26–NGF Conjugate Crosses Blood–Brain Barrier

To be effective, the OX-26–NGF conjugate must not only bind to the blood vessels, but also actually penetrate the BBB. We conducted a previously described (15, 29), two-site enzyme immunoassay (EIA) to determine the levels of NGF in host rat cerebellum. This brain area is especially suited for detection of exogenous NGF levels, because the normal endogenous NGF levels are low compared to other brain regions. Host rats are sacrificed 1, 4, 8, or 24 hr after receiving tail vein injections of OX-26–NGF, OX-26 alone, saline, or NGF alone. The cerebellum is dissected, and NGF levels are measured. The injection of OX-26–NGF conjugate elicits significant increases in cerebellar NGF levels, especially at 4 hr postinjection. None of the other compounds appears to have any effect on cerebellar NGF levels, as demonstrated in Fig. 6.

Capillary depletion experiments performed by Friden *et al.* (21) have shown that antibody–methotrexate conjugates and unconjugated antibodies to the transferrin receptor cross the BBB (20). The technique was also used to determine whether the OX-26–NGF conjugate could cross the BBB and accumulate in brain parenchyma. The results in Fig. 7 are consistent with those previously found for unconjugated antibody in that the radiolabeled NGF conjugate initially accumulated in the capillary fraction of the brain

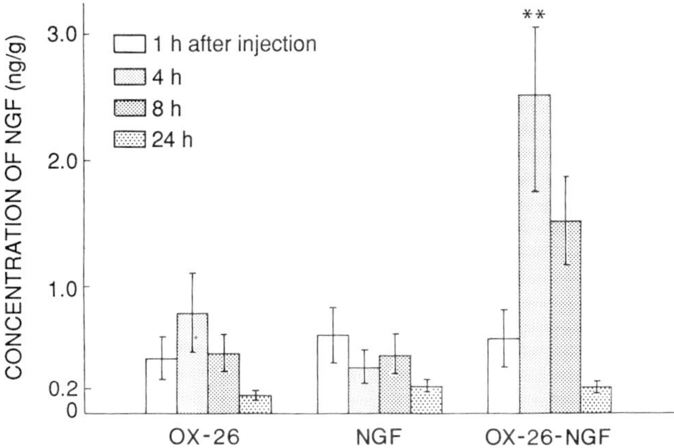

FIG. 6 Levels of NGF in host rat cerebellum, using a two-site enzyme immunoassay for NGF. OX-26–NGF, OX-26 alone, or NGF alone was injected into the tail vein of rats, and the animals were sacrificed 1, 4, 8, or 24 hr following injection. The cerebellum was dissected and NGF levels measured. Note that the injection of OX-26–NGF conjugate elicited significant increases in cerebellar NGF levels, whereas the other three injected compounds did not give rise to any significant changes. Comparison of the 4-hr OX-26–NGF value versus 4-hr levels of NGF alone gives a p value of $p < 0.01$. [Reproduced from Granholm *et al.* (25).] Copyright William & Wilkins, 1993.

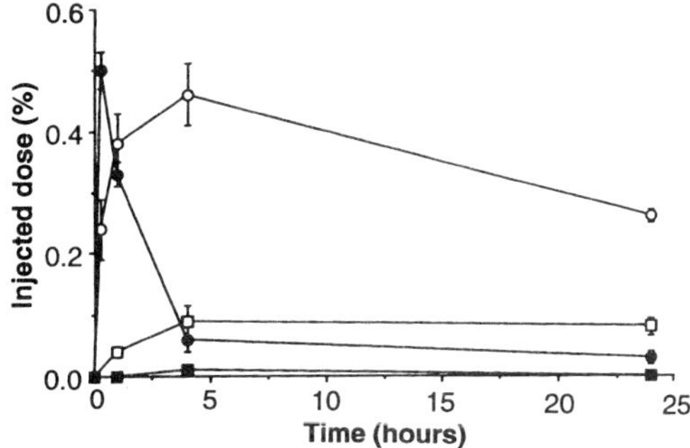

FIG. 7 Enhanced delivery of conjugated NGF across the BBB. Radiolabeled NGF, either as an OX-26–NGF conjugate or as a free protein, was injected intravenously into rats. Capillary depletion was performed on brains taken from the animals at various times after injection (time in hours on x axis). Results are expressed as the percentage of injected dose per brain in either the parenchyma or capillary fraction, and are shown as mean ± SEM (n = three animals per time). (○) OX-26–NGF in brain parenchyma; (●) OX-26–NGF in capillaries; (□) NGF in brain parenchyma; (■) NGF in brain capillaries. [Reproduced from Friden *et al., Science* **259,** 373–377 (1993). Copyright 1993 by the AAAS.]

(20). This is consistent with the antibody binding to and transferring across the capillary endothelial cells of the BBB (see Ref. 21). Over time the amount of conjugate associated with the capillaries decreased while the amount associated with the parenchyma increased (Fig. 7).

Effects of Physiological Doses of OX-26–NGF on Intraocular Transplants of Septal Tissue

It was previously demonstrated (26, 33) that growth of intraocular brain tissue transplants can be stimulated by injections of NGF directly into the anterior chamber of the eye. The anterior chamber of the eye provides an ideal site for noninvasive, continuous observation of growth and vascularization throughout the life of the transplant. We and others have demonstrated that these grafts develop a functional BBB as soon as 2 weeks after transplantation (24, 25). Figure 8 demonstrates development of a BBB in intraocular septal transplants 2 weeks postgrafting, as evidenced with intravenous Evans blue injections into the host rat tail vein (Fig. 8A), and development of transferrin receptors in grafted brain tissue blood vessels (Fig. 8B). Transplants may be viewed repeatedly through the cornea while rats are lightly anesthetized with metophane. A microscope with a reticule in the eye piece may be utilized for accurate determination of tissue size (Fig. 2). In this study, we have measured the area of each transplant through the cornea, and derived growth curves for each treatment group on the basis of these values. Figure 9 depicts evidence for the effect of the OX-26–NGF conjugate on septal transplants *in oculo*. Adult hosts received transplants *in oculo* of fetal forebrain tissue containing the septal nuclei, as described in detail above. In the first experiment, hosts were injected intravenously 2, 4, 6, and 8 weeks following transplantation with either OX-26–NGF at an NGF dose of 6.2 μg/injection, or an equivalent amount of OX-26 alone (Fig. 9a). In a second experiment, we tested peripheral injections of OX-26–NGF conjugate at the same dose (6.2 μg of NGF per injection) versus injections of saline, NGF alone, and OX-26 alone at equivalent doses, also at 2, 4, and 6 weeks after transplantation (Fig. 9b). Peripheral administration of the OX-26–NGF conjugate in both experimental series resulted in a significantly greater final graft size than the transplants in the groups receiving only the carrier OX-26 antibodies, saline, or NGF alone (Fig. 9a and b). In addition to these short-term effects of OX-26–NGF on septal transplant growth, we studied the long-term effects of OX-26–NGF injection on the growth of septal transplants. Animals with intraocular septal transplants received injections of OX-26–NGF, OX-26, or NGF alone at 2, 4, and 6 weeks postgrafting. There-

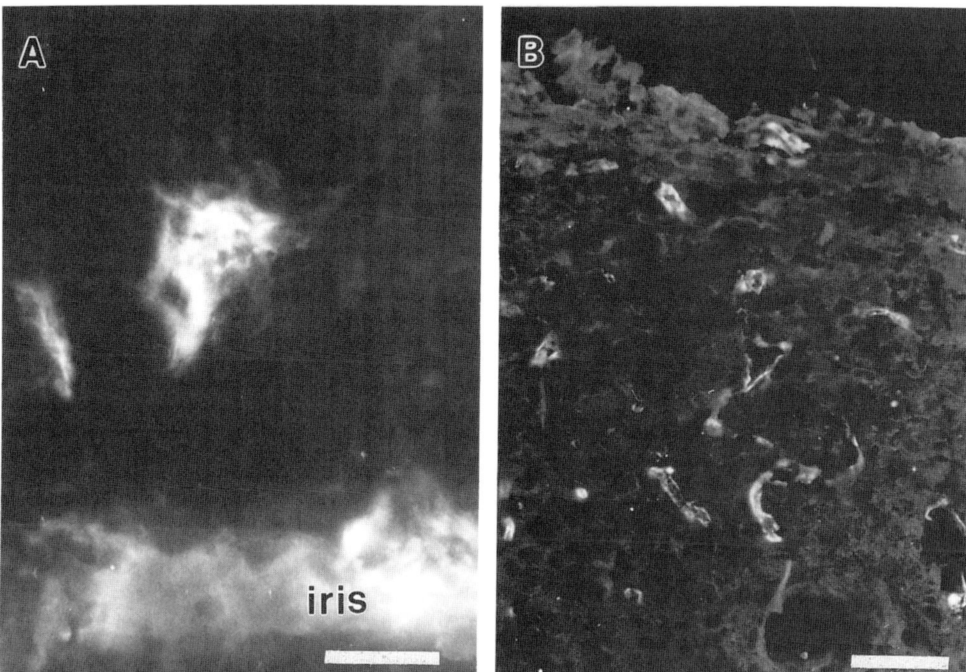

FIG. 8 Microphotographs illustrating the existence of a functional BBB in intraocular septal transplants 2 weeks after transplantation. (A) Stained blood vessels and iris after an intravenous injection of Evans blue into host rat 2 weeks after transplantation. Note that there is no staining in the graft parenchyma, indicative of an existing BBB in the graft blood vessels at this point. (B) Distribution of transferrin receptors on graft blood vessels in a septal graft 2 weeks after grafting, using immunohistochemistry with OX-26 antibodies. Note the wide distribution of thin-walled blood vessels with transferrin receptors throughout the graft neuropil. Bars: (A) 50 μm; (B) 100 μm. [Reproduced from Granholm *et al.* (25).] Copyright William & Wilkins, 1993.

after, the animals were left uninjected for 5 months (thus, 7 months postgrafting), and the growth of transplants was measured monthly during this period. The bar graph in Fig. 9c demonstrates that the transplants in the OX-26–NGF-injected group remained larger than the controls (NGF or OX-26 alone), even at 5 months following the last injection. Statistical analysis [analysis of variance (ANOVA)] showed a significant difference ($p < 0.05$) between OX-26–NGF group and the other two groups, even at this interval after the last injection.

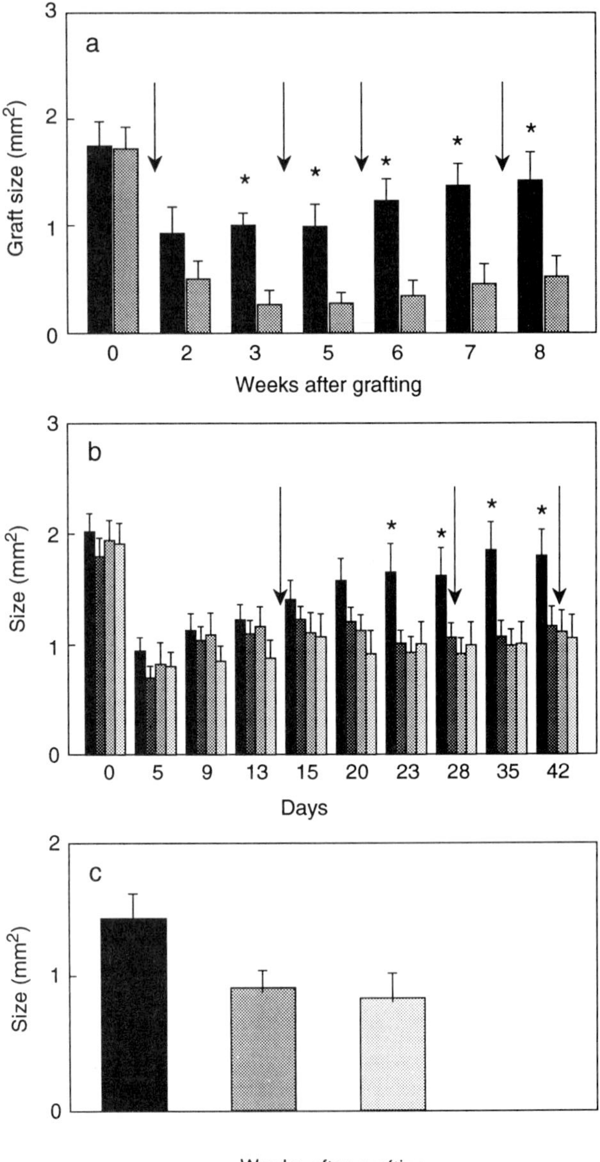

FIG. 9 The intraocular growth of medial forebrain transplants from the time of transplantation ($t = 0$). (a) The sizes of the grafts in the first experimental series, in which animals with septal grafts of embryonic day 18 (E18) tissue were injected intravenously at 2, 4, 6, and 8 weeks postgrafting with either OX-26–NGF (at an NGF dose of 6.2 μg/injection, solid bars) or OX-26 alone at equivalent doses (stippled

Transplant Size and Neural Structures

Although transplants in hosts that were injected with OX-26–NGF conjugate clearly exhibited size differences, as shown in Fig. 9, the overall densities of neural and glial structures did not appear to be altered (see Ref. 21). Intraocular septal transplants seemed to have similar vascularization patterns and cell density in all four groups studied (OX-26–NGF, NGF, OX-26, or saline), as evidenced by routine histology shown in Fig. 10. Further evidence for normal vascular development in all groups (OX-26–NGF, OX-26, NGF, and saline) came from experiments involving incubation of tissue sections with laminin antibodies. The overall distribution of laminin immunoreactivity in the grafts was similar in all four groups, indicative of a similar vascular development, regardless of the injected compounds (see Ref. 25). The immunoreactivity with antibodies directed against NGF, neurofilament, and glial fibrillary acidic protein (GFAP) was also investigated in these experiments. The overall distribution of intermediate filaments in grafted nerve cells, as evidenced with neurofilament antibodies (Fig. 11), as well as in glial cells (GFAP antibodies), was similar in all four groups (injected with OX-26–NGF, OX-26, NGF, or saline intravenously). These findings clearly suggest a specific effect on cholinergic neurons in the grafted forebrain tissue, because ChAT immunoreactivity was the only morphological marker evidently changed in the grafts injected with OX-26–NGF (see the next section, and Fig. 13). Immunohistochemistry with antibodies directed against β-NGF demonstrated accumulation of NGF-like immunoreactivity in transplants where hosts had been injected with OX-26–NGF (Fig. 12b), but could be found only in portions of the host iris and in blood vessels in grafts where hosts were injected with control substances (OX-26, NGF, or saline; Fig. 12a). This finding provided further evidence for transport of the OX-26–NGF conjugate across the BBB into the grafted brain tissue parenchyma. Nerve

---

bars). (b) Growth of septal transplants in the second experiment, in which hosts were injected at 2, 4, and 6 weeks postgrafting with OX-26–NGF (6.2 μg of NGF/injection; solid bar), OX-26 alone (narrow cross-hatching), NGF alone (wide cross-hatching), or saline (stippled bars) at equivalent doses, respectively. Vertical arrows in (a) and (b) demonstrate the times of injection. The y axis represents graft size in mm^2. [Reproduced from Friden *et al.* (21).] (c) The long-term effects of OX-26–NGF injection on the growth of septal transplants *in oculo*. The bar graph illustrates the mean size of transplants injected with OX-26–NGF (solid bar), NGF alone (striped bar), or OX-26 alone (stippled bar) 5 months following the last injection. Statistical analysis (ANOVA) showed a significant difference ($p < 0.05$*) between the OX-26–NGF group and the other group in all three experiments (a–c). [(c) was reproduced from Granholm *et al.* (25)]. Copyright William & Wilkins, 1993.

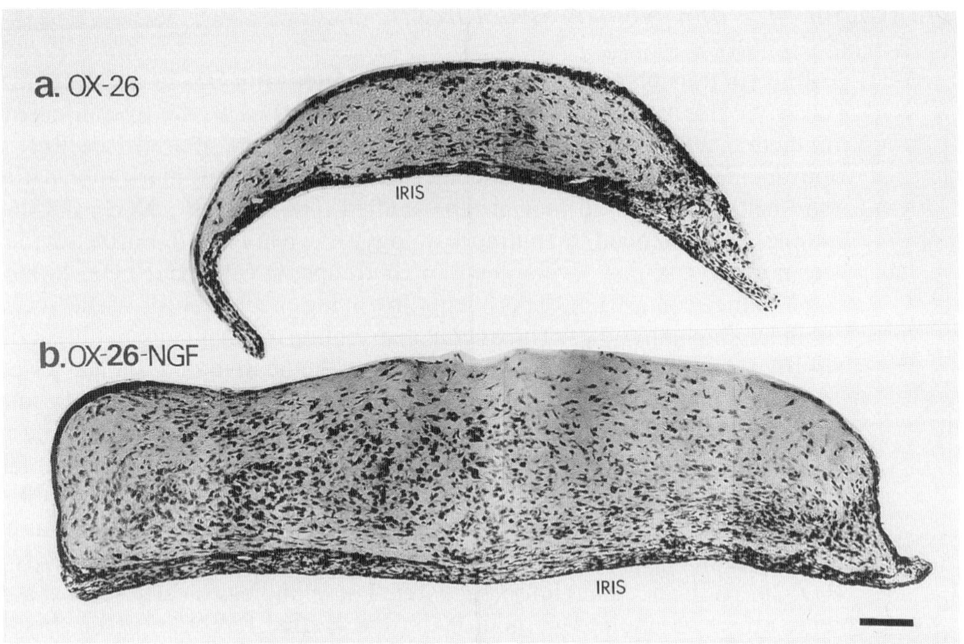

FIG. 10 Sections of intraocular septal transplants stained with toluidine blue. Iris is located in the lower portion of transplants. (a) Section from an OX-26-injected host; (b) section from an OX-26–NGF-injected host. Note that the overall density of cells in the two grafts seems to be approximately the same. Bar: 200 μm. [Reproduced from Friden *et al.*, *Science* **259,** 373–377 (1993). Copyright 1993 by the AAAS.]

growth factor immunoreactivity after OX-26–NGF injection was present only in grafts immediately after the last injection (4–10 hr), and was not seen in graft neuropil of any grafts 5 months after the last injection (see Ref. 25).

Specific Effects of Peripheral OX-26–NGF on Cholinergic Neurons in Intraocular Septal Grafts

Although no major changes in overall glial or neural components were observed in transplants from OX-26–NGF-injected hosts, a specific effect on cholinergic neurons could be found in both experimental series described above. Cryostat sections of intraocular grafts from all groups (injected 2, 4, 6, and 8 weeks postgrafting) were incubated with antibodies against ChAT (25), using the ABC (avidin–biotin complex) Vectastain Elite kit (Vector

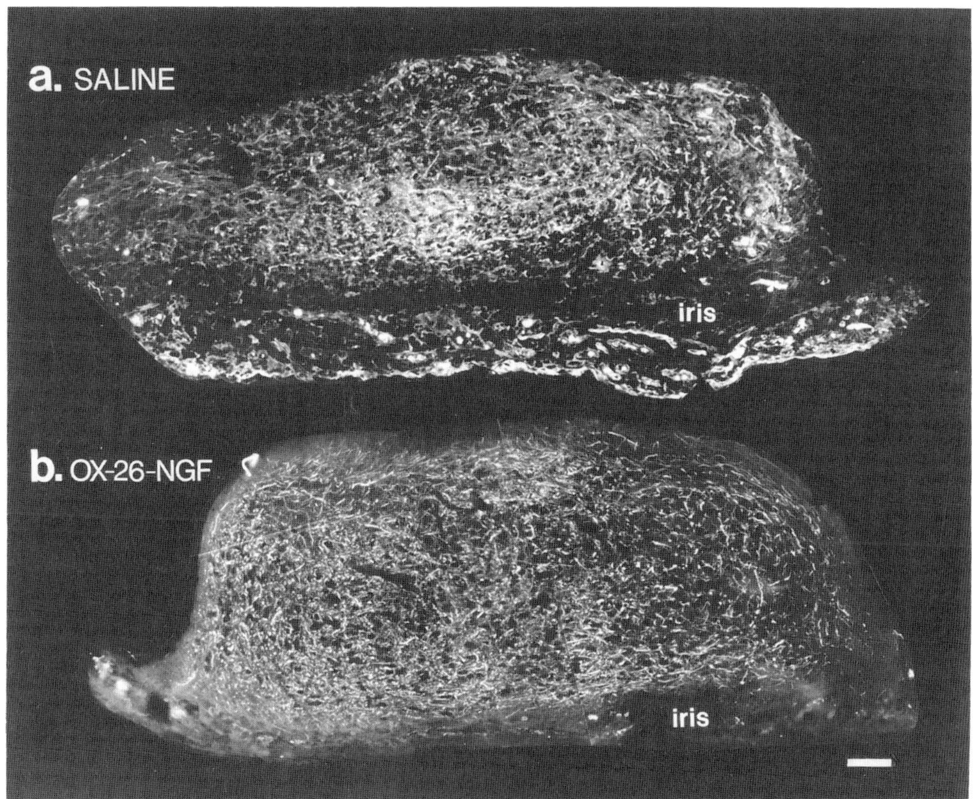

FIG. 11 Neurofilament immunoreactivity in sections from transplants in a saline-injected host (a) and an OX-26–NGF-injected host (b). Both density and distribution of neurofilament-positive elements appeared to be similar in all groups. Bar: 100 μm. [Reproduced from Granholm *et al.* (25).] Copyright William & Wilkins, 1993.

Laboratories, Burlingame, CA). Image analysis of cholinergic cell numbers and staining density was performed using a Joyce-Lobl Magiscan-Zeiss image analysis system (Carl Zeiss Inc., Tempe, AZ, 21). The number of ChAT-positive neurons was increased 3.5-fold in transplants in which the hosts were injected with OX-26–NGF (Fig. 13C), as compared to all three control groups (OX-26, NGF, or saline; Fig. 13D). Furthermore, the transplanted cholinergic neurons in the experimental group exhibited a more dense immunohistochemical staining, as well as an increased number of ChAT-positive processes within the grafted tissue (Fig. 13C). This offers further support for the hypothesis that the OX-26–NGF conjugate crossed the BBB and enhanced the postnatal survival of grafted cholinergic neurons. A similar

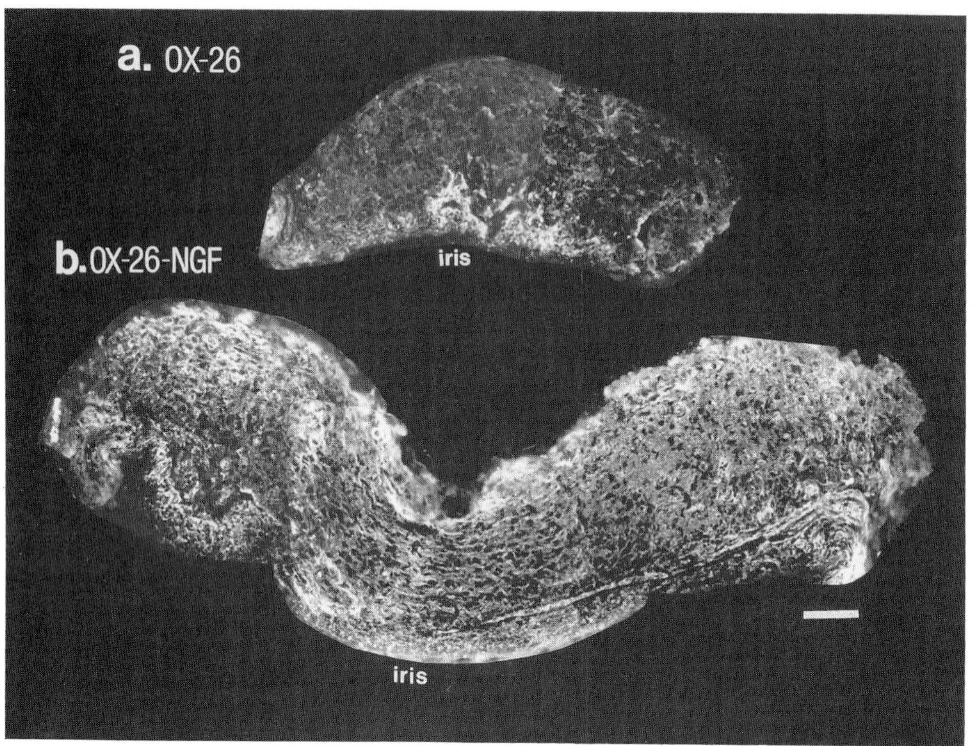

FIG. 12 Sections of septal transplants incubated with NGF antibodies. (a) Section from an animal injected with OX-26; (b) section from an animal injected with OX-26–NGF. Note the overall distribution of NGF-like immunoreactivity in the OX-26–NGF-injected graft, whereas the control graft contains NGF-like immunoreactivity only in the host iris (in lower portion of graft). The animals were sacrificed approximately 6 hr following the last injection. Bar: 100 μm. [Reproduced from Granholm *et al.* (25).] Copyright William & Wilkins, 1993.

relationship in surviving cholinergic neurons between the different groups was found in the long-term group (see Fig. 9c), in which hosts were injected at 2, 4, and 6 weeks postgrafting, and then left to mature for 5 months following the last injection. Figure 13A and B demonstrates transplants from this long-term group, injected with OX-26–NGF (Fig. 13A) and NGF alone (Fig. 13B), respectively.

Effects of OX-26–NGF Injections on Peripheral Systems

It is possible that injections of NGF using a protein vector delivery system could result in severe side effects on peripheral systems. Jeffries *et al.* (18), found the transferrin receptors to be located mostly in the endothelium of brain. They found low concentrations of transferrin receptors in the thymus, lymph nodes, spleen, heart, kidney, liver, pancreas, and small intestine (18). Therefore, it is believed that an antibody directed against this receptor could provide a selective vector for brain-targeted proteins. Nevertheless, we investigated the effects of the OX-26–NGF conjugate on peripheral systems. Specifically, we examined the effects of the OX-26–NGF conjugate on the adrenal gland, which contains chromaffin tissue, a tissue normally sensitive to NGF actions (34). Adrenal tissue from all four groups in experiment 2 (see page 80) (OX-26–NGF at 6.2 μg of NGF; OX-26, NGF or saline; see also Ref. 21) was sonicated in cold acetate buffer (pH 5.0) that contained dihydroxybenzylamine (DHBA) as an internal standard. Samples are centrifuged at 16,000 *g* for 10 min and 50 μl of supernatant is directly injected into the high-performance liquid chromatography system coupled with dual coulometric electrochemical detectors described by Hall *et al.* (35). The norepinephrine and epinephrine levels are detected with serial electrochemical detectors; chromatography peaks are identified by retention times and standard-addition protocols. Whole tissue levels are calculated using calibration curves for each compound and recovery is determined using the internal standard DHBA (35). Statistical comparison between groups is performed by ANOVA. Table I lists the data from experiments comparing saline, OX-26 alone, NGF alone, and OX-26–NGF injections on the wet weight, and norepinephrine and epinephrine content in the adrenals. Our results indicate that there were no hyperplastic effects in the adrenals, as evidenced by either wet weight or catecholamine content directly after the last injection or 5 months later (Table I). This seems consistent with the idea that a transferrin receptor antibody targets brain tissue selectively (25).

Formation of Antibodies against the Antibody–Drug Conjugate

A concern regarding injections of antibody–drug conjugates for therapeutic purposes is the formation of antibodies against the OX-26–NGF conjugate. We performed enzyme immunoassays for NGF antibodies in serum as described previously (15, 30). Immunoplates are coated with the purified mouse β-NGF (0.5 μg/ml) in 0.05 *M* carbonate buffer (pH 9.6). Each well received 50 μl and the dishes are incubated at 4°C overnight. The immunoplates are blocked for 1 hr at room temperature with 1% (w/v) bovine serum albumin in the same buffer. After washing with Tris-buffered saline [0.02 *M* Tris-HCl (pH 7.4), 0.5 *M* NaCl, 0.5% (v/v) Tween 20], different dilutions of serum from injected rats are added for overnight incubation (1 : 100 to 1 : 10 million) at 4°C. The plates are washed and incubated with biotinylated antibodies to rat IgG (0.5 μg/ml; Vector Laboratories) for 30 min. Finally, β-galactosidase

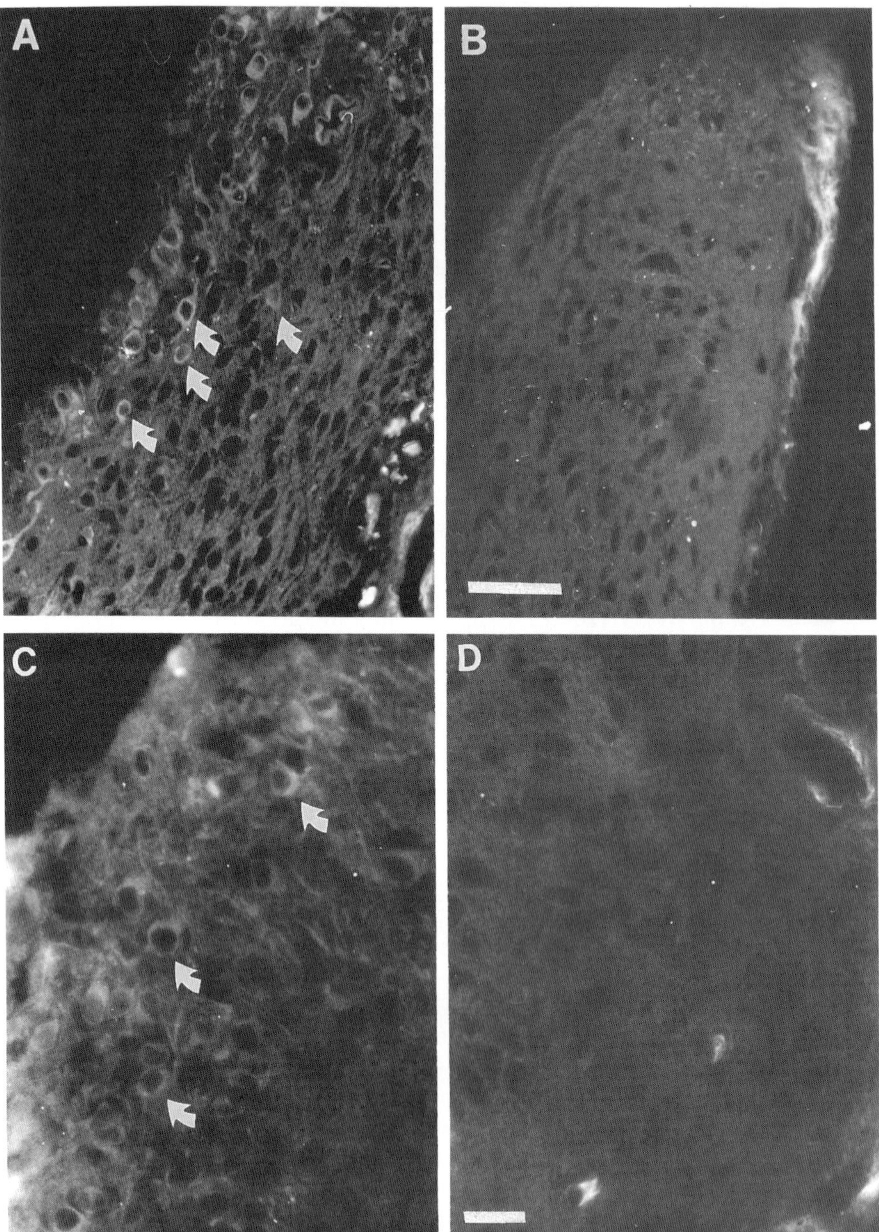

FIG. 13 Sections of septal transplants incubated with ChAT antibodies. (A and C) Sections from OX-26–NGF-treated hosts; (B and D) sections from NGF-treated

TABLE I Effects of Treatments on Adrenal Weight and Catecholamine Content[a,b]

	Injection[c]			
	Saline	OX-26	NGF	OX-26–NGF
Acute exposure	$N = 7$	$N = 7$	$N = 6$	$N = 7$
Weight (mg)	42 ± 9[d]	38 ± 3	45 ± 9	42 ± 3
Epinephrine (ng/mg)	261 ± 27	272 ± 17	226 ± 23	279 ± 18
Norepinephrine (ng/mg)	43 ± 5	51 ± 4	39 ± 3	47 ± 5
5 months postinjection	$N = 3$	$N = 6$	$N = 6$	$N = 7$
Weight (mg)	43 ± 5	40 ± 4	40 ± 5	41 ± 3
Epinephrine (ng/mg)	320 ± 78	403 ± 57	370 ± 48	355 ± 26
Norepinephrine (ng/mg)	48 ± 13	84 ± 19	48 ± 8	47 ± 7

[a] From Granholm *et al.* (25). Copyright William & Wilkins, 1993.
[b] Using a one-way ANOVA, no significant differences were seen between treatment groups either for acute exposure or 5 months after the last injection.
[c] N, number of animals.
[d] Values represented as mean ± SEM.

conjugated with streptavidin (1:1000; Bethesda Research Laboratories, Gaithersburg, MD) was added for 15 min. The plates are then washed and incubated with 4-methylum-belliferyl-β-galactoside (MUG) as detailed above. The resulting titers are given as a function of the serum concentration (25). Table II presents the NGF antibody titers in host blood, both directly after the last injection (8 weeks postgrafting) and 5 months following the last injection (7 months postgrafting). These data indicate that the NGF antibody titers were slightly elevated as compared to the controls directly following the last injection. However, the NGF antibody titers were back to control values (represented by saline-injected host in Table II) 5 months postinjection.

Concluding Remarks

The work presented here has demonstrated that NGF covalently conjugated to a protein vector delivery system, the OX-26 rat antibody against the transferrin receptor, can be successfully transported across the BBB in septal

hosts. The transplants in (A) and (B) were sacrificed 5 months following the last injection, and the transplants in (C) and (D) within 1 day of the last injection. Transplants in NGF-injected hosts contained few or no ChAT-positive neurons (B and D), whereas the OX-26–NGF-treated grafts contained numerous ChAT-positive neurons (A and C). Bars: (A and B) 100 μm; (C and D) 50 μm. [Reproduced from Granholm *et al.* (25).] Copyright William & Wilkins, 1993.

TABLE II Anti-Nerve Growth Factor Antibody Titers Determined by Enzyme Immunoassay in Rat Sera[a,b]

	Injection			
	Saline	OX-26	NGF	OX-26–NGF
Titer at end of injection period	1.0 ± 0.09	1.6 ± 0.22	0.8 ± 0.07	14.8 ± 3.06
Titer 5 months after injection period	1.0 ± 0.10	0.8 ± 0.22	1.7 ± 0.34	1.4 ± 0.28

[a] From Granholm *et al.* (25). Copyright William & Wilkins, 1993.

[b] Values are given as means of three determinations of sera from two to four rats from each group (relative to saline controls, SEM indicated). Rats immunized with adjuvant and mouse NGF normally reach titers in the range 600–1200X, and rabbits immunized with mouse NGF normally achieve titers of 8000–16,000×.

grafts *in oculo*. This antibody–NGF conjugate significantly improves survival of intraocular septal cholinergic neuron transplants for at least 5 months after cessation of treatment. The conjugate does not have any significant effects on other neural or glial structures in the grafts or in the peripheral host adrenal glands. In addition, the conjugate does not seem to stimulate the production of antibodies directed against NGF in the hosts. Furthermore, levels of NGF in the host cerebellum were significantly increased several hours following a single OX-26–NGF conjugate injection. These data indicate that delivery of large peptide neurotherapeutics, such as growth factors, into the brain may be possible utilizing the iron–transferrin transport mechanism.

Acknowledgments

The authors would like to express thanks to Ms. Lorie Gottshalk for assistance in preparing this chapter. The work was supported by USPHS Grants MH49661, AG12122, AG04418, and AG06434, funds from Alkermes, Inc., and in part by a small business innovation research (SBIR) grant, NS29601. Thanks are due to Dr. D. Dahl for providing the GFAP antibodies. The data in this chapter were gathered from two articles: Granholm *et al.* (25) and Friden *et al.* (21).

References

1. P. Whitehouse, D. Price, R. Struble, A. Clark, J. Coyle, and M. DeLong, *Science* **215,** 1237 (1982).

2. F. Hefti and B. Will, *J. Neural Transm. Suppl.* **24,** 309–315 (1987).
3. R. Levi-Montalcini, *Annu. Rev. Neurosci.* **5,** 341–362 (1982).
4. M. Schwab, U. Otten, Y. Agio, and H. Thoenen, *Brain Res.* **168,** 473 (1979).
5. M. McKinney, J. Coyle, and J. Hedereen, *J. Comp. Neurol.* **217,** 103–121 (1983).
6. B. Wainer, A. Levey, E. Mufson, and M. Mesulam, *Neurosci. Int.* **6,** 163–182 (1984).
7. K. Crutcher and F. Collins, *Science* **217,** 67–68 (1982).
8. S. Korsching, G. Auburger, R. Heumann, J. Scott, and H. Thoenen, *IMBO J.* **4,** 1389–1393 (1985).
9. U. Gasser, G. Weskamp, U. Otten, and A. Dravid, *Brain Res.* **376,** 351–356 (1986).
10. S. Whittemore, T. Ebendal, L. Lärkfors, and L. Olson, *Proc. Natl. Acad. Sci. U.S.A.* **83,** 817–821 (1986).
11. P. Rennert and G. Heinrich, *Biochem. Biophys. Res. Commun.* **138,** 813–818 (1986).
12. C. Ayer-Lelièvre, L. Olson, and T. Ebendal, *Science* **240,** 1339–1341 (1988).
13. F. Hefti, *J. Neurosci.* **6**(8), 2155–2166 (1986).
14. P. Friden, L. Walus, G. Musso, M. Taylor, B. Malfroy, and R. Starzyk, *Proc. Natl. Acad. Sci. U.S.A.* **88,** 4771–4775 (1991).
15. L. Olson, E. Backlund, T. Ebendal, R. Freedman, B. Hamberger, P. Hansson, B. Hoffer, U. Lindblom, B. Meyerson, I. Strömberg, O. Sydow, and Å. Seiger, *Arch. Neurol.* (*Chicago*) **48,** 373–381 (1991).
16. L. Olson, A. Nordberg, H. von Holst, L. Bäckman, T. Ebendal, I. Alafuzoff, K. Amberla, P. Hartvig, A. Herlitz, A. Lilja, H. Lundqvist, B. Långström, B. Meyerson, A. Persson, M. Viitanen, B. Windblad, and Å. Seiger, *J. Neural Transm.* **4,** P-D Sect., 79–95 (1992).
17. R. Roberts, A. Sandra, G. Siek, J. Lucas, and R. Fine, *Ann. Neurol.* **32,** Suppl., S43–S50 (1992).
18. W. Jeffries, M. Brandon, S. Hunt, A. Williams, K. Gatter, and D. Mason, *Nature* (*London*) **312,** 162–163 (1984).
19. W. Pardridge, J. Buciak, and P. Friden, *J. Pharmacol. Exp. Ther.* **259**(1), 66–70 (1991).
20. G. Goldstein and A. Betz, *Sci. Am.* **255,** 74–83 (1986).
21. P. Friden, L. Walus, P. Watson, S. Doctrow, J. Kozarich, C. Bäckman, H. Bergman, B. Hoffer, F. Bloom, and A.-C. Granholm, *Science* **259,** 373–377 (1993).
22. L. Olson, Å. Seiger, and I. Strömberg, *Adv. Cell. Neurobiol.* **4,** 407–411 (1983).
23. A-C. Granholm, *Methods Neurosci.* **7,** 327–345 (1991).
24. R. Knobler, J. Marini, D. Goldowitz, and F. Lublin, *J. Neuropathol. Exp. Neurol.* **51,** 36–39 (1992).
25. A.-C. Granholm, C. Bäckman, F. Bloom, T. Ebendal, G. Gerhardt, B. Hoffer, L. Mackerlova, L. Olson, S. Söderström, L. Walus, and P. Friden, *J. Pharmacol. Exp. Ther.* **268,** 448–459 (1993).
26. M. Eriksdotter-Nilsson, S. Skirboll, T. Ebendal, L. Hersh, J. Grassi, J. Massoulie, and L. Olson, *Exp. Brain Res.* **74,** 89 (1989).
27. S. Buxser, S. Vroegop, D. Decker, J. Hinzmann, R. Porrman, D. Thomsen, M.

Stier, I. Abraham, B. Greenberg, N. Hatzenbuhler, M. Shea, K. Curry, and C. Tomich, *J. Neurochem.* **56,** 1012 (1991).
28. T. Ebendal, L. Olson, Å. Seiger, and K.-O. Hedlund, *Nature (London)* **286,** 25–28 (1980).
29. T. Ebendal, L. Olson, Å. Seiger, and M. Belew, *in* "Cellular and Molecular Biology of Neuronal Development" (I. Black, ed.), pp. 231–242. Plenum, New York, 1984.
30. T. Ebendal, *Prog. Growth Factor Res.* **1,** 143–159 (1989).
31. S. Söderström, C. Hallböök, C. Ibañez, H. Persson, and T. Ebendal, *J. Neurosci. Res.* **27,** 665–677 (1990).
32. W. Pardridge, *Endocr. Rev.* **7,** 314–330 (1986).
33. M. Eriksdotter-Nilsson, S. Skirboll, T. Ebendal, and L. Olson, *Neuroscience* **30,** 755 (1989).
34. H. Thoenen and D. Edgar, *Science* **229,** 238–242 (1985).
35. M. Hall, B. Hoffer, and G. Gerhardt, *LC-GC* **7,** 258–265 (1989).

[6] Ferrotransferrin and Antibody against the Transferrin Receptor as Potential Vehicles for Drug Delivery across the Mammalian Blood–Brain Barrier into the Central Nervous System

Richard D. Broadwell, Belinda J. Baker, William A. Banks, Phillip Friden, Marjorie Moran, Constance Oliver, and Juan C. Villegas

Introduction

Determining an efficacious, noninvasive approach for delivering blood-borne, non-lipid-soluble therapeutics into the central nervous system (CNS) has occupied significant clinical and research attention for more than 50 years. Many chemotherapeutic molecules administered systemically to combat infections, tumors, toxins, and enzyme or neurotransmitter deficiencies associated with CNS disease or dysfunction fail to enter the CNS. This failure is due predominantly to two basic cell types providing for a blood–brain barrier (BBB). The cell types include the nonfenestrated endothelium (i.e., the cellular constituent of capillaries, arterioles, and venules) and phagocytes (e.g., macrophages, microglia, and pericytes) located within the perivascular and subarachnoid spaces. Contiguous BBB endothelia are joined by circumferential belts of tight junctional complexes that preclude bidirectional, extracellular passage of macromolecules (e.g., proteins and peptides) between blood and brain. The phagocytes provide for a first line of defense once the BBB is breached experimentally, pathologically, or, as is considered below, normally vis-à-vis extracellular and/or transcellular routes. The endothelial and phagocytic cells possess hydrolytic enzymes for degradation of many blood-borne macromolecules entering these cells; for the most part, the enzymes are lysosomal, whereas others are extralysosomal (e.g., monoamine oxidase). Characteristics of the mammalian BBB are detailed elsewhere (1).

The model of Rapoport *et al.* (2) for osmotic opening of the BBB has been applied clinically with some success for delivery of blood-borne antineoplastic agents to treat CNS tumors (3, 4; also see Neuwelt and Kroll [4], this volume). The osmotic approach has a major shortcoming insofar as it compromises the BBB in normal CNS sites far removed from tumor-occupying

Methods in Neurosciences, Volume 21

lesions. Although this widespread opening of the BBB can be argued as beneficial for CNS delivery of antineoplastic agents (5), the primary function of the BBB, that of maintaining the internal milieu of the CNS, is necessarily compromised or at the very least jeopardized.

The best approach for delivering exogenously administered blood-borne substances to the CNS would be one that successfully "harnesses" normally occuring cell biological events or processes. One potential cellular process is transendothelial transport or transcytosis. This process collectively involves cellular internalization or endocytosis of a given substance from outside the cell, transport of that substance through the cell, and subsequent secretion or exocytosis of the substance from the cell opposite the side of entry. Transcytosis of non-lipid-soluble molecules through BBB endothelia initially was believed to be restricted to the experimentally modified BBB or to CNS pathology (for a review, see Ref. 6). Morphological and pharmacological data now suggest the BBB endothelium normally participates in a recycling of its lumenal surface membrane and, thus, is involved with endocytosis and the potential for transcytosis of macromolecules (i.e., proteins and peptides) from blood into the CNS.

Transcytosis represents a highly specific event associated with specific cell surface receptors and their recognition by equally specific ligands. The event as a whole is referred to as *receptor-mediated transcytosis*. Of the receptors and affiliated ligands identified with BBB endothelia (7), a "harnessing" of the tranferrin receptor and/or its endogenous ligand, ferrotransferrin, may represent the most easily adaptable approach for successfully delivering blood-borne macromolecules and therapeutics into the brain across the noncompromised BBB. Although many cell types outside the CNS have transferrin receptors, the only blood vessels in the mammal possessing this receptor are cerebral vessels (8), or more precisely BBB vessels (9, and see below).

The cell biological role for transferrin and its receptor is to deliver iron from the blood into cells, a well-documented event in a variety of cell types (10). In the case of the central nervous system, we speculate that the delivery of iron into the brain parenchyma from the blood invokes the transcytosis of iron and transferrin through BBB endothelia. Morphological data obtained in our laboratory and compared to data derived from multiple control experiments suggest blood-borne ferrotransferrin does cross the intact BBB *in vivo* by receptor-mediated transcytosis. These data are considered below from the perspective of intracellular events associated with the endomembrane system of organelles and intraendothelial membrane trafficking. Additional consideration is directed to our data in support of the transendothelial transfer of blood-borne antibody against the ferrotransferrin receptor (11–13). Available evidence advocates both ferrotransferrin and antibody against its receptor as macromolecular vehicles for the CNS introduction of non-lipid-soluble macromolecules that otherwise fail to penetrate the intact cerebral, nonfenestrated, endothelial cell.

Iron, Transferrin, and Transferrin Receptor

Iron occupies a significant position in cellular metabolism as a cofactor for heme and non-heme-containing enzymes. The role of iron in the mitochondrial respiratory pathway and in adenosine triphosphate requirements of the neuron necessitates maintaining high levels of iron in the developing brain and in the adult brain to sustain normal cell function. Because of the toxicity of free iron radicals, special proteins for iron transport, uptake, and storage are mandated for iron utilization in cell metabolism and are critical components in controlling iron delivery to the CNS. The control is mediated by the interactions of iron with transferrin and of this ferrotransferrin with the transferrin receptor.

Transferrin is a serum, monomeric glycoprotein with a molecular weight of 80,000; it is synthesized and secreted predominantly by the liver. Transferrin exists in an iron-free or apo form and an iron-laden or ferro form. Apotransferrin becomes ferrotransferrin when the transferrin molecule binds two ferric (3+ charge) ions in the blood. Within the systemic circulation, ferrotransferrin is recognized by high-affinity, cell surface receptors that bind the ferro form, but not the apo form, of transferrin. Receptor binding of ferrotransferrin initiates internalization into the cell of this membrane receptor–ligand complex; the internalized cell surface membrane appears as receptor-mediated endocytic vesicles 40–70 nm in diameter. These vesicles are conveyed to endosomes, which serve as intracellular clearing centers for internalized cell surface membrane and endocytosed macromolecules (14). An acidic pH (5.5) within the endosome stimulates the dissociation of ferric ions from the transferrin molecule. In the vast majority of cells in which receptor-mediated endocytosis of ferrotransferrin has been investigated, the transferrin protein remains complexed to the membrane receptor subsequent to iron liberation in the endosome; the transferrin–membrane receptor complex then recycles as a whole from the endosome back to the cell surface, whereupon the neutral pH of the interstitial fluid stimulates release of apotransferrin from the membrane receptor for a rebinding of two additional ferric ions (15). The dissociated iron remaining in the cell is incorporated into mitochondrial and cytosolic ferritin, an iron-storing protein, or into hemosiderin as insoluble granules in secondary lysosomes.

The intracellular fate of iron and transferrin just described is well established in a variety of cell types, most notably the hepatocyte (16). If blood-borne iron and transferrin are recognized as breaching the BBB by receptor-mediated transcytosis, the event dictates the BBB endothelium differs from other cell types insofar as it does not adhere to conventional processing of internalized iron and associated receptor–ligand complex. This point is controversial in the BBB–transferrin literature (17–19). The BBB endothelium very likely engages in at least some recycling of the internalized transferrin receptor–ligand complex; however, quantitative assessment for recycling of the transferrin receptor–ligand complex versus that for possible transcytosis of ferrotransferrin requires greater scrutiny.

Preparation and Application of Ferrotransferrin and Antibody against the Ferrotransferrin Receptor

Ferrotransferrin and ascites fluid-derived antibody against the ferrotransferrin receptor (OX-26 antibody) employed in our investigations are commercially available (Pierce, Rockford,IL; Bioproducts for Science, Indianapolis, IN). Both proteins are conjugated to type VI horseradish peroxidase (HRP; Sigma Chemical Co., St. Louis, MO) in our laboratories to permit the intraendothelial fate and possible transendothelial transfer (transcytosis) of the two proteins to be studied ultrastructurally. OX-26 antibody *not* conjugated to HRP also has been used and is identified histologically by peroxidase immunohistochemistry. Ferrotransferrin–HRP (1 : 1; 4–6 mg in 0.5 ml of sterile saline solution), OX-26 conjugated to HRP (1 : 1; 300–750 μg in 0.5 ml of sterile saline solution), or native (unconjugated) OX-26 antibody (200–400 μg) is delivered into the systemic circulation of young adult (200–250 g) Sprague-Dawley rats; postinjection survival times range from 5 min to 6 hr. The ferrotransferrin–HRP conjugate must be administered into the carotid artery, which allows the ligand–HRP direct and rapid access to ferrotransferrin receptors on cerebral vessels. Immediate exposure to receptors on BBB vessels afforded by the arterial injection is an absolute prerequisite to obtain positive results; intravenous injection of the ligand conjugate necessarily results in total body distribution of the ferrotransferrin–HRP with subsequent exposure of the probe to ferrotransferrin receptors in multiple extracerebral sites, such as the liver and kidney. However, this problem is not encountered with the OX-26 antibody administered into the jugular vein.

Peroxidase Conjugation of Ferrotransferrin

Ferrotransferrin–HRP (M_r 120,000) is made by a disulfide exchange reaction (20, 21). Twelve milligrams of rat-derived transferrin (Calbiochem, San

Diego, CA) is dissolved in 0.25 *M* Tris buffer (pH 8.0) to which is added 2 μl of 10 m*M* sodium bicarbonate; 40 μl of 100 m*M* sodium nitrilotriacetate with 16.9 mg of ferric chloride also is added with stirring. The resulting solution is passed over a PD-10 column (Pharmacia, Piscataway, NJ), eluted with phosphate-buffered saline (PBS), and concentrated to 2.5 ml. Two hundred and fifty microliters of 1 *M* potassium phosphate, 25 μl of 10 m*M* ferric ammonium sulphate, and 25 μl of iminothiolane (13 mg/ml) are added to the diferric transferrin followed by incubation for 60 min at room temperature; this solution is passed over a PD-10 column. These conditions introduce one -SH group per transferrin molecule. Derivatized peroxidase is prepared by dissolving HRP (30 mg) in a solution of 1 ml of PBS, to which is added 13 mg of 2-iminothiolane-HCl (Pierce, Rockford, IL) in 100 μl of PBS. The resulting solution is incubated at room temperature for 2 hr and passed over a PD-10 column. Four milliliters of derivatized HRP is added to 20 μl of 0.1 *M* 5,5′-dithiobis(2-nitrobenzoic acid) (Sigma) dissolved in 1 *M* potassium phosphate (pH 7.0). After 5 min, the OD_{412} is measured to ensure only one -SH group is introduced per HRP moleule. Active HRP is separated from other reagents by passing the mixture over a PD-10 column. Two milliliters of derivatized transferrin is mixed with 2 ml of derivatized HRP and the solution incubated at room temperature for 2 hr. The reaction mixture is concentrated to 1 ml and the transferrin–HRP separated by passing the solution over a 1.0 × 57 cm Sephacryl S-200 column equilibrated with PBS. The eluate is collected in 0.5-ml aliquots, and material in the front half of the peak (OD_{280} and OD_{405}) is evaluated for purity by sodium dodecyl sulfate-polyacrylamide gel electrophoresis (SDS-PAGE). The fractions containing no free HRP are pooled and concentrated for experimental application. As a point of information, human ferrotransferrin conjugated to HRP is available commercially (Pierce); this conjugate is recognized by the rat ferrotransferrin receptor (our unpublished results, 1994).

To test the biological activity of the ferrotransferrin–HRP, rat basophilic leukemic cells (clone 2H3) are used (22). The cells are plated at 1×10^6 cells/35-mm dish in Eagle's minimum essential medium (EMEM) supplemented with 15% (v/v) fetal calf serum, penicillin, and streptomycin, and are maintained at 37°C in a humidified incubator with 5% CO_2. The cells are rinsed twice in EMEM containing 1% (v/v) BSA and returned to the incubator for 30 min. The cultures then receive ferrotransferrin–HRP (25 μl/ml in EMEM–BSA). The cells are permitted to incorporate the HRP conjugate for 30 min, or the cells are rinsed free of the conjugate after 10 min, fresh medium is added, and the cells are returned to the incubator for an additional 20 min. The cells are rinsed twice in PBS and fixed in 1% (v/v) glutaraldehyde–1% (v/v) formaldehyde (Ladd Research Industries, Burlington, VT) in 0.1 *M* cacodylate buffer (pH 7.4). The cells subsequently are rinsed in cacodylate buffer followed by buffer containing 0.1 *M* glycine. The fixed cells are incubated for 45 min at room temperature in diaminobenzidine–H_2O_2 medium (see below) to develop the peroxidase reaction product. After again rinsing the cells in cacodylate buffer, the cells are postfixed in 2% (v/v osmium tetroxide in cacodylate buffer, dehydrated through a graded series of ethanols, and embedded in Embed 812 (Electron Microscopy Sciences, Port Washington, PA). Ultrathin sections of the embedded cells are prepared and not poststained with heavy metals for examination in the electron microscope. The cells are scrutinized ultrastructurally to determine the intracellular location of the HRP conjugate and for the possibility of transcytosis of the conjugate through the cells. The ferrotransferrin–HRP conjugate is considered worthy of further experimental application if it has cleared the cells after a 20-min chase and is localized intracellularly only within endosomes in the 30 min of continuous labeling.

Ascites Antibody Preparation

Although OX-26 mouse monoclonal antibody against the rat ferrotransferrin receptor is available commercially (Bioproducts for Science, Indianapolis, IN), we have prepared in our laboratory quantities of the purified ascites antibody suitable for intravenous injection in the rat. F_1 hybrid mice derived from crossing BALB/c and DBA_2 mice strains are used for the preparation of OX-26 antibody. Adult F_1 hybrid mice are pretreated with an intraperitoneal injection (0.5 ml) of 2,6,10,14-tetramethylpentadecane (Pristane) 7 days prior to administering OX-26 hybridoma cells (5×10^6 cells; MRC Cellular Immunology Unit, Oxford University, Oxford, England) intraperitoneally. The mice develop distended abdomens, at which time the ascites fluid is harvested. Each mouse is sacrificed by cervical dislocation and then dipped into 70% ethanol. Ascites fluid is removed from the abdomen and transferred to centrifuge tubes. Drops (three or four) of 0.1 *M* ethylenediaminetetraacetic acid (EDTA) are added to each centrifuge tube, and the fluid is spun at 1200 rpm (100 *g*) for 10 min; the fluid subsequently is poured into fresh centrifuge tubes and spun at greater than 500 rpm for 15 min. The clear ascites fluid is removed with a Pasteur pipette and stored with a few grains of sodium azide at −20°C. The pellet of cells remaining after withdrawal of the ascites fluid is resuspended in 5 ml of PBS; 5×10^6 cells again are injected into Pristane-treated mice, and the procedure is repeated as above.

Purification of Ascites Antibodies

The method for purifying the ascites fluid antibody is adapted from that of Mason and Williams (23). The extracted ascites fluid is spun at 10,000 *g* (800 rpm) at 4°C for 20 min. Excess Pristane is removed, and the final volume is noted and labeled *a*. Sodium sulfate (18%, w/v) is added slowly to the ascites in the cold room, allowing each addition to dissolve. The solution is incubated at 37°C for 30 min and then spun at 8000 rpm for 25 min at 25°C using a Beckman (Fullerton, CA) JA-20 rotor. The supernatant is decanted and the pellet dissolved in Milli-Q water (Millipore, Bedford, MA) to 33% of the initial volume (*a*); this volume is noted and labeled volume *b*. Sodium sulfate (18%, w/v) is added slowly in the cold room, allowing each addition to dissolve as before. This solution is incubated for 30 min at 37°C and spun at 8000 rpm for 20 min at 25°C. The supernatant is decanted and the pellet redissolved in Milli-Q water at 20% of volume *b*. The solution is dialyzed for 2 days against 5 liters of 25 m*M* Tris buffer–50 m*M* NaCl, and the pH adjusted to 7.4 with HCl at room temperature.

The dialyzed ascites fluid is passed through a DEAE-Sephacel anion-exchange column. The column is prepared using a 10-ml syringe with a rubber-ended plunger. The syringe minus the plunger is clamped, and a small amount of glass wool is packed in the bottom and dampened with buffer (25 m*M* Tris–50 m*M* NaCl, pH 7.4). An outlet tube is placed on the end of the syringe and clamped. Diethylaminoethyl (DEAE)-Sephacel (Pharmacia) suspension is shaken and poured into the syringe to approximately three-fourths full. The suspension is left to settle, after which time a small amount of buffer (1 ml) is added. The rubber end of the plunger is removed, and an inverted 19-gauge × 1.5-in. needle is placed through the center of the inverted rubber bung. The inverted rubber bung is placed in the top of the syringe so that the needle end does not contact the buffer. The outlet is unclamped, and a small amount of buffer is drawn through. Tubing then is connected between the needle and a buffer reservoir, and 200 ml of buffer is permitted to run through to equilibrate the column.

An LKB (Bromma, Sweden) 2112 Redirac fraction collector is used to collect 30 drops (0.5 ml) per tube. When the column is equilibrated, the outlet tube is placed in the arm of the fraction collector. The tube then is transferred from the equilibration buffer to the tube containing ascites. When all the ascites fluid has passed into the tube, the fluid is transferred back into the buffer. The optical density (OD) of each fraction is assessed using a Pye Unicam SP6-500 ultraviolet (UV) spectrophotometer at 280 nm; buffer alone serves as the blank. The OD_{280} is plotted against the fraction tube number, and when the readings return to background level the outlet is clamped off. The peak and the arm are pooled separately as pools A and B, and each pool is read on the spectrophotometer and converted into protein concentration using Beer's law [Extinction (E) = k_{Protein}]:

$$\text{Extinction} = \text{OD}$$
$$k \text{ for IgG at } OD_{280} = 1.4$$

The outlet is unclamped and the tube transferred from 25 m*M* Tris–50 m*M* NaCl to 50 m*M* Tris–100 m*M* NaCl. The fractions are collected again and read on the spectrophotometer at 280 nm. When the readings return to background level the outlet is clamped off and the peak pooled is labeled pool C. The monoclonal antibody OX-26 is purified as above and comes off in pools A, B, and C. A salt gradient is prepared using two beakers joined by a tap. NaCl buffer (100 m*M*) is placed in the first beaker and 2 ml of this buffer is permitted to enter the second beaker. NaCl buffer (50 m*M*) is added to the second beaker so that the two beakers are at the same level. The second beaker is connected to the column, and the tap between the two beakers is opened. The second beaker is stirred continuously using a magnetic stirrer. When 100 ml of this gradient buffer passed through the column, the ascites pool is passed through the column followed by 50 ml of the gradient buffer. The fractions are collected and their OD read as before. The peak is pooled, and the OD read.

To assess the purity of the immunoglobulin fraction, the pooled material is analyzed by SDS-PAGE, using the following reagents.

Reagent A: Combine 30% (w/v) acrylamide and 0.8% (w/v) bisacrylamide (*N,N*,-methylamine bisacrylamide) (Sigma); this material is filtered and kept at 4°C

Reagent B: 0.75 *M* Tris-HCl, pH 8.8

Reagent C: 100 *M* Tris-HCl, pH 6.8

Reagent D: 10% SDS (lauryl sulfate) (Sigma)

Reagent E: 1% (w/v) ammonium persulfate (Sigma); this solution is made fresh prior to use

Running buffer: Combine 60.6 g of Tris and 288 g of glycine in 2 liters of distilled water (pH 8.3) and dilute 10× for use

Sample buffer: Combine 4.4 g (0.2 *M*) of Tris, 96.96 g of urea, and 4.6 g (2%, w/v) of SDS in 600 ml of distilled water

The gels are prepared using the following formula for each gel:

Ingredient	10% gel	3% gel
Reagent A	30 ml	2.4 ml
Reagent B	45 ml	
Reagent C		3.0 ml
Reagent D	0.9 ml	0.24 ml
Reagent E	4.5 ml	1.2 ml
Distilled water	9.6 ml	17.13 ml
TEMED (*N,N,N',N'*-tetramethylethylenediamine; Sigma)	60 μl	45 μl

The TEMED is added just before polymerizing the gels. The samples are reduced to break the sulfide bonds such that the heavy and light chains are separated.

Sample Preparation

Dithiothreitol (DTT), 31 mg/5 ml of sample buffer
Iodoacetamide (IAA), 123 mg/1 ml of water

Iodoacetamide prevents reformation of disulfide bonds by adding acetamide groups to -SH. Bromophenol blue (BPB; 20 μl) is added to visualize the gels. Equal volumes of DTT are added to the samples (maximum, 100 μl), which then are boiled for 2 min. Ten microliters of IAA is added to each, followed by boiling for 2 min. The standard (see below) is diluted 5 μl/100 μl in sample buffer, and 5 μl of DTT is added. Ten percent gel is formed, and a film of water is poured on top to prevent air contact. When the gel has set, 3% gel is poured gently on top and the well holes inserted. The 3% gel is a stacking gel to align the samples before they reach the 10% gel. When the 3% gel has set the well holes are removed. The complete unit is constructed and running buffer added. Ten to 15 μl of sample is added per well. Because 1.4 OD units = 1 mg/ml, 1.4/OD = X μl from sample tubes. For dilute samples (i.e., 10 μl or less) equal volumes of DTT are not possible. The current is run at 35 mA. The samples are added to each well and the gel run until the bromophenol blue marker line reaches 1 cm from the bottom. The gel is removed and stained for protein using the Coomassie blue stain for 1 hr.

Coomassie blue stain: Combine 1 g of Coomassie, 73.6 ml of acetic acid, 364 ml of methanol, and 364 ml of distilled water

The gel is destained with a solution containing 150 ml of acetic acid, 100 ml of methanol, and 170 ml of distilled water.

The standards used are derived from the electrophoresis calibration kit (Pharmacia):

Standard	Molecular weight
Phosphorylase *b*	94,000
Bovine serum albumin (BSA)	67,000
Ovalbumin	43,000
Carbonic anhydrase (carbonate dehydratase)	30,000
Soybean trypsin inhibitor	20,100
α-Lactalbumin	14,400

A few grains of sodium azide are added to the pools, which are frozen at −20°C.

Peroxidase Conjugation of OX-26 and IgG_{2a} Antibodies

OX-26 antibody is conjugated to type VI HRP in a multistep process that is a modification of that described by Goding (24). Type VI HRP is oxidized with sodium periodate (0.03 *M*) in 5 m*M* sodium acetate buffer (pH 4.0) for 15 min in the dark. Unreacted starting materials are removed and the buffer changed to 0.3 *M* sodium carbonate buffer (pH 9.5) by passing the reaction mixture over a 10-ml Sephadex G-25 column. Antibody at a minimum concentration of 5 mg/ml in the pH 9.5 buffer is mixed with the oxidized HRP at a ratio of 1 mg of HRP to 4 mg of antibody. The reaction is permitted to proceed for 1 hr at room temperature and then stopped by adding sodium borohydride to a final concentration of 80 μg/ml. This mixture is left to incubate for 1 hr at room temperature or overnight at 4°C. Unconjugated materials are separated from OX-26–HRP by size on a 10- to 12-ml Sephadex G-100SF column. The degree of substitution is determined by the ratio of A_{280} to A_{403}.

Immunohistochemical Staining

Brains from rats receiving an intravenous injection of OX-26 antibody not conjugated to HRP and brains from rats not so injected are prepared for light microscopic immunohistochemical detection of the ferrotransferrin receptor. Commercially available OX-26 antibody (Bioproducts for Science) represents the primary antibody for conventional, immunohistochemical staining of brain sections.

In preparation for immunohistochemical staining, rats are sacrificed by an overdose of sodium pentobarbital administered intraperitoneally. The brains are removed fresh and immersed in isopentane for freezing in liquid nitrogen. Cryostat sections 15 μm thick are mounted on glass slides and stained by the immunoperoxidase technique of Barclay (25). Mounted brain sections are fixed in ethanol followed by washing in PBS. Cryostat sections of brains obtained from rats *not* injected intravenously with ascites OX-26 antibody are incubated in OX-26 primary antibody (1 part OX-26: 2 parts PBS), washed, and exposed to HRP-conjugated rabbit anti-mouse polyclonal secondary antibody (Dako). Conversely, brain sections from rats injected intravenously with native OX-26 antibody (200–400 μg) and after perfusion with saline are incubated directly in the secondary antibody–HRP conjugate. The bound peroxidase-conjugated secondary antibody is revealed by peroxidase histochemistry. All sections are counterstained with toluidine blue.

Control Injections

Control experiments are instrumental for interpreting results obtained with ferrotransferrin–HRP and the ferrotransferrin receptor OX-26 antibody conjugated or not conjugated to HRP. Results with ferrotransferrin–HRP as a receptor-mediated phase marker are compared to results obtained with native HRP as a fluid-phase probe and with wheat germ agglutinin (WGA)–HRP (Sigma) as an adsorptive phase marker. Native HRP is delivered into the carotid artery (4–6 mg) or into the jugular vein (10–70 mg) of young adult rats; WGA–HRP (1.25 mg) is injected into the jugular vein. A nonspecific antibody, IgG_{2a} (UPC10; 2.4–5.5 mg/ml; Sigma), conjugated to HRP serves as an additional control and is injected intravenously. Postinjection survival times for the control rats are 10 min through 6 hr. Results for both blood-borne HRP and WGA–HRP have been published by Broadwell and colleagues (26–28) and share similarities with the ferrotransferrin–HRP results. A control antibody for our immunohistochemical staining is OX-27 (Bioproducts for Science), which is directed against and is specific for the major histocompatibility complex class I antigen of the PVG rat strain.

The perfusion–fixation process of rats injected intravenously with HRP-conjugated macromolecules and the general procedure for HRP cytochemistry, with diaminobenzidine (DAB) as the chromogen, for visualization of peroxidase reaction product at light and electron microscopic levels are provided in detail by us in other publications (29, 30); tetramethylbenzidine (TMB) is an alternative chromogen we have used for enhanced development of peroxidase reaction product at the light microscopic level (31).

Analyses of Potential Transcytosis of Blood-Borne, Receptor-Mediated Probe Molecules across the Blood–Brain Barrier

Our interpretation of results rests on the identification of peroxidase reaction product in histological sections prepared for light and electron microscopic analyses. Because no experimental approach is available to permit us to visualize either ferrotransferrin or antibody against the ferrotransferrin receptor directly, we must necessarily rely on the peroxidase conjugate and its reaction product to indicate where within the histological preparation the HRP-tagged macromolecule is located. In this regard, we are confident of two important points worthy of emphasis. First, the covalent linkage of HRP molecules with ferrotransferrin molecules or with the antibody molecules is

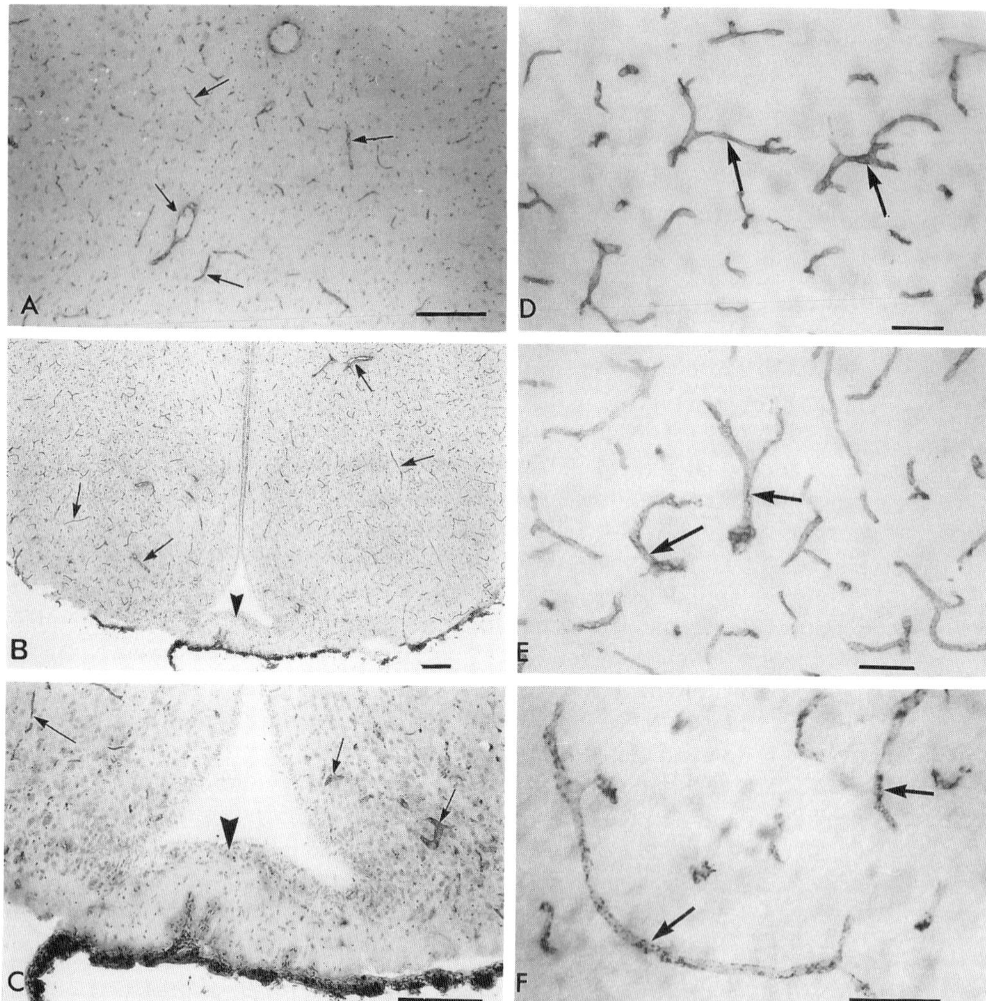

FIG. 1 (A–C) Immunohistochemical staining for the ferrotransferrin receptor, with OX-26 primary antibody (mouse anti-rat IgG) directed against the receptor and followed with HRP-conjugated rabbit anti-mouse immunoglobulin applied to cryostat sections of fresh-frozen rat brain, reveals a plethora of OX-26-positive, small- and large-caliber blood vessels (arrows) throughout the sections. The only CNS sites not harboring OX-26-positive blood vessels are circumventricular organs such as the median eminence (B and C; arrowheads); these sites do not possess BBB vessels. When OX-26 ascites fluid antibody is administered intravenously to rats sacrificed 10 min to 6 hr postinjection, cryostat brain sections immunostained with HRP-conjugated rabbit anti-mouse immunoglobulin demonstrate a network of OX-26-positive blood

particularly strong, so that we need not be concerned about the peroxidase probe separating from either molecule. Second, all unbound HRP is eluted from the peroxidase-conjugated macromolecule mixture, thus ensuring we have a pure conjugate not contaminated with unbound HRP to cloud our results. Despite this confidence, we remain unsure of the intraendothelial fate of the iron associated with the ferrotransferrin–HRP conjugate once the conjugate is channeled to endosomes following receptor-mediated endocytosis. We do not know if peroxidase reaction product is indicative of ferrotransferrin per se or of transferrin–HRP free of iron. For this report we will interpret the HRP reaction product as indicative of the presence of ferrotransferrin–HRP, although we believe iron ions are dissociated from transferrin once the intracellular endosome compartment is reached. Last, as concerns the peroxidase-conjugated antibody against the transferrin receptor, the probe macromolecule tells us nothing about the intraendothelial pathway or fate of the internalized cell surface receptor. Our interest, however, lies in ascertaining the intraendothelial pathway and fate of the peroxidase-conjugated antireceptor antibody.

Distinct similarities and dissimilarities exist among blood-borne ferrotransferrin-HRP, OX-26–HRP, and native OX-26 in the labeling of CNS cells and organelles at both light and electron microscopic levels. This statement also applies to results obtained with the receptor-mediated phase probes compared to those of control fluid-phase (e.g., native HRP, IgG_{2a}–HRP) and adsorptive-phase (e.g., wheat germ agglutinin) markers. The existent similarities mandate a scrutiny of control results for assessing the potential transcytosis of receptor-mediated phase macromolecules.

Light Microscopic Observations

The most demonstrable similarity histologically in a comparison of the receptor-mediated phase probes is cerebral blood vessel labeling, which is identical to that obtained with OX-26 antibody applied for immunohistochemical staining (Fig. 1). Highly fenestrated vessels, which are leaky to blood-borne protein and supply the various circumventricular organs (e.g., median eminence, choroid plexus, and area postrema) that lie outside the BBB, remain unlabeled when exposed to blood-borne ferrotransferrin–HRP and OX-26

---

vessels (D–F; arrows), except in the circumventricular organs. Blood vessel staining appears uniform or homogeneous at 10 min (D) but is demonstrably punctate at 2 hr (E) and 6 hr (F), suggesting the OX-26 antibody-tagged receptors have been internalized by BBB endothelia. Bars: (A–C) 2 mm; (D–F) 10 mm.

conjugated and not conjugated to HRP. These three blood-borne probes, when administered into the blood in the concentrations we use routinely, are observed consistently not to leak from fenestrated vessels. OX-26 antibody applied for immunohistochemical staining of brain sections also does not label circumventricular organ blood vessels (Fig. 1B and C). Immunostaining with control antibody against MHC class I antigen of the PVG rat strain fails to label cerebral endothelia in cryostat sections of the Sprague-Dawley rat CNS. Our results as a whole suggest the ferrotransferrin receptor within the mammalian CNS is affiliated predominantly if not exclusively with BBB vasculature. The labeling of BBB vessels is evident when DAB serves as the chromogen but is particularly striking with TMB.

Cerebral vessel staining with blood-borne OX-26–HRP and native OX-26 appears homogeneous initially (Fig. 1D) but becomes distinctly punctate with time (Fig. 1E and F). We believe the punctate labeling, which resembles that identified in neuronal cell bodies labeled with native HRP by retrograde axonal transport (29), is indicative of the endothelial internalization or recycling of the ferrotransferrin receptor; this pattern of endothelial cell labeling is not evident with blood-borne ferrotransferrin–HRP and native HRP. No labeling whatsoever is seen with the control IgG_{2a}–HRP antibody.

The widespread labeling of perivascular phagocytes is most obvious at the light level with blood-borne ferrotransferrin–HRP (less so with native OX-26) and not at all with either OX-26–HRP delivered intravenously or OX-26 antibody applied for immunohistochemical staining. We should emphasize at this point that the labeling of perivascular phagocytes with blood-borne probes is not bona fide evidence signaling the transendothelial transfer or transcytosis of the macromolecules. Native HRP, a fluid-phase probe, delivered intravenously in excess of a 10-mg concentration consistently labels perivascular phagocytes throughout the CNS (1, 6, 27, 28, 30, 31). Blood-borne native HRP and endogenous immunoglobulins are documented to enter the CNS extracellularly by way of circumventricular organs and permeable vessels inhabiting the pial surface/subarachnoid space (27); on gaining access to CNS perivascular spaces in these sites, blood-borne, fluid-phase macromolecules are speculated to be propelled deeper through the perivascular clefts in the brain by the pulsatile activity of arterioles in the live animal. Native HRP in a 6-mg concentration delivered into the carotid artery of rats does not label BBB vessels and perivascular phagocytes (when either DAB or TMB is used as the chromogen) and does not appear to escape leaky vessels in the circumventricular organs or on the surface of the CNS. In this regard, native HRP in a 6-mg dose is an important control for our purposes and adds credibility to our results and interpretation of data obtained with ferrotransferrin–HRP. Blood–brain barrier vessels and perivascular phagocytes label with ferrotransferrin–HRP in less than 1 hr after the intracarotid administration of 4–6 mg of the probe. OX-26–HRP labeling of perivascular phagocytes is not identified at the light level but is observed ultrastructurally (see below).

The concentration of the receptor-mediated probes injected into the blood is smaller than that of native HRP and more comparable to the concentration of WGA–HRP (1.25 mg) administered intravenously. Blood-borne WGA–HRP, which binds to specific oligosaccharides on the cell surface and enters cells by the process of adsorptive endocytosis, labels all cerebral vessels without distinguishing between BBB and leaky vessels. Perivascular phagocytes throughout the CNS label with blood-borne WGA–HRP after 3 hr postinjection; in the same time frame, cells and processes within the neuropil also sequester reaction product of blood-borne WGA–HRP. The WGA–HRP results suggest this macromolecular probe undergoes an adsorptive-phase transcytosis through BBB endothelia (1, 26, 28). As with our receptor-mediated phase probes, there is no evidence to suggest WGA–HRP enters the CNS extracellularly through inherently leaky vessels in the circumventricular organs or on the pial surface/subarachnoid space. The latter result and comparable results with 6 mg of HRP into the carotid artery strengthen our belief that most if not all of each of the receptor-mediated probes we deliver into the carotid artery bind to transferrin receptors on BBB endothelia, thereby leaving little of each probe free in the blood to enter the CNS by extracellular routes. For this reason, the labeling of CNS perivascular phagocytes with blood-borne ferrotransferrin–HRP, OX-26–HRP, and native ascites OX-26 is interpreted as initial support for the potential receptor-mediated transcytosis of these probes through the BBB.

Ultrastructural Observations

Endothelial organelles labeled with peroxidase reaction product following receptor-mediated endocytosis of blood-borne ferrotransferrin-HRP and OX-26–HRP are basically no different from those labeled with native HRP or WGA–HRP as control probe molecules. The labeled organelles include 40- to 70-nm wide endocytic vesicles, tubular profiles, endosomes (predominantly spherical bodies rimmed internally with peroxidase reaction product; tubular profiles also may represent a component of the endosome apparatus), and dense bodies inundated with reaction product (Fig. 2). Some dense bodies and tubular profiles within BBB endothelia are identified as secondary lysosomes with acid hydrolase cytochemistry (1, 6). Reaction product of OX-26–HRP (Fig. 3A) and of WGA–HRP additionally is localized within the innermost saccule of the Golgi complex. Vesicles harboring peroxidase reaction product of ferrotransferrin–HRP and OX-26–HRP lie in proximity to

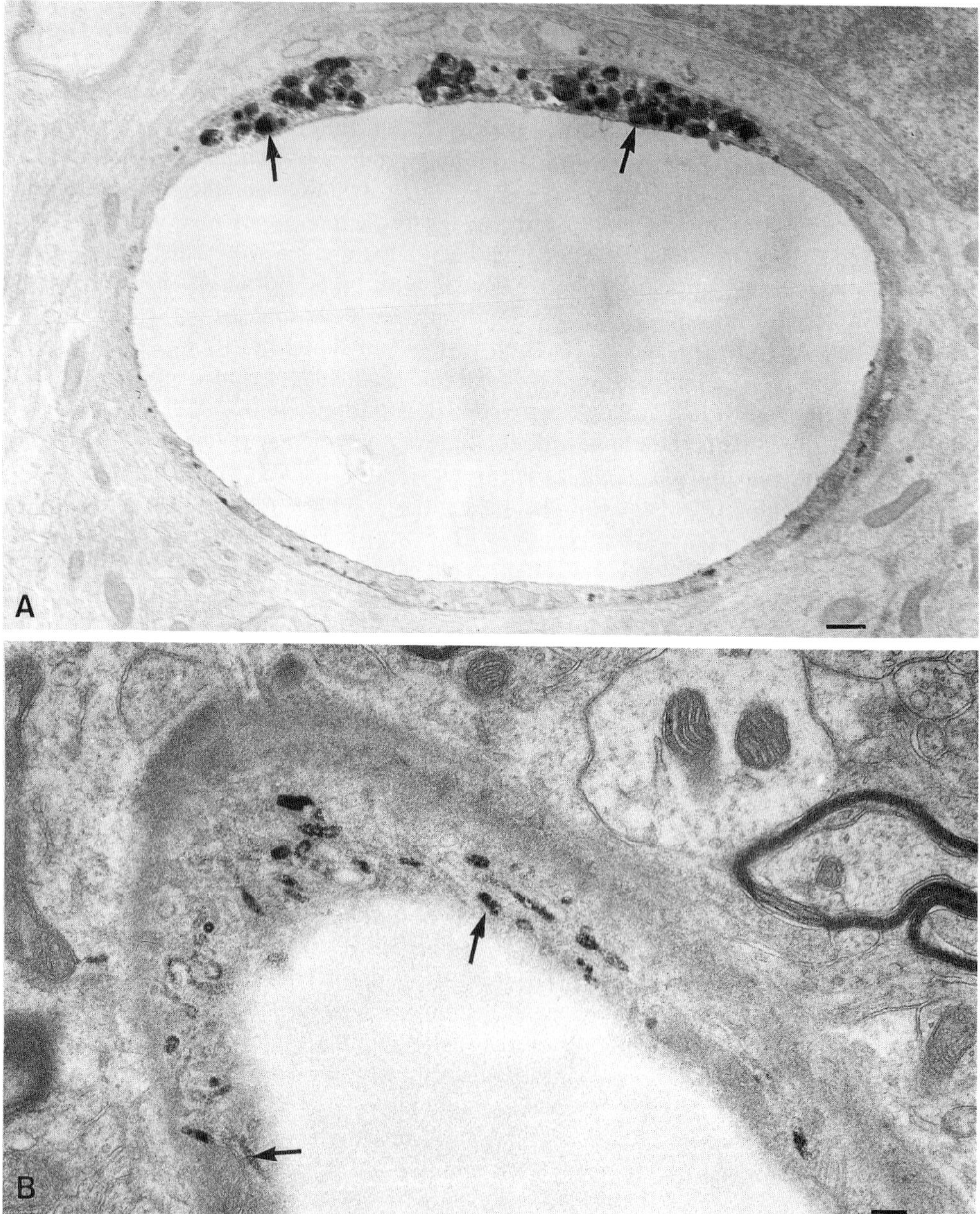

FIG. 2 Ferrotransferrin conjugated to HRP (A) and administered into the carotid artery of rats or OX-26 antibody-conjugated HRP (B) delivered intravenously binds to the lumenal plasmalemma of BBB endothelia and, within 1 hr postinjection, at

the ablumenal plasmalemma of a given BBB endothelial cell. Infrequently, possible vesicular profiles appear to establish membrane continuity with the ablumenal plasmalemma, thereby permitting exocytosis of vesicle content into the perivascular cleft (Fig. 3B–D). Reaction product of ferrotransferrin–HRP within the CNS perivascular clefts (Fig. 4) is far more conspicuous and widespread than that representing OX-26–HRP.

Endocytic vesicles and dense bodies of perivascular phagocytic cells exhibit reaction product for ferrotranferrin–HRP and for OX-26–HRP (Fig. 5A). In animals receiving ferrotransferrin–HRP into the carotid artery, peroxidase reaction product occupies endocytic vesicles, tubular profiles, endosomes, and dense bodies in cells and processes deep within the neuropil (Fig. 5B), suggesting blood-borne ferrotransferrin–HRP has moved into the CNS parenchyma beyond the BBB endothelium and perivascular cleft; indeed, in this preparation many parenchymal cells are well laden with peroxidase-labeled organelles. Some labeling of parenchymal cells also is evident with blood-borne WGA–HRP (1, 26, 28) but not to the extent identified with ferrotransferrin–HRP. Parenchymal cell labeling has not been observed with either blood-borne OX-26–HRP or native HRP. Although native HRP labels perivascular phagocytes, presumably moving through extracellular routes circumventing the BBB (27), reaction product has yet to be seen in perivascular clefts far removed from CNS sites deficient in a BBB. Reaction product of blood-borne IgG_{2a}–HRP as a control probe inhabits only BBB endothelia.

Transendothelial Pathways for Ferrotransferrin and Antibody against the Ferrotransferrin Receptor as Vehicles for Circumventing the Blood–Brain Barrier

Previous publications from our laboratory have argued against the likelihood of a direct transendothelial vesicular pathway from blood to brain (for reviews see Refs. 1 and 6), and our results with the ferrotransferrin and OX-26–peroxidase conjugates are compatible with this argument. The intraendothelial pathways we propose to be associated with the transfer of blood-borne ferrotransferrin–HRP and OX-26–HRP from blood to brain are summarized diagrammatically in Fig. 6.

---

the ultrastructural level, labels endothelial organelles such as 40- to 70-nm wide endocytic vesicles, dense bodies (A; arrows), and tubules (B; arrows); the latter two types of subcellular organelle may represent endosomes (a prelysosomal compartment) or secondary lysosomes. Bars: 1 μm.

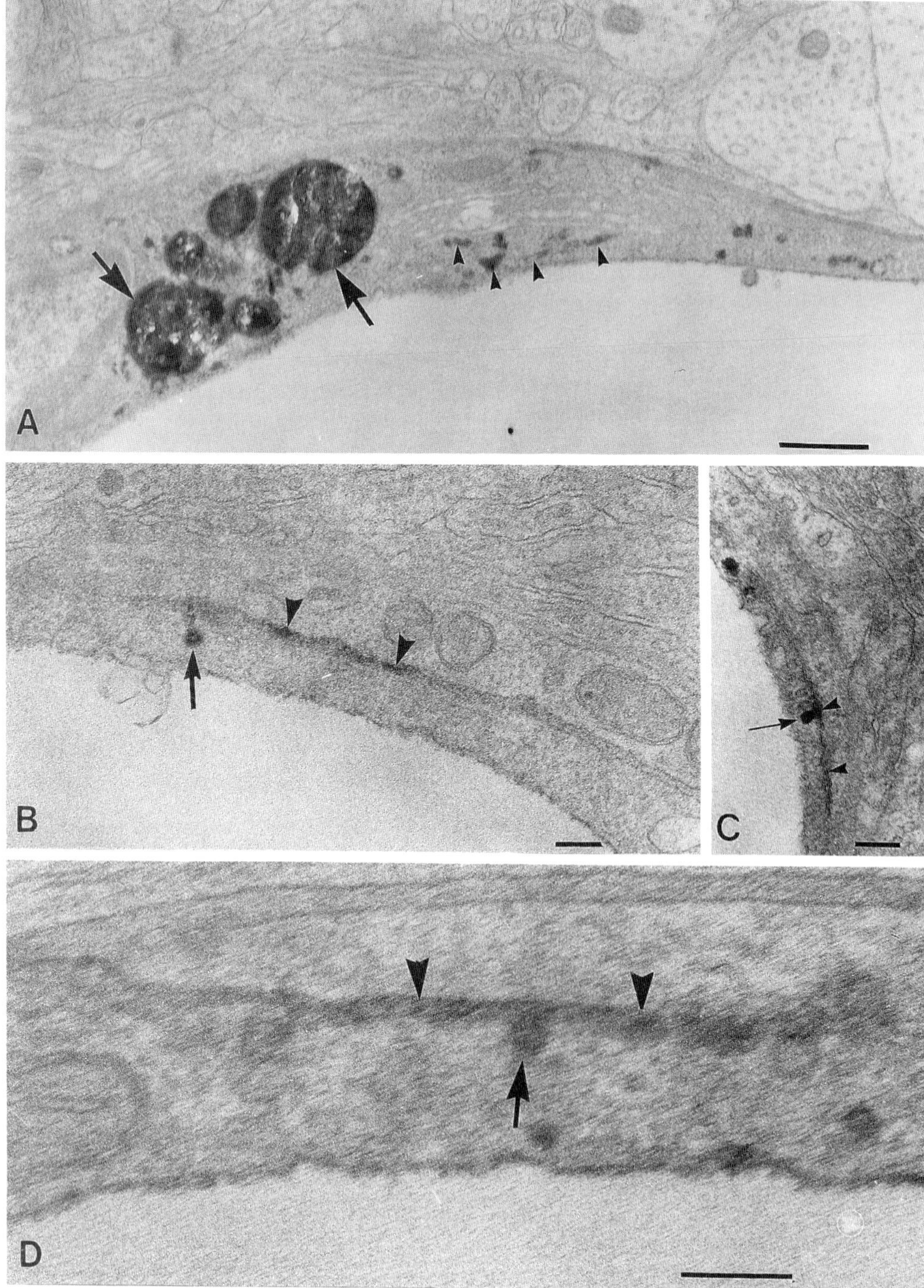
A
B
C
D

The endosome apparatus within the BBB endothelial cell conceivably represents the first intracellular stop for the internalized, cell surface ferrotransferrin receptor and attached ligand (i.e., ferrotransferrin or antibody against the receptor). Endothelial vesicular transport from cell surface to endosome is indeed compatible with the proposed function of the endosome apparatus and proposed manner by which iron is introduced to cells in general (15, 16).

The "efferent" pathways from the endosome apparatus are difficult to define with confidence histologically and ultrastructurally. Dogmatic statements are ill advised when attempting to reconstruct dynamic intracellular events based on two-dimensional, static electron micrographs. This same argument applies equally well to interpreting and identifying the act of exocytosis at the ablumenal front of BBB endothelia. The identified "vesicular profile" speculated to be engaged in exocytosis at the ablumenal plasmalemma may not be an exocytic vesicle at all but rather a static pit or caveola in that cell surface membrane (1, 6, 27). Nevertheless, the transendothelial pathway from lumenal surface to endosome and from endosome to ablumenal surface *a priori* appears the most logical route for delivering iron and transferrin, albeit indirectly, from blood to brain. We cannot exclude the possibility that the Golgi complex may serve as an additional intracellular intermediary in this transendothelial pathway. Our ferrotransferrin–HRP data do not suggest a recruitment of the Golgi complex in traversing the BBB. Snider and Rogers (32) have demonstrated that in cultured cell lines if either transferrin or its receptor is desialylated, the internalized receptor-ligand complex may be diverted to the transmost Golgi saccule for resialylation.

The involvement of the Golgi complex in the transcellular transfer of blood-borne WGA–HRP across the BBB endothelium is documented by morphological and pharmcological analyses (26, 28, 33). The antibody against the ferrotransferrin receptor now represents an additional ligand that may depend on the Golgi complex for conveyance through the BBB from blood

FIG. 3 Although blood-borne OX-26 antibody-conjugated HRP (A and B) and ferrotransferrin conjugated to HRP (C and D) are endocytosed by BBB endothelia and label endothelial dense bodies predominantly (A; arrows), only the OX-26 conjugate is identified to be sequestered within the innermost saccule (A; arrowheads) of the Golgi complex. Peroxidase reaction product indicative of the OX-26 conjugate or of the transferrin conjugate labels portions of the albumenal plasmalemma/perivascular clefts (B–D; arrowheads) of BBB endothelia and may occupy transcytotic vesicles (B–D; arrows) that have established membrane continuity with the albumenal plasmalemma for exocytosis of the conjugates into the perivascular clefts. Bars: 1 μm.

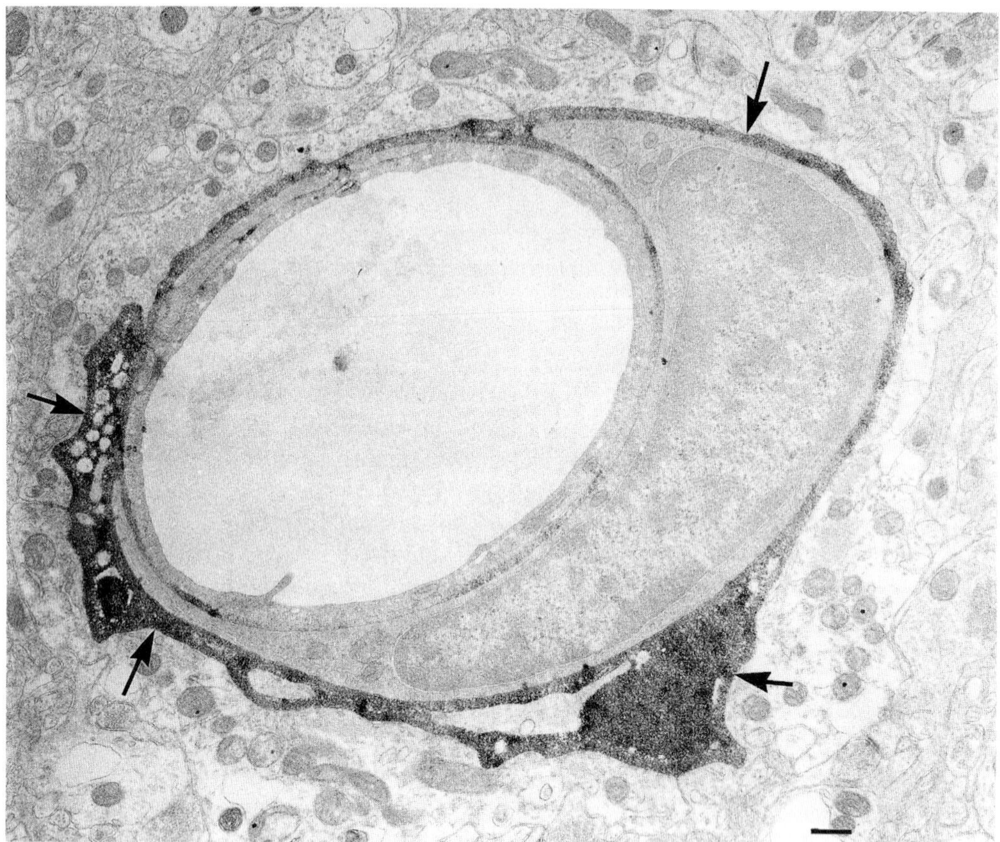

FIG. 4 Flooding of BBB endothelial perivascular clefts and basal lamina with HRP reaction product (arrows) in rats receiving a carotid injection of ferrotransferrin conjugated to HRP is conspicuous ultrastructurally and can be fairly widespread within the rat brain at 1 hr postinjection. This observation suggests transendothelial transfer of blood-borne ferrotransferrin into the rat CNS may be a demonstrable event. Bar: 1 μm.

to brain. Whereas the "efferent pathways" from the innermost saccule of the Golgi complex are known in the cell biological literature and incorporate the exocytic route (34), identifying the "afferent pathway" to the Golgi complex from the cell surface is more difficult. In our OX-26–HRP preparations, as with WGA–HRP, the peroxidase labeling of Golgi saccules on a time scale follows that of the endosome apparatus; therefore, we cannot state with confidence if OX-26–HRP (or WGA–HRP) associated with internalized

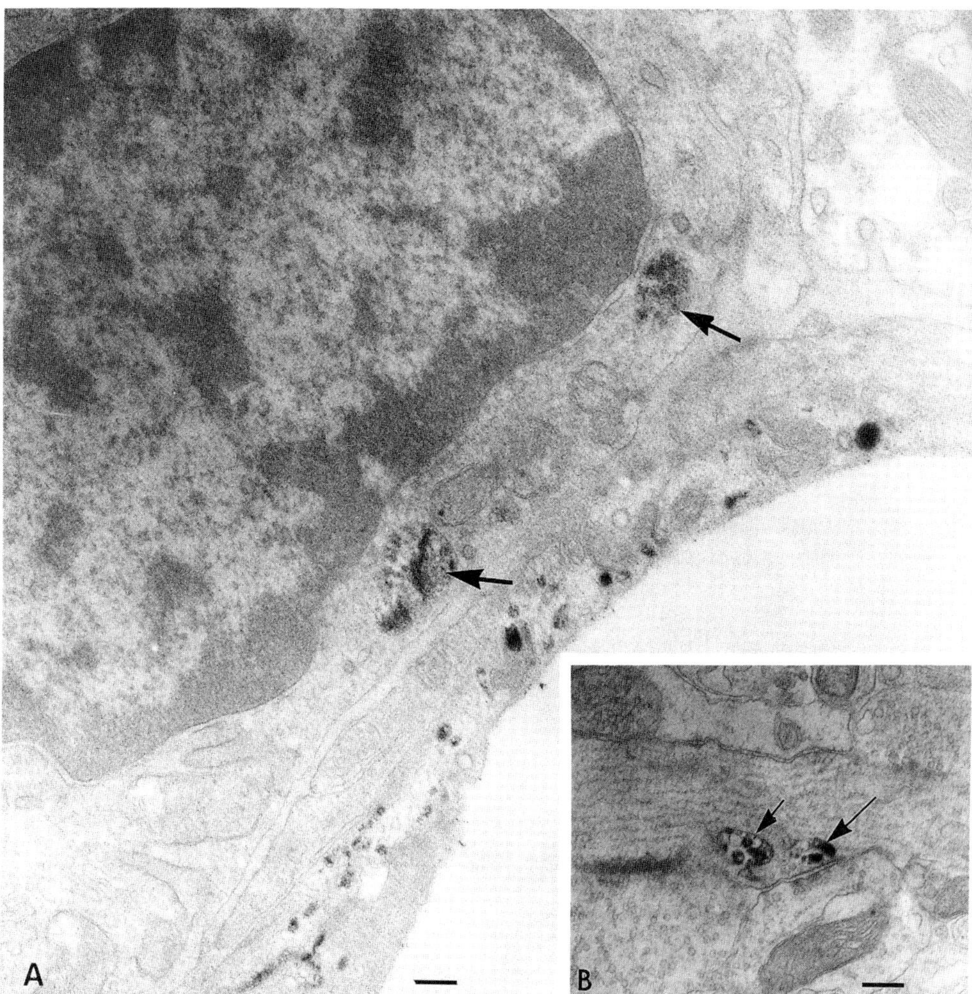

FIG. 5 Additional evidence advocating the transendothelial transfer of ferrotransferrin conjugated to HRP (A) and of OX-26 conjugated to HRP from blood to brain in the rat is the ultrastructural identification of peroxidase-labeled endosomes and dense bodies within perivascular phagocytes (A; arrows). Similar peroxidase-labeled organelles are evident in cell bodies and processes of neurons (B; arrows) and glia deep in the brain parenchyma behind the BBB in rats receiving ferrotransferrin–HRP. Bars: 1 μm.

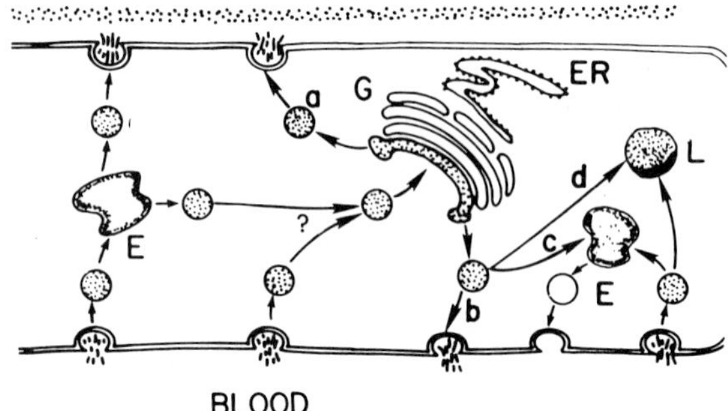

FIG. 6 Blood-borne ferrotransferrin–HRP and OX-26 conjugated to HRP enter blood–brain barrier endothelia within vesicles derived from the lumenal plasmalemma by the process of receptor-mediated endocytosis. The protein-laden endocytic vesicles may be directed to endosomes (E), a prelysosomal compartment, or to secondary lysosomes (L) for subsequent degradation. Alternatively, the endocytic vesicles may be channeled to the innermost saccule of the Golgi complex (G) directly from the lumenal plasmalemma or indirectly from endosomes. Available data suggest the Golgi pathway involves the OX-26–peroxidase conjugate but not the ferrotransferrin–HRP conjugate. Transport vesicles derived from the endosome compartment may function to complete a transendothelial or transcytotic pathway (a) by conveying the ferrotransferrin–HRP and OX-26–HRP to the albumenal plasmalemma for exocytosis to commence. Transport vesicles of endosomal origin may be directed to the lumenal plasmalemma where exocytosis also can occur; this pathway could involve the recycling of the transferrin receptor and subsequent exocytosis of the apo form of the transferrin molecule. A second transendothelial pathway is envisioned for transport vesicles (a) derived from the inner Golgi saccule. Other Golgi transport vesicles may follow a pathway (b) to the lumenal plasmalemma where exocytosis can occur, or they may function as primary lysosomes that convey acid hydrolase enzymes to (c) the endosome compartment or to (d) secondary lysosomes.

lumenal surface membrane in the BBB endothelial cell is channeled directly to the Golgi complex or indirectly by way of transfer vesicles taking origin from the endosome compartment. Perhaps the more important question to ask is, why should OX-26–HRP, or WGA–HRP for that matter, be channeled to the Golgi complex at all? One plausible answer is that the cell surface or endosome route to the Golgi complex may represent a secondary intracellular pathway related to the physical size of the OX-26–HRP molecule (M_r 165,000). Available data suggest the normal intracellular pathway for internalized transferrin conjugates is altered when the ferrotransferrin receptors are cross-linked by the probe molecule (35). Alternatively, the endosome compartment may be incapable of dissociating the ferrotransferrin receptor membrane from the OX-26–HRP conjugate, whereupon the membrane receptor with attached ligand is redirected to the Golgi complex, where the task is accomplished.

OX-26–HRP directed to the inner face of the Golgi complex would be packaged for export in vesicles derived from the inner Golgi saccule. Figure 6 indicates the exocytic pathway to the ablumenal side of the BBB endothelium is one of four intracellular pathways Golgi-derived vesicles, in which OX-26–HRP would be packaged for export, may follow. This dilution and widespread distribution of OX-26–HRP could explain why OX-26–HRP labeling of perivascular phagocytes, perivascular clefts, and brain parenchymal cells seen in our preparations is not as demonstrable as that with ferrotransferrin–HRP. The apparent difference in CNS labeling between the two probes also can be attributed to intravenous delivery of OX-26–HRP versus carotid injection of ferrotransferrin–HRP.

Summary and Conclusions

The potential for receptor-mediated transcytosis of blood-borne ferrotransferrin and antibody against the ferrotransferrin receptor (OX-26) through the endothelial cell of the BBB in the rat has been analzyed qualitatively with peroxidase-based cytochemical approaches at light and electron microscopic levels. The endothelial cell receptor for ferrotransferrin appears by immunohistochemical analysis to be restricted to BBB vessels and recognizes both ferrotransferrin and antibody against the receptor conjugated to the 40K protein tracer horseradish peroxidase. That the two blood-borne ligands successfully ferry HRP into the brain parenchyma in less than 1 hr following their administration into the blood is a testimony to the potential of both molecules to serve as vehicles for the delivery of additional non-lipid-soluble substances into the CNS. This statement, with respect to OX-26, is supported by the capillary depletion experiments of Friden and colleagues (12, 13), who have demonstrated the blood-to-brain entry of OX-26 conjugated to methotrexate and nerve growth factor. Intraendothelial membrane trafficking associated with blood-borne OX-26–HRP appears to involve a sorting process through the Golgi complex, whereas ferrotransferrin–HRP is suggested to undergo transendothelial transfer more efficiently by way of the endosome apparatus only. The efficiency is translated into CNS neurons and supporting cells exhibiting peroxidase reaction product related to ferrotransferrin–HRP administration. The proposed membrane trafficking of blood-borne ferrotransferrin through the BBB endothelium is at odds with the conventional interpretation for the recycling of the transferrin receptor with ferro vs. apo forms of transferrin. Nevertheless, our data do suggest histochemically demonstrable ferrotransferrin–HRP does enter the CNS from the blood, a finding that requires a quantitative reassessment of the reportedly low to nil transendothelial transfer of blood-borne transferrin into the CNS (18, 19).

Acknowledgments

This study was supported by U.S. Public Health Service Grant #NS18030 from NINDS, NIH (to R.D.B.) and by Alkermes, Inc. (Cambridge, MA). The authors thank Drs. Aizik Wolf and Paul Ebert and Mr. Musa Tangoren for technical assistance.

References

1. R. D. Broadwell and W. A. Banks, Cell Biological Perspective for the Trancytosis of Peptides and Proteins through the Mammalian Blood–Brain Fluid Barriers. *In* "The Blood–Brain Barrier" (W. M. Partridge, ed.), p. 165. Raven Press, New York, 1993.
2. S. I. Rapoport, K. Matthews, and H. K. Thompson, *Brain Res.* **136,** 23 (1977).
3. E. A. Neuwelt, P. A. Barnett, and M. Glasberg, *Cancer Res.* **43,** 5278 (1988).
4. E. A. Neuwelt, D. L. Goldman, and S. A. Dahlborg, *J. Clin. Oncol.* **9,** 1580 (1991).
5. E. A. Neuwelt, "Implications of the Blood-Brain Barrier and Its Manipulation: Clinical Implications," Vol. 2. Plenum Press, New York, 1989
6. R. D. Broadwell, *Acta Neuropathol.* **79,** 117 (1989).
7. W. M. Pardridge, "Peptide Drug Delivery to the Brain." Raven Press, New York, 1991.
8. W. A. Jefferies, M. R. Brandon, S. U. Hunt. A. F. Williams, K. C. Gatter, and D. Y. Mason, *Nature* (*London*) **312,** 162 (1984).
9. R. D. Broadwell, B. J. Baker, P. Ebert, and W. F. Hickey, *Micros. Res. Tech.* **27,** 471 (1994).
10. P. Aisen, *Ann. Neurol.* **32,** S62 (1992).
11. W. M. Pardridge, J. L. Buciak, and P. M. Friden, *J. Pharm. Exp. Therapeut.* **259,** 66 (1991).
12. P. M. Friden, L.R . Walus, G. F. Musso, M. A. Taylor, B. Malfroy, and R. M. Starzyk, *Proc. Natl. Acad. Sci. U.S.A.* **88,** 477 (1991).
13. P. M. Friden, L. R. Walus, P. Watson, S. R. Doctrow, J. W. Kozarich, C. Backman, H. Burgman, B. Hoffer, F. Bloom, and A. Granholm, *Science* **259,** 373 (1993).
14. A. Helenius, I. Mellman, D. Wall, and A. Hubbard, *Trends Biochem. Sci.* **8,** 245 (1983).
15. A. Dautry-Varsat, A. Ciechanover, and H. F. Lodish, *Proc. Natl. Acad. Sci. U.S.A.* **80,** 2258 (1983).
16. A. Dautry-Varsat and H. F. Lodish, *Sci.Am.* **250,** 52 (1984).
17. J. B. Fishman, J. B. Rubin, J. B. Handrahan, J. R. Connor, and R. E. Fine, *J. Neurosci. Res.* **18,** 299 (1987).

18. R. Roberts, A. Sandra, G. C. Siek, J. J. Lucas, and R. E. Fine, *Ann. Neurol.* **32,** S43 (1992).
19. C. M. Morris, A. B. Keith, J. A. Edwardson, and R. G. L. Pullen, *J. Neurochem.* **59,** 300 (1992).
20. M. C. Willingham, J. A. Hanover, R. B. Dickson, and I. Pastan, *Proc. Natl. Acad. Sci. U.S.A.* **81,** 175 (1984).
21. D. P. Fitzgerald, *Methods Enzymol.* **151,** 139 (1987).
22. E. L. Barsumian, C.Isersky, M. G. Petrino, and R. P. Siraganian, *Eur. J. Immunol.* **11,** 317 (1987).
23. D. W. Mason and A. F. Williams, *Biochem. J.* **187,** 1 (1980).
24. J. W. Goding, "Monoclonal Antibodies: Principles and Practice," 2nd Ed. Academic Press, London, 1986.
25. A. N. Barclay, *Immunology* **42,** 593 (1981).
26. J. Villegas and R. D. Broadwell, *J. Neurocytol.* **22,** 67 (1993).
27. R. D. Broadwell and M. V. Sofroniew, *Exp. Neurol.* **120,** 245 (1993).
28. W. A. Banks and R. D. Broadwell, *J. Neurochem.* **62,** 2404 (1994).
29. R. D. Broadwell and M. W. Brightman, *Methods Enzymol.* **103,** 187 (1983).
30. B. J. Balin, R. D. Broadwell, M. El-Kalliny, and M. Salcman, *J. Comp. Neurol.* **251,** 260 (1986).
31. R. D. Broadwell, H. M. Charlton, B. J. Balin, and M. Salcman, *J. Comp. Neurol.* **260,** 47 (1987).
32. M. D. Snider and O. C. Rogers, *J. Cell Biol.* **100,** 826 (1985).
33. R. D. Broadwell, B. J. Balin, and M. Salcman, *Proc. Natl. Acad. Sci. U.S.A.* **85,** 632 (1988).
34. A. Dautry-Varsat and H. F. Lodish, *Trends Neurosci.* **6,** 484 (1983).
35. M. R. Neutra, A. Ciechanover, L. S. Owen, and H. F. Lodish, *J. Histochem. Cytochem.* **33,** 1134 (1985).

[7] DepoFoam-Mediated Drug Delivery into Cerebrospinal Fluid

Sinil Kim

Introduction

Many of the drugs, peptides, and proteins potentially useful in the central nervous sytem (CNS) do not pass through the blood–brain or blood–cerebrospinal fluid (CSF) barriers. One obvious approach for providing therapeutic access to the brain for such molecules is a direct injection method. Direct injection approaches, such as lumbar punctures, Ommaya reservoir for intraventricular injections,and epidural catheter systems, are being used clinically in the treatment or prophylaxis of human patients against leptomeningeal metastasis and for CNS delivery of anesthetics and narcotics. However, because most molecules have relatively short half-lives in the CNS, frequent, multiple injections are necessary to maintain therapeutic concentrations. Such frequent and multiple injections into Ommaya reservoirs and epidural catheters are associated with increased risk of infections and frequent lumbar punctures are uncomfortable for the patients. We have developed a lipid-based drug delivery system, DepoFoam (1), that can deliver a variety of water-stable molecules into the CSF over a prolonged period following a single injection.

DepoFoam is composed of microscopic spherical particles, each enclosing multiple nonconcentric aqueous chambers bounded by a single-bilayer lipid membrane (2). These particles are made from nontoxic synthetic lipids identical to those naturally found in cell membranes and generally regarded as safe. DepoFoam particles have advantages over other drug delivery systems in that the multiple internal lipid membranes result in high stability during storage, good control over the drug release rate, highly efficient entrapment of hydrophilic molecules, and production that is relatively easy to scale up (1, 3–5).

This chapter describes encapsulation of four drugs, that is, cytarabine (ara-C), methotrexate (MTX), morphine sulfate, and interferon α (IFN), into DepoFoam; the results of *in vivo* animal studies; and early clinical trial results of DepoFoam-encapsulated ara-C (DTC 101) in humans.

Methods in Neurosciences, Volume 21

Synthesis of DepoFoam-Encapsulated Ara-C (DTC 101)

One milliliter of a 20-mg/ml ara-C solution in water (pH = 1.1 with HCl) is placed into a 1-dram vial containing 9.3 μmol of dioleoyl lecithin, 2.1 μmol of dipalmitoyl phosphatidylglycerol, 15 μmol of cholesterol, 1.8 μmol of triolein, and 1 ml of chloroform (3). The vial is capped tightly and attached horizontally to the head of a Vortex mixer (Baxter Diagnostics, Inc., McGaw Park, IL) and shaken at the maximum speed for 6 min. Each half of the resulting "water-in-oil" emulsion is individually pushed rapidly through a narrow-tip Pasteur pipette into 1-dram vials, each containing 2.5 ml of water, glucose (3.2 g/100 ml), and free-base lysine (40 mM), and then shaken on the Vortex mixer for 3 sec at the "5" setting to form chloroform spherules. The chloroform spherule suspensions in the two vials are combined into the bottom of a 250-ml Erlenmeyer flask containing 5 ml of water, glucose (3.2 g/100 ml), and free-base lysine (40 mM). A stream of nitrogen gas at 7 liters/min is flushed through the flask to evaporate chloroform for 10 to 15 min at 37°C. The DTC 101 particles are then isolated by centrifugation at 600 g for 5 min and washed three times with a 0.9% (w/v) NaCl solution.

Preparation of DepoFoam-Encapsulated Methotrexate (Depo/MTX)

A method similar to that described above for DTC 101 is used. The discontinuous aqueous phase consists of 2-hydroxypropyl-β-cyclodextrin solution (100 mg/ml), HCl (0.1 N), and methotrexate (10 mg/ml) (6). One milliliter of the discontinuous aqueous phase is placed into a 1-dram vial containing 13.9 μmol of dioleoyl lecithin, 3.15 μmol of dipalmitoyl phosphatidylglycerol, 22.5 μmol of cholesterol, 2.7 μmol of triolein, and 1 ml of chloroform. The rest of the procedure is virtually identical to that for DTC 101 above.

Preparation of Depo/Morphine

Again, a method almost identical to that for DTC 101 is used. One milliliter of discontinuous aqueous phase containing morphine sulfate (18 mg/ml) and HCl (0.1 N) is placed into a 1-dram vial containing 9.3 μmol of dioleoyl lecithin, 2.1 μmol of dipalmitoyl phosphatidylglycerol, 15 μmol of cholesterol, 1.8 μmol of triolein, and 1 ml of chloroform (7). The rest of the procedure is identical to that for DTC 101.

Following the subcutaneous (sc) administration of 1 mg of Depo/Morphine in mice, the total amount of morphine remaining at the sc injection site decreases with a first-order kinetic $T_{1/2}$ of 2.6 ± 0.2 days (mean ± SD;

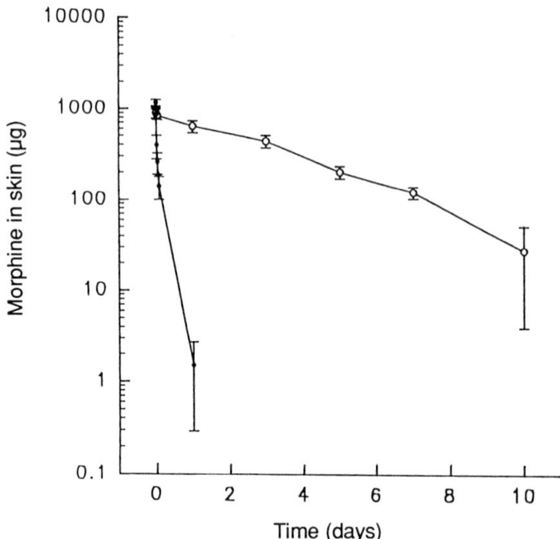

FIG. 1 Amount (μg) of morphine remaining at injection site following sc injection of 1.0 mg of unencapsulated morphine (●) or Depo/Morphine (○). Each point represents the mean and SD from four to five mice. (Reproduced with permission, from Ref. 7.)

$r^2 = 0.98$), compared to a $T_{1/2}$ of 0.46 ± 0.04 hr (mean ± SD; $r^2 = 0.97$) for unencapsulated morphine (Fig. 1). Plasma morphine (native drug plus metabolites) concentration rises to a maximum of 1.2 ± 0.4 μg/ml (mean ± SD) within 1 hr with Depo/Morphine and then decreases monoexponentially with a $T_{1/2}$ of 8.3 ± 2.1 days (mean ± SD; $r^2 = 0.86$; Fig. 2). Unencapsulated morphine injection yields a maximum plasma concentration of 19 ± 5 μg/ml (mean ± SD) within 30 min, which then decreases rapidly with a $T_{1/2}$ of 0.45 ± 0.21 hr (mean ± SD; $r^2 = 0.90$) (7).

Synthesis of Depo/IFN

One milliliter of discontinuous aqueous phase [human IFN-α_{2b} (hIFN-α-2b), 1.1 million IU/ml; mannitol, 40 mg/ml; sodium acetate, 2.5 mM; glycine, 12 mM; Na_2HPO_4, 7 mM; NaH_2PO_4, 2 mM; Tween 80, 0.01 mg/ml; HCl, 0.1 N; human serum albumin, 0.04 mg/ml] is placed into a 1-dram vial containing 13.9 μmol of dioleoyl lecithin, 3.15 μmol of dipalmitoyl phosphatidylglycerol, 22.5 μmol of cholesterol, 2.7 μmol of triolein, and 1 ml of chloroform (8). Steps virtually identical to those for DTC 101 are used for the rest of the encapsulation procedure.

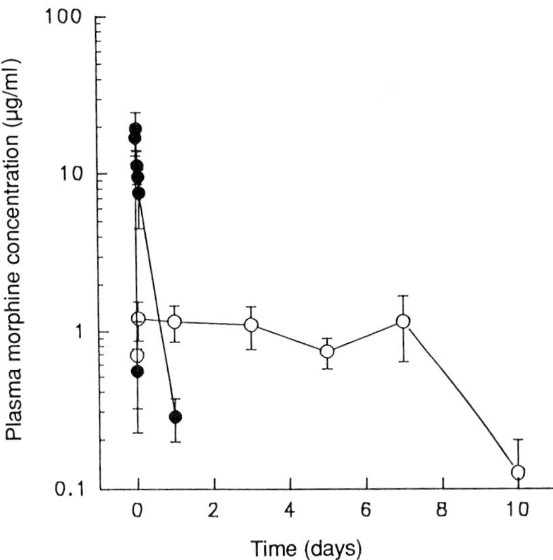

FIG. 2 Plasma concentrations of morphine following sc injection of 1.0 mg of unencapsulated morphine (●) or Depo/Morphine (○). Each point represents the mean and SD from four to five mice. (Reproduced with permission, from Ref. 7.)

Following injection of Depo/IFN into murine peritoneal cavity, the total interferon concentration in peritoneal cavity initially increases eightfold during the first 8 hr. Thereafter, the intraperitoneal concentration declines slowly with a half-life of 20 hr (8). This is in contrast to a half-life of 1.5 hr for unencapsulated interferon.

Central Nervous System Pharmacokinetic Analysis

Pharmacokinetic curves are fitted to a biexponential function $C(t) = Ae^{-\alpha t} + Be^{-\beta t}$, where $C(t)$ is the concentration at time t, A and B are coefficients, and α and β are the initial and terminal rate constants respectively. The RSTRIP computer program (MicroMath Scientific Software, Salt Lake City, UT) is used for curve fitting by iterative nonlinear regression. The area under the curve (AUC) is determined by linear trapezoidal rule up to the last measured concentration and then extrapolated to infinity. Cerebrospinal fluid clearance of the drug is calculated by dividing the dose of ara-C by the AUC. The initial volume of distribution of injected drug in CSF (V_d) is calculated by dividing the total dose administered by the maximum CSF concentration achieved.

Intraventricular Pharmacokinetics of DTC 101 in Rats

This procedure (3) generally employs male Sprague-Dawley rats (3 to 5 months old, weighing 360 to 460 g). Animals are anesthetized with sodium pentobarbital [45 mg/kg, intraperitoneal (ip)] and mounted on a stereotaxic frame (David Kopf Instruments, Tujunga, CA). The dorsal surface of the skull is exposed with a midline scalp incision. A 1-mm hole is drilled through the calvarium at a point 0.4 mm rostral and 1.8 mm lateral to the bregma. The dura is torn with a sharp needle, and a 30-gauge blunt needle tip is lowered into the brain to a point 4.2 mm below the skull surface into a lateral ventricle. Placement of the needle tip can be validated in a separate group of rats by infusion of Evans Blue dye. Fifty microliters of free unencapsulated drug in 0.9% (w/v) NaCl solution or 50 μl of DTC 101 suspension, both containing 1 mg of ara-C, is injected over 25 min, using a syringe infusion pump. At the end of the injection, the needle is removed, the skull hole is immediately closed with bone wax, the skin is stapled, and 30,000 U of benzathine penicillin are given intramuscularly (im).

At appropriate time points, three rats are sacrificed with sodium pentobarbital (100 mg/kg ip), the blood specimens obtained with cardiac puncture, and the animals exsanguinated. The skin overlying the calvarium is dissected away and, using a bone rongeur, the calvarium is removed carefully without disturbing the underlying dura. A small tear is made in the dura in the frontal area without tearing the dural sinuses, and a capillary pipette is used to obtain 20-μl specimens of cerebrospinal fluid. The fluid is diluted with 100 μl of 0.9% NaCl solution and immediately spun in a Microfuge centrifuge (Brinkmann Instruments, Westbury, NY) for 1 min, and the supernatant (containing free drug) is separated from the pellet (containing DepoFoam particles) before storage at -20°C. The brain is lifted out of the cranial cavity with a spatula, and the cranial vault is washed thoroughly with 0.9% NaCl solution to collect all the drug in the cranial compartment. The spinal cord is extruded forward into the cranial vault by inserting in the rostrad direction a 19-gauge hypodermic needle in the low lumbar spinal canal at a point 2.5 cm rostrad to the base of the tail and pushing 0.9% NaCl solution into the canal at high pressure. The empty spinal canal is washed thoroughly with 0.9% NaCl solution to collect all the drug in the spinal canal. The brain compartment specimens are collected separately from the spinal canal specimens. The specimens are homogenized on ice with distilled water using a Dounce (Wheaton, Millville, CT) manual tissue grinder, sonicated to disrupt intact DepoFoam particles, and filtered through ultrafiltration membrane (YMT membrane No. 4104; Amicon Corp., Danvers, MA). The ultrafiltrates are analyzed with a Waters and Associates (Milford, MA) high-performance liquid chromatograph system with a 280-nm ultraviolet (UV) detector.

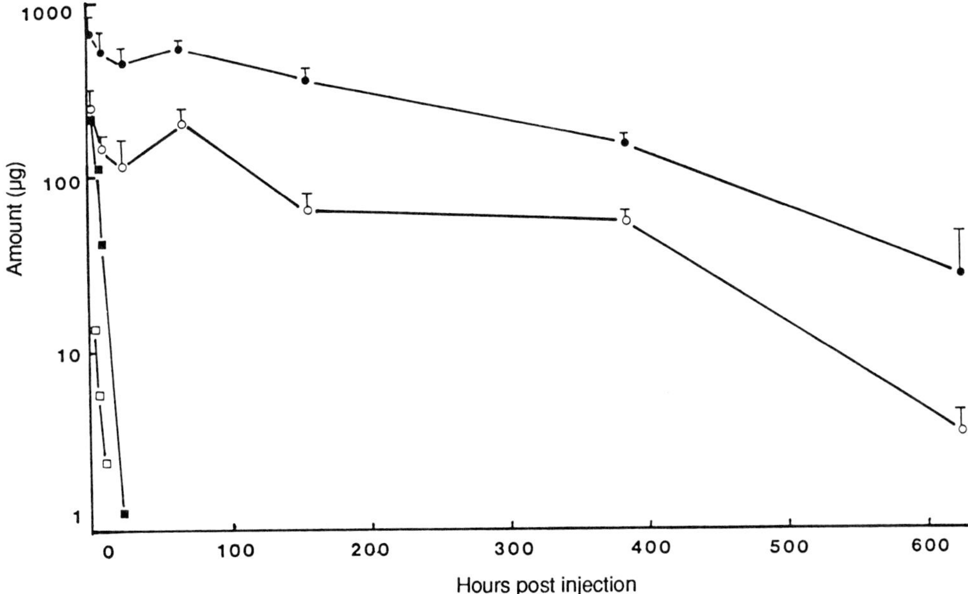

FIG. 3 The amounts of ara-C remaining within cranial and spinal compartments following a single 1-mg intraventricular injection of DTC 101 in rats. (●) Amount in cranial compartment and (○) amount in spinal compartment, after the injection of DTC 101, each point representing the mean from three rats. Error bars represent the SD. (■) Amount in cranial compartment and (□) amount in spinal compartment, after injection of unencapsulated ara-C, each point from a single rat. (Reproduced with permission, from Ref. 3.)

Figure 3 shows the pharmacokinetic result following intraventricular injection of 1 mg of DTC 101. The half-life of the drug (in micrograms) within the cranial compartment is 148 hr for DTC 101, which is about 55-fold higher than that for standard ara-C (3).

Intralumbar Pharmacokinetics of DTC 101 in Monkeys

Adult male rhesus monkeys (*Macaca mulatta*) weighing 9 to 12 kg are used for intrathecal (intralumbar) pharmacokinetic studies (9). Animals are anesthetized with ketamine and xylazine. After sterilization of the lumbosacral area skin, a 22-gauge spinal needle is inserted into the subarachnoid space at the L5–L6 intervertebral space. A CSF sample for zero time point is obtained through the spinal needle. Two milligrams of DTC 101 is injected intrathecally followed by a 0.4-ml flush of Elliotts B solution. A separate control animal is given a 2-mg intralumbar dose of unencapsulated area-C. Cerebrospinal fluid samples are obtained from the lumbar thecal sac under anesthesia at 0.33, 24, 48, 96, 120, 192, 336, 504, and 672 hr in the animals injected with DTC 101 and at 0.25, 0.5, 1, 2, 3, 4, 6, and 8 hr in the control animal injected with unencapsulated ara-C. The DepoFoam particles in CSF are separated by centrifugation in an Eppendorf Microfuge for 5 min. The supernatant is separated from the pellet and both are kept frozen until assayed. A simultaneous blood sample is obtained in a heparinized tube. To prevent degradation of ara-C, all blood and CSF samples are collected into tubes containing 40 m*M* (final concentration) tetrahydrouridine. The concentration of ara-C in monkey CSF is determined in triplicate by radioimmunoassay (9).

Figure 4 shows the CSF concentration curves of ara-C following intrathecal injection of a single 2-mg dose of DTC 101 ($n = 6$) and the curve following injection of unencapsulated ara-C ($n = 1$). The DTC 101 concentration in CSF decreases in a biexponential fashion, with an initial half-life of 14.6 hr and a terminal half-life of 156 hr. The free drug concentration remains above the minimal cytotoxic level of 0.1 μg/ml or 0.4 μM for greater than 672 hr. In contrast, the free ara-C CSF concentration in the control animal (injected with unencapsulated ara-C) decreases in a biexponential fashion, with an initial half-life of 0.13 hr (8 min) and a terminal half-life of 0.74 hr (44 min). The ara-C concentration remains above the minimum cytotoxic level for 11 hr in the control animal.

Intracisternal Pharmacokinetics with Depo/MTX in Rats

In this procedure (6) animals are anesthetized with ketamine-HCl (90 mg/kg) and acetopromazine maleate (2.2 mg/kg) intramuscularly, and mounted in a stereotaxic frame. A midline cutaneous incision is made from the occipital crest to just behind the ears, approximately 1 cm in length. The muscle ligament along the occipital crest at the skull is detached for 4 mm on either side of the midline. The muscle is gently freed from the occipital bone down to the atlas/occipital membrane and retracted away from the atlantooccipital membrane. Either 20 μl of unencapsulated drug in 0.9% NaCl solution or 20 μl of Depo/MTX suspension, both equal doses of 100 μg (0.22 μmol) of methotrexate, are injected over 20 sec via a 30-gauge needle through the membrane. The skin is then sutured with 3-0 silk, and the animal is given 10 ml of lactated Ringer's solution subcutaneously for hydration.

At appropriate time points postinjection, the previous method for exposing the atlantooccipital membrane is carried out with injected rats and a sample of cerebrospinal fluid is obtained through a 19-gauge needle. Samples are

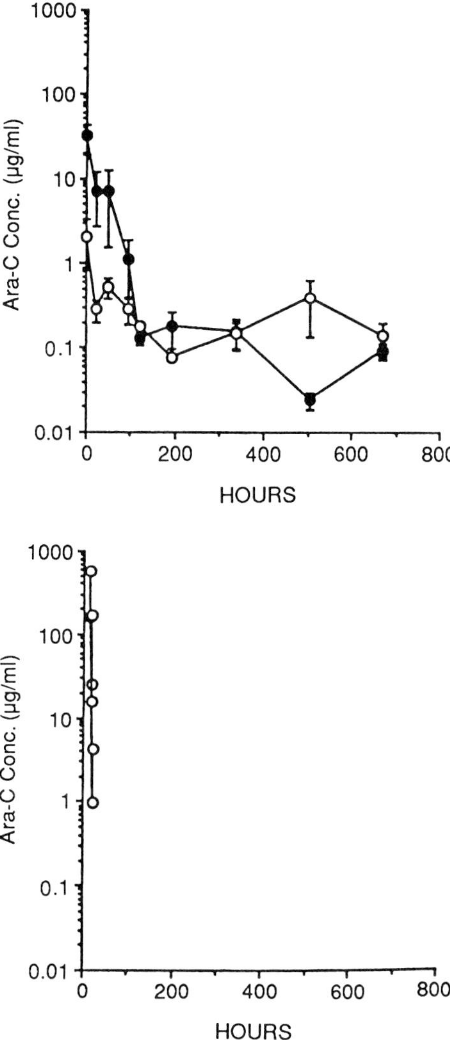

FIG. 4 Cerebrospinal fluid pharmacokinetics after a single 2-mg intralumbar dose of DTC 101 (top) and unencapsulated ara-C (bottom) in monkeys. (●) DTC 101 concentration; (○) free ara-C concentration. Data from six monkeys for DTC 101 group and one animal for unencapsulated ara-C. The error bars represent the SEM. (Reproduced with permission, from Ref. 9.)

obtained at 1 min and at 4, 24, and 48 hr postinjection with unencapsulated methotrexate, and at 1 min and at 1, 3, 7, 14, and 21 days postinjection with Depo/MTX. The CSF samples obtained are diluted with 70 μl of 0.9% NaCl solution and immediately centrifuged in a Microfuge for 1 min and supernatant is separated from the pellet. Fifty microliters of methanol and 50 μl of sterile water are sequentially added to the pellet and vortexed to break the Depo/MTX particles. The CSF samples are kept frozen at -20°C until analysis. The CSF samples are analyzed with a high-performance liquid chromatography (HPLC) system.

Following the CSF sampling, the animals are sacrificed with an overdose of ketamine (90 mg/kg) and acetopromazine (20 mg/kg) intraperitoneally. Blood samples are obtained via cardiac puncture, and the animals are exsanguinated completely. The brain and spinal compartment samples are obtained as described above (see Intraventricular Pharmacokinetics of DTC 101 in Rats, above).

The homogenized contents of brain and spinal canal compartments are analyzed by HPLC. A 500-μl aliquot of homogenate is placed in a glass centrifuge tube and 100 μl of theophylline aqueous solution (2.0 mg/ml), 250 μl of trichloroacetic acid solution (10% in water), and 250 μl of glacial acetic acid are added. After mixing well, 5 ml of ethyl acetate is added and mixed

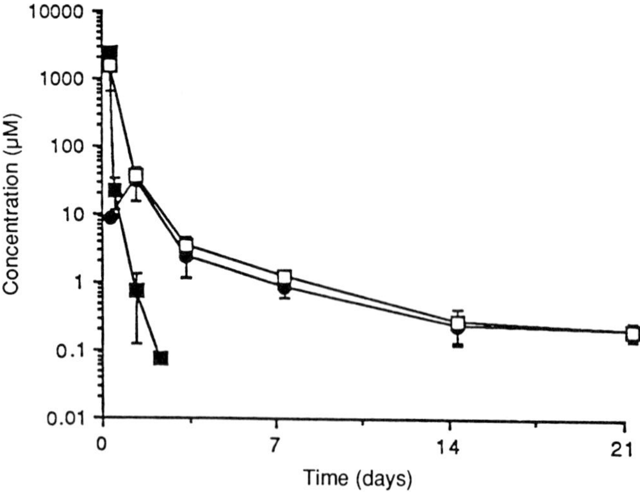

FIG. 5 The cerebrospinal concentrations of methotrexate after intracisternal injection of 100 μg (0.22 μmol) of methotrexate as unencapsulated drug (■) and encapsulated into DepoFoam particles (●, free; □, total). Each point represents the mean and standard deviation from a group of three rats. (Reproduced with permission, from Ref. 6.)

well again. The two immiscible phases are allowed to separate; ethyl acetate is decanted and evaporated under nitrogen at 60°C. The residue is dissolved in 200 μl of mobile phase and a 100-μl volume is injected into the HPLC system. A mobile phase consisting of H_3PO_4 (10 mM) : KH_2PO_4 (10 mM) : methanol in a 180 : 540 : 280 ratio (final pH 3) is pumped at a flow rate of 1 ml/min with a Waters model 510 pump through a Beckman (Fullerton, CA) ultrasphere ODS 5μ × 4.6 mm × 25 cm solumn. Methotrexate is detected at 303 nm with a Waters model 490 programmable multiwavelength detector. The retention times of theophylline and methotrexate are 5 and 7 min, respectively. The limit of detection is 5 pmol of methotrexate injected.

Figures 5 and 6 depict the CSF pharmacokinetics (in terms of CSF concentration and CNS amount) of Depo/MTX and encapsulated methotrexate. After intracisternal injection of Depo/MTX, the CSF concentration of free methotrexate reached a maximum on day 1 and then decreased in a biexponential fashion, with an initial half-life of 0.41 days and terminal half-life of 5.4 days (6). In contrast, injection of unencapsulated methotrexate resulted in an initial half-life of 0.024 days and a terminal half-life of 0.30 days.

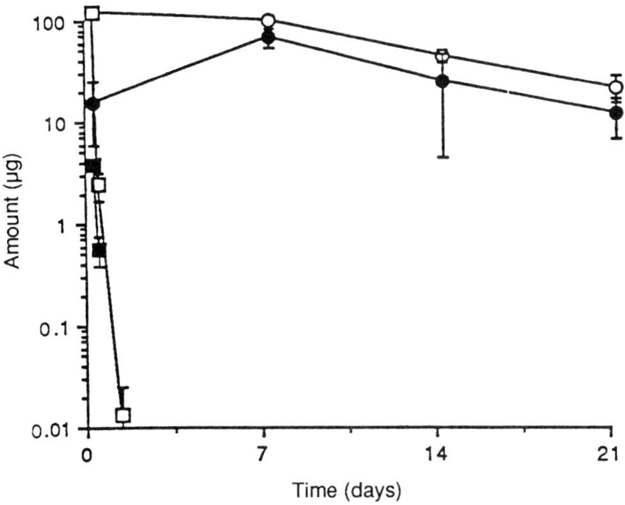

FIG. 6 The amounts of methotrexate remaining within the CNS after intracisternal injection of 100 μg of methotrexate as unencapsulated drug (□) and encapsulated into DepoFoam particles (○). The amounts of methotrexate remaining within the cranial compartment after injection of unencapsulated drug (■) and Depo/MTX (●). Each point represents the mean and standard deviation from a group of three rats. (Reproduced with permission, from Ref. 6.)

Intraventricular Pharmacokinetics of DTC 101 in Humans

Informed consent is obtained from human patients with a histologically proven diagnosis of cancer and radiological or cytological evidence of neoplastic meningitis (1, 5). Human investigation in the United States must be performed with written approval of the institutional review board and the U.S. Food and Drug Administration (FDA) under an Investigational New Drug Exemption (IND).

An Ommaya reservoir is placed in the right lateral ventricle by a neurosurgeon. Therapy consists of DTC 101 suspended in a preservative-free, 0.9% NaCl solution administered intraventricularly as a single injection once every 2–3 weeks. Following DTC 101 administration and at each CSF sampling, the reservoir or spinal needle is flushed with autologous CSF.

The treatments are given until disease progression or until a maximum of seven doses has been administered. Initial work-up includes history and physical examination, including a neurological examination; complete blood count (CBC) and platelet count; CSF sample for cytology; serum chemistries; computerized tomography (CT) or magnetic resonance imaging (MRI) brain scan with and without appropriate contrast agents and [^{111}In]diethylenetriaminepentaacetic acid ([^{111}In]DTPA)– CSF flow studies. Before each cycle of chemotherapy, neurological history and examination, blood counts, and chemistries are performed, and CSF samples are obtained for cytological examination. Complete cytological response is defined as two consecutive negative CSF cytology examinations at least 1 week apart; anything less than a complete cytological response is considered as no response. Changes in parenchymal CNS lesions or lesions outside the CNS are not used as part of the response determination because these are not expected to be influenced by intra-CSF therapy.

Ventricular CSF and blood samples are obtained immediately before injection, at 1 hr, and at 1, 2, 4, 7, 14, and 21 days following injection. All CSF and blood samples are collected in tubes containing tetrahydrouridine at a final concentration of 40 μM to inhibit conversion of ara-C to uracil arabinoside (ara-U) by cytidine deaminase. The heparinized blood samples are immediately placed on ice and plasma is separated from blood cells by centrifugation. The CSF samples are centrifuged at 600 g for 5 min to separate DepoFoam particles from the free ara-C fraction. The DepoFoam pellet is lysed by vortexing sequentially in 200 μl of methanol and in distilled water. The free ara-C fractions of CSF are analyzed without further processing. The plasma is ultrafiltered (YMT membrane No. 4104; Amicon Corp.). The CSF and plasma samples are stored frozen at −20°C until analysis. The samples are analyzed on a high-performance liquid chromatography system (Waters Associates) with 254- and 280-nm UV detectors, two Pecosphere

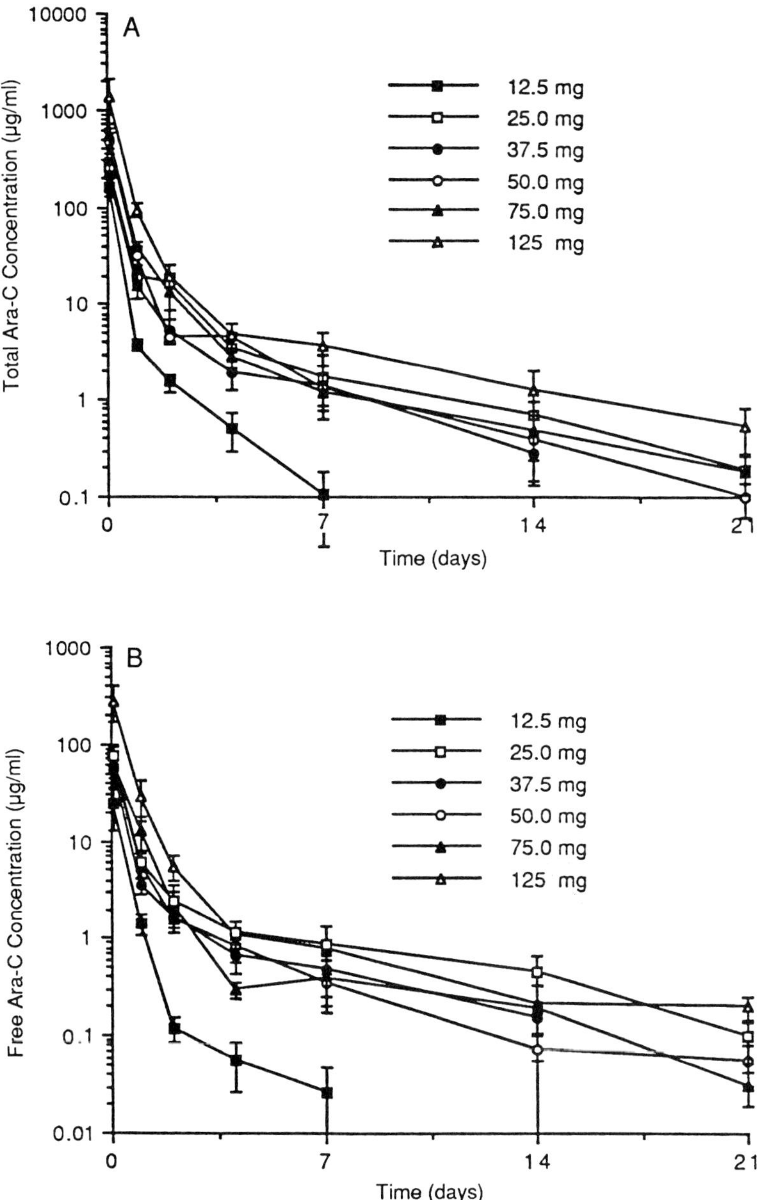

FIG. 7 Ventricular CSF pharmacokinetics of intraventricularly administered DTC 101 as a function of dose from 12.5 to 125 mg. DTC 101 was administered into the lateral ventricle and the CSF samples were obtained from the same ventricle. (A) Total ara-C concentration; (B) free ara-C concentration. Each data point is an average from at least three courses and the error bars represent standard errors of mean. (Reproduced with permission, from Ref. 1.)

C_{18} reversed-phase columns (3 × 3C cartridge; Perkin-Elmer, Norwalk, CT) in tandem, and a 6.7 m*M* potassium phosphate/3.3 m*M* phosphoric acid mixture (pH 2.8) as an isocratic mobile phase at a flow rate of 1.0 ml/min. Retention time for ara-C is 6 min and that for the major metabolite, ara-U, is 7 min. There are no interfering peaks.

Figure 7 shows the CSF pharmacokinetics of ara-C following intraventricular administrations of DTC 101 at various doses ranging from 12.5 to 125 mg, where CSF samples were obtained from the same ventricle into which DTC 101 had been injected. Following intraventricular administration of the maximum tolerated dose (75 mg), the ventricular concentration of free ara-C (ara-C that had been released from DepoFoam particles into the CSF) decreased biexponentially with an average initial (α) half-life of 9.4 ± 1.6 hr (SEM), and terminal (β) half-life of 141 ± 23 hr (SEM). This is in contrast to a terminal (β) half-life of only 3.4 hr for unencapsulated ara-C (10).

Nine of 12 patients had a positive CSF cytology immediately prior to treatment. Seven of these 9 cytologically evaluable patients cleared their CSF of malignant cells with DTC 101 treatment. Responders included one each of patients with breast cancer, non-small-cell lung cancer, melanoma, primitive neuroectodermal tumor, chronic myelogenous leukemia in blast crisis, AIDS-related non-Hodgkin's lymphoma, and multiple myeloma (1).

Summary

With the advances in basic neurosciences and growth of biotechnology, the blood–brain and blood–CSF barriers are increasingly being recognized as major stumbling blocks in CNS drug development. We have demonstrated in animal models and in human clinical trials the feasibility of using DepoFoam as a practical drug delivery system into the CNS. Following intraventricular injection in a rat model, DepoFoam encapsulation increased the half-life of ara-C more than 50-fold, from 2.7 to 148 hr. In a monkey model, the terminal half-life was increased more than 200-fold, from 0.74 to 156 hr following intralumbar administration. In humans, the terminal half-life was increased more than 40-fold, from 3.4 to 141 hr following intraventricular administration through an Ommaya reservoir. Furthermore, therapeutic intraventricular and intralumbar drug concentrations can be achieved and maintained following intralumbar administration (1), which could possibly eliminate the need for the expensive and invasive Ommaya reservoir placement. In addition to ara-C, methotrexate, morphine, and interferon α have been encapsulated and tested in animal models. DepoFoam appears to be a promising system for drug delivery of a broad range of water-stable molecules into the central nervous system.

Acknowledgments

DepoFoam, Depo/MTX, Depo/IFN, and Depo/Morphine are trademarks of DepoTech Corporation. Dr. Sinil Kim is a shareholder and an officer of DepoTech Corporation.

References

1. S. Kim, E. Chatelut, J. C. Kim, S. B. Howell, C. Cates, P. Kormanik, and M. C. Chamberlain, Extended cerebrospinal-fluid cytarabine exposure following intrathecal administration of DTC 101. *J. Clin. Oncol.* **11,** 2186–2193 (1993).
2. S. Kim and S. B. Howell, Multivesicular liposomes containing cytarabine entrapped in the presence of hydrochloric acid for intracavitary chemotherapy. *Cancer Treat. Rep.* **71,** 705–711 (1987).
3. S. Kim, D. J. Kim, M. A. Geyer, and S. B. Howell, Multivesicular liposomes containing 1-beta-D-arabinofuranosylcytosine for slow-release intrathecal therapy. *Cancer Res.* **47,** 3935–3937 (1987).
4. S. Kim, S. Scheerer, M. A. Geyer, and S. B. Howell, Multivesicular liposomes for CSF delivery of retroviral agent ddC. *J. Infect. Dis.* **162,** 750–752 (1990).
5. M. C. Chamberlain, S. Khatibi, J. C. Kim, S. B. Howell, E. Chatelut, and S. Kim, Leptomeningeal metastasis with intraventricular Depo/Ara-C; as phase I study. *Arch. Neurol. (Chicago)* **50,** 261–264 (1993).
6. E. Chatelut, T. Kim, and S. Kim, A slow-releasing methotrexate formulation for intrathecal therapy. *Cancer Chemother. Pharmacol.* **32,** 179–182 (1993).
7. T. Kim, J. Kim, and S. Kim, Extended release formulation of morphine for subcutaneous administration. *Cancer Chemother. Pharmacol.* **33,** 187–190 (1993).
8. A. Bonetti and S. Kim, Pharmacokinetics of an extended-release human interferon alpha-2b formulation. *Cancer Chemother. Pharmacol.* **33,** 258–261 (1993).
9. S. Kim, S. Khatibi, S. B. Howell, C. McCully, F. Balis, and D. G. Poplack, Prolongation of drug action in CSF by encapsulation into multivesicular liposomes. *Cancer Res.* **53,** 1596–1598 (1993).
10. S. Zimm, J. M. Collins, J. Miser, D. Chatterji, and D. G. Poplack, Cytosine arabinoside cerebrospinal fluid kinetics. *Clin. Pharmacol. Ther.* **35,** 826–830 (1984).

Section IV

Polymeric Release Systems for the Central Nervous System

[8] Interstitial Drug Delivery to the Central Nervous System Using Controlled Release Polymers: Chemotherapy for Brain Tumors

Rafael J. Tamargo, Robert Langer, and Henry Brem

Introduction

The prognosis for patients with malignant brain tumors remains poor despite numerous advances in neurosurgical operative techniques and in adjuvant chemotherapy and radiotherapy. In the United States, about 15,600 individuals develop primary brain tumors every year (1). More than half of these tumors originate from transformed glial cells and are recognized histopathologically as glioblastomas multiforme, anaplastic astrocytomas, astrocytomas, oligodendrogliomas, or mixed gliomas (2). Surgical resection of a glioblastoma multiforme, the most aggressive of the malignant gliomas, leaves patients with a predicted median survival of only 14 weeks (3). The administration of radiotherapy after surgical resection increases the median survival to 36 weeks (4). The addition of systemic chemotherapy with 1,3-bis(2-chloroethyl)-1-nitrosourea (BCNU)—the most effective chemotherapeutic agent against malignant astrocytomas (5)—to surgical resection and radiotherapy increases the median survival of patients with malignant astrocytomas to only 51 weeks, with less than a 6% chance of survival at 5 years (2, 4).

The blood–brain barrier has limited the adjuvant treatment of malignant brain tumors with chemotherapeutic agents administered systemically. This physiological and pharmacological barrier results from tight junctions between endothelial cells of the capillaries in the central nervous system (6). In general, only small, electrically neutral, lipid-soluble molecules can penetrate this capillary endothelium (7), and most chemotherapeutic agents do not fall in this category. As a result, only a few cytotoxic agents, such as the nitrosoureas, have been useful in the treatment of brain tumors. These agents have been delivered systemically in high doses to reach therapeutic levels in the central nervous system. This approach has had a modest impact on the survival of patients with malignant gliomas, but has also resulted in systemic side effects (5).

We have explored the possibility of delivering chemotherapeutic agents interstitially within the brain parenchyma using controlled release polymers. This approach has two major potential advantages. The first advantage is

Methods in Neurosciences, Volume 21

that interstitial drug delivery bypasses the blood–brain barrier. Using this approach, any drug that can be released from a polymer can be administered into the central nervous system. The second advantage is that this form of drug delivery can result in high levels of drug concentration at the site of pathology with minimal leakage of the drug into the systemic circulation. Thus, unwanted side effects of a cytotoxic agent could be minimized.

In this chapter we review the rationale and techniques that we have employed in the development of interstitial chemotherapy for brain tumors using controlled release polymers. Our criteria for selection of controlled release polymers, chemotherapeutic agents, and tumor models are discussed. We then describe the techniques for polymer fabrication, drug incorporation into the polymer, and surgical implantation of the polymers. Finally, we review the techniques and results of our pharmacokinetic, biocompatibility, toxicity, and efficacy studies. We conclude this chapter by describing the results of our ongoing clinical trials of interstitial chemotherapy for malignant gliomas and by commenting on the wide applications of this approach for the treatment of pathology of the central nervous system.

Methods

Selection of Controlled Release Polymer

A wide variety of synthetic polymers capable of controlled release of drugs is currently available (8). Only a few, however, are inert or minimally inflammatory, nontoxic, and capable of releasing drugs with both high and low molecular weights. Controlled release polymers can be broadly categorized as diffusion-regulated or degradation-regulated devices. The diffusion-regulated polymers are typically nonbiodegradable. A drug incorporated into this type of polymer is released by diffusion from the polymeric matrix. The degradation-regulated polymers are usually biodegradable and disintegrate gradually in the presence of a solvent such as water. A drug incorporated into a biodegradable polymer is released as the polymeric matrix degrades. For our experiments, we selected ethylene–vinyl acetate copolymer (EVAc), a diffusion-regulated polymer, and poly[bis(*p*-carboxyphenoxy)]propane–sebacic acid copolymer (PCPP–SA), a degradation-regulated polymer. Both the diffusion-regulated and degradation-regulated polymers have advantages and disadvantages.

The advantages of a diffusion-regulated polymer such as EVAc are that it is inert and that its release kinetics are highly reproducible (9–11). Because drug release is dependent on diffusion alone, the release kinetics are dependent on a limited number of variables such as the physicochemical properties of the drug (e.g., particle size and lipid solubility), the polymeric composition of the matrix, and the size and shape of the polymer. A disadvantage of EVAc is that it does not degrade and is therefore a permanent implant.

The major advantages of a degradation-regulated polymer such as PCPP–SA are that it is biodegradable and that, in the case of PCPP–SA, the degradation rate of the matrix—and therefore the release rate of the drug—can be modified by changing the proportions of the two monomers (12). The anhydrous polymer protects the drug from hydrolysis and enzymatic destruction until it is released. Studies show that the degradation of PCPP–SA initially occurs slightly more slowly *in vivo* than *in vitro*. The presence of a tumor or BCNU does not affect the degradation rate of the polymer (13).

There are, however, some disadvantages of this type of polymer. Although the release kinetics of a polymer such as PCPP–SA should theoretically be a function of only the degradation rate of the matrix, when water-soluble drugs are incorporated into the polymer matrix at loadings greater than 10%, then its release kinetics are a result of both drug diffusion and matrix degradation. This may result in complex release kinetics that may be difficult to modify. Another disadvantage is that the degradation of PCPP–SA evokes a mild inflammatory response in the surrounding tissues (14).

When we initiate a controlled release project, we generally prefer to start with a diffusion-regulated polymer such as EVAc. Once we understand the release kinetics and efficacy of the drug as it is released from EVAc, and if the ultimate clinical applications of the drug may be facilitated with the use of a biodegradable implant, then we develop the pharmacokinetics, biocompatibility, and efficacy studies with the degradation-regulated polymer. In some cases, however, there are no theoretical or practical considerations that require a shift to a biodegradable polymer.

Selection of Chemotherapeutic Agent

In theory, any drug is a potential candidate for delivery with controlled release polymers. In practice, however, one must evaluate each drug individually and either confirm or reject one's predictions by careful pharmacokinetics studies, because the release rate of the drug may not fulfill the physiological parameters required for the drug to be effective.

Drugs that require metabolic activation may not be candidates for local, controlled release therapy. For instance, cyclophosphamide, an alkylating agent widely used in oncology, has poor cytotoxic and mutagenic activity.

Once cyclophosphamide is administered systemically and is processed by the cytochrome *P*-450 oxidase system of the liver, it is metabolized into 4-hydroxycyclophosphamide (4-HC) and aldophosphamide, both of which are highly cytotoxic agents. Therefore, intracranial implantation of the polymer loaded with cyclophosphamide would result in minimal, if any, cytotoxic activity against a brain tumor. By contrast, interstitial delivery of 4-HC would be effective.

Another major consideration in selecting a drug for controlled release is its affinity for aqueous or lipid media. Hydrophilic drugs generally have rapid release rates and hydrophobic drugs tend to have slow release rates. This physicochemical property of a drug is expressed as its partition coefficient between octanol and water; hydrophilic compounds have low partition coefficients and hydrophobic (or lipophilic) compounds have high partition coefficients (6, 15). If one wishes to release a drug over a long period of time, such as years, one should select a hydrophobic drug with a high partition coefficient. By contrast, if one desires to release a drug in a burst that lasts only a few hours or days, it would be better to choose a hydrophilic drug with a low partition coefficient.

Before initiating a controlled release project, one must have evidence that a drug is biologically active. In neurooncology, this means that a drug is cytotoxic against tumor cells, as evidenced by *in vitro* assays in which neoplastic cells are exposed to the drug, or by *in vivo* assays in which a tumor growing outside of the central nervous system responds to systemic administration of the drug. In addition, one should have evidence that the drug is selective in its cytotoxicity and that it will spare the normal cells in the region of a tumor.

The best candidates for controlled release therapy against brain tumors are drugs that do not cross the blood-brain barrier, have significant systemic toxicity, and are selectively cytotoxic against neoplastic cells. Nevertheless, cytotoxic drugs that do cross the blood–brain barrier and have minimal systemic toxicity could be considered for intracranial controlled release therapy because this form of drug delivery can achieve high drug levels in the region of the tumor without the difficulties associated with systemic chemotherapy.

Biological response modifiers, many of which are large proteins that do not cross the blood–brain barrier (16), can be incorporated into polymers and released intracranially. Both diffusion-regulated and degradation-regulated polymers are capable of controlled release of macromolecules such as immunoglobulins.

We chose BCNU for our initial experiments because of its known activity against both experimental and human malignant gliomas and the extensive pharmacological experience with this drug.

Selection of Tumor Model

A comprehensive discussion of animal tumor models in neurooncology is beyond the scope of this chapter. The basic principles, however, are described below.

An animal tumor model, as the term implies, never replicates perfectly the biological behavior of the human tumor that it resembles. Tumors that grow in tissue culture or in laboratory animals have undergone a screening process that, ultimately, may select for nothing more than the ability of the tumor to divide under laboratory conditions. During this process, even tumors that are subcultured from human neoplasms may lose the biological features of the parent tumor and be no closer to the tumor of origin than any other tumor.

We chose to use only cell lines derived from glial tissue, because we are interested in malignant gliomas. We then had to decide between human or animal tumor lines and between a syngeneic or heterogeneic animal host for the tumor. After several passages, most human cell lines drift away from their tumors of origin and lose many of the biological features that made them relevant initially. For instance, in one study, as many as 70% of the human glioma-derived cell lines studied were unable to generate tumors when injected into athymic nude mice (17). We also felt that, for the purposes of our studies, a syngeneic host would be preferable. Heterogeneic tumor transplants require immunocompromised hosts, such as nude mice or rats, which are delicate and expensive. We therefore selected the 9L gliosarcoma, a brain tumor syngeneic to Fischer 344 rats and originally induced in these animals by weekly injections of *N*-nitrosomethylurea (18–21). This tumor is well characterized and grows vigorously both in tissue culture and in Fischer 344 rats. The C6 glioma, a similar tumor also induced in rats by *N*-nitrosomethylurea injections, was induced in "randomly bred Wistar rats," which seem to be genetically different from the modern, commercially available Wistar rats (18, 22). In our laboratory, the C6 glioma does not survive more than two or three passages in Wistar rats.

We obtained the 9L gliosarcoma in 1985 from M. Barker (Brain Tumor Research Center, University of California, San Francisco, CA). The cells are grown in minimum essential medium (Eagle's) with 10% (v/v) fetal bovine serum, L-glutamine (398 μg/ml), penicillin (base) (80.5 U/ml), and streptomycin (80.5 μg/ml) (all products from GIBCO Laboratories, Grand Island, NY) in a humidified atmosphere of 5% CO_2 at 37°C. The cells are grown to confluence, changing the medium every 2–3 days, detached with trypsin [0.25% (v/v) in Hanks' balanced salt solution without calcium and magnesium] (GIBCO Laboratories), and resuspended in medium. A solid tumor can be established by injecting the cell suspension in the flanks of Fischer

344 male rats (Harlan Sprague-Dawley, Inc., Indianapolis, IN). In our laboratory, the cell line has been propagated for a limited number of passages as a solid tumor in the flank. To transfer the tumor, the flank of the carrier is shaved and prepared with 70% ethyl alcohol and povidone–iodine solution. Under sterile conditions, the tumor is excised, minced into pieces of approximately 0.5 cm^3, and dissociated into smaller fragments by pressing it through a 40 mesh (380-μm) screen in a Cellector tissue sieve (Bellco Glass, Inc., Vineland, NJ). The tumor homogenate is then suspended in Hanks' balanced salt solution without calcium or magnesium. The flank of the recipient is similarly prepared for the injection of the tumor homogenate. The tumors must be transferred approximately every 2 weeks. The tumor samples used in our experiments had undergone about 10 passages at the time of implantation into the experimental animals.

Polymer Fabrication and Drug Incorporation

The ethylene–vinyl acetate copolymer (EVAc) [40% vinyl acetate by weight; Elvax 40P] was obtained from the Du Pont Company (Wilmington, DE). Before proceeding with drug incorporation, EVAc must be washed in absolute ethyl alcohol to extract its inflammatory impurities, mainly the antioxidant butylhydroxytoluene (BHT). The polymer beads are poured into a glass beaker with ethyl alcohol [1 : 10 (w/v) EVAc to ethyl alcohol] and stirred continuously, with total ethyl alcohol volume changes every 24–48 hr. The presence of BHT in the wash is monitored spectrophotometrically at 230 nm and the washes continued until the absorbance falls below 0.03 units. This typically takes 30–50 days. The polymers are then dried in a vacuum desiccator over 4–5 days. We prefer this technique over the acetone wash because a significant amount of polymer is lost during the acetone wash. The acetone wash procedure, however, has the advantage of being faster.

1,3-Bis(2-chloroethyl)-1-nitrosourea was obtained from the Drug Synthesis and Chemistry Branch, Division of Cancer Treatment (National Cancer Institute, but it is also commercially available. To make BCNU–EVAc polymers, BCNU and EVAc are dissolved in methylene chloride [1 : 9 (w/v), EVAc to methylene chloride] in a 3 : 7 BCNU-to-EVAc ratio. This solution yields dry polymers 30% loaded (w/w) with BCNU. The solution is then poured into cylindrical glass molds at −70°C. The resulting polymer cylinders are transferred to glass plates at −30°C and allowed to dry for about 7 days. The 30% BCNU–EVAc cylinders are then cut into disks for implantation in the rats either subcutaneously or intracranially. Empty EVAc cylinders can be fabricated using the same procedure as described above. All the disks are exposed to ultraviolet irradiation for 1–2 hr prior to implantation.

A copolymer of bis(*p*-carboxyphenoxy)propane (PCPP) and sebacic acid (SA), poly[bis(*p*-carboxyphenoxy)propane–sebacic acid] copolymer (PCPP–SA), is synthesized by melt polycondensation and formulated into disks by compression molding as previously described (12). The prepolymers are obtained by mixing the two monomers in a 1 : 4 (or "20 : 80") (PCPP : SA) ratio with acetic anhydride. A polymer made entirely of PCPP degrades slowly over a period of years. By contrast, a polymer made entirely of sebacic acid degrades rapidly over a few days. By mixing the monomers in different ratios, one can adjust the rate of degradation of the copolymer. The 20 : 80 PCPP–SA copolymer degrades over 5 weeks (14). After copolymerization, PCPP–SA is available as a powder that is mixed with BCNU in a 3 : 7 (BCNU : PCPP–SA) ratio. The resulting mixture is then homogenized by dissolving it in methylene chloride. This solution (both PCPP–SA and BCNU are soluble in methylene chloride) is poured on a plate at room temperature and placed in a vacuum desiccator overnight. The dry polymer–drug mixture is then scraped from the plate, sieved through a 90- to 150-μm mesh to obtain a uniform particle size,and loaded into a cylindrical mold and compressed. A typical PCPP–SA disk used for the efficacy experiments measures 3 mm in diameter and weighs about 10–15 mg. The polymers are then kept at −35°C until the day of implantation and sterilized by exposure to UV light for about 1 hr.

Pharmacokinetic Studies

The release rates of the polymers can then be determined *in vitro*. The EVAc and PCPP–SA polymers loaded with BCNU are placed in 3 ml of 0.2 *M* sodium phosphate buffer (pH 7.4) and incubated at 37°C. The polymers are then sequentially transferred into new vials with phosphate buffer. The amount of BCNU released into the solution is then assayed by scanning the buffer solution either spectrophotometrically (23) or chromatographically (24).

Once the release profile of the drug is evaluated *in vitro,* one can proceed to more complicated *in vivo* studies in which the polymers are implanted in animals and their tissues and blood samples are harvested for spectrophotometric, chromatographic, or autoradiographic determinations of drug concentrations (23–25). Intracranial implantation in rats of EVAc polymers 30% loaded with BCNU results in delivery of the total dose in approximately 9 days (23).

Biocompatibility and Toxicity Studies

As determined by the rabbit cornea assay—one of the most sensitive biocompatibility assays available (26)—EVAc is inert, and causes minimal, if any, inflammation in the surrounding tissues (9, 11). The neural biocompatibility of PCPP–SA (20 : 80) was evaluated in the brains of rats (14) and monkeys (27). In the rat experiments, PCPP–SA, oxidized regenerated cellulose (Surgicel), or absorbable gelatin sponge (Gelfoam) was implanted in the frontal cortices of 56 animals. Surgicel and Gelfoam are hemostatic agents routinely used in neurosurgical procedures and placed in contact with neural tissues. PCPP–SA was found to be slightly more inflammatory than Gelfoam, but less so than Surgicel. The PCPP–SA implants degraded completely over 5 weeks (14). In the monkey experiments, PCPP–SA polymers were implanted in the frontal cortex of each animal. Histologically, subacute inflammatory response was observed 16 days after implantation and a mild chronic inflammatory response was seen 72 days after implantation (27).

The local and systemic toxicity associated with the controlled release of BCNU in the brain was similarly tested in rats (28) and monkeys (27). In the rat experiments, EVAc polymers containing 30% BCNU by weight were implanted in the brains of one group of rats. The same total BCNU dose contained in the intracranial polymer (14 mg/kg) was administered intraperitoneally to another group of rats. The mean survival of the intracranial group was 92.7 days and that of the intraperitoneal group was 63.3 days (28). A lower BCNU dose of 3 mg/kg was used in the monkey experiments. Eight monkeys underwent intracranial implantation of PCPP–SA polymers containing 1.9% BCNU by weight. Of these eight monkeys, three underwent radiation therapy as well. The animals were evaluated with serial computerized tomography (CT) and magnetic resonance imaging (MRI) as well as with full autopsies 16 and 72 days after implantation. No neurological or systemic toxicity was seen in any of the animals (27).

Efficacy Studies

Once the biocompatibility, toxicity, and release kinetics of the polymers containing BCNU were elucidated, we proceeded to an efficacy study to evaluate the effect of the controlled release of BCNU in 9L gliosarcomas growing in the flanks of rats. After demonstrating an effect on tumor growth in the flank, we proceeded to studies evaluating the effect of interstitial release of BCNU in 9L gliosarcomas growing in the brains of Fischer 344 rats.

Fischer 344 male rats weighing about 200–250 g were anesthetized with an intraperitoneal injection of a 2- to 4-ml/kg stock solution containing ketamine hydrochloride (25 mg/ml), xylazine (2.5 mg/ml), and 14.25% ethyl alcohol in normal saline.

For the subcutaneous tumor growth experiments, the flanks of 90 rats were shaved and prepared in sterile fashion. The tumor was induced by the subcutaneous injection of 0.1 ml of 9L gliosarcoma homogenate. Tumor growth was documented twice weekly by measuring the length and width of the tumors with dial calipers and a tumor volume was calculated from these measurements. The treatment with BCNU was initiated when the tumors reached a volume of about 600 mm^3. For this purpose, the animals were anesthetized, both flanks were shaved and prepared in sterile fashion, and small incisions were made above the tumor on the left flank and on a similar location on the contralateral flank. To evaluate the controlled delivery of BCNU, 30% BCNU–EVAc disks were implanted either adjacent to the tumor or in the contralateral flank. Empty EVAc disks were used as controls. To evaluate the systemic delivery of the same dose of BCNU, an intraperitoneal injection of 0.1 ml of an ethyl alcohol–normal saline solution (1 : 1, v/v) containing BCNU (30 mg/ml) was administered to one group (28).

For the intracranial tumor growth and survival experiments, 9L gliosarcoma fragments measuring approximately $2 \times 2 \times 1$ mm^3 were excised at the time of implantation and, using microsurgical technique, a midline incision was made on the posterior aspect of the head and the periosteum swept laterally to expose the sagittal, coronal, and lambdoidal sutures. A 3-mm burr hole was made over the left parietal region with its center 5–6 mm behind the coronal suture and 3–4 mm lateral to the sagittal suture. The dura was opened and the underlying cortex was aspirated until the vascular junction between the posterior thalamus and the anterior superior colliculus was exposed. Cortical bleeding was controlled by cauterization with a silver nitrate applicator. The tumor fragment was transferred into the cortical defect over the brainstem and the wound was irrigated copiously before closing the skin with surgical clips. The rats in the control groups underwent the same intracranial procedure but did not receive tumor implants.

On the fourth day after tumor implantation, the rats were randomized to one of eight experimental groups for initiation of treatment and implantation of the polymeric disks. The wound was reopened and the polymer disks were inserted through the craniotomy defect into the cerebral cortex. An intraperitoneal injection of 0.2 ml of an ethyl alcohol–normal saline (1 : 1, v/v) solution containing BCNU was administered to two groups and the same volume of the vehicle was administered to the six other groups.

The rats were examined twice daily, giving particular attention to behavioral changes manifested by decreased alertness, passivity, impaired grooming and unkempt appearance, restlessness, irritability, or fearfulness, and to neurological deficits as manifested by focal motor deficits or gait disturbances. In this model, 12–24 hr prior to death from the intracranial tumor, the animals become lethargic, passive, develop scruffy coats, develop lacrimal debris around the eyes, manifest an ataxic gait, or, in the advanced stages, display extensor posturing of the hind legs. The animals were sacrificed when at least four of these six signs appeared and a full autopsy was conducted to determine the cause of neurological deterioration. The brain, lungs, liver, stomach–duodenum, and kidneys were placed in buffered formalin for 10–14 days, embedded in paraffin, sectioned with a microtome, and stained with hematoxylin and eosin for histological examination.

Results

Both EVAc and PCPP–SA are biocompatible polymers. The biocompatibility of EVAc has been well established since the early 1970s and repeatedly confirmed in numerous laboratories, including our own (9, 11, 24, 29). Indeed, in our opinion, EVAc biocompatibility is the standard against which new polymers should be measured. We have found that PCPP–SA is also biocompatible, although its degradation evokes a mild, benign inflammatory response in the surrounding tissues (14). In the case of tumor therapy, this inflammatory response is innocuous and may even be advantageous. Cer-

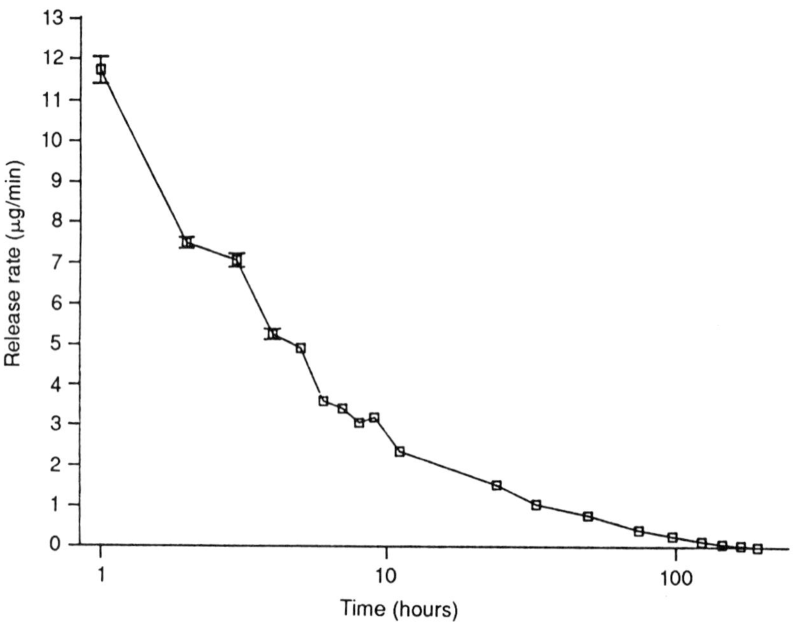

FIG. 1 Release rates of BCNU from EVAc into phosphate buffer over a period of 195 hr. The time scale is logarithmic (five polymers; bars, SEM).

tainly no adverse effects were demonstrated in rats, rabbits, monkeys, or humans that underwent intracranial implantation of this polymer (14, 27, 30, 31).

Both EVAc and PCPP–SA release BCNU in a controlled fashion, protecting the drug from degradation until the time it is released. The *in vitro* pharmacokinetics studies of EVAc loaded with BCNU showed that active drug was released over the course of 195 hr (Fig. 1). When BCNU–EVAc polymers were implanted in the brain of rats, BCNU was detected in high concentrations in the hemisphere where the polymer was implanted, yet a minimal amount of drug was detected in the contralateral hemisphere and in the sytemic circulation during the first 24 hr of the study (Fig. 2) (23). The BCNU concentration achieved with this delivery mode is 17 times higher than can be obtained when the same amount of drug is delivered systemically (23). We considered this controlled release profile of several days (as opposed to weeks or months) optimal for BCNU, given that previous work had demonstrated that the administration of a single dose of BCNU was preferable to multiple doses (32, 33).

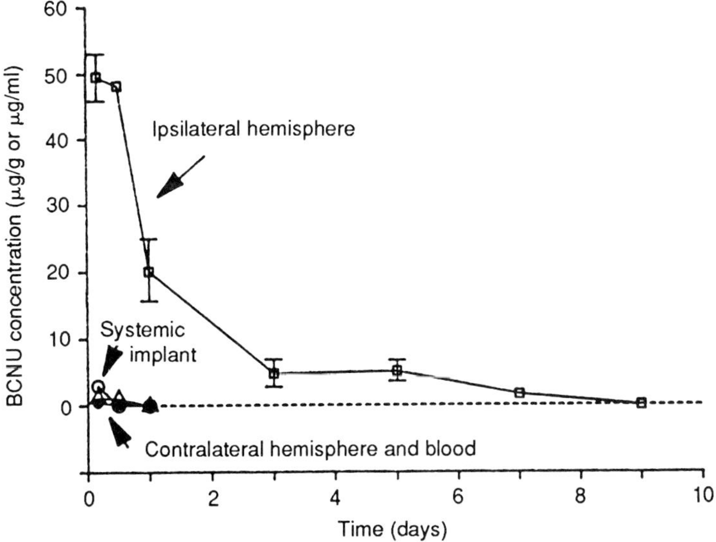

FIG. 2 BCNU concentration in the ipsilateral hemisphere (□), contralateral hemisphere (△), and blood (●) of rats receiving 15-mg BCNU–EVAc implants intracerebrally (ic). In a separate experiment, the BCNU concentration was measured in the left hemisphere (○) of rats receiving 15-mg BCNU–EVAc implants intraperitoneally (ip). Similar or lower concentrations were measured in the right hemisphere and blood. The results were normalized for animal weight (225 g) and polymer weight (15 mg) (three rats; bars, SEM).

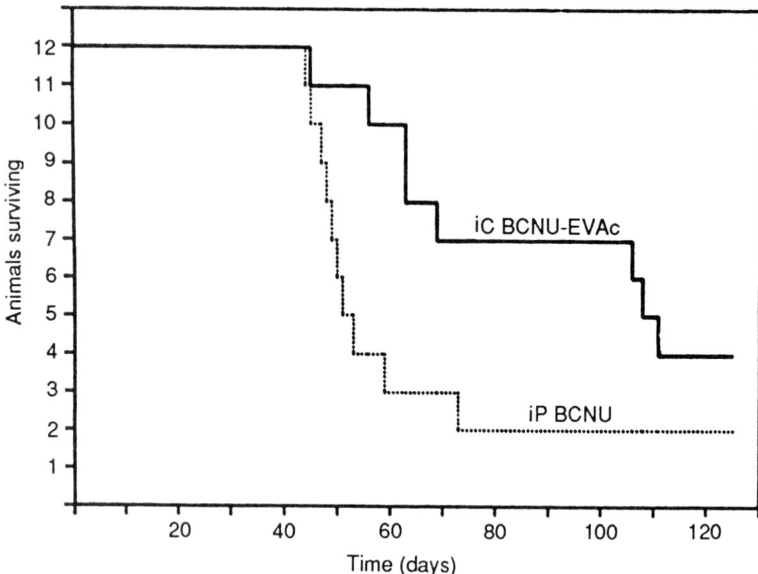

FIG. 3 Survival curves of the groups exposed to BCNU systemically (ip BCNU) or interstitially (ic BCNU–EVAc).

The interstitial, controlled release of BCNU in the brain is associated with toxicity that is significant at BCNU levels of 14 mg/kg in rats and negligible at levels of 3 mg/kg in monkeys (27, 28). Even in rats, where an interstitial, polymer-delivered dose of 14 mg of BCNU per kilogram resulted in a mean survival of 92.7 days, the systemic administration of the same BCNU dose intraperitoneally was associated with a higher toxicity manifested by a mean survival of only 63.3 days (Fig. 3) (28). In the monkey experiments, no significant toxicity was associated with the interstitial, intracranial polymer delivery of BCNU (3 mg/kg) (27).

In rats, the intracranial, controlled release of BCNU to treat the 9L gliosarcoma resulted in a significant 5.4- to 7.3-fold increase in survival, whereas the sytemic administration of the same dose of BCNU resulted in a 2.4-fold increased survival (Table I and Fig. 4) (28). Although no long-term cures were obtained in the group treated with BCNU systemically, 17 and 42% long-term cures were seen in the groups treated with BCNU interstitially using PCPP–SA and EVAc polymers, respectively (Table I and Fig. 4) (28). Therefore, the intracranial, interstitial delivery of BCNU using controlled release polymers appears more efficacious and less toxic than the systemic administration of the same dose of this drug.

We would like to emphasize the importance of proceeding in a systematic fashion from pharmacokinetic release studies, to toxicity studies, and finally

TABLE I Survival Values of Rats Treated Systemically with BCNU[a]

Group label	9L[b] glioma	Intracranial polymer implant	Intraperitoneal injection	Survival (days)
9L/EVAc	Yes	Empty EVAc	Vehicle	10.9 ± 0.8
9L/PCPP:SA	Yes	Empty PCPP–SA	Vehicle	11.6 ± 0.7
9L/BCNU (ip)	Yes	Empty EVAc	BCNU	27.3 ± 3.1
9L/BCNU–EVAc	Yes	BCNU in EVAc	Vehicle	80.0 ± 11.6
9L/BCNU–PCPP:SA	Yes	BCNU in PCPP–SA	Vehicle	62.3 ± 9.9
Control	No	Empty EVAc	Vehicle	(125)
BCNU (ip)	No	Empty EVAc	BCNU	63.3 ± 8.0
BCNU (ic)	No	BCNU in EVAc	Vehicle	92.7 ± 8.9

[a] Each group had 12 rats. Survival values are presented as mean ± SEM. Two rats that died perioperatively (one from an intracranial hemorrhage and the other from an intracranial abscess) were excluded from the study.

[b] 9L, ic implantation of the 9L gliosarcoma at first operation; empty EVAc, ic implantation at second operation of an 11.5-mg EVAc disk; vehicle, ip injection at second operation of 0.1 ml of ethyl alcohol and 0.1 ml of normal saline; empty PCPP–SA, ic implantation at second operation of an 11.5-mg PCPP–SA disk; BCNU, ip injection at second operation of 3.5 mg of BCNU in 0.1 ml of ethyl alcohol and 0.1 ml of normal saline; BCNU in EVAc, ic implantation at second operation of an 11.5-mg EVAc disk containing 3.5 mg of BCNU (30% loading of BCNU); BCNU in PCPP–SA, ic implantation at second operation of an 11.5-mg PCPP–SA disk containing 3.5 mg of BCNU.

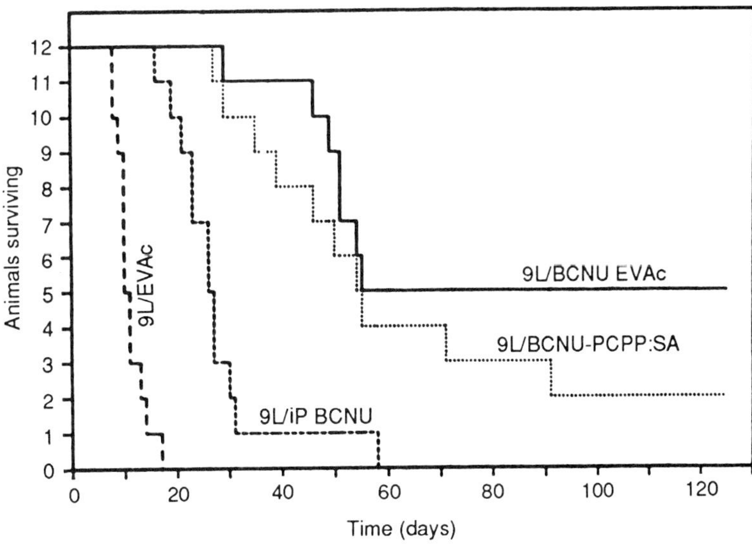

FIG. 4 Survival curves of the groups bearing ic tumors treated with either systemic (9L/ip BCNU) or interstitial ic (9L/BCNU–EVAc and 9L/BCNU–PCPP:SA) BCNU.

to efficacy experiments when investigating a drug as a candidate for interstitial, controlled release. It is discouraging to initiate a costly and time-consuming efficacy study only to have it fail either because the drug is released from the polymer too rapidly or too slowly, or because the interstitial delivery of the drug results in immediate or delayed animal toxicity. This toxicity may preclude the evaluation of the effect of the drug on tumor growth and animal survival.

Although we have described the applications of the interstitial, controlled release of a chemotherapeutic agent for the treatment of brain tumors, this approach can be easily generalized and applied to a wide range of drugs to treat local and even systemic pathology of most organ systems. The studies described here have led to a phase I–II and a phase III multiinstitutional clinical trial for the treatment of patients with malignant astrocytomas with PCPP–SA polymers containing BCNU. In the phase I–II study, 21 patients with recurrent malignant astrocytomas were treated by implanting polymers at the time of surgery. No adverse effects associated with this treatment were identified in serial examinations, blood tests, or radiological studies (31). The phase III study involving 222 patients treated in 27 medical institutions further demonstrated the safety of this approach as well as a significant prolonged survival in the treatment group.

Conclusions

Controlled release polymers could be used to treat a wide range of disorders in the central nervous system. For instance, steroids could be released interstitially to control edema (24) and adrenergic/cholinergic agents could be delivered with polymers to treat movement disorders such as Parkinson's disease and Huntington's chorea (34, 35). We are currently investigating the controlled release of anticonvulsants for epilepsy (36) and the controlled release of vasodilators for posthemorrhagic vasospasm. Another promising area is that of the controlled release of biological response modifiers, such as angiogenesis inhibitors (24, 29), for the treatment of tumors. In summary, there are many potential uses for controlled release technology in the central nervous system and we anticipate many exciting developments in this field in the coming years.

References

1. B. E. Henderson, R. K. Moss, and M. C. Pike, *Science* **254,** 1131 (1991).
2. M. E. Berens, J. T. Rutka, and M. L. Rosenblum, *Neurosurg. Clin. North Am.* **1,** 1 (1990).

3. M. D. Walker, E. Alexander, Jr., W. E. Hunt *et al., J. Neurosurg.* **49,** 333 (1978).
4. M. D. Walker, S. B. Green, D. P. Byar *et al., N. Engl. J. Med.* **303,** 1323 (1980).
5. P. L. Kornblith and M. D. Walker, *J. Neurosurg.* **68,** 1 (1988).
6. R. J. Tamargo and H. Brem, *Neurosurg. Q.* **2,** 259 (1992).
7. D. P. Rall and C. G. Zubrod, *Annu. Rev. Pharmacol.* **2,** 109 (1962).
8. R. Langer, *Science* **249,** 1527 (1990).
9. R. Langer and J. Folkman, *Nature (London)* **263,** 797 (1976).
10. W. D. Rhine, D. S. T. Hsieh, and R. Langer, *J. Pharm. Sci.* **69,** 265 (1980).
11. R. Langer, H. Brem, and D. Tapper, *J. Biomed. Mater. Res.* **15,** 267 (1981).
12. K. W. Leong, B. C. Brott, and R. Langer, *J. Biomed. Mater. Res.* **19,** 941 (1985).
13. M. P. Wu, J. A. Tamada, H. Brem, and R. Langer, *J. Biomed. Mater. Res.* (in press) (1994).
14. R. J. Tamargo, J. I. Epstein, C. S. Reinhard *et al., J. Biomed. Mater. Res.* **23,** 253 (1989).
15. A. Leo, C. Hansch, and D. Elkins, *Chem. Rev.* **71,** 525 (1971).
16. M. J. Hawkins, D. F. Hoth, and R. E. Wittes, *Semin. Oncol.* **13,** 132 (1986).
17. D. E. Bullard, S. C. Schold, S. H. Bigner, and D. D. Bigner, *J. Neuropathol. Exp. Neurol.* **40,** 410 (1981).
18. P. Benda, K. Someda, J. Messer, and W. H. Sweet, *J. Neurosurg.* **34,** 310 (1971).
19. H. H. Schmidek, S. L. Nielsen, A. Schiller, and J. Messer, *J. Neurosurg.* **34,** 335 (1971).
20. M. Barker, T. Hoshino, O. Gurcay *et al., Cancer Res.* **33,** 976 (1973).
21. M. Barker, T. Hoshino, K. T. Wheeler, and C. B. Wilson, *JNCI, J. Natl. Cancer Inst.* **54,** 851 (1975).
22. P. Benda, J. Lightbody, G. Sato, *et al., Science* **161,** 370 (1968).
23. M. B. Yang, R. J. Tamargo, and H. Brem, *Cancer Res.* **49,** 5103 (1989).
24. R. J. Tamargo, A. K. Sills, Jr., C. S. Reinhard, *et al., J. Neurosurg.* **74,** 956 (1991).
25. S. A. Grossman, C. Reinhard, O. M. Colvin, *et al., J. Neurosurg.* **76,** 640 (1992).
26. M. A. Gimbrone, R. S. Cotran, S. Leapman, and J. Folkman, *J. Natl. Cancer Inst. (U.S.)* **52,** 413 (1974).
27. H. Brem, R. J. Tamargo, A. Olivi, *et al., J. Neurosurg.* **80,** 283 (1994).
28. R. J. Tamargo, J. S. Myseros, J. I. Epstein, *et al., Cancer Res.* **53,** 329 (1993).
29. R. J. Tamargo, K. W. Leong, and H. Brem, *J. Neuro-Oncol.* **9,** 131 (1990).
30. H. Brem, A. Kader, J. I. Epstein, *et al. Sel. Cancer Ther.* **5,** 55 (1989).
31. H. Brem, M. S. Mahaley, Jr., N. A. Vick, *et al., J. Neurosurg.* **74,** 441 (1991).
32. M. L. Rosenblum, D. A. Dougherty, and C. B. Wilson, *Br. J. Cancer* **41,** Suppl. 4, 253 (1980).
33. M. L. Rosenblum, M. A. Gerosa, D. V. Dougherty, and C. B. Wilson, *J. Neurosurg.* **58,** 177 (1983).
34. M. J. During, B. A. Freese, B. A. Sabel, *et al., Ann. Neurol.* **25,** 351 (1989).
35. M. A. Howard, A. Gross, M. S. Grady, *et al., J. Neurosurg.* **71,** 105 (1989).
36. R. J. Tamargo, L. A. Rossell, B. M. Tyler, and J. J. Aryanpur, *J. Neurosurg.* **80,** 372 (1994).

[9] Sustained Intracerebral Delivery of Nerve Growth Factor with Biodegradable Polymer Microspheres

Alejandro Mendez, Paul J. Camarata, Raj Suryanarayanan, and Timothy J. Ebner

Introduction

The potential application of nerve growth factor (NGF) and other nervous system trophic factors in the therapy of neurological diseases is a growing area of interest (1). Prolonged administration of NGF has been demonstrated to have a therapeutic action in several models of degenerative neurological diseases, including Alzheimer's disease (AD), and in augmenting the survival of adrenal medullary grafts in Parkinson's disease (PD). Given the accelerating rate of discovery of new neural growth factors, many with highly specific and powerful actions (2), the therapeutic attractiveness of these agents will undoubtedly grow.

Penetration of the blood–brain barrier by these protein growth factors is limited in their naturally occurring state (3). To increase intracerebral distribution, local drug delivery strategies have been developed, including local infusion with mechanical (4) and osmotic pumps (5) and local synthesis and delivery by genetically modified cells (6) and NGF-producing tumor cells (7). Another approach has been the use of biocompatible, biodegradable polymers (8). In this chapter we describe the methodology for encapsulation of NGF in poly(L-lactide)coglycolide microspheres, using a modified triple-phase solvent evaporation technique (9). The *in vitro* and *in vivo* evaluation of NGF release from this polymer is described and the effects of NGF delivered from polymer microspheres on the functional outcome of adrenal medullary grafts in parkinsonian rodents is analyzed.

Biology of Nerve Growth Factor

Described by Levi-Montalcini in 1954 (for review see Ref. 10), NGF is the best characterized member of an expanding family of polypeptide neurotrophic factors (1). Initially NGF was recognized for its key role in the embryonic and early postnatal survival and differentiation of peripheral

Methods in Neurosciences, Volume 21

sympathetic neurons and mediodorsal sensory neurons of dorsal root ganglia (10). However, the actions of NGF are not limited to the developing neural tissue. Nerve growth factor and NGF receptors have a widespread distribution, including central and peripheral nervous systems and nonneuronal tissue (11). It is now clear that this neurotrophic factor also plays a key role in the regeneration of postnatal nervous tissue and in the maintenance of the differentiated phenotype of mature neurons. In the central nervous system, NGF is important in the embryonic development of the septohippocampal cholinergic projection, basal forebrain, nucleus basalis, olfactory bulb, posterior pituitary gland and cerebellum (11, 12). In the adult central nervous system, it maintains a neurotrophic effect on cholinergic neurons, with the highest levels found in the cortex and hippocampus, targets of the cholinergic basal forebrain system (12, 13). In the adult peripheral nervous system, NGF plays an important role in the regeneration of peripheral nerves (14). With this widespread distribution and numerous trophic actions, NGF could have considerable therapeutic uses.

Potential Clinical Uses of Nerve Growth Factor

Of the potential clinical uses of NGF and other trophic factors, one particularly promising area is its use in Alzheimer's disease. The intraventricular infusion of NGF prevents the degeneration of cholinergic septal neurons in the fimbria–fornix transection rodent and primate models of AD (15). This beneficial effect occurs even with delayed infusion of NGF following the lesion (16). In the aged rat NGF modifies the morphology of frontal cortex pyramidal cells (17), partially reverses the atrophy of cholinergic cell bodies, and improves spatial memory retention (18). The first human AD patient receiving intraventricular infusion of NGF showed a persistent increase in positron emission tomography (PET)-measured cortical blood flow, a decrease in electroencephalogram (EEG) slow wave activity, and improvement in verbal episodic memory. Other possible therapeutic uses include NGF neuroprotective action in noncholinergic neurons, including neurons of the visual cortex and lateral geniculate nucleus after monocular deprivation (20), CA1 hippocampal neurons after global ischemia (21), and striatal and hippocampal neurons after intracerebral injection of neurotoxic levels of glutamate agonists and other excitatory amino acids (22). Similarly, NGF facilitates peripheral nerve regeneration (19) and prevents peripheral toxic neuropathy (23). The observations that NGF receptors are sometimes found on neuronal tumors and that NGF can stimulate neoplastic cells to differentiate suggest a role in tumor therapy (24).

Nerve Growth Factor Augmentation of Adrenal Medullary Grafts in Parkinson's Disease

One of the intriguing possibilities for NGF therapy is to improve the outcome of neural grafts for Parkinson's disease. Initial experimental results using adrenal medullary grafts in the 6-hydroxydopamine (6-OHDA) rat model of PD documented an amelioration of the behavioral deficit and an increase in dopamine levels at the graft site (25). These experimental studies prompted trials of adrenal medullary grafts in human parkinsonism. However, graft survival was poor, with less than 5% of the grafted cells surviving long term in rats (26), nonhuman primates (27), and humans (28). The vast majority of adrenal medullary cells grafted into the striatum die within a few hours after the transplantation (29). It is not surprising that the initial clinical results met with limited success, with only 20–30% of the grafted patients improving partially (30).

The low survival rate of grafted chromaffin cells as well as the lack of phenotypic change is hypothesized to be related to the low concentration of NGF in the striatal parenchyma (31). Both *in vitro* (32) and *in vivo* (5), adrenal chromaffin cells undergo a transformation from endocrine to neuronal morphology if exposed to NGF in the absence of corticosteroids. This transformation occurs in fetal, young postnatal, and adult chromaffin cells (33) derived from different species, including humans (34). The importance of NGF was demonstrated by the study of Stromberg *et al.* (5), in which solid, adult adrenal medullary (AM) grafts were transplanted to the striatum of 6-OHDA-lesioned rats and combined with an intrastriatal delivery of NGF using a miniosmotic pump. Morphological transformation of the endocrine cells to the neuronal phenotype and formation of extensive networks of catecholaminergic nerve fibers were described. A marked increase in chromaffin cell survival for up to 1 year was documented with a significant improvement in behavioral outcome when compared to non-NGF-supplemented grafts. In AM chromaffin cell cultures in which normally less than 10% of the cells survive (33), NGF increases the survival rate to 30%, and to 50% when cocultured with C6 glioma cells, which secrete NGF and other trophic factors. These findings led to the first trial of NGF infusion with a stereotaxic putaminal AM graft in human PD (4). The NGF was infused into the striatum for 3 months through a polyurethane catheter connected to an external pump. Unlike the previous experience of this group with AM grafts, this patient showed sustained and progressive improvement for up to 11 months of follow-up. These studies suggest that NGF augments adrenal medulla graft survival and improves the functional outcome.

Intracerebral Administration of Nerve Growth Factor

Nerve growth factor β (β-NGF) is a dimeric polypeptide (MW 26,518) that does not permeate the blood–brain barrier (BBB). Of the strategies developed for intracerebral administration, one novel method is the conjugation of NGF to an antibody to the transferrin receptor, allowing for the transport of this complex across the BBB (3). Using this technique, labeled biologically active NGF was recovered in the brain parenchyma. Although this is an extremely interesting form of administration for drugs with low BBB penetration, the consequences of the systemic administration of NGF should not be overlooked. Nerve growth factor receptors have been found on chromaffin adrenergic cells, some adult mesenchymal tissue, neonatal tumors, and on hematopoietic cells (11). In the latter, NGF induces the proliferation and degranulation of mast cells (35). Nerve growth factor enhances the glutamate toxicity in PC-12 cells (36) and NGF receptors have been identified on the cell surface and nucleus of different carcinoma cell lines, including the A875 melanoma and SKBr5 breast carcinoma lines (37) (stimulating the cell proliferation of the latter). Therefore, caution should be exercised concerning the systemic effects of NGF. Also, the transferrin complex delivery method provides no ability to target the site of NGF delivery.

Of the local delivery strategies, the continuous intracerebral or intraventricular infusion of NGF with osmotic pumps (5) has the advantage of controlled and localized delivery for a defined period of time. Disadvantages of this technique include the requirement for an invasive procedure, the need for repeated refilling of the pump, and the evidence of pump-derived toxins (38). In humans, pumps require exteriorization with the obvious risks of infection (4). Another local delivery strategy is to use cografts of peripheral nerve (39), or grafting genetically modified cells capable of secreting NGF (6). These technqiues depend on graft survival for the production of NGF. At present the amount of NGF delivered cannot be controlled (6) and the delivery cannot be terminated. The issue of the neoplastic or tumorogenic potential of the grafts remains unresolved.

Sustained-release biodegradable polymeric formulations have been used successfully for the prolonged systemic delivery of different drugs such as antibiotics, chemotherapeutic agents, and contraceptives (40). This approach has several advantages. In these formulations, the drug release kinetics can be controlled (41), permitting highly accurate drug delivery. With the development of techniques that permit encapsulation of small quantities of drugs (42), sustained delivery in specific areas of the brain can be accomplished. These polymers have been used for intracerebral administration of dopamine, bethanechol, 1,3-bis(2-chloroethyl)-1-nitrosourea (BCNU), and corticosteroids (43). The first human trials of biodegradable polymers involved the intracerebral delivery of BCNU for malignant gliomas (44). A copolymer of carboxyphenoxypropane and sebacic acid (20 : 80 molar ratio) was used that provided sustained intracerebral delivery of BCNU for over 3 weeks. The BCNU–polymer implants increased survival time compared with controls and showed no systemic toxicity.

Polymer systems have been used for the sustained delivery of proteins, including NGF (45). It is essential that the preparation method not alter the biological activity of the protein. The preparations of some polymeric dosage forms require heating which could result in protein denaturation. Ethylene–vinyl acetate has been used for the sustained delivery of NGF (45), but this polymer is not biodegradable. The most promising polymers are the polyesters, such as homo- and copolymers of lactic and glycolic acid. These polymers have been used to encapsulate proteins in microspheres and in polymer matrix preparations, with preservation of biological activity and delivery over prolonged periods of time (46). Encapsulation and delivery of high molecular weight proteins have also been achieved (46). These polymers have been used extensively as biodegradable sutures with proven biocompatibility (47). The tissue reaction induced is minimal, with no known deleterious effects in experimental animals (48) or humans (49). Because the polymers are biodegradable, there is no need to remove the implants. Their degradation occurs by hydrolysis, yielding glycolic and lactic acid, which are eliminated (47). Because diffusion through the polymer matrix is negligible for compounds of high molecular weight, drug release occurs as a result of erosion of the matrix, and a delivery period of weeks to months can be achieved. Overall, these polymers are excellent candidates for delivery of trophic factors.

Methods

Microsphere Preparation

Microspheres are prepared with poly(L-lactide)coglycolide (PLGA), using a modification of the method originally described by Ogawa *et al.* (9, 50). In brief, this technique involves the use of three phases: (1) an inner water phase (W1) containing the drug to be incorporated, (2) an intermediate oily phase consisting of the polymer dissolved in an organic solvent, and (3) an outer water phase (W2) containing an emulsifying agent. In the first step, a microfine water-in-oil (W/O) emulsion is prepared. Because of its high water solubility, NGF will be partitioned into the aqueous phase. In the second step, the outer water phase containing an emulsifying agent is added to form a (W/O)/W emulsion. As the organic solvent evaporates, the polymeric wall of the microspheres hardens, yielding microspheres with incorporated drug.

Microspheres are prepared with NGF loads ranging from 0.001 to 0.050% (w/w). A known amount of NGF (2.5S NGF from mouse submaxillary gland; Boehringer-Mannheim, Indianapolis, IN) is dissolved in 500 μl of a 2% (w/v) bovine serum albumin solution in sterile phosphate-buffered saline (pH 7.4). Gelatin (100 mg) is slowly added to the NGF solution, vortexed for 3 min, and the solution incubated at 35°C for 30 min with frequent vortexing. This is the inner aqueous phase (W1). The oily phase is prepared by dissolving 2 g of poly(L-lactide)coglycolide (75 : 25) (MW 80,000; Medisorb Technologies International, Cincinnati, OH) in 5 ml of methylene chloride. The outer aqueous phase (W2) is 200 ml of 0.5% (w/v) polyvinyl alcohol solution. W1 is slowly added with a micropipette into the oily phase while mixing with a Vortex mixer (Scientific Products, McGaw, IL). The resulting water-in-oil emulsion is cooled to 20°C and slowly poured into W2 maintained at 15°C while stirring vigorously with a magnetic bar. The organic solvent is removed in a rotary evaporator (Buchi 011; Buchi, Geneva, Switzerland) at 35°C. The complete removal of the solvent is accomplished in 3 hr. The microspheres are collected by centrifugation, washed three times in deionized H_2O, lyophilized (Lyph Lock 18), and stored at −80°C.

Structure and Size of Microspheres

Microsphere size distribution is analyzed with a particle size analyzer (model 2010; Brinkmann, Westbury, NY). The shape, size, and structure are also studied by optical and scanning electron microscopy (8).

In Vitro Release

The *in vitro* release of NGF is quantified by a 2.5S enzyme-linked immunosorbent assay (ELISA). Approximately 100 mg of microspheres [NGF load, 0.013% (w/w)] is suspended in 1 ml of a 0.5% (w/v) bovine serum albumin solution (pH 7.4) maintained at 37°C in a microstirring module (Reacti-therm Biotech, Inc., Worcester, MA). Periodically, the suspension is centrifuged and the supernatant frozen until analyzed. The microspheres are then resuspended in fresh buffer. Nerve growth factor content in release medium is quantified by a sandwich-type ELISA technique (8). The limit of detection is 5 pg/ml.

The biological activity of the released NGF is determined by the chick dorsal root ganglion assay (51). Dorsal root ganglia dissected from 8- to 11-day-old chick embryos are incubated in a plasma clot made of 25 μl of fresh chicken plasma (Cocalico Biologicals, Ephrata, PA), 25 μl of the sample medium, and 25 μl of thrombin (1000 U/ml) diluted 10:1 with Dulbecco's modified Eagle's medium. The cultures are incubated for 20 hr at 37°C in a 95% O_2/5% CO_2 incubator. These ganglia have an absolute requirement for NGF to survive, and biologically active NGF is detected by the appearance of neurite outgrowth from the ganglia. The neurite response is dose dependent and bell shaped for concentrations of NGF in a range from 1 to 10 ng/ml (51).

In Vivo Release

A qualitative analysis of *in vivo* release of NGF from microspheres is performed by detecting NGF reactivity by an indirect immunofluorescence technique. Microspheres are stereotaxically implanted into the corpus striatum of Sprague-Dawley rats. Animals are sacrificed after 1 and 4.5 weeks with an intracardiac perfusion of paraformaldehyde–picric acid fixative solution. The brains are sectioned at 15-mm intervals on a cryostat and selected sections are mounted on gelatin-coated slides. The sections are rehydrated and covered with 10% (v/v) normal goat serum in phosphate-buffered saline (PBS) for 30 min. Rabbit anti-mouse 2.5S NGF antiserum (Collaborative Research, Bedford, MA) is used as the primary antibody, diluted 1:200 in a 0.3% (v/v) Triton X-100 solution in PBS. The sections are incubated overnight at 4°C with the primary antibody, washed with PBS, and incubated for 1 hr at room temperature with a fluorescein isothiocyanate-conjugated goat anti-rabbit secondary antibody (Boehringer-Mannheim). Sections are examined by epifluorescence microscopy.

In Vivo Effect of Microsphere-Delivered Nerve Growth Factor on Adrenal Medullary Grafts

The 6-OHDA rodent model of Parkinson's disease is used (52). The neurotoxin 6-OHDA is unilaterally injected into the substantia nigra and medial forebrain bundle of Sprague-Dawley rats. The subsequent immediate degeneration of dopaminergic neurons leads to spontaneous ipsilateral rotation and upregulation of striatal dopaminergic receptors (53). Any therapy that reestablishes striatal dopamine concentration reduces the number of apomorphine-induced rotations.

Preoperative rotational behavior in response to subcutaneous apomorphine (0.1 mg/kg) is determined weekly for a period of 4–6 weeks. After grafting, rats are challenged with apomorphine every other week. The rotational response in 38-cm diameter flat-base cylinders is quantified for 70 min each session, using a computerized, video-based movement analyzer (Videomex-V; Columbus Instruments, Columbus, OH). Animals are randomly assigned to four treatment groups. These groups receive (a) blank microspheres ($n = 7$), (b) NGF-loaded microspheres ($n = 7$), (c) dissociated adrenal medullary cells ($n = 8$), and (d) adrenal medullary cells and NGF microspheres ($n = 8$).

Dissociated adrenal medulla (AM) cell suspensions are prepared from young donor rats (100–150 g). The AM is completely separated from adrenal cortex and incubated for 10 min at 37°C in 5 ml of Hank's balanced salt solution (HBSS) with collagenase (0.125%, w/v; Sigma, St. Louis, MO), dispase (0.05%, w/v; Sigma), and DNase (0.015%, w/v; Sigma). The AM is mechanically disrupted by gentle pipetting. The enzymatic reaction is terminated with 10% fetal calf serum at 4°C. Cells are collected by centrifugation at 1000 rpm for 10 min and resuspended in HBSS. Cell count and viability are determined using 0.2% (w/v) trypan blue in a hemacytometer, using optical microscopy. Usually 10^5 viable cells are obtained from every gland. Cells are concentrated to 10^5 cells/5 μl HBSS and immediately grafted.

Two intrastriatal targets per animal are selected as grafting sites. Coordinates from bregma are as follows: AP, +0.15 mm; L, 0.25 mm; V, 0.55 mm; and (b) AP, 0.00 mm; L, 0.25 mm; V, 0.55 mm. The tip of a cut No. 20 spinal needle is stereotaxically positioned 0.5 mm ventral to the target. Five microliters of microsphere suspension (10 mg/10 μl) is injected at a rate of 1 μl/min. The spinal needle (with its occluder) is left in place for 5 min and slowly retracted 1 mm. A 26-gauge Hamilton syringe is passed through the spinal needle, its tip placed at the target. Five minutes later, 5 μl of the cell suspension is injected at a rate of 0.5 μl/min. The spinal needle is left in place for 5 min, and an additional 5 μl of microsphere suspension is slowly injected. The spinal needle is left in place an additional 5 min before slowly removing it. The total volume injected is 15 μl in all animals. In animals receiving only microspheres (containing NGF or blank), 5 μl of saline solution is injected through the Hamilton instead of the cell suspension. In animals receiving only cells, 10 μl of saline solution is injected instead of the microsphere suspension, using the described sequence. As the volume injected is significant, only one target site is injected per procedure, and the two procedures are performed at least 4 days apart.

After 10 or 20 weeks of postgrafting behavioral evaluation, animals are sacrificed under deep barbiturate anesthesia with intracardiac infusion of 4% paraformaldehyde with 0.2% glutaraldehyde. The brains are removed, sectioned on a vibratome, and processed for cresyl violet staining and glial fibrillary acidic protein (GFAP) immunohistochemistry.

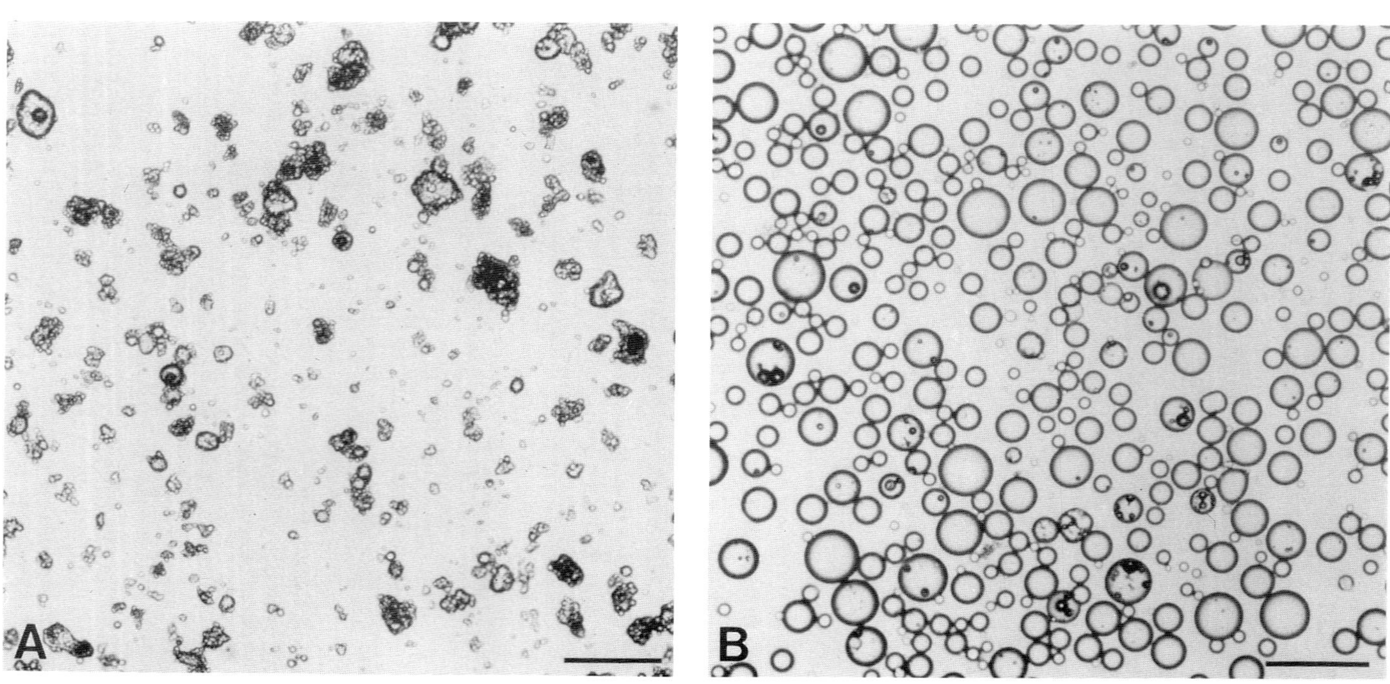

FIG. 1 Example of microspheres prepared by stirring in a homogenizer (A) and by using vortexing and magnetic stirring (B). Vortex-prepared microspheres have a more uniform shape and size. Bars: 100 μm.

Results

Microsphere Characteristics and Release Process

The two emulsions (W1/Oil and W1/Oil/W2) were initially prepared by stirring in a homogenizer, but this caused a significant increase in temperature, thereby facilitating evaporation of the organic solvent. Consequently the viscosity of the polymer solution increased, and the handling of the system became difficult. This not only decreased the microsphere yield but also resulted in microspheres of varying sizes (Fig. 1A). The use of a vortex mixer (W1/Oil emulsion) and magnetic stirring (to prepare W1/Oil/W2 emulsion) did not raise the sample temperature. As a result microspheres of uniform size and shape were obtained (Fig. 1B).

The average diameter of the microspheres was 17.2 μm (SD = 12.5 μm), with 75% of the microspheres in the 7- to 33-μm size range. Scanning electron micrography revealed a smooth external polymer surface (Fig. 2A). When placed in an aqueous medium, the formation of pores in the polymer wall is apparent (Fig. 2B and C). These pores result from the erosion of the polymeric matrix (9). This can be seen 1 week after suspension of the microspheres in buffer solution. The progressive erosion of the matrix caused an increase in the size of the pores (Fig. 2B). Four weeks after incubation, there were few remaining structures resembling microspheres (Fig. 2C and D). The polymer degradation rate can be modified by changing the lactide-to-glycolide ratio as well as by changing the molecular weight of the polymer (9, 41), with resultant delivery periods that range from 2 weeks to 6 months or more for PLGA.

In Vitro and in Vivo Release

It is difficult to quantify the total amount of NGF incorporated in the microspheres, as this would entail the dissolution of the microspheres in an organic solvent and the subsequent extraction of NGF into an aqueous medium. This might result in a significant loss of NGF activity due to protein denatur-

---

FIG. 2(A) and (B) Scanning electron micrographs of microspheres after incubation for varying intervals. (A) Prior to incubation the spheres have smooth external surfaces (×2500). (B) After 1 week of incubation the surfaces exhibit some irregularities (×2500). In (A) and (B) the bar in the right-hand corner is 10 μm. [Reproduced with permission from Camarata *et al.* (8).]

FIG. 2(C) and (D) (C) The surfaces have become porous and irregular after 2 weeks of incubation (×5000). (D) Spherical form is lost by 4 weeks, with most of the polymer dissolved (×1000). In (C) the bar in the right-hand corner is 1 μm whereas in (D) it is 10 μm. [Reproduced with permission from Camarata *et al.* (8).]

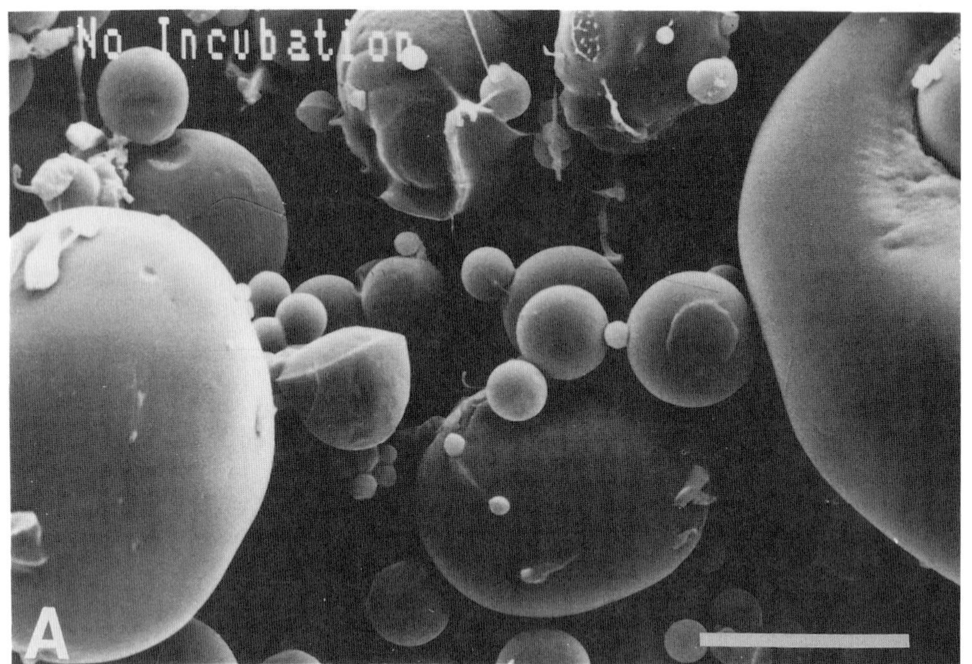
No Incubation
A

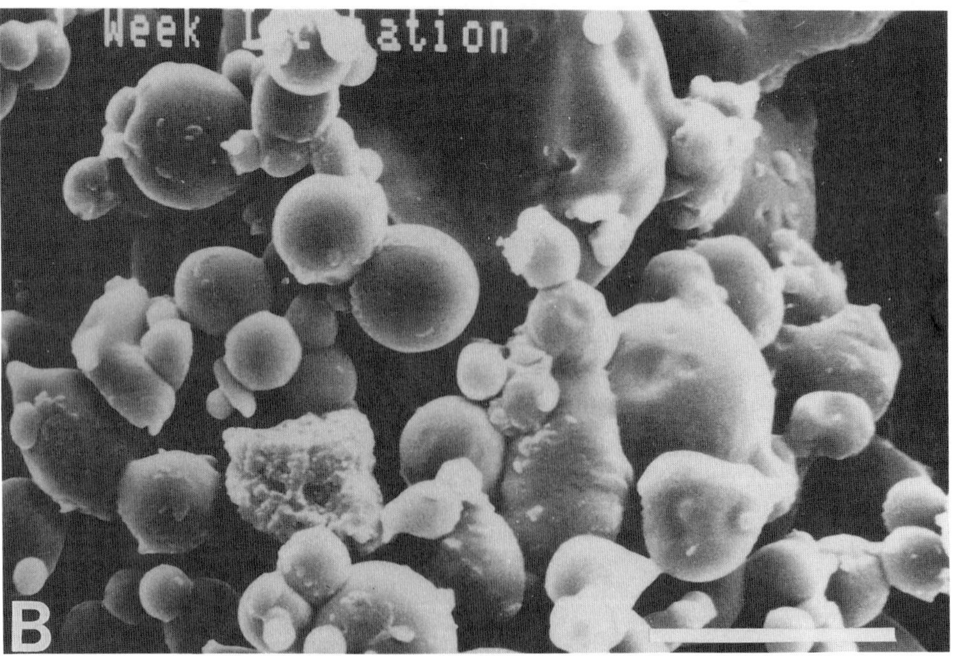
Week
B

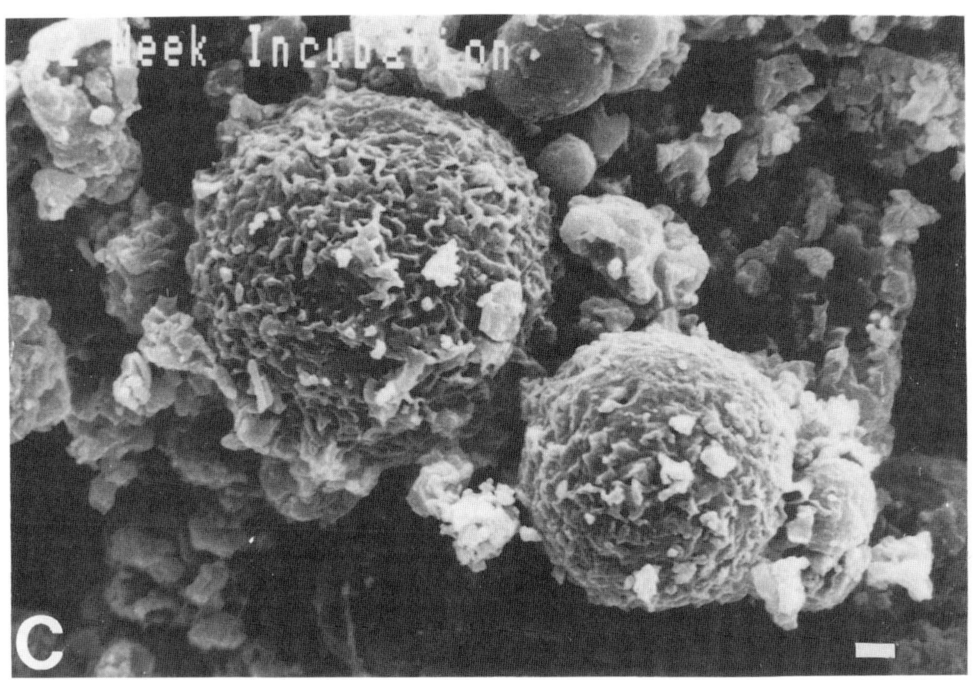
C

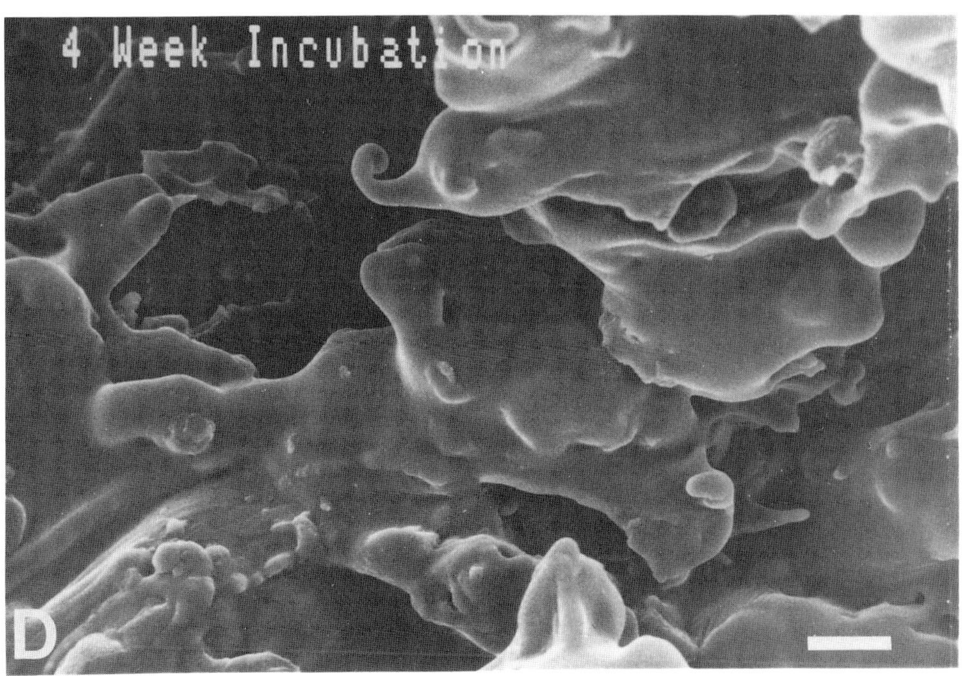
4 Week Incubation
D

ation. *In vitro* release studies [NGF load, 0.013% (w/w)] revealed significant NGF release during the 5-week sampling period. Therefore, the release of NGF from these microspheres incubated in buffer solution at 37°C was assayed with ELISA. Significant amounts of NGF were detected throughout the 5-week sampling period (Fig. 3).

It was also necessary to ensure that the NGF released from the microspheres was biologically active. Following the incubation of the microspheres [NGF load, 0.013% (w/w)], the release medium was collected and added to dorsal root ganglion explants. This produced a halo of neurite outgrowth. Microspheres were also used directly in the culture assay. The microspheres were first incubated in buffer for 24 hr and then placed directly in the tissue culture plasma clot, and this also resulted in abundant neurite outgrowth. Adding rabbit anti-2.5S NGF antibody to the culture completely blocked neurite outgrowth, demonstrating the specificity of the response to NGF released from the microspheres (8).

In vivo release of NGF was demonstrated by stereotaxically implanting microspheres into the striatum. One week after implantation, NGF immunoreactivity was abdundantly present in the microspheres and surrounding tissue (Fig. 4A). After 4.5 weeks, the area of fluorescent microspheres was markedly thinner, presumably because of the degradation of the polymer (Fig. 4B).

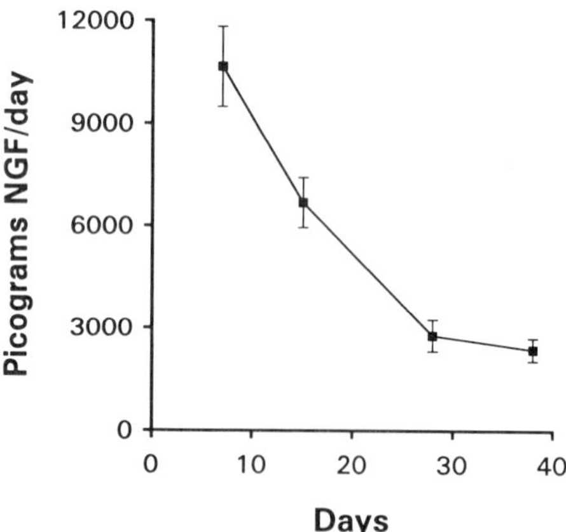

FIG. 3 Amount of NGF released per day from microspheres as determined by NGF ELISA. One hundred milligrams of microspheres [0.013% (w/w) NGF] was maintained in 1 ml of buffer for 5 weeks. Progressive decrease in NGF release occurs over the 5-week period.

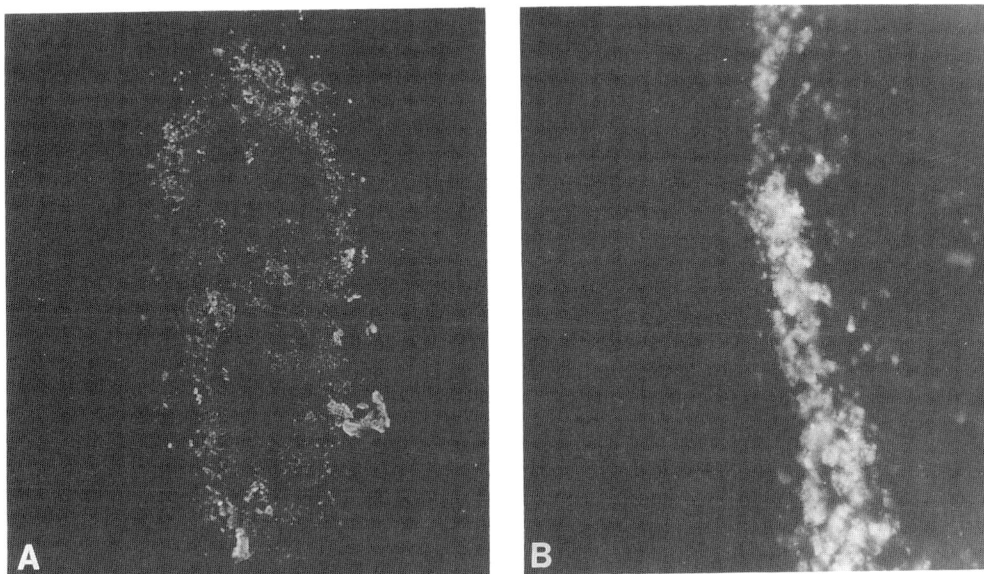

FIG. 4 Photomicrographs of rat brain slices through the basal ganglia of implanted NGF microspheres. Sections stained with fluorescent antibody to NGF. (A) One week after implantation. (B) Four and a half weeks after implantation. [Reproduced with permission from Camarata *et al.* (8).]

Effect of Microsphere-Delivered Nerve Growth Factor on Adrenal Medullary Grafts

The tissue reaction observed in the striatum of rats receiving polymer microspheres was minimal. GFAP immunostaining revealed a mild reactive astrocytosis, with few macrophages in the vicinity of the grafts. The tissue reaction was similar in groups receiving solely cells as compared to those receiving microspheres.

A statistically significant (two-tailed paired Student's t test; $p < 0.01$) decrease in apomorphine-induced rotations occurred only in the rats receiving both adrenal medullary cell suspension and NGF-loaded microspheres (Fig. 5A). This treatment produced a 40.5% reduction in rotations compared to baseline pretreatment rotations. All eight animals demonstrated a decrease in their rotatory behavior, ranging from 21 to 64% for individual animals. Animals receiving adrenal medullary cells did not show a statistically significant improvement as a group but did have the second largest reduction of

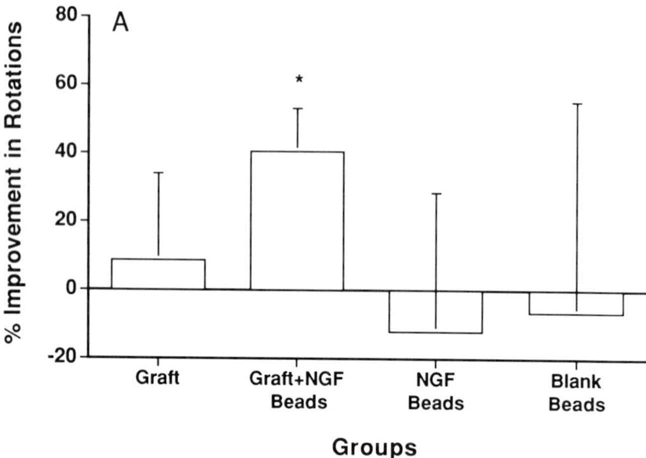

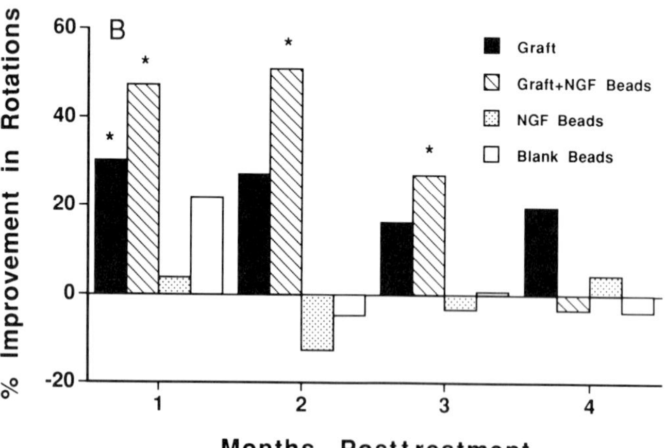

FIG. 5 Changes in apomorphine-induced rotations in the four different groups of 6-OHDA rats. An improvement in rotations, that is, a decrease in the number of rotations toward the lesioned side, is denoted by a positive number. (A) Overall effect on rotation behavior averaged over the 4-month period. Only the graft plus NGF polymer group had a significant reduction in the number of rotations. (B) Time course of the rotational behavior. The decrease in rotations was statistically significant for 3 months in the graft plus NGF polymer group. For the graft group the reduction in rotation was significant only for the first month.

19.6%. This degree of reduction is similar to previously published results (5, 25). In this group there was a reduction of rotations in only four of the eight animals. Animals that received only the adrenal medullary cells showed a range of 18% increase to 68% decrease in apomorphine-induced rotations. The other two groups, receiving NGF microspheres and blank microspheres, had nonsignificant increases in apomorphine-induced rotations.

The time course of the behavioral responses is shown in Fig. 5B. The rotations were significantly reduced in the first 3 months [repeated measurements by analysis of variance (ANOVA); $p < 0.05$] following transplantation among rats receiving adrenal medullary cells plus NGF microspheres. The behavioral improvement gradually diminished, with no significant difference found by the fourth month when compared to preoperative baseline rotations. A similar time course for the behavioral response was observed for the group receiving only adrenal medullary grafts. The other two groups showed no clear temporal trends in their rotational behavior.

Although these results show a statistically significant behavioral improvement when dissociated adrenal medullary cells are grafted with NGF microspheres, this response lasted only 2 months. This finding is not fully consistent with previous reports (5), in which a 1-month administration of NGF resulted in prolonged functional and histological improvement. This discrepancy may be related to several factors. First, we used dissociated adrenal medullary cells, not solid adrenal grafts. The enzymes used to dissociate the tissue could potentially alter the NGF cell surface receptor, modifying the long-term response to NGF. Second, the amount of NGF delivered with microspheres in our study was less than delivered by a miniosmotic pump by Stromberg *et al.* (5). It is possible that long-term effects of NGF are dose dependent. *In vitro* studies suggest that after NGF induces a change in the morphology of adrenal medullary cells toward the neuronal phenotype, the deprivation of NGF results in dedifferentiation of these cells in culture (54). Our results are compatible with these findings, suggesting that NGF was locally delivered for 2 to 3 months, as anticipated from the polymer composition used.

Summary

We have demonstrated that the microencapsulation of biologically active NGF is possible. With this technique, sustained delivery of NGF occurred with minimal trauma and tissue reaction. Moreover, local targeted delivery of this factor can be attained, reducing the exposure of nontargeted tissue. The supplementation of adrenal medullary grafts with NGF delivered from these biodegradable microspheres resulted in a marked behavioral improvement compared to non-NGF-supplemented grafts. This difference persisted during a period of time in which NGF was probably being released from the microspheres. These studies demonstrate that biodegradable, biocompatible polymers for the local intracerebral administration of macromolecules is a viable strategy for providing pharmacological access to the brain.

Acknowledgments

We wish to thank Joan Aanderud for typing the manuscript and Mike McPhee for the graphics. We also wish to thank Keyvan Abtin for his help at the beginning of this study. This study was funded in part by the United Parkinson's Disease Foundation, the Minnesota Medical Foundation, and a gift from Mary Meidl. Dr. Camarata was funded by an American College of Surgeons Scholarship and NIH Grant T32-NS07361.

References

1. T. Ebendal, *J. Neurosci. Res.* **32,** 461 (1992).
2. L. H. Lin, D. H. Doherty, J. D. Lile, S. Bektesh, and F. Collins, *Science* **260,** 1130 (1993).
3. P. M. Friden, L. R. Walus, P. Watson, S. R. Doctrow, J. W. Kozarich, C. Backman, H. Bergman, B. Hoffer, F. Bloom, and A. C. Granholm, *Science* **259,** 373 (1993).
4. L. Olson, E. O. Backlund, T. Ebendal, R. Freedman, B. Hamberger, P. Hansson, B. Hoffer, U. Lindblom, B. Meyerson, and I. Stromberg, *Arch. Neurol. (Chicago)* **48,** 373 (1991).
5. I. Stromberg, M. Herrera-Marschitz, U. Ungerstedt, T. Ebendal, and L. Olson, *Exp. Brain Res.* **60,** 335 (1985).
6. D. M. Frim, M. P. Short, W. S. Rosenberg, J. Simpson, X. O. Breakefield, and O. Isacson, *J. Neurosurg.* **78,** 267 (1993).
7. G. Bing, M. F. Notter, J. T. Hansen, C. Kellogg, J. H. Kordower, and D. M. Gash, *Neuroscience* **34,** 687 (1990).
8. P. J. Camarata, R. Suryanarayanan, D. A. Turner, R. G. Parker, and T. J. Ebner, *Neurosurgery* **30,** 313 (1992).
9. Y. Ogawa, M. Yamamoto, S. Takada, H. Okada, and T. Shimamoto, *Chem. Pharm. Bull.* **36,** 1502 (1988).
10. R. Levi-Montalcini, *Science* **237,** 1154 (1987).
11. M. Bothwell, *Curr. Top. Microbiol. Immunol.* **165,** 55 (1991).
12. F. H. Gage, M. H. Tuszynski, K. S. Chen, A. M. Fagan, and G. A. Higgins, *Curr. Top. Microbiol. Immunol.* **165,** 71 (1991).
13. R. A. Bradshaw, *Annu. Rev. Biochem.* **47,** 191 (1978).
14. A. Derby, V. W. Engleman, G. E. Frierdich, G. Neises, S. R. Rapp, and D. G. Roufa, *Exp. Neurol.* **119,** 176 (1993).

15. M. H. Tuszynski, H. Sang, K. Yoshida, and F. H. Gage, *Ann. Neurol.* **30,** 625 (1991).
16. T. Hagg, M. Manthorpe, H. L. Vahlsing, and S. Varon, *Exp. Neurol.* **101,** 303 (1988).
17. R. F. Mervis, D. Pope, R. Lewis, R. M. Dvorak, and L. R. Williams, *Ann. N. Y. Acad. Sci.* **640,** 95 (1991).
18. W. Fischer, K. Wictorin, A. Bjorklund, L. R. Williams, S. Varon, and F. H. Gage, *Nature* (*London*) **329,** 65 (1987).
19. L. Olson, A. Nordberg, H. von Holst, L. Backman, T. Ebendal, I. Alafuzoff, K. Amberla, P. Hartvig, A. Herlitz, A. Lilja A, *et al., J. Neural Transm. Park. Dis. Dement. Sect.* **4,** 79 (1992).
20. N. Berardi, L. Domenici, V. Parisi, T. Pizzorusso, A. Cellerino, and L. Maffei, *Proc. R. Soc. London* **251,** 17 (1993).
21. T. Shigeno, T. Mima, K. Takakura, D. I. Graham, G. Kato, Y. Hashimoto, and S. Furukawa, *J. Neurosci.* **11,** 2914 (1991).
22. J. M. Schumacher, M. P. Short, B. T. Hyman, X. O. Breakefield, and O. Isacson, *Neuroscience* **45,** 561 (1991).
23. S. C. Apfel, J. C. Arezzo, L. Lipson, and J. A. Kessler, *Annu. Neurol.* **31,** 76 (1992).
24. M. J. Yaeger, A.Koestner, K. Marushige, and Y. Marushige, *Acta Neuropathol.* **83,** 624 (1992).
25. W. J. Freed, F. Karoum, E. Spoor, J. M. Morihisa, L.Olson, and R. J. Wyatt, *Brain Res.* **269,** 184 (1983).
26. A. K. Shetty, G. Gopinath, and P. N. Tandon, *J. Neural Transplant. Plast.* **2,** 175 (1991).
27. J. M. Morihisa, R. K. Nakamura, and W. J. Freed, *Exp. Neurol.* **84,** 643 (1984).
28. J. H. Kordower, E.Cochran, R. D. Penn, and C. G. Goetz, *Ann. Neurol.* **29,** 405 (1991).
29. I. Stromberg, M. Herrera-Marschitz, L. Hultgren, U. Ungerstedt, and L. Olson, *Brain Res.* **297,** 41 (1984).
30. C. G. Goetz, W. Olanow, W. C. Koller, R. D. Penn, D. Cahill, R. Morantz, G. Stebbins, C. M. Tanner, H. L. Klawans, K. M. Shannon, C. L. Comella, T. Witt, C. Cox, M. Waxman, and L. Gauger, *N. Engl. J. Med.* **320,** 337 (1989).
31. S. G.Korsching, R. Auburger, R. Heumann, J. Scott, and H. Thoenen, *EMBO J.* **4,** 389 (1985).
32. A. S. Tischler, J. C. Riseberg, M. A. Hardenbrook, and V. Cherington, *J. Neurosci.* **13,** 1533 (1993).
33. M. F. D. Notter, J. T. Hansen, S. Okawara, and D. M. Gash, *Exp. Brain Res.* **76,** 38 (1989).
34. A. S. Tischler, R. A. DeLellis, B. Biales, G. Nunnemacher, G. M. Morse, V. Carabba, and H. J. Wolfe, *Lab. Invest.* **43,** 399 (1980).
35. M. Tomioka, R. H. Stead, L. Nielsen, M. D. Coughlin, and J. Bienenstock, *J. Allergy Clin. Immunol.* **82,** 599 (1988).
36. D. Schubert, H. Kimura, and P. Maher, *Proc. Natl. Acad. Sci. U.S.A.* **89,** 8264 (1992).

37. E. M. Rakowicz-Szulczynska, *J. Cell. Physiol.* **154,** 64 (1993).
38. H. L. Vahlsing, S. Varon, T. Hagg, B. Fass-Holmes, A. Dekker, M. Manley, and M. Manthorpe, *Exp. Neurol.* **105,** 233 (1989).
39. I. Date, S. Asari, A. Nishimoto, and D. Felten, *No Shinkei Geka* **19,** 919 (1991).
40. T. R. Tice and D. R. Cowsar, *Pharm. Technol.* **8,** 26 (1984).
41. G. E. Visscher, J. E. Pearson, J. W. Fong, G. J. Argentieri, R. I. L. Robison, and H. V. Maulding, *J. Biomed. Mater. Res.* **22,** 733 (1988).
42. J. Murray, L. Brown, and R. Langer, *Cancer Drug. Delivery* **1,** 119 (1984).
43. R. Langer, *J. Controlled Release* **16,** 53 (1991).
44. H. Brem, S. Mahaley, N. A. Vick, K. L. Black, S. C. Schold, P. C. Burger, A. H. Friedman, I. S. Ciric, T. W. Eller, J. W. Cozzens, and J. N. Kenealy, *J. Neurosurg.* **74,** 441 (1991).
45. E. M. Powell, M. R. Sobarzo, and W. M. Saltzman, *Brain Res.* **515,** 309 (1990).
46. S. Cohen, T. Yoshioka, M. Lucarelli, L. H. Hwang, and R. Langer, *Pharm. Res.* **8,** 713 (1991).
47. R. K. Kulkarni, K. C. Pani, C. Neuman, and F. Leonard, *Arch. Surg. (Chicago)* **93,** 839 (1966).
48. R. J. Tamargo, J. I. Epstein, C. S. Reinhard, M. Chasin, and H. Brem, *J. Biomed. Mater. Res.* **23,** 253 (1989).
49. D. L. Wise, T. D. Fellmann, J. E. Sanderson, and R. L. Wentworth, *in* "Drug Carriers in Biology and Medicine" (G. Gregoriadis, ed.), Chapter 12. Academic Press, London, 1979.
50. Y. Ogawa, M. Yamamoto, H. Okada, T. Yashiki, and T. Shimamoto, *Chem. Pharm. Bull.* **36,** 1095 (1988).
51. A. Zanini, P. Angeletti, and R. Levi-Moltalcini, *Proc. Natl. Acad. Sci. U.S.A.* **61,** 835 (1968).
52. U. Ungerstedt, *Eur. J. Pharmacol.* **5,** 107 (1968).
53. C. Pifl, H. Reither, and O. Hornykiewicz, *Brain Res.* **572,** 87 (1992).
54. K. Unsicker, T. J. Millar, and H. D. Hofmann, *Dev. Neurosci.* **5,** 412 (1982).

[10] Polymeric Drug Carrier Systems in the Brain

Abraham J. Domb and Israel Ringel

Introduction

The blood–brain barrier (BBB), a tightly tiled lining of the vascular system in the brain, presents a formidable obstacle in the delivery of drugs to the brain. Drugs may gain access to the brain interstitial space either by passive diffusion through the lipid membrane of the brain endothelial cells or by one of three transport mechanisms: carrier mediated (e.g., nutrients, thyroid hormones), receptor mediated (e.g., peptides), and plasma protein mediated (e.g., steroidal hormones and lipid-soluble compounds) (1–3).

The need for an effective and efficient delivery of therapeutic agents to specific sites in the brain is self-evident. The basic requirements for effective drug delivery to the central nervous system (CNS) are that the effect of the drug should be localized and that the drug have access to the brain, be stable for the duration of action, be nontoxic and safe, and give a sustained and controlled effective dose at the site. These requirements are partially fulfilled by lipophilic drugs that can passively diffuse into the brain: lipid microparticulate systems such as liposomes and emulsions (4), reversible lipophilic prodrug systems that cross the BBB (5), and implanted infusion pumps that deliver drugs in a controlled fashion through an intraventricular catheter (6, 7). These pumps have been used for the treatment of chronic pain, spasticity, brain tumors, and Alzheimer's disease. The subcutaneously implanted Ommaya reservoir system, which delivers drugs in a controlled fashion through an intraventricular catheter, has been used in treating cancer patients. The use of mechanical pumps for direct delivery to the brain is often associated with a high rate of infection, technical problems, limited reliability, high cost, and patient inconvenience. Another method for brain drug delivery is the temporary disruption of the BBB by, for example, hyperosmotic pressure (8). Except for the pumps, these methods are aimed at crossing the BBB, which still does not provide a solution for controlled localization of the drug to a target site within the brain. This can probably be solved by using an implantable controlled release polymeric implant. An excellent review on the methods for drug delivery to the brain has been published by Tamargo and Brem (9).

Methods in Neurosciences, Volume 21

This chapter reviews developments on the use of polymer-based implantable systems for the delivery of drugs to the brain. Implantation of drug-loaded polymeric devices directly into the brain provides effective drug concentrations into the diseased tissue and minimizes problems associated with systemic delivery of the drug, such as systemic side effects, peripheral drug inactivation, poor drug absorption, serum protein binding, inadequate BBB penetration, and poor patient compliance. In addition, the implants can be placed in specific regions of the brain, thereby avoiding undesirable distribution of the drug throughout the brain, which is frequently a problem with administration into the cerebrospinal fluid (CSF). However, there are potential disadvantages associated with the use of polymer implants. Once in place, discontinuation of the therapy is difficult, requiring a surgical procedure for the removal of the implant, which is sometimes hard to retrieve. In addition, dose adjustments are difficult once the polymer containing the drug is in place. For chronic long-term release, repeated implantations are required. This is the promise and challenge of polymeric brain implants.

Polymers for Drug Delivery

The use of polymers for local controlled drug delivery has been extensively reviewed (10–18). The devices can be divided into three groups: nondegradable polymers, biodegradable polymers, and drug-conjugated polymers. Nondegradable polymers are those that are stable in biological systems. The common polymers that are used as drug carriers are polysilicones, poly(ethylene–vinyl acetate) (EVAc), various acrylate-based hydrogels, and segmented polyurethanes, all of which are used as components of implantable devices. Synthetic and natural bioerodible products that are eliminated completely from the body. Examples of these polymers are poly (lactide–glycolide), polyanhydrides, poly(orthoesters), polyphosphazenes, collagen, fibrin, gelatin (Gelfoam, The Upjohn Company, Kalamazoo, MI), and oxidized cellulose (Surgicel, Ethicon, Inc., Somerville, NJ). Polymers for drug conjugation include degradable polymers containing functional groups available for drug attachment via hydrolyzable ester or amide bonds. Examples of common polymeric carriers for drug attachment are polysaccharides such as dextrans, modified cellulose and amylose, synthetic polyamides such as polyglutamic acid and polylysine, polyvinyl alcohol, and polyphosphazenes.

The desirable characteristics of any polymer system used for drug delivery are minimal tissue reaction after implantation, high polymer purity and reproducibility, a reliable drug release profile, and (for biodegradable polymers) *in vivo* degradation at a well-defined rate to nontoxic and readily excreted degradation products. Other considerations in developing polymer-based drug delivery systems include drug loading and uniformity, duration and rate of drug release, pharmacokinetics of drug and polymer degradation products, route of administration, drug stability in the polymer, storage stability, and sterilization method. The main advantage of using a biodegradable polymer over a nondegradable implant is that it need not be removed after the drug has been depleted. The advantages and disadvantages of these systems have been discussed elsewhere (14).

The drug release from implant and distribution in brain tissue has been reviewed (19–21). The drug release from a polymer implant into the brain tissue can be characterized by the following three steps: (a) drug release from the polymer matrix, (b) drug diffusion into the aqueous environment just outside of the matrix, and(c) drug distribution into the surrounding tissue. Many detailed studies have been published on each of the three aspects of the transport process (19–21). These studies include developing and modeling novel polymeric implantable systems, examining the transport of drug through an unstirred fluid, and studying the fate of drugs following release and distribution into the surrounding tissue (19). The drug release rate from these polymer implants can be generally described as zero order, first order, and square root of time release kinetics. As the drug is transported to the implant surface it must penetrate the stagnated layer to reach the desired site of action. Diffusion of a drug through a fluid may be critical in determining ideal implant characteristics. For example, a drug must move through the extracellular space away from an implant in dense tissue to produce its pharmaceutical effect. Measuring and predicting diffusion through this unstirred layer can be described by Fick's laws. Devices implanted directly into brain tissue have demonstrated the ability to deliver a variety of compounds from a polymer implant (19–21). Models were developed to predict drug distribution in the rat brain (19–21). These models have predicted that to maximize the extent of drug distribution, a candidate drug should be a water-soluble, slowly eliminated molecule with a high diffusion coefficient in the brain tissue.

Polymeric direct delivery to the brain has been used extensively for the delivery of chemotherapeutic agents and neurotransmitters and neuromodulators. This chapter reviews the delivery systems for these agents for the treatment of brain cancer and brain disorders.

Nondegradable Implants for Treatment of Brain Cancer

Several chemotherapeutic agents have been impregnated in biodegradable and nondegradable polymers and used for direct delivery in the brain. Compressed tablets of bleomycin and lactose coated with ethyl cellulose or an acrylic polymer were implanted into the cerebellum of dogs (22). Following implantation, detectable CSF levels of bleomycin were measured for 20 days. These tablets released the drug for 7 to 30 days *in vitro*. On the basis of these results, the formulation was tested clinically in six patients with craniopharyngioma. In one case, the recurrence was greatly delayed (23). The nondegradable poly(methyl methacrylate) (PMMA) (24, 25) was used to deliver a series of anticancer drugs including mitomycin, Adriamycin (doxorubicin) ACNU (minustine), and 5-fluorouracil (5-FU). The polymeric pellet was implanted into the remaining tumor at the time of excision or into the tumor by a computer tomography-guided stereotactic method. The reported survival rate was 47% in glioblastoma at 12 months and 91% in anaplastic astraocytoma at 18 months. Methotrexate-loaded PMMA pellets implanted into rat brain tumor showed a reduction in tumor size and an increase in survival rate compared to untreated animals (25).

Biodegradable Implants for Treatment of Brain Cancer

Bioerodible polymeric implants have been used for the delivery of a range of anticancer drugs (10–18). These devices are more favorable for clinical use because the device is eliminated from the brain after the drug has been depleted. Most studies were conducted by Brem and co-workers (16, 18, 26–39) using two polymers: poly(1,3-*p*-carboxyphenoxypropane–sebacic acid) [P(CPP–SA)] and poly(fatty acid dimer–sebacic acid) [P(FAD–SA)].

The biocompatibility and elimination processes of these polymers have been extensively studied and found to be biocompatible and biodegradable in the brain (11, 26–28, 40). The inflammatory reaction elicited by these polymers when implanted in the brains of rat, rabbit, and monkey was compared with that elicited by clinically used implants of Surgicel (oxidized regenerated cellulose) and Gelfoam (absorbable gelatin sponge) (11, 26–28, 40). In all experiments, there was no evidence of neovascularization or corneal edema, with acceptable minimal inflammatory reaction or necrosis confined to the surrounding tissue around the implant, as confirmed by histological examination. All materials were degraded and eliminated from the implant site within 8 to 12 weeks after implantation. The FAD–SA polymer was also extensively tested in rats, rabbits, and dogs for its biocompatibility when implanted in bone or muscle. These studies were part of preclinical studies on a gentamicin-releasing bone implant for the treatment of osteomyelitis (41). The polymer has been shown to be biocompatible and was allowed for use in phase I clinical trials.

The metabolic disposition and elimination process of P(CPP–SA) (20 : 80) implanted in rat brain was studied (42). Two polymers were prepared, one with [^{14}C]SA and unlabeled CPP, and the other copolymer with [^{14}C]CPP and unlabeled SA. Using two polymers, the metabolic disposition of each monomer after polymer degradation was studied. Polymer wafers loaded with 1,3-bis(2-chloroethyl)-1-nitrosourea (BCNU) or without the drug were implanted in the rat brain.

For the rats implanted with the [^{14}C]SA-labeled polymer, approximately 40% of the radioactivity was found in the expired CO_2, 10% in the urine, about 2% in the feces, and about 10% remained in the device over a 7-day period after implantation. On the other hand, only about 4% of the [^{14}C]CPP monomer was eliminated by urine and feces during this period. The drug-loaded polymer degraded faster than the reference polymer. Nearly all the radioactivity in each polymer was excreted by the 4-week time point and the device was completely eliminated from the implant site 4 weeks after implantation. This study demonstrated that the polymer is a biodegradable material useful for specific delivery of drugs directly into the brain with continued release over a period of time, while minimizing systemic exposure to potent chemotherapeutic agents. A similar study on rabbits resulted in similar data (43).

The elimination process of the FAD–SA polymer was studied in conjunction with the development of a gentamicin polymer implant for the treatment of osteomyelitis (41, 44). In these studies, the polymer was implanted in the bone or muscle of dogs and the polymer elimination from the implantation site was followed for 26 weeks. At each time point (4, 8, 12, and 26 weeks) three dogs were sacrificed and the polymer remnants were collected and analyzed and the surrounding tissue was examined histologically. The conclusion of this study was that the polymer is biocompatible and well tolerated both in bone and muscle and that the polymer biodegrades faster in bone than in muscle. The polymer implant was progressively degraded and disappeared from the site; by 8 weeks postimplantation most of the polymer had been eliminated and the remnants consisted mostly of the FAD monomer. After 12 weeks more of the polymer was eliminated and by 26 weeks the polymer was completely eliminated in most of the dogs. The elimination rate for this polymer in the brain is expected to be similar, which means complete elimination within 6 months postimplantation, with about 90% having gone after 8 weeks (41).

The general experimental procedure for the evaluation of the antitumor activity of polyanhydrides loaded with anticancer agents is as follows (29): male Fischer 344 rats weighing 200–250 are anesthetized with an intraperitoneal injection of a mixture of ketamine hydrochloride and xylazine in alcohol–saline solution. The anesthetized animal is shaved and the skull is exposed with a midline incision and a 3-mm burr hole drilled through the skull 5 mm posterior and 3 mm lateral to the bregma. The cortex and the white matter are resected with suction until a superior aspect of the brainstem is visualized. A 1-mm^3 piece of rat tumor tissue (either 9L or F98 gliosarcoma, depending on the evaluated drug) is introduced into the cranial defect and placed on the brainstem and the wound is irrigated with wound clips. Surgery is performed 5 days later to implant the polymer chemotherapy device (10 mg, 2.5 $\times$ 1 mm in size). The original incision is reopened aseptically, the device is put in place, and the wound is reclosed with surgical staples. The rats are followed daily and the time of death recorded. In some experiments 10^5 tumor cells, instead of the tumor tissue, are injected in the site to induce tumor growth. The polymer disks containing the drug are prepared either by compression molding of a mixture of polymer powder and the drug, or by mixing the drug in the polymer melt and casting the polymer–drug melt into a 1-mm film, which is then cut into 2.5-mm disks.

The first biodegradable implant ever used clinically in the brain was the P(CPP–SA) disk loaded with BCNU for the treatment of glioma multiforma. A number of review articles have been published describing the developmental process of this implant (9, 11, 15, 16, 18, 30, 31). On the basis of the satisfactory results with the BCNU-loaded P(CPP–SA) (20 : 80) in animals and in humans, a number of anticancer agents have been incorporated in this polymer and tested in rats for the treatment of brain cancer.

Carboplatin (CB), a cisplatin analog with significantly less ototoxicity, renal toxicity, and nephrotoxicity compared to cisplatin, was the second drug to be incorporated into a polyanhydride and implanted in the rat brain (32). Carboplatin was dispersed in P(FAD–SA) by melt mixing and tested against F98 rat glioma. Tissue distribution of CB in the rat brain followed for 6 weeks showed high platin concentration at the implant site, with a gradual decrease in tissue concentrations as a function of the distance from the implant site. Disks loaded with 5% carboplatin were implanted into the brain of Fischer 344 rats 5 days after inoculation with F98 rat glioma cells. The median survival of the carboplatin-implanted rats was 52 days, whereas the control animals implanted with the blank polymer had a median survival of 16 days. Histological examination of the carboplatin-implanted rats revealed a significant inhibition of tumor growth in the vicinity of the polymer (32).

4-Hydroperoxycyclophosphamide (4HC) is an active derivative of cyclophosphamide that does not need to be activated by the hepatic cytochrome *P*-450 system. The efficacy of 4HC incorporated in P(FAD–SA) disks against F98 rat glioma was studied (33, 34). The 20% loaded disks implanted in rats bearing F98 glioma model had a median survival of 35 days compared to only 22 days for the blank polymer. The *in vivo* concentration of 4HC released from the polymer showed cerebral drug peaks between 5 and 20 days after implantation whereas the cerebral drug concentration after systemic delivery fell rapidly by 48 hr after injection. Brain levels of 4HC were significantly higher than the blood drug levels at all time points.

Methotrexate (MTX) conjugated to dextran was suggested for direct delivery to the brain from a polymer matrix. The purpose of these conjugates was to increase MTX penetration and retention in the brain by increasing drug hydrophilicity (45). Methotrexate was conjugated to dextran via a spacer molecule either by an ester or an amide bond. The MTX dissociation from the carrier was dependent on the linkage chemistry, the amide-bonded MTX–dextran having a longer half life in phosphate buffer (20 days) than the ester-bonded derivative (3 days). The MTX–dextran conjugates were effective in killing human brain tumor cells; on a per MTX molecule basis, the cytotoxicity of MTX–dextran was as effective as MTX. The MTX conjugates were incorporated in a polyanhydride matrix and the drug release and effectiveness were determined in three-dimensional cell culture. These conjugates were able to penetrate and kill cells within a three-dimensional culture and thus can be used for the treatment of solid tumors in the central nervous system. In another study, biodegradable disks loaded with 5 to 20% MTX were implanted in rats bearing 9L or F98 tumors and the survival rate was compared to rats implanted with blank polymers. A minor increase in the survival rate was found for the 5% loaded MTX disks, whereas the higher loading disks were toxic and decreased the survival rate.

Targeting of MTX to the brain by conjugating MTX to carboxymethyl chitosan and administering the conjugate intraarterially in the external carotid artery was studied by Gallo and co-workers (46, 47). The conjugate and free MTX were at an MTX dose of 1 mg/kg. Animals were sacrificed at various times after administration and the MTX brain concentration was measured. Brain MTX concentrations were 18- and 12-fold greater at 15 min and 3 hr, respectively. This study suggests that MTX–chitosan conjugates can penetrate the BBB to deliver MTX to the brain without physically placing a device in the brain. However, the mechanism for the increase in MTX concentration in the brain was not reported.

Taxol is a novel antitumor agent that has demonstrated an anticancer activity against ovarian, breast, and nonsmall cell lung cancers. It has been shown to inhibit glioma xenograft growth subcapularly in nude mice (48) and act as a radiation enhancer for glioma cells *in vitro* (49). However, it penetrates the blood–brain barrier poorly, as evident from pharmacokinetic clinical trials and animal experiments. To evaluate the antitumor activity of taxol against brain tumors, taxol was incorporated in polyanhydride matrices and implanted intracranially in a rat model of malignant glioma (35). Taxol was incorporated into the CPP–SA polymer at loadings of 20 to 75% by weight in a 10-mg pellet and implanted in the 9L glioma rat model using the general procedure described above. Efficacy studies in rats demonstrated that the taxol–polymer implant successfully extended survival in rats (Fig. 1). The taxol-loaded polymers doubled (38 days, 40% taxol loading) and tripled (61 days, 20% taxol loading) the median survival of rats relative to control rats (19.5 days). The taxol release rate from the polymer into a buffer solution was determined either by high-performance liquid chromatography (HPLC) or by using ^{14}C- or ^{1}H-labeled taxol (Fig. 2). Drug loading of 20–40% showed significant release of drug measured for over 40 days, with 50–80% of the drug initially loaded in the polymer released into solution. Measurements of the intracerebral distribution of drug released from matrices implanted intracranially in rats showed a taxol concentration of 75–125 ng of taxol/mg tissue (100–150 μM taxol) and 4 ng/mg within a 2- and 8-mm radius of the disk, respectively. These concentrations are 2–3 logs higher than the 90% lethal dose (LD_{90}) values for taxol versus rat and human malignant brain tumors.

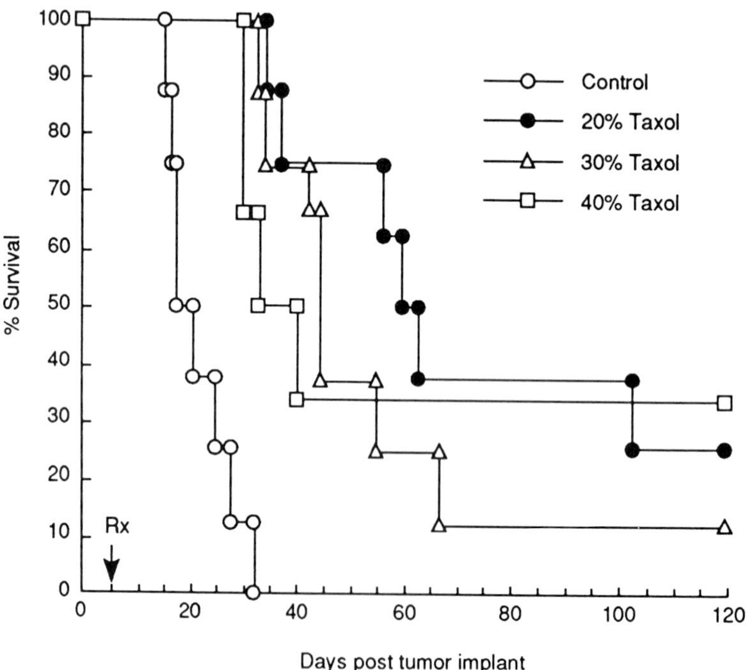

FIG. 1 Kaplan–Meier survival curves for taxol-loaded polymer disks. Rats received an intracranial 9L gliosarcoma tumor implant on day 0 and were treated on day 5 with an intratumoral implant consisting of a 10-mg disk of poly(CPP–SA) (20 : 80) implant loaded with 20, 30, or 40% taxol by weight. Control animals received a 10-mg blank polymer implant. [From Walter *et al.* (35).]

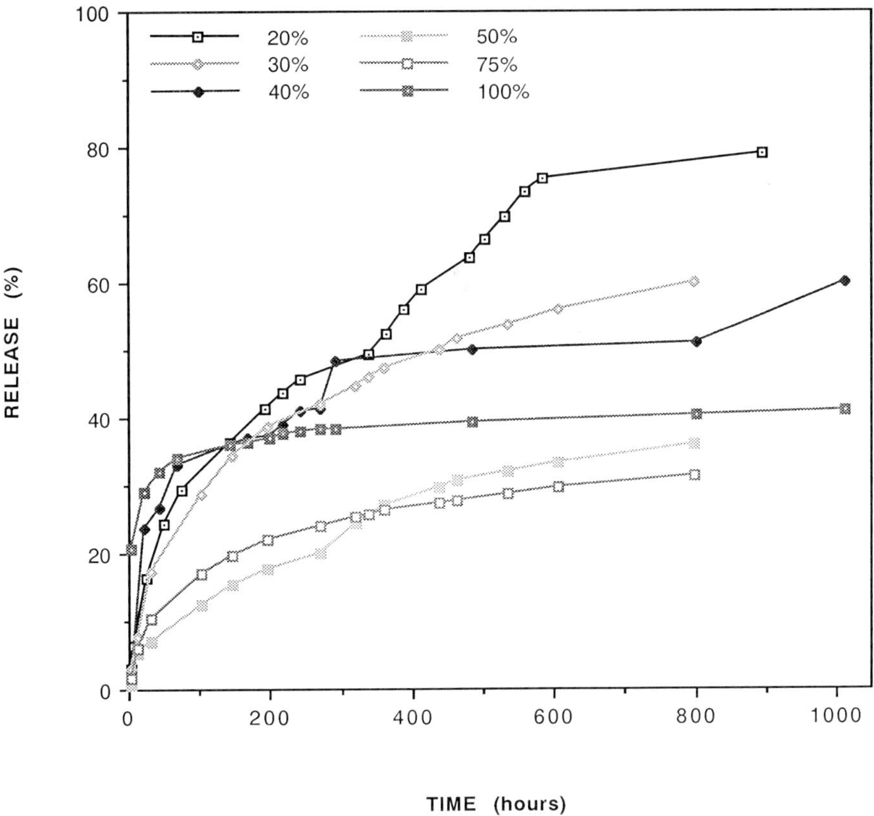

FIG. 2 *In vitro* release profiles of poly(CPP–SA) (20 : 80) loaded with 20 to 100 wt% taxol. The 100% taxol disks contained no polymer. Results are an average of three independent experiments. [From Walter *et al.* (35).]

Camptothecin, a topoisomerase I inhibitor, was tested for its local activity against brain cancer when applied by a polymer implant (36). This drug caused systemic toxicity and presented a low antitumor activity in clinical studies. It was hypothesized that local delivery would allow effective tumor concentrations without the observed systemic side effects and low activity. Systemic administration (by injection once daily for 4 days) did not extend survival compared to controls. Local delivery by polyanhydrides or EVAc extended survival and resulted in 40–70% long-term survivors. This study demonstrates that gliomas are sensitive to camptothecin and that camptothecin is effective when delivered locally.

Angiogenesis inhibitors such as heparin, cortisone, and minocycline have been tested for their activity against tumor growth when administered locally. Angiogenesis inhibition has been shown to restrict the growth of a tumor by disrupting its vascular supply (37, 38). Heparin and cortisone, delivered in a biodegradable or in a nondegradable polymer, reduced neovascularization induced by the tumor (37, 38) and retarded the growth of 9L gliosarcoma tumor implants in the rat flank.

The effect of biological response modifiers delivered locally in combination with anticancer drugs on the growth of brain tumors was studied by Weingart and Brem (39). BCNU was tested in combination with minocycline, a collagenase and angiogenesis inhibitor, in the rat brain. The combination of minocycline and BCNU delivered locally resulted in a significant extension of median survival to 56 days compared to BCNU alone (29 days) and to controls (13 days). When delivered alone either systemically or locally, minocycline had no effect on survival, which emphasizes that the combination of angiogenesis inhibitors may act synergistically with antineoplastic agents.

Delivery of Neurotransmitters and Neuromodulators

The role of neurotransmitters, neuropeptides, and neurotrophic factors in neurological disease and how they might be treated by polymeric controlled release techniques have been revealed by Byrd (17). The application of polymeric implants for treating CNS disorders has been a focus of several investigators. Implantation of drug-loaded polymeric implants directly into the brain can effectively deliver neuroactive agents to a specific location within the brain in a controlled and prolonged fashion without risk of infection due to indwelling cannulas.

The implantation of polyanhydride microspheres containing excitatory amino acids in proximity to brainstem motor nuclei has been investigated (50–52). The purpose of this investigation has been to determine the efficacy of slow-release L-glutamate to stimulate increased activity of trigeminal motoneurons and the masticatory muscles they supply, and thereby change the biomechanical forces generated by those muscles that alter growth patterns of facial, calvarial, and mandibular bones of the skull (52). Stereotactic implantation of glutamate microspheres on 33- to 38-day-old rats resulted in facial asymmetries, in which their snouts were redirected toward the side of the microsphere implant. It was concluded that the greater implant-side incisor wear was due to increased activity of implant-side masticatory muscles relative to their nonimplant side antimers. Another drug, thyrotropin-releasing hormone (TRH), is now being investigated using the same microsphere system for the regulation of mastication.

Polyanhydride microsphere systems were also used for the delivery of cholinergic agents as a potential treatment for Alzheimer's disease. Howard *et al.* (53) incorporated bethanecol, a potential cholinergic agonist, into microspheres of a polyanhydride and then implanted them into the hippocampus of rats lesioned by bilateral stereotactic fimbria–fornix transections. The animals that received the polymer containing bethanechol demonstrated a marked improvement in performance that lasted for at least 50 days.

Another polyanhydride microsphere system was developed to deliver [^{3}H]acetylcholine (ACh) to brain parenchyma (54). Drug-loaded microspheres were implanted bilaterally into the hippocampus of 25 rats, and brain sections processed for autoradiography in groups of 5 animals at 2, 5, 10, 20, and 40 days. By densitometric analysis, the concentration of radiolabeled ACh in polymer and adjacent hippocampus rapidly decreased between 2 and 5 days, after which a gradual decrease in ACh was observed for up to 40 days. The spread of labeled ACh into adjacent brain parenchyma showed a similar temporal relationship, with initially wider dispersion at 2 days, then a linear decrease in dispersion over the remaining period, suggesting bulk flow of the radiolabel into hippocampus. Brain parenchyma showed only a minimal inflammatory reaction to the polymer over all time periods.

A potential treatment for Parkinson's disease using injectable microspheres was described by Mason *et al.* (55) and McRae Deguerce *et al.* (56, 57). Parkinson's disease is characterized by a decrease both in the brain levels of dopamine and in the number of dopaminergic neurons in the brain. Dopamine was incorporated into poly(DL-lactide-coglycolide) biodegradable microspheres. The *in vitro* dopamine release from these microspheres showed a rapid release of about 90% of the loaded drug within 30 min. However, it appeared that the release *in vivo* was much slower. Rats were unilaterally lesioned in the ascending median forebrain bundle, using 6-hydroxydopamine. In these rats, a dopaminergic agonist such as apomorphine produces stereotypical turning behavior. Animals were stereotactically implanted with either dopamine-loaded or placebo microspheres in two sites in the lateral striatum. Animals implanted on the contralateral side demonstrated no turning behavior, nor did sham-operated animals implanted on the other side. However, animals implanted with dopamine polymer on the ipsilateral side demonstrated turning behavior comparable to that elicited by apomorphine, lasting for over 3 hr. It appears that direct delivery of dopamine to the brain can restore function for prolonged periods using bioerodible polymer.

Nondegradable, biocompatible EVAc matrix was used for dopamine delivery to the brain (58, 59). *In vitro* dopamine release was proportional to the square root of time. Matrices coated with a thin layer of EVAc provided a constant drug release from 15 to 50 days, depending on the initial loading of dopamine into the matrix. These matrices were implanted adjacent to the corpus striatum in rats (59). The striatal extracellular fluid concentrations of dopamine were over 200-fold greater than the control values (59). A similar dopamine–EVAc releasing system was also described by Åebischer *et al.* (60). Rods loaded with dopamine were coated with EVAc and showed a 2-week constant drug release *in vitro*. The rods were implanted in the denervated striatum of the rat and the dopamine and apomorphine levels were monitored. The results showed a significant decrease in apomorphine-induced rotational behavior in lesioned animals treated with this device. On removal of the device, the effect gradually reversed after 2 weeks and reached the preimplant control value 4 weeks after removal.

Attempts were made to use polymeric implants for brain tissue repair. In one study, cross-linked collagen sponge was used for wound healing and tissue ingrowth (61). The results show that neural tissue and elements of extracellular matrices penetrated the collagen hydrogel sponge.In another study, EVAc matrices containing nerve growth factor (NGF) were developed to provide a 1-month controlled release of NGF (62). Nerve growth factor stimulated neurite sprouting in cultured PC-12 cells, thus demonstrating the possible use of an implant in the treatment of Alzheimer's disease. Exogenous NGF has been shown to enhance the rate of regeneration and to prevent degeneration and death of the lesioned neurons (63–65). These studies have used biodegradable polyurethane-based nerve guides for bridging gaps in rat sciatic nerve. The guides were found on histological grounds to be superior to autologous nerve grafts (65). There was also an increase in the number of myelinated axons in the regenerated segment when adrenocorticotropic hormone (ACTH) was instilled in the nerve guide (65). Several other substances have been examined as factors which may enhance regeneration and functional recovery following peripheral nerve trauma. Several studies have focused on ciliary neurotropic factor (CNTF), originally isolated from chick eye extract (66). Locally applied CNTF prevented degeneration of motoneurons in the facial nucleus following facial nerve transection in neonatal rats (67).

The use of polymers for constant release of neurological peptides was demonstrated by the release of vasopressin from hollow polyethylene fibers (68, 69). Vasopressin was released for a period of 50 days *in vitro*. The device was implanted in the rat brain and released the drug for at least 1 week.

Concluding Remarks

The studies reviewed here demonstrate the usefulness of direct delivery of bioactive agents to the human brain, using biodegradable polymeric implants. Available stereotactic neurosurgery techniques combined with computerized tomography (CT) scan methods permit the accurate placement of these polymeric implants at specific locations in human patients. Several bioerodible polymer carriers including polyanhydrides and poly(lactide–glycolide) have shown good biocompatibility and biodegradability in animals and in the human brain. Bioerodible polymers are most useful for acute treatment of brain disease such as brain cancer, for which the drug is delivered for periods of several weeks to months.

References

1. L. P. Rowland, M. E. Fink, and L. Rubin, *in* "Principles of Neural Science" (E. R. Kandell, J. H. Schwartz, and T. M. Jessell, eds.), Elsevier, New York, 1991.
2. N. H. Greig, *in* "Implications of the Blood–brain Barrier and Its Manipulation" (E. A. Neuwelt, ed.), p. 311. Plenum, New York, 1989.
3. P. M. Friden, L. R. Walus, P. Watson, S. R. Doctrow, J. W. Kozarich, C. Backman, H. Bergman, B. Hoffer, F. Bloom, and A. C. Granholm, *Science* **259,** 373 (1993).
4. A. Kito, J. Yoshida, N. Kageyama, N. Kojima, and K. Yagi, *J. Neurosurg.* **71,** 382 (1989).
5. N. Bodor, *Ann. N.Y. Acad. Sci.* **507,** 289 (1987).
6. R. E. Harbaugh, R. L. Saunders, and R. Reeder, *Neurosurgery* **23,** 693 (1988).
7. V. A. Levin, C. S. Patlak, and H. D. Landahl, *J. Pharmacokinet. Biopharm.* **8,** 257 (1980).
8. D. R. Groothuis, P. C. Warkne, P. Molnar, G. D. Lapin, and M. A. Mikhael, *J. Neurosurg.* **72,** 441 (1990).
9. R. J. Tamargo and H. Brem, *Neurosurg. Q.* **2,** 259 (1992).
10. A. J. Domb, M. Maniar, and R. Langer, eds., "Absorbable Polymers for Site-Specific Drug Delivery," Spec. Issue, Vol. 3, No. 6, Wiley, Chichester, 1992.
11. A. J. Domb, S. Amselem, R. Langer, and M. Maniar, *in* "Designed to Degrade Biomedical Polymers" (S. Shalaby, ed.). Carl Hauser Verlag (in press).
12. A. J. Domb, *in* "Polymer Site-Specific Pharmacotherapy" (A. J. Domb, ed.), p. 1. Wiley, Chichester, 1994.
13. R. Langer and M. Chasin, "Polymers as Drug Delivery Systems." Dekker, New York, 1990.
14. A. J. Domb, S. Amselem, and M. Maniar, *in* "Polymeric Biomaterials" (S. Dumitriu, ed.), Ch. 13. Dekker, New York, 1993.
15. A. J. Domb, M. Maniar, S. Bogdansky and M. Chasin, *CRC Crit. Rev. Ther. Drug Carrier Syst.* **8,** 1 (1991).
16. H. Brem, K. A. Walter, R. J. Tamargo, A. Olivi, and R. Langer, *in* "Polymer Site-Specific Pharmacotherapy" (A. J. Domb, ed.), p. 117. Wiley, Chichester, 1994.
17. K. E. Byrd and E. L. Hamilton-Byrd, *in* "Polymer Site-Specific Pharmacotherapy" (A. J. Domb, ed.), p. 141. Wiley, Chichester, 1994.
18. H. Brem, K. A. Walter, and R. Langer, *Eur. J. Pharm. Biopharm.* **39,** 2 (1993).

19. G. Lapin, *in* "Polymer Site-Specific Pharmacotherapy" (A. J. Domb, ed.), p. 69. Wiley, Chichester, 1994.
20. M. W. Radomsky, *in* "Polymer Site-Specific Pharmacotherapy" (A. J. Domb, ed.) (in press).
21. W. A. Saltzman and M. W. Radomsky, *Chem. Eng. Sci.* **46,** 2429 (1991).
22. R. Katakura, T. Mori, K. Mineura, and J. Susuki, *No Shinkei Geka.* **8,** 1057 (1980).
23. R. Katakura, T. Mori, and J. Susuki, *No Shinkei Geka.* **10,** 941 (1982).
24. O. Kubo, H. Himuro, N. Inoue, Y. Tajika, *et al., No Shinkei Geka.* **14,** 1189 (1986).
25. B. Rama, T. Mandel, J. Jansen, E. Dingeldein, and H. D. Mennel, *Acta Neurochir.* **87,** 70 (1987).
26. H. Brem, A. Kader, J. I. Epstein, R. J. Tamargo, A. Domb, R. Langer, and K. Leong, *Sel. Cancer Ther.* **5,** 55 (1988).
27. H. Brem, A. J. Domb, D. Lenartz, C. Dureza, A. Olivi, and J. I. Epstein, *J. Controlled Release* **19,** 325 (1992).
28. R. J. Tamargo, J. I. Epstein, C. S. Reinhard, M. Chasin, and H. Brem, *J. Biomed. Mater. Res.* **23,** 253 (1988).
29. M. B. Yang, R. J. Tamargo, and H. Brem, *Cancer Res.* **49,** 5103 (1989).
30. L. F. Langer, H. Brem, and R. Langer, *Technol. Rev.* **63,** February/March (1991).
31. Y. Madrid, L. F. Langer, H. Brem, and R. Langer, *Adv. Pharmacol.* **22,** 299 (1991).
32. A. J. Domb, A. Olivi, K. Judy, M. L. Pinn, M. G. Ewend, J. H. Goodman, and H. Brem, *Polym. Prepr., Am. Chem. Soc., Div. Polym. Chem.* **32,** 219 (1991).
33. K. D. Judy, A. Olivi, A. J. Domb, O. M. Colvin, and H. Brem, *Congr. Neurol. Surgeons,* Orlando, FL, 1991.
34. K. G. Buahin, K. D. Judy, A. J. Domb, C. Hartke, M. Maniar, O. M. Colvin, and H. Brem, *Polym. Adv. Technol.* **3,** 311 (1992).
35. K. A. Walter, M. A. Cahan, A. Gur, B. Tyler, J. Hilton, O. M. Colvin, A. Domb, and H. Brem, *Cancer Res.* (in press).
36. J. Weingart, B. Tyler, O. M. Colvin, and H. Brem, *Drug Discovery & Dev. Symp., 3rd,* San Diego (1993).
37. C. Guerin, R. J. Tamargo, A. Olivi, and H. Brem, *in* "Angiogenesis in Health and Disease" (M. E. Maragoudakis, ed.), pp. 265–273. Plenum, New York, 1992.
38. R. J. Tamargo, R. A. Bok, and H. Brem, *Cancer Res.* **51,** 672 (1991).
39. J. Weingart and H. Brem, *Drug Discovery & Dev. Symp., 3rd,* San Diego (1993).
40. C. Laurencin and H. Elgendy, *in* "Polymer Site-Specific Pharmacotherapy" (A. J. Domb, ed.), p. 27. Wiley, Chicester, 1994.
41. A. J. Domb and S. Amselem, *in* "Polymer Site-Specific Pharmacotherapy" (A. J. Domb, ed.), p. 243. Wiley, Chichester, 1994.
42. A. J. Domb, M. Rock, C. Perkin, B. Proxap, J. G. Villemure, *Biomaterials* (in press).
43. A. J. Domb, M. Rock, C. Perkin, B. Proxap, J. G. Villemure, submitted for publication (1993).
44. A. J. Domb and R. Nudelman, *58th Annu. Meet. Isr. Chem. Soc., 1993* (1993).
45. W. Dang, O. M. Colvin, and W. M. Saltzman, *Proc. Int. Symp. Controlled. Release Bioact. Mater.* **20,** 196 (1993).

46. Y. D. Sanzgiri, C. D. Blanton, and J. M. Gallo, *Polym. Adv. Technol.* **3,** 317 (1992).
47. E. E. Hassan and J. M. Gallo, *J. Drug Targeting* **1,** 70 (1993).
48. J. Riondel, M. Jacrot, M. Fessi, and F. Puisieux, *In Vivo* **6,** 23 (1992).
49. E. K. Rowinsky, W. P. McGuire, and R. C. Donehower, *Princ. Pract. Gynecol. Oncol. Update* **1,** 1 (1993).
50. E. L. Hamilton-Byrd, A. J. Sokoloff, A. J. Domb, L. Terr, and K. E. Byrd, *Polym. Adv. Technol.* **3,** 337 (1992).
51. K. E. Byrd, A. J. Domb, A. J. Sokoloff, and E. L. Hamilton-Byrd, *Polym. Adv. Technol.* **3,** 337 (1992).
52. E. L. Hamilton-Byrd, A. J. Sokoloff, A. J. Domb, L. Terr, and K. E. Byrd, *Soc. Neurosci. Abstr.* **16,** 647 (1990).
53. M. A. Howard, A. Gross, M. S. Grady, R. Langer, E. Mathiowitz, H. R. Winn, and M. R. Mayberg, *J. Neurosurg.* **71,** 105 (1989).
54. A. S. Gross, R. Langer, E. Mathiowitz, and M. R. Mayberg, *J. Neurosurg.* (in press).
55. D. W. Mason, A. McRae-Deguerce, D. L. Dillon, R. M. Gilley, and T. R. Tice, *Proc. Int. Symp. Controlled Release Bioact. Mater.* **15,** 170 (1988).
56. A. McRae-Deguerce, D. L. Dillon, R. M. Gilley, and T. R. Tice, *Soc. Neurosci. Abstr.* **13,** 569 (1987).
57. A. McRae-Deguerce, A. Hajorth, D. L. Dillon, D. W. Mason, and T. R. Tice, *Neurosci. Lett.* **92,** 303 (1988).
58. A. Freese, B. A. Sabel, W. M. Saltzman, M. J. During, and R. Langer, *Exp. Neurol.* **103,** 234 (1989).
59. M. J. During, A. Freese, B. A. Sabel, W. M. Saltzman, A. Deutch, R. H. Roth, and R. Langer, *Ann. Neurol.* **25,** 351 (1989).
60. S. R. Winn, L. Wahlberg, P. A. Tresco, and P. Åebischer, *Exp. Neurol.* **105,** 244 (1989).
61. S. Woerly, R. Marchand, and C. Lavallee, *Biomaterials* **11,** 97 (1990).
62. E. M. Powell, M. R. Sobarzo, and W. M. Saltzman, *Brain Res.* **515,** 309 (1990).
63. J. P. Hollowell, A. Villadiego, and K. M. Rich, *Exp. Neurol.* **110,** 45 (1990).
64. H. Horie, Y. Bando, H. Chi, and T. Takenaka, *Neurosci. Lett.* **121,** 125 (1991).
65. P. H. Robinson, B. van der Lei, H. J. Hoppen, J. W. Leenslag, A. J. Pennings, and P. Nieuwenhuis, *Microsurgery* **12,** 412 (1991).
66. G. Barbin, M. Manthorpe, and S. Varon, *J. Neurochem.* **43,** 1468 (1984).
67. M. Sendtner, G. M. Kreusberg, and H. Thoenen, *Nature (London)* **345,** 440 (1990).
68. G. J. Boer, T. P. van der Woude, J. Kruisbrink, and J. van Heerikhuize, *J. Neurosci. Methods* **11,** 281 (1984).
69. G. J. Boer and J. Kruisbrink, *Biomaterials* **8,** 265 (1987).

Section V

Using Pump Delivery Devices within the Brain

[11] Using Osmotic Minipumps for Intracranial Delivery of Amino Acids and Peptides

Jeffrey D. White and Michael W. Schwartz

Concomitant with the revolution in molecular biological techniques applied to neurobiology has come an ever-increasing appreciation of the roles that peptides and amino acids play in the development, maintenance, and function of the nervous system. For example, the nerve growth factor family of neurotrophins, insulin and the insulin-like growth factors, fibroblast growth factor, and transforming growth factors are all known to play an integral role in both the developing nervous system and in adults. Amino acids, or their derivatives, are implicated as the "fast" or "classic" transmitter in most central nervous system (CNS) synapses and disturbances of transmission in these systems are associated with diseases ranging from excitotoxicity to depression. Similarly, it is now understood that colocalization of one or more neuropeptides with a classic transmitter is the norm rather than the exception in CNS neurons. Because virtually all neuropeptide receptors (apart from growth factor receptors) belong to the G protein-linked superfamily of receptors, neuropeptides can modulate intracellular protein kinase signaling cascades as well as influence neuronal excitability by altering conductance properties of ion channels. Thus, from this brief introduction it should be apparent that any understanding of the functions of and interactions between cells in the central nervous system must involve studies of peptides and amino acids.

For the investigator interested in peptide or amino acid neurobiology *in vivo,* it is important to optimize the approach to studying and/or perturbing these systems. How does one introduce peptides, amino acids, or pharmacological agents for their receptors into the CNS? One option is the peripheral administration of a particular compound. The existence of saturable blood–brain barrier (BBB) transport systems for amino acids is well documented and it appears that there are also saturable transport systems for some peptides [see Section III of this volume, and Schwartz *et al.* (1)]; however, some compounds do not pass and the extent to which these systems are effective for most peptides is unclear. Moreover, it is not always experimentally desirable or economically feasible to administer peptides peripherally in doses that are sufficient to achieve pharmacological activity centrally. Therefore, it is necessary to devise a method for introducing these compounds directly into the brain. To this end, osmotic minipump delivery systems have been used successfully for over 15 years for direct administration of peptides and amino acids into the brain. In this chapter we summarize the experiences from our laboratories and review the work of others in which osmotic minipumps have been used to infuse peptides, amino acids, and drugs through indwelling cannulas into the cerebral ventricles or into specific CNS tissue sites. In the course of these discussions we emphasize technical considerations for using minipump delivery systems and highlight potential limitations, pitfalls, and controls to consider when using these systems.

Intracerebroventricular Injection versus Microinjection into Brain

General Considerations

Brain Interstitial Fluid and Cerebrospinal Fluid Formation and Movement
Early investigators believed the blood–brain barrier to be impermeable to virtually all solutes, and the cerebrospinal fluid (CSF) to be the principal vehicle for nutrient delivery to the brain (2). A common misconception stemming from this belief was that brain interstitial fluid (ISF) is derived from CSF, and that intracerebroventricular (icv) administration results in effective distribution of a drug throughout the brain. It is now evident, however, that circulating nutrients are provided to the CNS principally via transport across the BBB endothelium, and that CSF, in fact, is a relatively ineffective vehicle for solute delivery to many brain areas. Moreover, brain ISF and CSF differ in their origin, nutrient and electrolyte content, pattern of flow, and clearance mechanisms. These considerations emphasize the important differences in distribution of agents following icv administration versus direct infusion into brain tissue.

The microvasculature of the CNS is characterized by an endothelium with many unique features. First, the barrier function of brain vasculature is attributable to the extensive network of tight junctions (zonula occludens) that characterize this endothelium (3). Second, the many nutrient transport systems (e.g., glucose and amino acid transporters) expressed by brain microvascular endothelium are vital to the normal functioning of neural and glial elements within the CNS (4, 5). The formation of brain ISF represents a third specialized feature of the BBB endothelium (6). Once formed, brain ISF flows along perivascular interstitial channels, ultimately draining into cervical lymphatics, with a small fraction entering the CSF (7, 8).

This pattern of brain ISF production, flow, and removal is distinctive, having little in common with the movement of CSF. In contrast to brain ISF, CSF formation occurs largely within the choroid plexus (9, 10). This specialized organ, composed of a vascular tuft invested by a tightly opposed epithelium (the "blood–CSF barrier"), is present in lateral, third, and fourth cerebral ventricles. The CSF formed at the choroid plexus is the product of an energy-dependent secretory process (11). A smaller contribution to CSF formation is provided by bulk movement of ISF out of the brain and into subarachnoid and ventricular CSF (12). It is noteworthy that solute concentrations are not in equilibrium between brain ISF and CSF; rather, there is a net movement of most solutes from brain ISF to CSF down a concentration gradient, and few solutes are delivered to the brain via the CSF under physiological circumstances. Once formed, CSF flows about the subarachnoid and ventricular surfaces of the brain in a rostral-to-caudal direction (13), and is removed principally across arachnoid villi that project into venous sinuses draining the brain.

Solute Removal from Cerebrospinal Fluid

That CSF volume and pressure remain constant over time reflects the equal rates at which CSF formation and removal occur. In the rat, this rate represents a complete turnover of the CSF volume (0.15 ml) every 1–2 hr, such that the half-life of most CSF solutes is ~0.75 hr (9). Cerebrospinal fluid removal occurs via bulk flow, and solutes are generally cleared from CSF with the same rate constant regardless of size. Exceptions to this rule include certain neuropeptides and neurotransmitters, for which high-affinity receptors or enzymatic clearance mechanisms are present on the surface of the brain. In such cases, clearance from CSF may occur much more rapidly. Angiotensin II, for example, has a CSF half-life of <1 min, owing to enzymatic degradation (14).

Sink Action of Cerebrospinal Fluid and Solute Diffusion into Brain Tissue

What, then, is the fate of intraventricularly administered peptides and amino acids? The rapid rate of bulk flow CSF turnover relative to the rate of diffusion of solutes from CSF into the brain creates a "sink effect" (9), which has important consequences for intraventricularly administered agents. Because CSF-borne solutes penetrate brain tissue by diffusion, the efficacy of the intraventricular route of administration is critically dependent on the distance of the target site within the brain from the ventricular or subarachnoid surface (6). Because the CSF-to-brain concentration ratio falls exponentially with increasing distance from the ependymal surface of the brain, it is now clear that many brain areas are exposed to trivial fractions of CSF solute concentrations. In addition to distance from the CSF, other factors that limit solute penetration from CSF to brain include high molecular size, sequestration and/or inactivation by brain cells, and high permeability across cell membranes, which result in more rapid solute clearance from

CSF into the circulation (6). In the case of biologically active peptides, it is estimated that structures located >1 mm from CSF are exposed to levels that may be <0.1% of the CSF concentration (6). Even if this estimate is inaccurate by an order of magnitude, it is clear that during icv administration, pharmacological levels of peptides must be present in CSF to provide physiological concentrations in many brain regions.

The above considerations influence not only the level of a CSF-borne peptide or amino acid to which a given brain area is exposed, but also the time necessary for this exposure to occur. The time interval required for a peptide to travel from CSF to a given brain area is determined by the same factors that influence its concentration in brain tissue; for example, the distance from the ependymal surface and the diffusability of the agent. Whereas sodium diffuses 3 mm in <1.5 hr, for example, albumin requires more than a day to travel the same distance (6). It may be anticipated, therefore, that if the efficacy of a large peptide hinges on delivery to a brain area situated at a considerable distance from the CSF (e.g., deep within the cerebral cortex or caudate nucleus), several hours may pass following icv administration before any exposure to the peptide occurs. Conversely, agents that elicit a rapid response on icv injection (e.g., angiotensin II-induced drinking behavior) may be safely assumed to be acting at a site near the ependymal surface of the brain.

Implications for Efficacy of Intracerebroventricular Delivery versus Microinjection

The preceding discussion of fluids and their movements in the CNS emphasizes both the limited distribution of peptides and amino acids following icv administration and the nonphysiological nature of this approach. As highlighted by Pardridge (6), in order to achieve significant peptide concentrations in brain tissue 2 mm removed from CSF, the required CSF concentration could result in blood levels that paradoxically exceed those achieved in brain.

Despite these limitations, the icv route has proved useful in the hands of many. Third ventricular infusion of insulin in the rat, for example, results in reduced food intake (15) and altered neuropeptide gene expression within the hypothalamic arcuate nucleus (1, 16) at doses that do not significantly affect circulating insulin or glucose levels (<3 mU/24 hr). This outcome may reflect the close proximity of the arcuate nucleus to the ependyma of the third ventricle, which facilitates exposure to insulin during intraventricular infusion. Nonetheless, the observation that direct intrahypothalamic insulin infusion yields comparable effects on food intake at doses two to three orders of magnitude lower than those required during icv infusion reiterates the nonphysiological nature of the icv route for administering peptides to the brain.

In contrast to the icv method, administration of peptides or amino acids directly into brain by either microinjection or continuous infusion reliably yields high local concentrations in the area surrounding the injection site. The injection volume impacts significantly on the radius of drug distribution about the injection site. For studies involving brain areas where many sensitive structures reside in close proximity to one another, small injection volumes are critical for mapping responses to peptides. For example, Stanley has reported orexigenic effects of neuropeptide Y to be highly localized within the rat hypothalamus (17) by using microinjection volumes of 10 nl, rather than the larger volumes (500 nl) traditionally used. Microinjection of this smaller volume limited distribution of the peptide to within 0.8 mm of the injection site. Moreover, although more technically demanding, this approach evidently facilitated identification of discretely responsive hypothalamic areas undetected in previous studies using larger injection volumes.

Minipump Delivery Systems

Advantages and Disadvantages

As with any experimental system, there are benefits and limitations to the use of osmotic minipump delivery paradigms. Foremost among the advantages is that a substance can be administered with no intervention from the investigator or disturbance to the animal once the pump has been implanted. This implies that all treatments can be performed on conscious, freely moving animals. Obviously, this is a requirement for any behavioral study (e.g., feeding, reproductive, or learning paradigms), but is also advantageous for *in vivo* studies in general because stress of handling is minimized. In addition, long-term studies are facilitated by minipump systems and help eliminate variables such as different injection times, depending on the investigator's schedule and different skills in administering compounds by different laboratory workers. Furthermore, continuous infusion avoids peaks and troughs of concentrations of administered agents, so that a steady state concentration can be achieved. Last, minipump infusions can generally be accomplished with a minimum of tissue damage at the site of cannula placement.

There are also several limitations to minipump infusions that must be considered carefully. In prolonged infusion paradigms it must be determined that the peptide, amino acid, or pharmacological agent to be infused is stable at 37°C for the period of the experiment. Thus, preliminary experiments must be conducted in which the compound to be infused is incubated at 37°C for an appropriate period, after which its chemical identity or biological activity verified. Similarly, a common problem for peptides is precipitation at concentrations used for infusion when stored in saline or artificial CSF. Therefore, at the end of the infusion period it is important to verify the concentration and biological activity of the peptide in the infusate, e.g., by radioimmunoassay (RIA) or bioassay.

The minipump paradigm is not totally intervention free because minor surgery is required at the time of pump implantation. Thus, although usually not a problem in rodents, investigators must monitor animals for signs of infection and stress as the result of surgery and must allow sufficient time for the animal to recover from effects of anesthesia before beginning an experiment. It is important to carry out parallel experiments with animals receiving infusion only of vehicle to control for effects that are due solely to pump or cannula implantation or vehicle infusion. When infusions are performed directly into brain tissue, it is also important to verify the extent of any tissue damage due to the infusion. Thus, in behavioral paradigms, microscopic analysis of the infusion site should be performed at the end of the experiment. In experiments in which such post hoc analysis is not possible, for example, when the end point is the assay of brain tissue extracts, preliminary or parallel experiments should be performed in which microscopic analysis is performed on similarly cannulated and infused tissue. Some authors have found that in prolonged perfusion paradigms, pump-derived cytotoxins reach concentrations sufficient to ablate a area of tissue 1–3 mm in diameter (18). This difficulty does not appear to represent a significant problem in shorter term experiments and may be obviated in long-term experiments by modifications to the minipumps to reduce flow rates [see Hagg, this volume, and Hagg *et al.* (19)]. Yet another concern is that infusion paradigms are rarely ideal in that icv peptide infusions may have limited delivery to the brain area of interest (see above) or, conversely, may exert nonspecific or confounding effects on brain structures unrelated to the hypothesis being tested. On the other hand, direct tissue infusion is limited in its effectiveness by the degree of diffusion from the tissue site, so that the concentration of infused agent will fall off as an exponential function of the distance from the infusion site. For small brain areas such as hypothalamic nuclei, this latter concern is usually not a problem but in larger brain areas such as cortex or hippocampus, experiments must be confined to the region of diffusion. For example, Kasamatsu *et al.* (20) estimated a 500-fold dilution of infused agent at a 3-mm distance from the infusion cannula. For a discussion of methods to determine tissue concentrations of infused agent, the reader is referred to the section Practical Considerations, below.

The continuous nature of minipump infusion can also be problematic because a variety of neuronal and neuroendocrine systems are believed to be regulated in a pulsatile fashion. Therefore, continuous infusion would not mimic the true *in vivo* nature of peptide or amino acid interaction in that system. This difficulty has been addressed by some authors by filling tubing alternately with a dose of drug to be infused separated by a small volume of air. This paradigm is applicable when pulses occur over 1- to 2-hr time spans but would be unsuitable for circadian-type experiments. These latter experiments would require that infusion in the intervening time be with vehicle that could be separated from agent by a small air pocket. Again, in using any type of pulsatile infusion paradigm it would be necessary to verify that air infusion did not lead to significant tissue damage.

Last, investigators must be cognizant of the potential for infusion failure either due to an occluded cannula (see below) or minipump failure. In long-term studies, it is simple to remove any remaining fluid from the pump chamber and determine that the volume remaining corresponds to the initial volume added minus the volume calculated to be delivered. In short-term experiments in which infusion is performed for only a few hours, it is often desirable to load the agent to be infused into polyethylene (PE) tubing (rather than directly into the minipump), then load the minipump with saline containing a dye such as bromophenol blue. Successful infusion is then verified when the blue dye is pumped into the PE tubing to displace the infusate. Knowing the distance the dye is pumped into the tubing and the volume of the tubing, one can easily determine if the desired volume of infusate was delivered.

Examples

Examples of studies in which osmotic minipumps have been used to deliver peptides, amino acids, or associated drugs are given in Table I. Even in this abbreviated list, it can be seen that minipump delivery systems have been used successfully to address numerous neurobiological problems with a variety of agents.

Practical Considerations for Cannulation and Minipump Use

Procedure for Third Ventricular Cannulation and Minipump Placement in Rat

We prefer to induce and maintain general anesthesia via inhalation of halothane vaporized with 100% oxygen, as it affords minute-to-minute control

TABLE I Peptides, Amino Acids, and Drugs Infused Using Osmotic Minipumps

Compound infused[a]	Site	Experimental paradigm	References[b]
Insulin	icv	Feeding	1, 2
	icv	Feeding, gene expression	3
Nerve growth factor	Hippocampus	Reinnervation	4
	icv	Memory	5
Fibroblast growth factor		Cell death	6
Horseradish peroxidase	Lateral geniculate	Cell labeling	7
Neuropeptide Y	icv	Feeding	8
Corticotropin-releasing factor	icv	Feeding, obesity	9, 10
Cholecystokinin	icv	Feeding	11
Leupeptin	icv	Long-term potentiation	12
Angiotensin II, III	icv	Blood pressure	13
Neurotensin, substance P, TRH	icv	Dopamine receptor regulation	14
Enkephalin, β-endorphin, morphine	icv	Dependence	15
Interleukin 3	icv	Trophic factor	16
Glucose	icv	Feeding	17, 18
Glutamate, aspartate, GABA	Striatum, hippocampus		19
GABA	Visual cortex		20
APV	Visual cortex	Cortical plasticity	21
Ibotenic acid	Visual cortex	Lesion mapping	22
Dopamine, dopamine agonist	icv	Experimental parkinsonism	23
MPP^+	Substantia nigra	Experimental parkinsonism	24
Norepinephrine	Visual cortex	Cortical plasticity	25, 26
	Hypothalamus	Feeding	27

Histamine	Suprachiasmatic nucleus	Feeding	28
$[^3H]$Pro, -Leu	Hypothalamus, striatum	Peptide biosynthesis	29, 30
$[^{35}S]$Met, -Cys	Hypothalamus, hippocampus, striatum	Peptide biosynthesis	30–32
Morphine	icv	Pulsed delivery	33

[a] TRH, Thyrotropin-releasing hormone; GABA, γ-aminobutyric acid; APV, 2-amino-5-phosphonovaleric acid; MPP^+, *N*-methyl-4-phenylpyridinium cation.

[b] Key to references: (1) H. Ikeda, D. B. West, J. J. Pustek, D. P. Figlewicz, M. R. Greenwood, D. Porte, Jr., and S. C. Woods, *Appetite* **7,** 381 (1986); (2) K. Nagai, T. Mori, T. Nishio, and H. Nakagawa, *Biomed. Res.* **3,** 175 (1982); (3) M. W. Schwartz, A. J. Sipols, J. L. Marks, G. Sanacora, J. D. White, A. Scheurink, S. E. Kahn, D. G. Baskin, S. C. Woods, D. P. Figlewicz, and D. Porte, Jr., *Endocrinology (Baltimore)* **130,** 3608 (1992); (4) T. Hagg, H. L. Vahlsing, M. Manthorpe, and S. Varon, *J. Neurosci.* **10,** 3087 (1990); (5) W. Fisher, A. Bjorklund, and F. H. Gage, *J. Neurosci.* **11,** 1889 (1991); (6) K. J. Anderson, D. Dam, S. Lee, and C. W. Cotman, *Nature (London)* **332,** 360 (1988); (7) A. J. Weber and R. E. Kalil, *J. Comp. Neurol.* **220,** 336 (1983); (8) B. Beck, A. Stricker-Krongrad, J.-P. Nicolas, and C. Burlet, *Int. J. Obesity* **16,** 295 (1992); (9) F. Rohner-Jeanrenaud, C.-D. Walker, R. Grecco-Perotto, and B. Jeanrenaud, *Endocrinology (Baltimore)* **124,** 733 (1989); (10) K. Arase, N. S. Shargill, and G. A. Bray, *Am. J. Physiol.* **256,** R751 (1989); (11) R. R. Schick, C. W. Stevens, T. L. Yaksh, and V. L. W. Go, *Brain Res.* **448,** 294 (1988); (12) U. Staubli, J. Larson, O. Thibault, M. Baudry, and G. Lynch, *Brain Res.* **444,** 153 (1988); (13) K. Katahira, H. Mikami, T. Ogihara, K. Kohara, A. Otsuka, Y. Kumahara, and M. C. Khosla, *Am. J. Physiol.* **256,** H1 (1989); (14) S. M. Simasko and G. A. Weiland, *Eur. J. Pharmacol.* **106,** 653 (1984); (15) E. Wei and H. Loh, *Science* **193,** 1262 (1976); (16) M. Kamegai, K. Niijima, T. Kunishita, M. Nishizawa, M. Ogawa, M. Araki, A. Ueki, Y. Konishi, and T. Tabira, *Neuron* **2,** 429 (1990); (17) J. D. Davis, D. Wirtshafter, K. E. Asin, and D. Brief, *Science* **212,** 81 (1981); (18) J. Panksepp and J. Rossi, III, *Behav. Brain Res.* **3,** 381 (1981); (19) R. M. Mangano and R. Schwarcz, *Brain Res. Bull.* **10,** 47 (1983); (20) S. Brailowsky, C. Silva-Barrat, C. Menini, D. Riche, and R. Naquet, *Electroencephalogr. Clin. Neurophysiol.* **72,** 147 (1989); (21) M. F. Bear, A. Kleinschmidt, Q. Gu, and W. Singer, *J. Neurosci.* **10,** 909 (1990); (22) M. R. Dursteler, R. H. Würtz, and W. T. Newsome, *J. Neurophysiol.* **57,** 1262 (1987); (23) J. G. de Yebenes, S. Fahn, V. Jackson-Lewis, P. Jorge, M. A. Mena, and J. Reiriz, *J. Neural Transm.* **27,** suppl., 141 (1988); (24) D. J. S. Sirinathsinghji, R. P. Heavens, S. J. Richards, I. J. M. Beresford, and M. D. Hall, *Neuroscience* **27,** 117 (1988); (25) J. D. Pettigrew and T. Kasamatsu, *Nature (London)* **271,** 761 (1978); (26) T. Kasamatsu, T. Itakura, and G. Jonsson, *J. Pharmacol. Exp. Ther.* **217,** 841 (1981); (27) T. Shimazu, M. Noma, and M. Saito, *Brain Res.* **369,** 215 (1986); (28) N. Itowi, K. Nagai, H. Nakagawa, T. Watanabe, and H. Wada, *Physiol. Behav.* **44,** 221 (1988); (29) J. E. Krause, J. P. Advis, and J. F. McKelvy, *Endocrinology (Baltimore)* **111,** 344 (1982); (30) J. E. Krause, A. J. Reiner, J. P. Advis, and J. F. McKelvy, *J. Neurosci.* **4,** 775 (1984); (31) J. D. White, J. E. Krause, and J. F. McKelvy, *J. Neurosci.* **4,** 1262 (1984); (32) J. D. White, C. M. Gall, and J. F. McKelvy, *Proc. Natl. Acad. Sci. U.S.A.* **83,** 7099 (1986); (33) V. C. Rayner, I. C. A. F. Robinson, and J. A. Russell, *J. Physiol. (London)* **396,** 319 (1988).

over the anesthesia level and facilitates rapid postoperative recovery, although other methods may be used effectively.

Cannulation of the third ventricle is described here in detail. The first step is to insert a guide sleeve; the cannula itself is inserted through the guide sleeve at the time of pump implantation. Our method calls for stereotaxic insertion of a 22-gauge stainless steel guide sleeve (model C313G; Plastics One, Roanoke, VA) through the midline of the brain into the third ventricle. The coordinates are calculated as follows: the anterior–posterior (A–P) coordinate is calculated as 0.20 times the difference between the bregma A–P and the interaural (IA) line A–P coordinates. The dorsal–ventral (D–V) coordinate is calculated as 0.68 times the difference between the superior sagittal sinus D–V and the IA line D–V coordinates. Following the removal of a small (0.625 cm^2) piece of overlying skull, the cannula guide sleeve is inserted through the sagittal midline of the brain after visualizing and gently retracting the superior sagittal sinus. The guide sleeve is then fixed into place with dental acrylic and the overlying skin sutured to enclose all but the proximal 1 cm of the guide sleeve. An obturator is inserted at the conclusion of the surgical procedure and maintained in position during the subsequent recovery period.

After at least 1 week of postoperative recovery, the animals should be ready for entry into a study protocol. Animals are lightly reanesthetized, using halothane prior to surgical implantation of the osmotic minipump into the interscapular subcutaneous space. Prior to implantation, the osmotic minipump (model 2001; Alzet, Palo Alto, CA) and connecting PE tubing are primed by submersion in isotonic saline for 12 hr at room temperature. It is important to realize that icv infusion (and hence the study protocol) begins immediately on connection of the PE tubing from the primed pump to the infusion cannula (model C313, 26 gauge; Plastics One), which is inserted into the guide sleeve. To minimize variability in measured parameters on initiation of the study protocol, it is essential to minimize surgical and anesthetic stress at the time of pump implantation.

Dosing calculations are based on the desired infusion rate, which has been standardized at 1 μl/hr at 37°C for most products. Therefore, if one desires a continuous infusion of a peptide at a rate of 1 μg/hr, the pump should be filled (usual pump volume is 200 μl) with a solution containing 1 μg/μl of the peptide of interest.

Verifying Cannula Placement and Patency

Correct placement of the cannula can be assessed in two ways prior to pump implantation. The first is simply to look for reflux of CSF following insertion of the infusion cannula, which is evident in the majority of successful cannulations. The second approach is to inject angiotensin II through the infusion cannula (30 ng in 3 μl of saline) in the unanesthetized rat and monitor for a drinking response (>5 ml in 30 min) (21). This drinking response is transient, as angiotensin II has an extremely short half-life, and adverse effects have not been observed in our hands with this approach. In general, we find this test to be both specific and sensitive for establishing intraventricular location of the cannula prior to study, although quantitative data are not available.

At the time of sacrifice, patency of the infusion system and verification of cannula placement may be confirmed by injection of methylene blue dye (5 μl) through the PE tubing and internal cannula, and into the third ventricle. Resistance to flow indicates obstruction of the infusion system; if there is no resistance to flow, but blue staining does not appear in the third ventricle (which can be determined by visual examination of the ventral surface of the brain), cannulation of the third ventricle was likely unsuccessful. This staining procedure does not interfere with histochemical methods such as *in situ* hybridization. However, such a lack of interference should be confirmed for more specialized anatomical analyses. Finally, assay of CSF sampled from the cisterna magna at the time of sacrifice for determination of the level of infused peptide or amino acid may help to verify successful infusion. However, cisternal levels of biologically active peptides may not be in equilibrium with levels present in the third ventricle, if CSF clearance occurs independent of bulk flow. Nonetheless, cisternal levels should be higher in experimental animals receiving icv peptide infusion than in vehicle-treated controls.

Estimates of Tissue Concentrations Using Radiolabeled Compounds

For some studies, in which compounds are infused directly, it may be critically important to derive an estimate of the tissue concentration of the infused amino acid, peptide, or homologous drug, for example, to demonstrate that a peptide produces physiological effects in the concentration range that is optimal for specific receptor interaction. Bear *et al.* (18) have effectively approached this problem by coinfusion of tracer amounts of labeled APV (an *N*-methyl-D-aspartate [NMDA] receptor antagonist) and experimentally relevant amounts of unlabeled APV. At the end of the infusion period, the animal is deeply anesthetized, and the brain is then exposed and frozen *in situ,* using liquid nitrogen. The brain is then removed as rapidly as possible and, with as little thawing as practical, 500-μm tissue sections are prepared from the region surrounding the infusion site, using a McIlwain tissue chopper. Each slice is placed into 1 ml of water and sonicated to disrupt the tissue. One-half of the sonicate is removed for protein content determination and from the protein content an estimate of tissue wet weight is derived.

(Preliminary control experiments using noninfused tissue permit a wet weight determination to be made prior to sonication, which is then correlated with protein content to allow derivation of wet weight per milligram protein from infused tissue.) The remaining sonicate is then used for determination of total radioactivity and, knowing the specific activity of the total labeled and unlabeled compound infused, a value for nanomoles of compound per milligram tissue (wet weight) is derived.

The value derived for tissue radioactivity (or nanomoles of compound) per milligram tissue (wet weight) represents the combination of free extracellular compound, receptor-bound compound, and, perhaps, internalized compound or radioactivity. It therefore becomes necessary to construct a standard curve in which tissue radioactivity can be related to the extracellular level of compound. This standard curve can be constructed by incubating tissue slices in known concentrations of labeled compound. After determining the length of time for tissue radioactivity levels to stabilize, which may be as long as 12–18 hr, it is then known that the free extracellular concentration of labeled compound is equal to the bath concentration. The slices are then removed, filtered rapidly with nylon mesh to remove the bath radioactivity and tissue protein, and radioactivity levels determined as above. By incubating tissue slices in a range of radiolabeled compound concentrations, it is possible to construct a standard curve for nanomoles of compound per milligram tissue protein (or wet weight) vs extracellular compound concentration. From this standard curve, the value derived for nanomoles of infused compound per milligram tissue (wet weight) is used to calculate free extracellular concentrations of infused compound.

This method can be used to derive an estimation for extracellular tissue concentrations of infused drugs as a function of distance from the cannulation site or in a given brain region following icv infusion. For either icv or direct infusion, this determination relies on the infusion time being of sufficient duration for the tissue concentration of the infused compound to reach equilibrium. For shorter duration infusions, the derived tissue concentration will not be absolutely accurate but nevertheless will yield a rough estimation of concentrations for the investigator. A second, and significant, caveat to this method is that it is optimally suited for drugs that are not significantly metabolized by brain tissue. If this method is to be used for determining local peptide concentrations, the initial experiments using brain slices must also include a method such as high-performance liquid chromatography purification of radiolabeled peptide at the end of the incubation period to determine what fraction of radioactivity represents intact peptide. Naturally, with a steady state bath incubation method, the peptide will achieve an equilibrium in which the total tissue radioactivity represents the balance between diffusion of peptide into the tissue from the bath and the sum of extracellular intact peptide, extracellular degraded peptide, receptor-bound peptide, and internalized peptide. When the amount of intact peptide radioactivity is determined and compared to total tissue radioactivity, this same ratio can then be applied to values derived from infusion experiments (provided they are of sufficient duration to estimate a steady state reasonably). This method should not be used for radiolabeled amino acids, the incorporation of which into protein yields an additional difficulty in interpretation.

Summary

Osmotic minipump delivery systems can be designed to deliver virtually any compound into the CNS via indwelling cannulas for administration via the CSF or into specific tissue sites. When used with appropriate care and recognizing the limitations to conclusions derived from the data obtained, these systems can be used to approach a wide variety of behavioral, physiological, and biochemical questions.

Acknowledgments

This work was supported by Grants NIMH MH42074 and NSF BNS 9007573 to J.D.W. J.D.W. is the recipient of a Research Scientist Development Award from NIMH. M.W.S. is the recipient of a Career Development Award from the Veterans Administration and a Research Associate of the Department of Veterans Affairs.

References

1. M. W. Schwartz, D. P. Figlewicz, D. G. Baskin, S. C. Woods, and D. Porte, Jr., *Endocr. Rev.* **13,** 387 (1992).
2. L. Stern and R. Gautier, *Arch. Intern. Physiol.* **17,** 391 (1922).
3. M. W. B. Bradbury, *Cir. Res.* **57,** 213 (1985).
4. C. Crone, *J. Physiol.* (*London*) **181,** 103 (1965).
5. Q. R. Smith, *in* "Implications of the Blood–Brain Barrier and Its Manipulation" (E. Neuwelt, ed.), p. 85. Plenum, New York, 1990.
6. W. M. Pardridge, "Peptide Drug Delivery to the Brain," p. 111. Raven Press, New York, 1991.
7. M. W. B. Bradbury, H. F. Cserr, and R. J. Westrop, *Am. J. Physiol.* **240,** F329 (1981).
8. H. F. Cserr, D. N. Cooper, and P. K. Suri, *Am. J. Physiol.* **240,** F319 (1981).
9. H. Davson, "Physiology of the Cerebrospinal Fluid," p. 55. Churchill, London, 1967.

10. C. E. Johanson, *in* "Neuromethods: The Neuronal Microenvironment" (A. A. Boulton, G. B. Baker, and W. Walz, eds.), p. 33. Humana Press, Clifton, NJ, 1988.
11. H. Davson, K. Welch, and M. B. Segal, "The Physiology and Pathophysiology of the Cerebrospinal Fluid," p. 201. Churchill-Livingstone, London, 1987.
12. G. A. Rosenberg, "Brain Fluids and Metabolism." Oxford Univ. Press, New York, 1990.
13. R. A. Fishman, "Cerebrospinal Fluid in Diseases of the Nervous System." Saunders, Philadelphia, 1980.
14. J. W. Harding, M. S. Yoshida, R. P. Dilts, T. M. Woods, and J. W. Wright, *J. Neurochem.* **46,** 1292 (1986).
15. H. Ikeda, D. B. West, J. J. Pustek, D. P. Figelwicz, M. R. Greenwood, D. Porte, Jr., and S. C. Woods, *Appetite* (*London*) **7,** 381 (1986).
16. M. W. Schwartz, A. J. Sipols, J. L. Marks, G. Sanacora, J. D. White, A. Scheurink, S. E. Kahn, D. G. Baskin, S. C. Woods, D. P. Figlewicz, and D. Porte, Jr., *Endocrinology* (*Baltimore*) **130,** 3608 (1992).
17. B. G. Stanley, W. Magdalin, A. Seirafi, W. J. Thomas, and S. F. Leibowitz, *Brain Res.* **604,** 304 (1993).
18. M. F. Bear, A. Kleinschmidt, Q. Gu, and W. Singer, *J. Neurosci.* **10,** 909 (1990).
19. T. Hagg, H. L. Vahlsing, M. Manthorpe, and S. Varon, *J. Neurosci.* **10,** 3087 (1990).
20. T. Kasamatsu, T. Itakura, and G. Jonsson, *J. Pharmacol. Exp. Ther.* **217,** 841 (1981).
21. A. Johnson and A. Epstein, *Brain Res.* **86,** 399 (1975).

[12] Continuous Central Nervous System Infusion with Alzet Osmotic Pumps

Theo Hagg

Introduction

Treatment of human central nervous system (CNS) disorders and investigation of neurobiological questions in experimental animals require in many cases the establishment of a therapeutic concentration of an agent in the CNS itself. As described in other chapters of this volume, several approaches are considered to reach that goal. Direct intra-CNS delivery by invasive cannulation may be the method of choice in many experimental paradigms and also for select human conditions. Proteins usually cannot cross the blood–brain barrier unless it is breeched (see elsewhere in this volume). Perhaps more importantly, intracerebral or intraspinal administration allows the establishment of high concentrations in particular regions of the CNS, which is especially useful for agents that have peripheral or systemic actions and could cause general negative side effects. Moreover, in experimental investigations, intra-CNS administration can establish whether an agent acts directly in the CNS and not through their peripheral action, that is, through induction of different or modified agents (in liver, kidney, etc.) that in turn affect the CNS. Another indication for the use of direct intra-CNS administration is the possibility to vary agents and/or concentrations in time, including the termination of the treatment, in contrast to some other treatment strategies.

The rationale for continuous infusions rather than repeated injections for long-term treatments is that more stable and higher concentration can be reached and that fewer interventions are involved in the treatment. On the other hand, repeated injections are essential for labile substances, which would be degraded in an implanted container (pump). Substances could be injected repeatedly into a pump reservoir with an interval that is consistent with their half-life. One type of pump that has proved especially useful for animal experimentation is the Alzet osmotic pump (Alza Corporation, Palo Alto, CA).

This chapter is based on work in the University of California, San Diego (La Jolla, CA)-based neurobiology research group, which has included at different times investigators such as L. R. Williams, M. Manthorpe, S. Varon, H. L. Vahlsing, and myself. We have over many years developed

Methods in Neurosciences, Volume 21

the continuous infusion technique to a state-of-the art method suitable for routine use. The detailed description of the procedures and some of the background or underlying theoretical considerations was chosen to facilitate the startup procedure for novices, as well as to provide helpful hints to the experts. This chapter emphasizes the use of custom-made infusion devices and all measurements are for adult rats. We have found that the effort to establish this refined and apparently cumbersome technique is rewarded by overall better experimental results and the ability to design and execute experiments that would otherwise not have been possible.

Construction of Infusion Devices

The Alza Corporation produces CNS infusion kits that consist of a metal cannula (0.36-mm diameter), plastic rings that allow cannula placement up to 5 mm at incremental 0.5-mm depths into the brain, and a line that connects the cannula to the osmotic pumps. These infusion kits have been successfully used by many investigators to administer agents into the brain.

The rest of this section describes the construction of custom-made devices [a more detailed description is available from the author; see also Vahlsing *et al.* (1)]. In short, the infusion device consists of a metal or polyvinyl cannula of variable length, which is connected to the pump by a coiled line reservoir that contains the fluid to be infused (infusate) (Fig. 1A and B). The cannula is embedded/encased in a dental acrylic stabilization platform that is preformed over a plaster mold of the skull or any other bony structure to which it will be attached in the animal.

Cannula The cannula can be made from flexible, kink-resistant polyvinyl line (e.g., Bolab intravenous tubing V-1, 0.64-mm o.d., or larger in some cases; Bolab, Inc., Lake Havasu City, AZ), which is suitable for insertion into the subdural space for brain superfusion or intrathecally for applications around the spinal cord. Intrathecal placement of such lines can be achieved over large distances by pushing the line caudally along the cord from another vertebral level (e.g., C1–2 or the lumbosacral junction) where the thecal space is accessible. Cannulas intended for stereotaxic placement at specific coordinates in the CNS are best made from stainless steel tubing (e.g., 0.30-mm o.d., 0.15-mm i.d.; Small Parts, Inc., Miami Lakes, FL). The inner diameter should not be smaller because such cannulas are prone to obstruction by brain tissue (possibly also through ingrowth of scar tissue). A larger outer diameter has been used by many investigators but causes much more damage to the surrounding tissue, for example, in the parenchymal tissue or in the lateral ventricle at the level of the medial septum, where such cannulas destroy the ventricular lining and part of the surrounding tissue.

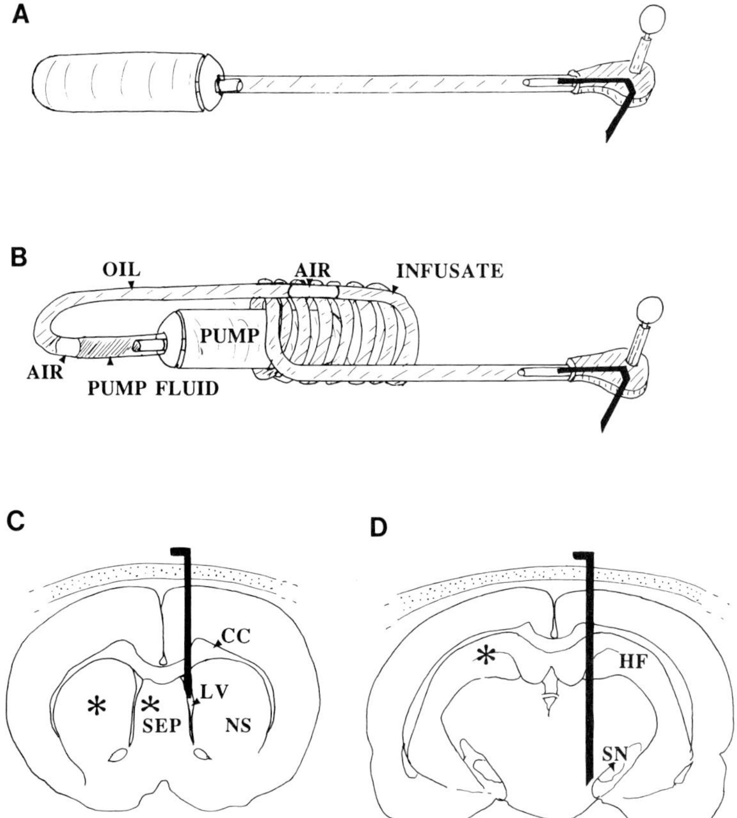

FIG. 1 Infusion device for continuous infusions into the CNS. (A) Device consisting of a cannula embedded in a dental acrylic platform, connected to the flow moderator of an Alzet osmotic pump via a straight polyvinyl line. Infusate is loaded directly into the pump. (B) Infusion device in which the connecting line is replaced by a coiled polyvinyl line serving as a reservoir for the infusate, which is separated from the colored pump fluid by a mineral oil spacer. (C) Coronal sections through the septum (SEP) and (D) hippocampal formation (HF) and rostral pole of the substantia nigra (SN), illustrating various cannula positions that are described in text. CC, corpus callosum; LV, lateral ventricle; NS, neostriatum or caudate-putamen.

Pieces of steel tubing (~10 mm longer than the intended depth of the cannula) can best be cut with a fresh grinding wheel (e.g., mounted on a Dremel drill). To ensure stability of the metal cannula inside the dental acrylic platform and after adhesion to the skull or other bony structures (see Platform, below), a 6-mm piece of its pump end is first bent 90–110°, to a position perpendicular to the long axis of the bone plate. A second angle is made 2–3 mm away from the first one, so that the pump end is positioned toward the final location of the pump, that is, toward the neck of the animal in the case of a skull placement. Collapse of the steel tubing at the angles, which would obstruct outflow, is prevented by inserting a thin steel wire into the tubing before bending and removing it afterward. Metal debris in the pump end of the cannula should be removed with a thin wire or a 30-gauge syringe needle (a dissection microscope is essential). After the cannula has been encased in the platform (see Platform, below) the CNS end of the cannula is beveled to the appropriate length with a rotating fresh grinding wheel under a dissection microscope, with the bevel facing the direction of intended outflow. Remaining metal debris is again removed to ensure proper outflow. If necessary, a smaller outer diameter can be achieved by buffing the outside of the cannula with a rotating rubber wheel to approximately 32 gauge.

Connection The connection between the cannula and the pump can be a straight piece of polyvinyl line (intravenous kink-resistant line V-4, 0.72-mm i.d., 1.22-mm o.d.; Bolab) as long as is necessary to allow appropriate placement of the pump (e.g., between the shoulders in rats for brain cannulas). A 7-mm piece of V-1 line is placed around the short pump end of the cannula, inserted completely into the V-4 line, and glued into place with a small drop of cyanoacrylic superglue [Elmar's Wonderbond Plus (Borden, Inc., Columbus, OH), long-term storage at 4°C], taking care that the glue does not exceed the length of the V-1 step-down line. Overuse of superglue causes the polyvinyl line to become brittle and potentially breakable after repeated movement inside the ambulant animal. Superglue polymerizes, that is, it does not dry, which is difficult with large volumes, and smaller volumes secure pieces together better and more rapidly. A cautionary note: superglue can glue skin together instantaneously; there are commercially available reagents that can dissolve the glue. The short end of the metal flow moderator that is supplied with the Alzet pumps is placed into the other end of the line and glued into place with a small amount of superglue. Afterward, the patency of the cannula can be tested by injecting water through the flow moderator and checking for a regular and unobstructed water jet from the tip of the cannula.

A variation on the straight connection line is the "coiled line reservoir." This coil replaces the Alzet pump as a reservoir for the infusate (which is pushed by the pump fluid but is separated from it by an oil spacer; see Infusate). The coil reservoir has several important advantages. First, the length of the line/reservoir can be chosen, allowing a variable reservoir volume rather than the fixed volume of the Alzet pump (200–230 μl, model 2002; Alzet). This is advantageous in cases of a short infusion period, especially with expensive or scarce agents. Conversely, if (stable) agents are to be infused over periods longer than the infusion capability of the pumps, a large reservoir volume can be expressed by replacing spent pumps with fresh ones. Second, by using colored (blue) pump fluid, the final infused volume can be calculated by its advance inside the coil reservoir. Third, the inside of the reservoir line can be coated to protect agents that would adhere or be modified by the line material. Last, as described in Infusion/Treatment Protocols in more detail, the coil reservoir allows sequential treatments with different substances without removal of parts of the assembled infusion device. The coil reservoir is made by winding a piece of V-4 polyvinyl line around a glass rod (outer diameter determined by the outer diameter of the Alzet pump that will later fit into the coil, e.g., a 5-ml glass pipette), excluding a 65-mm piece of line at the pump end of the coil and a 60-mm piece on the other end (or as long as is necessary between the coil and the cannula). The coil is glued together by small amounts of superglue along its axis, and the two loose ends are bent across the coil in an opposite direction and glued to all but the outside coil windings. The length of the coil line depends on the volume of the infusate plus an extra 60-mm length for the oil spacer. Different batches of polyvinyl Bolab line have different inner diameters and their volume per length should be measured routinely.

Platform Cannulas and electrodes in many laboratories are secured into place by applying freshly made and fluid/viscous dental acrylic directly on the skull or vertebra. However, the curing or hardening of the acrylic is slow and lengthens the surgical procedure. We therefore encase the cannula into a dental acrylic platform before the filling of the infusion device and surgery. The cannula (already glued into the line or coil) is placed into a hole in a petroleum jelly-coated plaster mold of the skull or vertebral column. This hole should ideally be drilled at a vertical angle, making later stereotaxic placement easier, and can be chosen according to the final coordinates. A freshly made fluid mixture of Coe-rect rigid denture liner (Coe Laboratories, Chicago, IL) is placed over of the cannula and the beginning of the polyvinyl line so that a small (4- to 5-mm diameter for skull or smaller for vertebrae) platform forms. The platform will harden completely in a few hours, and can be taken from the plaster mold and trimmed according to specific needs. The ventral side of the platform will have the shape of the bony structure to which it will be glued in the animal. A ball-headed pin is glued vertically to the platform with a piece of polyvinyl line around the metal pin, and will serve as an attachment for stereotaxic placement. Two or three pieces of straight polyvinyl line are attached between the platform and the coil reservoir, to reinforce the infusion device. By making these pieces slightly shorter than the piece of infusate line that connects the coil and cannula, the latter does not undergo excessive pull in the animal, which would cause its breakage. Again, small amounts of glue are best.

Siliconization In the case of infusion of proteins or other charged substances that might adhere to the polyvinyl line or metal parts of the device, the whole assembly can be siliconized by pulling a 1% solution of silicon (Prosil-28; PCR, Inc, Gainesville, FL) through the cannula. This is readily done by placing a piece of V-4 line, connected to a vacuum flask or syringe, over the flow moderator and then leaving the silicon inside the device for 1 min (repeat three times for good coating). Afterward, the inside of the device is rinsed by dipping the cannula 15 times in water while having vacuum on the flow moderator (i.e., intermittent water and air) and leaving water inside the line for 1 min (repeat three times for complete removal of excess silicon). The infusion device is dried by rinsing its inside with 95% ethanol and subsequent incubation in an anhydrous $CaSO_4$ desiccant (Drierite; W. A. Hammond, Xenia, OH)-containing vacuum bowl for several hours. The devices are placed in petri dishes with holes in the lids, held in place with a piece of poster putty, placed in sterilization pouches and sterilized with ethylene oxide gas (if not readily available, check with local hospitals). The temperature reached during sterilization by autoclaving is detrimental to the device.

Preimplantation Preparation of Pumps and Infusion Devices

The Alzet osmotic pump consists of a semipermeable hard outer shell, a compressible inner bag that will contain the pump fluid, and a substance with high osmolarity between the two. Consequently water can diffuse across the outer shell and the resulting increased volume will compress the inner bag. To reach a stable and maximum outflow rate [0.5 μl/hr for the 2002 model (Alzet)] the pumps are incubated for 4 hr in sterile phosphate-buffered saline (PBS) at 37°C (e.g., in a 15-ml capped tube) before filling of the pump and implantation in the animal. The pump volume and outflow rate can be chosen according to the animal species or the length of infusion. The pumps are generally too large for smaller animals (model 2002 is mostly used in adult rats with a potential infusion time of 14–18 days at 0.5 μl/hr). The outflow rate can be lowered by coating part of the outer pump casing with melted paraffin (or potentially by other substances). Coating of the side of the pump opposite the outflow hole over a 16- to 18-mm length will result in a steady and reliable flow rate of ~0.2 μl/hr and prolong the infusion time to 30–35 days. The new flow rate can be determined by attaching a long line of known volume to the flow moderator and measuring the daily output of the pump placed in PBS in a 37°C incubator. Care should be taken to use clean paraffin to prevent cracks from occurring in the coating, which would result in a higher flow rate. Also, the preincubation time in PBS at 37°C should at least be doubled. The inner diameter of the coiled line reservoir should be adjusted so that the coated pump fits easily inside without the possibility of stripping off the coat.

Infusate On the day of implantation (or potentially before with stable infusate reagents) the infusion devices are filled, preferably in a sterile laminar flow hood (tissue culture hoods). The use of rubber gloves and flaming of instruments will minimize contamination of the infusate and infusion device. For intra-CNS infusion, the basic infusate or vehicle can be any buffered solution, but preferably artificial cerebrospinal fluid [ACSF (g/liter): NaCl, 8.71; $CaCl_2$, 0.2; $MgSO_4 \cdot 7H_2O$, 0.296; glucose, 1.8; KH_2PO_4, 0.068; $K_2HPO_4 \cdot 3H_2O$, 0.342]. Addition of gentamicin sulfate (0.1 mg/ml) is essential and will prevent bacterial growth, which would degrade proteins in the infusate. In the case of proteins or other charged molecules that could bind to any surface area, a 1-mg/ml solution of serum albumin of the same species (fraction V for rats; Sigma, St. Louis, MO) should be added. After preparation of the infusate it should be filter sterilized (Acrodisc 0.45- or 0.22-μm pore size sterile filters; Gelman Sciences, Ann Arbor, MI). In the case of proteins, care should be taken that these filters, although weak in terms of protein binding, do not nonetheless sequester them. It is useful to flush or condition these filters with 1 ml of albumin-containing vehicle before sterilization of the final infusate. Similarly, syringes or ampoules and tubes can be precoated with sterile albumin-containing vehicle. Alternatively, stock solutions of the protein can be filter sterilized and added after sterilization of the vehicle.

In the case of a straight line infusion device the pump is completely filled with infusate through the Alzet filling needle (supplied with the pumps) placed all the way into the outflow hole of the pump. Often, the needle will obstruct the hole, which can be prevented by pushing against the pump in a direction perpendicular to its long axis. During injection, the air inside the pump will be forced out by the fluid. Air pockets inside the pump should be prevented, because they impair pump performance. Next, the flow moderator, which is connected to the polyvinyl line or reservoir, is inserted into the pump, and the infusion line allowed to fill until a small droplet forms at the tip of the cannula. The flow moderator should be inserted only approximately two-thirds at this time. In case the line does not fill up completely, future ones can be prefilled with infusate by injecting the flow moderator through a connecting piece of sterile polyvinyl V-4 tubing, using a 21-gauge blunt needle.

In the case of the coiled line reservoir, the pump is filled with a colored sterile PBS solution (e.g., cresyl violet) and placed inside the coil before injection of the infusate (a later placement could result in stretching of the coil and expulsion of some infusate). Next, the required volume of infusate is injected through the flow moderator up to approximately 70 mm from the tip of the cannula. Next, filter-sterilized mineral oil (e.g., intestinal lubricant) is injected after the infusate over a 50- to 60-mm length of the line, leaving a small air bubble between the infusate and the oil, until the infusate front reaches approximately 20 mm from the cannula. Before insertion of the flow moderator into the pump, a small air bubble is injected to serve as a separator between the oil and the pump fluid, which would otherwise mix. The flow moderator is inserted approximately two-thirds of the way, until a small droplet forms at the tip of the cannula. When using small amounts of infusate, the oil spacer and infusate can be advanced by injecting pump fluid until the infusate reaches a distance of 20 mm from the cannula, after which the flow moderator is inserted into the pump. In case the procedure fails to expel fluid from the cannula tip, the coil can be squeezed until the infusate reaches the end of the cannula and new infusate can be drawn up from a droplet of infusate placed on any low protein binding surface.

After loading, the infusion device–pump assembly is placed back into the PBS-containing, 15-ml tube and placed into a sterile 50-ml capped tube (at room temperature) for transportation and/or until the time of implantation into the animal.

Infusion/Treatment Protocols

As described above, the custom-made infusion device can accommodate infusion protocols for short term or longer term (>14 days) treatments. In addition, the infusion device can be exchanged for a fresh one by inserting a metal needle connector close to the cannula over which the line is secured by suture and glue. At the end of the first period, the straight or coiled line can be disconnected and replaced by a newly filled one. In the case of stable reagents, a coil reservoir doubled (or more) in volume could be served by renewing paraffin-coated pumps every 4 weeks. A treatment can be interrupted by disconnecting the line from the cannula or by pulling the cannula from its skull or vertebral position. An infusion can start before or with a delay after another experimental condition such as traumatic, ischemic, or toxic lesions. In studies in which the protective activity of agents against lesion-induced neurological damage is investigated, a 2-day pretreatment may provide better results by establishing a sufficiently high concentration before the lesion. In the case of a delayed treatment, the wound area is vascularized, which can make the implantation of an infusion device more difficult. Use of a cauterizer is advised. A special case of infusion protocol, which requires a rigorous preliminary study, involves the use of the coil reservoir for sequential administration of different agents or intermittent treatment with the same one. The length of the individual treatment periods is determined by the sequential insertion into the coil of a given volume per agent. To prevent mixing of the fluids, an air bubble is inserted between each agent. Because air is resorbed in the vehicle over time, the volume of the individual air spacers can be designed so that the air spacer will have disappeared just before the next agent reaches the cannula for its infusion into the CNS.

Stereotaxic Surgery

These procedures are based on the use of the infusion devices in adult rats and can be adapted to larger species. Visualization of the several delicate surgical techniques through a surgical microscope is invaluable. The rats should be anesthetized with the appropriate anesthesia. We routinely use an intramuscular (im) injection of a mixture of ketamine (62.5 mg/kg body weight), acepromazine (0.62 mg/kg), and xylazine (3.25 mg/kg). This immobilizes and anesthetizes the animals for up to 2 hr with essentially no loss of life. The head of the rat is shaved and aseptically prepared with betadine and/or 70% ethanol and placed in a Kopf stereotaxic apparatus with symmetrical ear bars, and the tooth bar is set at an appropriate setting. After incision of the skin, a sterile surgical cloth with a slit to allow access to the wound is placed over the animal and attached with wound retractors to create an aseptic field. Instruments should be flamed regularly and items such as gauze should be sterile before surgery. Next, muscles and fascia are spread to expose the bony surface, which is cleaned by scraping and/or repeated application of 5% H_2O_2. After stereotaxic determination of the mediolateral and rostrocaudal coordinates, a small hole is drilled in the skull or vertebra while taking care not to rupture the dura. Bleeding can be stopped with PBS-soaked Gelfoam. After further cleaning, the bony surface is allowed to air dry. The ball-headed pin and the attached infusion device are placed and tightened in a wire prong holder (Small Parts, Inc.) attached to the micromanipulator of the Kopf stereotaxic apparatus with the pump–coil assembly resting on the sterile cloth. The flow moderator is inserted further into the pump until a small droplet forms at the tip of the cannula, assuring that the infusate will immediately start flowing and preventing otherwise potential obstruction by blood clots. The distance of the colored fluid into the line should be recorded at this time. Next, the metal cannula is manipulated to a vertical position and moved to the appropriate coordinates. Flexible line cannulas can be positioned or inserted by hand, also under visual guidance.

After assuring that the platform will not touch wet surfaces, the infusion device is lowered until the platform just touches the bony surface. Immediately, a drop of superglue (Wonderbond) is placed between the platform and the bone, taking care not to glue the polyvinyl infusate line. The polymerization of the glue is greatly accelerated by sprinkling sodium bicarbonate onto the fresh glue. The pH change causes an instantaneous polymerization and securing of the platform. Second or third layers of glue and sodium bicarbonate will further strengthen the bond between the platform and the bone and should be applied as deemed necessary.

After securing of the platform, the pump–coil part is placed under the skin in a preformed subcutaneous pocket, taking care that the polyvinyl line to the pump is not kinked. The ball-headed pin can be removed by making vertical incisions on four sides of the polyvinyl line around the pin. The pocket and wound are flushed twice with 3 ml of sterile PBS to remove debris and blood, and 2 ml of gentamicin sulfate (0.1 mg/ml in PBS) is injected into the pocket and wound. In addition, 0.2% soluble Nitrofurazone powder (Fermenta Animal Health Company, Kansas City, MO) can be sprinkled into the wound. The skin is closed with metal wound staples or appropriate suture and the animal returned for postoperative recovery.

A few problems that may occur at different times after the surgery include (a) the formation of an abscess around the infusion device, which is likely caused by lack of aseptic conditions or by forgetting the gentamicin solution, (b) formation of a sterile fluid cyst around the pump–coil part, which is probably due to chemical and/or mechanical irritation by the device, and can be drained by transcutaneous insertion of a needle, and (c) line breakage at the point of entrance into the platform, mostly due to excess glue or to pull because of improperly placed reinforcement lines.

Post Vivo Analysis

After the infusion period, the infusion device can be checked for patency by noting and calculating the advance of the colored pump fluid into the line and by squeezing the coil lightly to see if a droplet forms at the tip of the cannula. A more refined method involves the measurement of fluid output into a polyvinyl line or glass capillary placed over the cannula over a 24-hr period of incubation in PBS at 37°C. In addition, the stability of biological activity of the remaining infusate can be determined by comparing it to the activity of the infusate at the time of loading. Histological analysis of tissue sections to assure correct cannula placement and to assess the tissue reaction to the cannula can include classic stains (e.g., cresyl violet) and immunochemical detection of glial fibrillary acidic protein (GFAP) in astrocytes or markers for inflammatory cells.

Experimental Examples

The osmotic pumps have been utilized extensively for infusions of proteins into the CNS, in particular to investigate the protective effects of trophic factors against trauma-induced degeneration of central neurons. The cannulation sites have included intraventricular, intraparenchymal, and subdural placements. The choice of such sites should be based on the intended extent of the treatment region (e.g., ventricular or subdural placements result in widespread diffusion through the CNS) and the diffusion capacity of the particular protein. For instance, although nerve growth factor (NGF) and brain-derived neurotrophic factor (BDNF) are sequentially and structurally related, BDNF can cross the intact ventricular wall with much less efficacy than NGF. In such a case, an intraparenchymal placement is preferable. Large proteins such as IgGs also do not cross the ventricular lining well. An important consideration for ventricular administration is the fact that CSF is produced and thus turned over at a rate of approximately 2 μl/min (2). Intraparenchymal infusions result in a more localized, more contained treatment region, depending on the diffusion distances of the individual agents, and probably result in a higher concentration in the tissue. Intraparenchymal NGF can reach effective concentrations up to 4–7 mm, depending on the responses measured.

The following are a few examples of studies in which the effects of trophic factors were investigated (Fig. 1C and D) (3). The cholinergic medial septum neurons that innervate the hippocampal formation can be axotomized by transection of the fimbria–fornix tract. Starting on the day of the lesion, factors have been infused into different locations in the lateral ventricles (a) at the level of the rostral septum, where the narrow width of the ventricle requires precise stereotaxic technique (1, 4), and (b) at the level of the fimbria–fornix transition, where the ventricular space is larger and where correct cannula placement is more consistent (5). In the latter case, the distance of the infusion site to the medial septum is greater and may result in a lower concentration in the septum. On the other hand, it is still unknown whether trophic factors act through receptors on the interrupted axons or on the cell body. Intraseptal infusions of factors has been used (6). Investigations of trophic factor roles for the axonal regeneration of these injured cholinergic neurons have utilized intraseptal (7), intrafornix (7), and intrahippocampal (8) infusions over periods of up to 1 month. These intraparenchymal infusions generally do not result in excessive tissue necrosis beyond the cannula tract. The dopaminergic neurons of the substantia nigra have also been treated with trophic factors. Intraventricular infusions would probably be effective by their action in the striatum, the innervation territory of these neurons. Factors have been infused intraparenchymally into the striatum and above the normal substantia nigra (9) or between a transection lesion of the nigrostriatal pathway and the substantia nigra (10). Intraventricular suprathalamic infusions have been used to protect anterior thalamic neurons from axotomy-induced degeneration (11). Trophic factors have also been administered to the spinal cord. The responses of injured peripheral sensory neurons (12) and regeneration of their intraspinal axons (13) have been investigated by intrathecal infusions with flexible line cannulas and more recently by the author's group by intraspinal infusions with permanent metal cannulas for periods of up to 1 month.

Conclusion

The Alzet osmotic pump has clearly facilitated and expanded the possibilities of experimental approaches in the investigation of the CNS. Their combination with customized infusion devices, such as those described in this chapter, has provided a powerful tool for administration of agents into the CNS. The use and further development of these devices has resulted in many elegant studies that would otherwise not have been possible. The protocols described here should serve those who are just becoming familiar with the infusion techniques but are also intended to stimulate further improvement and designing of custom-made devices that are particularly suited for a chosen experimental condition. However, direct infusions may have only a short-lived or small part in the treatment of chronic human neurological diseases. Such conditions should probably be approached by exogenous stimulation of production of endogenous proteins by local cells in the CNS, or by the development of external "homing" techniques to direct the distribution of agents toward particular CNS regions or neural cell groups.

Acknowledgments

The design and development of the infusion devices and techniques described here was made possible by the expert participation of H. Lee Vahlsing. I also wish to thank Michael Spencer, Martin Oudega, and Scott Dale for their ideas and help in the refinement of the design of these devices.

References

1. H. L. Vahlsing, S. Varon, T. Hagg, H. B. Fass, A. Dekker, M. Manley, and M. Manthorpe, *Exp. Neurol.* **105,** 233 (1989).
2. R. A. Fishman, "Cerebrospinal Fluid in Disease of the Nervous System." Philadelphia, Saunders, 1992.
3. T. Hagg, J. C. Louis, and S. Varon, *in* "Neuroregeneration" (A. Gorio, ed.), p. 265. Raven Press, New York, 1992.
4. T. Hagg, H. B. Fass, H. L. Vahlsing, M. Manthorpe, J. M. Conner, and S. Varon, *Brain Res.* **505,** 29 (1989).
5. V. E. Koliatsos, M. D. Applegate, B. Knusel, E. O. Junard, L. E. Burton, W. C. Mobley, F. F. Hefti, and D. L. Price, *Exp. Neurol.* **112,** 161 (1991).
6. J. K. Morse, S. J. Wiegand, K. Alderson, Y. You, N. Cai, J. Carnahan, J. Miller, P. S. DiStefano, C. A. Altar, R. M. Lindsay, and R. F. Alderson, *J. Neurosci.* **13,** 414b (1993).
7. T. Hagg and S. Varon, *Exp. Neurol.* **119,** 37 (1993).
8. T. Hagg, H. L. Vahlsing, M. Manthorpe, and S. Varon, *J. Neurosci.* **10,** 3087 (1990).
9. C. A. Altar, C. B. Boylan, C. Jackson, S. Hershenson, J. Miller, S. J. Wiegand, R. M. Lindsay, and C. Hyman, *Proc. Natl. Acad. Sci. U.S.A.* **89,** 11347 (1992).
10. T. Hagg and S. Varon, *Proc. Natl. Acad. Sci. U.S.A.* **90,** 6315 (1993).
11. R. E. Clatterbuck, D. L. Price, and V. E. Koliatsos, *Proc. Natl. Acad. Sci. U.S.A.* **90,** 2222 (1993).
12. V. M. Verge, W. Tetzlaff, M. A. Bisby, and P. M. Richardson, *J. Neurosci.* **10,** 2018 (1990).
13. E. Fernandez, R. Pallini, and D. Mercanti, *Neurosurgery* **26,** 37 (1990).

[13] Injection of Biologically Active Substances into the Brain

Paul M. Carvey, Terrence J. Maag, and Donghui Lin

Introduction

The injection of biologically active substances into the brain is an important technique in the field of neuroscience. Injection directly into the brain can circumvent numerous problems associated with systemic delivery of biologically active compounds. These problems may be described as follows.

1. The systemically administered agent does not readily penetrate the blood–brain barrier (BBB). Most of the brain is protected from the systemic circulation by the BBB. Quaternary amines, charged compounds, proteins, highly lipid- or water-soluble compounds, or cells that may be administered systemically would therefore not enter the brain readily. Direct injection thus affords probable access to brain parenchyma of compounds that would otherwise not enter the brain when administered by any other route.
2. The biologically active agent may be capable of penetrating the BBB but becomes deactivated on systemic delivery. This applies to many drugs that might be catabolized in the liver or elsewhere, leaving little compound available for entry into the central nervous system (CNS).
3. The systemically administered agent readily enters the brain but induces global brain effects that might mask the effect being sought. Regional specificity can therefore be achieved, in most cases, by simply injecting the agent into the brain region of interest.
4. The systemically administered drug readily enters the brain but peripheral actions of the drug complicate its study. This problem can be circumvented given that an agent that does not cross the BBB is available to antagonize the peripheral actions of the drug under study. However, barring the availability of such a compound, a selective CNS response can be obtained only when the agent is injected directly into the target structure.

Despite the advantages of injection directly into brain, one also has to appreciate that there are certain limitations to injection techniques that must also be considered. These may be described as follows.

1. The diffusion of solutions in brain is limited. The brain has the least extracellular space of any organ in the body. This decreased extracellular

Methods in Neurosciences, Volume 21

space therefore limits diffusion. Diffusion is further hampered by the numerous physical barriers that have ostensibly evolved to facilitate specificity within the brain. Synaptic regions are often protected by ensheathing glial processes that reduce diffusion of materials into the synapse. Cell bodies may receive literally millions of terminal boutons that physically limit access of an injected substance to its potential site of action. Numerous catabolizing enzymes and high-affinity as well as low-affinity uptake sites reduce extracellular concentrations, thereby reducing diffusion gradients, which in turn further limits diffusion distance. The continuous production of cerebrospinal fluid (CSF) and the tendency of drugs injected near the ventricular system to diffuse into the CSF can produce a "sink" for an injected agent, drawing drug out of the brain parenchyma faster than anticipated and thereby limiting diffusion. These phenomena, as well as others, restrict the spread of material away from the injection site. A rule of thumb we have developed in our laboratory is that most injected substances will diffuse a maximum of 2 mm away from the injection site.

These limitations on diffusion do not absolutely mean that substances cannot be distributed further than 2 mm. There appear to be a number of circumstances under which broad distribution of an injected compound may occur. Substances infused into the ventricular system can be dispersed throughout the brain but will predominantly affect brain parenchyma adjacent to the ventricular system. Substances may be taken up by neurons and retrogradely or anterogradely transported away from the injection site. The parallel extracellular spaces that are found in white matter tracts can allow diffusion of substances for reasonably long distances. Therefore, the limitations on diffusion distance will depend, in part on where in the brain a substance will be delivered, as well as on the unique characteristics of the agent under study.

2. Although diffusion distance is limited within the brain, diffusion that does occur can have adverse effects under certain circumstances.If, for instance, the intention is to influence the activity of a small nuclear region within the brain, diffusion out of that region and into an adjacent region can be a problem. This is especially true if the activity of the structure into which the injected substance diffuses influences the activity of the target structure under study.

Injection into the brain therefore has advantages as well as limitations. Determine up front what is to be accomplished in terms of the science and then pay considerable attention to the practical advantages, as well as limitations, associated with injection studies. The remainder of this chapter focuses on the practical, "how-to" aspects of injecting biologically active agents into the brain. There are topics that will not be covered; however, the principles that are discussed will touch on most of the basics and should therefore be applicable to almost any injection technique.

Getting Started

Suppose a target site within the brain has been chosen, and the next step is to order animals: consider bringing in two additional animals to be used to establish stereotaxic coordinates empirically. We have found that verification of coordinates using animals from the same delivery batch saves time, money, and aggravation. Even though extra animals are purchased for this purpose, the savings, in terms of the overall number of animals that will eventually be needed to complete a project, will far outweigh the cost of these extra two animals, due to the increased success rate of the procedure. Prior to establishing stereotaxic coordinates empirically, for example, our success rate in generating unilateral 6-hydroxydopamine (6-OHDA) mesencephalic lesions was around 70%. We now average around an 85% success rate and have had batches where we successfully lesioned 95% of the animals. The only change in our protocol has been the use of animals to establish empirical coordinates with each animal batch. One must remember that the stereotaxic coordinates published in the various atlases are for very young animals from one particular vendor. As the animal grows or vendors and strains change, optimal coordinates can move. Without *a priori* knowledge of this fact, a batch of animals whose stereotaxic coordinates are off by 10% could be generated for a study. It is not unusual for us to generate 400 6-OHDA-lesioned animals a year. Moving from a success rate of 70 to 90% saves 80 animals a year.

The procedure we use to verify coordinates prior to the implementation of a brain injection protocol is straightforward and relatively easy. On the basis of experience with a given procedure as well as the coordinates suggested by an atlas, we choose four sets of coordinates (two for each side of the brain). These coordinates vary on all three axes around what we feel is the most optimal coordinate (we use the bregma for the lateral and anterior–posterior coordinate reference and the surface of the skull for the depth reference; see below). We then perform four needle passes into the brain of the animal, euthanize it, remove the brain (do not perfuse), freeze it, mount it on a cryostat chuck, and then coronally section it. When sectioning, adjust the orientation of the cuts so that they conform to those listed in the atlas being used. This will provide a frame of reference. (Remember, it is important not only to adjust the left–right symmetry, but the superior–inferior symmetry as well.) In the absence of perfusion, the fresh needle tracks induce injury with associated bleeding. One can then visualize the injection path by looking for the red needle tracks on the freshly sectioned brain. On the basis of structures surrounding the target of interest, choose the set of coordinates that appear optimal, then repeat the procedure. The verification of coordinates in two animals takes only 3 hr to perform but saves considerable time, aggravation, and money in the long run. If animals are always ordered in the same manner (i.e., the same vender, strain, sex, age, and time period prior to surgery) then the variation between batches is minimized and reverification of coordinates may need doing only once or twice a year.

Preparing Guide Cannula and Stylet

The injection of chemical substances into brain parenchyma is a common technique. There is considerable flexibility with this technique. The target of the injection can be as big as the striatum or as small as the subthalamic nucleus. A single injection or multiple injections can be made. The time course of the injections can be acute or chronic. The tools used to deliver the chemical substances can be a Hamilton syringe or a stainless steel cannula attached to polyethylene tubing. For multiple injections, a guide cannula is generally placed permanently in the skull. For long-term chronic injection, an osmotic pump attached to a cannula is often used. Regardless of the technique employed, an appropriate portal of entry into the brain must be correctly prepared in order to avoid problems later on.

If a single injection is intended, and the animals will be sacrificed within 24 hr and no behavioral profile or brain activity is being monitored, then a single, open burr hole in the skull can be used followed by stereotaxic delivery of the drug. However, if the experiment involves the monitoring of behavior or a brain activity that may be influenced by the surgical procedure or anesthesia, then consider implanting a guide cannula, sealing it with a removable, snug-fitting stylet and cap, and performing the experiment the following week. Even if the plan is to chronically inject a chemical into the brain using a minipump, it is probably best to implant the cannula, wait 7 days, and then attach the minipump to the cannula at that time. This strategy avoids potential interactions between the injected drug and surgery or anesthetic as well as the impact of acute-phase inflammatory processes on the brain region under study. These factors can significantly influence experimental outcome in some cases. Separating the effects of surgery from effects of the injection reduces the potential for interaction among these effects, thereby enhancing the reliability as well as the validity of the study.

Once the coordinates are chosen, the cannulas, stylets, and injection needles should be prepared prior to surgery. The guide cannulas as well as the needle for injection must be stainless steel. Tubings or needles that are not stainless steel can leach contaminants into brain, especially during chronic studies. Stainless steel will also not react with the chemicals you are using. A wide assortment of tubings and stylets can be purchased (Plastics One, Inc., Roanoke, VA or any stainless steel tubing supply company). We prefer to use manufactured guide cannulas with plastic threaded collars and screw caps already in place (see Fig. 1). This assembly is particularly useful for chronic multiple injections. The outside diameter of the guide cannula is generally chosen for a given application to be as small as possible while still giving adequate internal clearance for the stylet or injection needle (see below for additional considerations). For most of our applications we use a stainless-steel guide cannula [23 gauge (0.64-mm o.d.)]. One must be careful not to choose a wall thickness that is so thin that it easily bends or crimps when manipulated. We have found that the wall thickness should be at least 0.1016 mm. Likewise, the stylet used should fill the bore of the cannula completely to prevent contaminants, especially bacteria, from entering the brain in between injections. For the 23-gauge cannula described above we use a 0.30-mm o.d. stylet. However, we have found that a stylet that requires some force to insert into the guide cannula may be almost impossible to pull out after it has been in the animal for 7 days. The stylet should therefore be snug but not tight.

Once the guide cannula and stylet have been chosen, they can be prepared for use. If cannulas without plastic collars are being used, cut them at least 2 cm longer than normal in order to facilitate handling during polishing, and then trim the proximal end (end outside of the brain) to the appropriate length once they have been polished. If an acute, 1-day procedure is to be done using a guide cannula, consider cutting the cannula long enough to

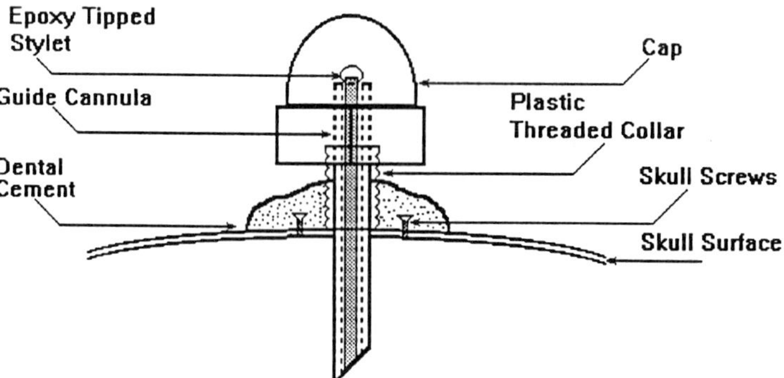

FIG. 1 Schematic depicting a guide cannula–stylet assembly with a screw cap in place in the skull. The whole assembly is embedded in dental cement placed around screws inserted in the skull to hold the cement in place.

actually mount in the stereotaxic frame. The stylet should, of course, be longer than the cannula so that it can be grasped and removed at the appropriate time. The proximal end of the stylet can simply be bent at a 60° angle to hold it in place. Alternatively, a drop of epoxy or other type of glue can be applied at the proximal end of the stylet so that the stylet length is fixed. The use of an epoxy-tipped stylet is especially useful when the plastic threaded collars are used, because they will easily fit under the screw cap. We feel it is best to insert the stylet into the cannula before it is cut. We then cut the distal end (the end in the brain) of the stylet and guide cannula together, using a Dremmel high-speed drill with a fine-toothed saw appropriate for stainless steel (see manufacturer specifications). If guide cannulas with plastic screw collars are used, the distal end must be cut reasonably close to the depth needed for the application, allowing adequate clearance for beveling and polishing (see below) and the thickness of the skull. The stylet and guide cannula should be held firmly in place with a small vise while being cut. Cutting the tubing with the guide cannula in place prevents collapse of the distal end of the guide cannula while it is being cut. The stylet also reduces the chance that small flecks of stainless steel, produced when the cannula is cut, will be trapped in the bore of the cannula or be pushed into the brain when a stylet or needle are subsequently inserted.

It is our belief that the guide cannula–stylet assembly should have a beveled tip (see Fig. 1). We feel that a beveled tip (~60°) cuts and separates tissue when inserted, producing less tissue trauma then that observed when a blunt-ended cannula is inserted. With the stylet still in the tubing, the end of the cannula–stylet assembly is filed and polished to a pointed bevel using a wet polishing stone (purchased at any hardware store). Because the stylet is held in place inside the cannula during this procedure, the distal tip of the cannula and stylet will have the same bevel, creating a smooth surface minimizing tissue damage with insertion. One alternative to this procedure is to insert the guide cannula without a stylet present. A tissue plug, however, can end up inside the cannula during insertion. Subsequent insertion of the stylet then pushes this tissue into the injection site, producing damage and necrosis that could influence the activity of the injected substance or the target structure. The other alternative is to implant a guide cannula–stylet assembly that is not beveled. This type of "blunt" dissection is often used in other applications. However, within the context of stereotaxic surgery, in which the cannula tip cannot be "wiggled" as it is inserted, tissue is torn or compressed. This procedure extends the diameter of tissue damage around the insertion route or, alternatively, compresses tissue into the eventual injection site, which again could adversely affect the diffusion of the injected substance.

The depth of the guide cannula–stylet assembly, once implanted, should be at least 1 mm above the coordinates selected for the injection. It is true that gliosis and tissue damage, which could influence the distribution and action of the injected substance, will occur around the injury site made by the insertion of the guide cannula–stylet assembly; however, because the guide cannula never reaches the injection site, the effects of gliosis and tissue damage at the injection site are minimal. When the injection needle is actually inserted into the target it will, of course, induce damage as it extends beyond the tip of the guide cannula. Because the distance penetrated by the injection needle is only ~1 mm and a small-caliber needle is used, the damage produced is less than that seen if the guide cannula penetrated all the way to the injection site.

After the guide cannula and stylet are made, prepare the actual needle that will be used to make the injections. Once the guide cannula is complete it will be clear exactly how long the needle must be to reach the actual target site. It is best to optimize the length so that the needle extends beyond the distal beveled tip of the guide cannula no more than 2 mm, and 1 mm is probably best. As the length the needle will extend beyond the guide cannula increases, so does tissue damage, as does the risk of needle deviation away from the target. The distance the needle extends beyond the guide cannula fixes the depth coordinates that must be used for cementing the guide cannula in place (see other considerations for guide cannula insertion depth in the next section). The next decision that needs to be made is whether or not to bevel the injection needle (see Injecting Solutions, below). Once these decisions have been made, the depth that the needle can be inserted into the guide cannula must be fixed. The most reliable strategy, of course, is to fix that depth using a stereotaxic frame. Thus, when the injection actually commences, the animal is placed back in the stereotaxic frame and the cannula is lowered to the appropriate depth. If there is any concern about anesthesia interaction or if several injections are being made (and a stereotaxic frame is just not practical), an alternative strategy is necessary. We feel it is easiest to manufacture the needle with the guide cannula and then fix the insertion depth by placing an epoxy collar on the injection needle. Place a drop of epoxy around the needle and then let it dry. Then, with the needle inserted in the guide cannula with the epoxy collar butting up against the proximal end of the guide cannula, cut or polish the distal end of the needle until the correct length is achieved. If a Hamilton syringe is to be used for the actual injections, the same technique can be employed. The epoxy can be scraped off after the injection so that the syringe can be used again. Once the guide cannula, stylet, and injection needle are completed, they should be soaked in a 70% ethanol solution, rinsed, and sterilized prior to use.

Inserting Guide Cannula–Stylet Assembly

Most stereotaxic coordinates employ the use of the bregma as the reference point. Scraping the cranium with a spatula or other blunt object and then wetting it with a sterile saline solution helps to identify the bregma more readily. We use the bregma for our lateral and anterior–posterior coordinates. Our experience has taught us that the depth coordinates are best determined by using the skull surface right above the entrance of the cannula as a reference point. Some laboratories use the surface of the brain as the depth reference. However, it is often difficult to identify the surface of the brain, especially if only a small opening is made in the cranium. Another alternative strategy uses the level of the ear bars as the reference point. We feel that this approach is subject to the nuance of animal-to-animal variation in the external auditory meatus. We have found that using the surface of the skull at the point of entry into the brain increases the success rate of procedures by at least 10–15%.

An electric drill (Dremmel or other high-speed dental drill) is used to open the skull most of the time. The hole in the skull should be big enough to ensure that the cannula will not touch the edge of the hole, because even a slight deflection of the needle at the level of the skull will cause the cannula to deviate considerably from deep targets. For the study of the cortex, it is wiser to use a manual drill because the heat generated by an electric drill can damage the superficial cortical tissue.

The dental cement that will be used to anchor the assembly to the skull does not provide adequate grip and can therefore loosen. To prevent this occurrence, place three stainless steel screws in the skull around the burr hole (a triangular array is best). Using a drill with a bit smaller than the external diameter of the screw, make three holes as far away from the burr hole as possible (at least 0.75 to 1 cm). Ideally, the screw holes should be as deep as possible without penetrating the skull completely. If they do penetrate the skull, they should not penetrate the dura. However, one must be careful not to make the holes too shallow, which would increase the risk of the screws coming loose. Then simply screw the screws in. Make sure they are secure but not flush up against the skull. Being flush against the skull defeats their purpose. Also, the distal end of the screws should never extend beyond the internal surface of the skull. If this were to occur, the dura may be irritated, which can lead to unforseen complications.

Once the burr hole has been completed and the screws are in place, the dura mater must be pierced before the guide cannula can be inserted. One can purchase a special tool called a dura-hook for this purpose. We simply use a 21-gauge beveled needle, which we tap lightly on the counter to bend the beveled tip. The bent tip (~70°) serves as a sharp hook. The needle is used to pierce the dura; then, with a lifting and twisting motion, the dura is torn. As is true of the size of the burr hole, the dura must be torn adequately to allow free, unimpeded passage of the cannula or injection needle. If the dura is not pierced adequately, the dura could deviate the cannula as it is lowered into the brain. The guide cannula may now be inserted.

The carpenter's rule applies next: that is, "measure twice, cut once." Just prior to insertion of the guide cannula, check the stereotaxic coordinates again to make sure that all of the calculations are correct. Then begin inserting the cannula. Make sure the stylet is in place and flush with the bevel of the guide cannula. The insertion of the cannula should be slow to reduce damage to the tissues (~2–3 mm/30 sec). This is especially true as the target depth coordinate is approached. If using cannulas with plastic screw collars, make sure that the base of the collar will not touch the surface of the skull once the guide cannula is inserted to its appropriate depth. If adequate clearance is not given (1–2 mm is best), the collar could impede the insertion of the guide cannula to the appropriate depth. If this were to occur, the procedure would have to be repeated. In such a case it is probably not wise to use the same animal twice, as excessive tissue damage following a second insertion would occur.

Once the guide cannula is stereotaxically implanted to the appropriate depth, the entire assembly is then fastened in place with dental cement. While applying the dental cement, make sure it fills the area under the head of the screws. Also, make sure that the dental cement is not piled so high around the assembly that it would interfere with pulling the stylet out, or prevent screwing on the plastic screw cap provided with the premanufactured cannula plastic screw collar (one should be able to make two full turns). If the screw caps are used, it is generally a good idea to screw the cap on in order to scrape off any cement that is in the threads. Do not, however, leave the cap on. Take it off again until the cement is completely dry (see Fig. 2).

After the guide cannula–stylet assembly is secured in place and the cement is dry, the skin flap can be secured back around the dental cement. It is always a good idea to sprinkle an antibiotic powder into the site prior to closing. A variety of these powders is available through your pharmacy. Ideally, the animal should be allowed to recover for a week before the actual injection starts.

Injecting Solutions

Neuroscientists often use the term *infusion* to describe the injection of solutions. To infuse means to deliver by gravity. Because a mechanical force

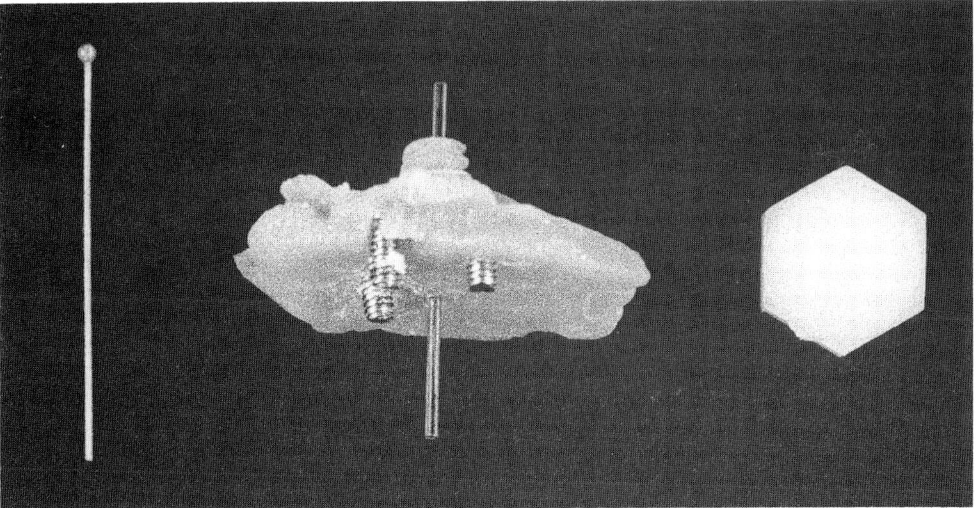

FIG. 2 Picture of a guide cannula embedded in dental cement with a triangular array of screws (center). Note the amount of cement used and the fact that cement is present under the screw heads, between the bottom of the screw head and the surface of the skull (not shown). Although the cement covers a large surface area, it is not piled so high as to cover the last two threads of the plastic portion of the assembly. The plastic screw top for the plastic-threaded, premanufactured, nonbeveled cannula is shown on the right. A stylet with an epoxy tip to ensure proper depth placement appears on the right.

such as is supplied by an injection needle, a pump, or an osmotic minipump is used to deliver the substance, the correct term is *injection*.

The chemical substances for injection can be held in a syringe or tubing. Many laboratories use Hamilton syringes for the actual injection. Several sizes are available to fit the needs of the experiment. Another option is to use a piece of clear tubing attached to a syringe on the proximal end and an appropriate size injection needle on the distal end. This strategy is particularly useful if an injection pump is used to deliver the solution or if small volumes are delivered (see below). The use of a small injection needle is also a useful strategy because the length of the needle can be manufactured accurately when the guide cannula is made. Having the injection needle length calibrated prior to the actual injection saves time, thereby reducing the duration of the injection procedure. Remember to consider the stability of the chemical under study and change solutions appropriately if several injections from the same solution batch are to be made. Consideration must also be given to the oncotic pressure of the solution. If the oncotic pressure of the solution to be injected is inappropriate for brain tissue, cell swelling or shrinkage can occur. If the solution has an unusual ionic composition, you run the risk of having the solution hyperpolarize or depolarize the target structure, which may complicate the interpretation of the study. Finally, the pH of the solution should be as close to 7.4 as possible. Having a pH below 7 or above 7.8 is probably not wise. Artificial CSF solutions are probably the best.

Clean the cannula thoroughly prior to removing the stylet, so as not to run the risk of pushing bacteria into the brain when the needle is inserted. Then insert the needle. Again, slow insertion reduces damage. Injection can now proceed. The final depth coordinate should be in the superior region of the target depending, of course, on the size of the target. If injecting into a small target, using the center of that target as the final depth coordinate may spare the superior region of the target unless this strategy is used. Although a delivered fluid will reflux slightly up the side of the injection needle, the majority of the fluid will be directed downward. Using a beveled cannula, the injected solution will be directed down and slightly to the side apposing the bevel. This strategy can be useful if the experiment involves injecting fluid into a target that is in close proximity to another structure whose activity can interfere with the activity in the target under study. Directing the flow away from the adjacent structure reduces the probability of flow into that structure (1).

The injection speed should be slow to avoid excess damage to the tissue. A maximum 1-μl/min injection rate is a good rule of thumb. A slow injection rate allows the solution to be absorbed into the surrounding tissue, leaving room for the injection of additional material. A rapid injection rate may distend the injection site and therefore increase tissue damage. For lesioning of the medial forebrain bundle with the dopamine (DA) neurotoxin 6-hydroxydopamine (6-OHDA), for example, we use a 1-μl/min infusion rate. However, if the target structure is small, it may be wise to lower the injection rate even farther. If one assumes that injecting a solution creates a positive pressure at the injection site, an increased pressure will "force" the fluid into surrounding tissues. This force will increase diffusion distances. Reducing the injection rate therefore reduces diffusion distance. For injection into a small target such as the subthalamic nucleus, we inject only 200 nl/min.

Injecting small volumes can present a problem in delivery. Our experience has taught us that the calibrated tubing strategy is the most reliable method for delivering small volumes. A small piece of clear plastic tubing (PE-50) is attached to a Hamilton syringe. Fill the tubing with distilled water. Draw 10 μl of distilled water into the syringe, push out 10 μl, attach the syringe securely to the tubing, draw in 1 μl of air into the tubing, and then 9 μl of water (this assumes a tubing capacity of approximately 25 μl; ~25 cm). The

1-μl air bubble should be clearly visible about 9 cm from the end of the tubing. Next, tape a piece of fine-ruled graph paper onto a flat surface and then tape the tubing containing the air bubble over the paper. Push some fluid out of the needle so that the water fills the entire length of the needle. Line the air bubble up with one of the lines on the graph paper and mark that point with a pencil. Preweigh a piece of wax weighing paper or, better yet, tare it on a microbalance. Then, holding the distal end of the tubing over the weighing paper, which is on a microbalance (propping the tubing is better because it leaves both hands free), deliver the desired volume to the scale (1 nl equals 1 ng at room temperature). Once the appropriate volume has been delivered, again mark the graph paper at the new location of the air bubble. Perform this procedure several times to confirm the calibration. Then, when the solution is to be injected into the brain, mark the graph paper where the air bubble is, mark the appropriate distance, and then move the air bubble to that mark to deliver an exact, small volume. Make sure the tubing and the syringe are flushed with the drug solution before drawing up the solution that will actually be injected. If any component of the solution binds to the tubing or any other part of the system, flushing the system prior to use will saturate those sites. Then, when the actual solution for injection into the tubing is drawn, the concentration delivered will be exact.

We believe this delivery system is more accurate and reliable for two reasons. First, attempting to deliver 200 nl out of a 5-μl syringe is not reliable and is tedious. The distance that the plunger must be moved to deliver this volume is short and therefore easy to misread. Use of a calibrated piece of tubing magnifies the distance the column of fluid must move to deliver a given volume, making it easier to read and therefore more reliable. Second, compliance within a delivery system can often accommodate small volumes. Thus, moving the plunger on a syringe the appropriate distance does not necessarily mean that a small volume has actually been delivered. Watching a bubble move 2 mm over a piece of graph paper at an even rate suggests smooth, unimpeded delivery of the column of fluid to the injection cannula, thereby increasing confidence that a 200-nl injection has actually been made.

On the other hand, injecting large volumes also has its problems. Delivering large volumes can induce damage no matter how slowly it is injected. Delivering large volumes can also increase intracranial pressure. The high end is probably around 10 μl when injecting directly into brain parenchyma. Larger volumes can be delivered into the ventricular system (see the next section).

After the injection, the needle and cannula should be left in place for at least 3 min. This time interval allows the injected solution to be absorbed into the surrounding tissue. Then withdraw the injection needle slowly. Withdrawing too fast creates suction, which will draw some of the solution up the needle track. If solution was injected with a needle attached to tubing, never disconnect the tubing prior to needle withdrawal. The suction created by withdrawal will draw fluid remaining in the injection needle into the brain, resulting in higher than anticipated delivery.

For multiple injections, the stylet should be replaced to avoid blockage of the guide cannula in between injections. The interval between the injections should be based not only on the half-life of the chemical, but also on the total number of the injections. Injecting too frequently might sensitize the animals.

If you plan on injecting nonanesthetized animals, handling the animal during the injection can be a problem. We have found that wrapping the animal in a towel with just its head exposed works well. Before actually administering the injection solution, allow the animal to become accustomed to the procedure three or four times. After several exposures to the towel, the animal will often go along with the procedure without a struggle. The only problem is that two people must be present for the injection, one to hold the animal and the other to make the injection.

Injecting Solutions into Ventricular System

There are times when injecting solutions into the ventricular system is the more desired strategy. The ventricular system may be used to distribute drug to a wider area of the brain than that achieved with intraparenchymal injections, although only tissue adjacent to the ventricular system will be affected. We inject 6-OHDA into the lateral ventricle to induce a bilateral lesion of the DA neurons in the mesencephalon. In general, significantly higher concentrations must be used when injecting intraventricularly, due to the dilutional effect of the CSF. When we induce unilateral lesions of the mesencephalon by injecting into the medial forebrain bundle just rostral to the substantia nigra (see the next section), we inject 8 μg of 6-OHDA in a 4-μl solution. To induce a comparable bilateral lesion following intraventricular lesions we inject 300 μg of 6-OHDA in a 10-μl solution 1 hr following intraperitoneal (ip) injection of the norepinephrine reuptake inhibitor desipramine (25 mg/kg) to prevent uptake into noradrenergic neurons. The dilutional effects the CSF has on an injected drug will depend on the drug being used and the target of that drug. These data may have to be established empirically, as we did with 6-OHDA.

Although not intuitively obvious, injection into one lateral ventricle can result in drug concentrations in the contralateral ventricle. Thus, diffusion into the contralateral lateral ventricle does occur and drugs delivered into one lateral ventricle can produce bilateral effects. Therefore, do not assume that delivery of a solution into one lateral ventricle can be used as a technique to induce unilateral effects.

The coordinates used for injection into the lateral ventricle should target the largest expanse of the lateral ventricle [−0.8 mm in the Paxinos and Watson rat brain atlas (2)]. Most of the time, insertion of a cannula into the ventricle yields a reflux of CSF, which verifies that the ventricle has been hit. Not seeing a CSF return does not mean that the animal cannot be used. Even if the cannula is located in parenchyma adjacent to the ventricle, once injection has started, the path of least resistance is generally into the ventricle and the bulk of the injected solution will end up in the ventricular system.

Unilateral 6-Hydroxydopamine Lesions

One of the more commonly encountered injection techniques is to unilaterally lesion the dopamine (DA) cell bodies in the mesencephalon. The result of this lesion is an animal with ipsilateral DA receptor site proliferation that can be used to study a variety of dopaminergic drugs or cell transplant techniques.

When we first started experimenting with this model, we did not have good success. Evaluation of our strategy revealed that we were not taking appropriate advantage of the medial forebrain bundle and the ability of that bundle to distribute the toxin to the DA cell bodies. If one targets the intuitively appropriate rostral–dorsal region of the substantia nigra compacta (SNc), the limited diffusion of the injected solution yields only partial lesioning of the target. This is an important consideration for any large brain target. Injection of solutions into a large structure such as the striatum will not diffuse throughout the entire structure and will therefore influence only a portion of the striatum. Because the striatum is a heterogeneous structure, it is difficult to interpret the results because only a selected region of the structure will be affected. To lesion the majority of the striatum with kainic acid, for instance, we therefore make at least two injections. Likewise, if one attempts to target the SNc and injects only into the SNc, only a partial lesion of that structure is created unless multiple injections are made. In fact, this strategy has been successfully used to generate selective lesions of the SNc while sparing the ventral tegmental area (VTA) (1).

We therefore tried injecting 6-OHDA into the medial forebrain bundle just rostral to the point where the fibers from the SNc and VTA merge (see Fig. 3). (For a 270- to 300-g animal, these coordinates are approximately A–P 4.3; L 1.2; D 8.3 from skull surface). Using these coordinates, we found a significantly higher lesion rate and an almost complete lesion pattern in both the SNc and VTA. This dramatic improvement probably stems from the fact that injection into the fiber bundle distributes the solution up and down that bundle. The fibers thus act as unimpeded pathways for the distribution of

a

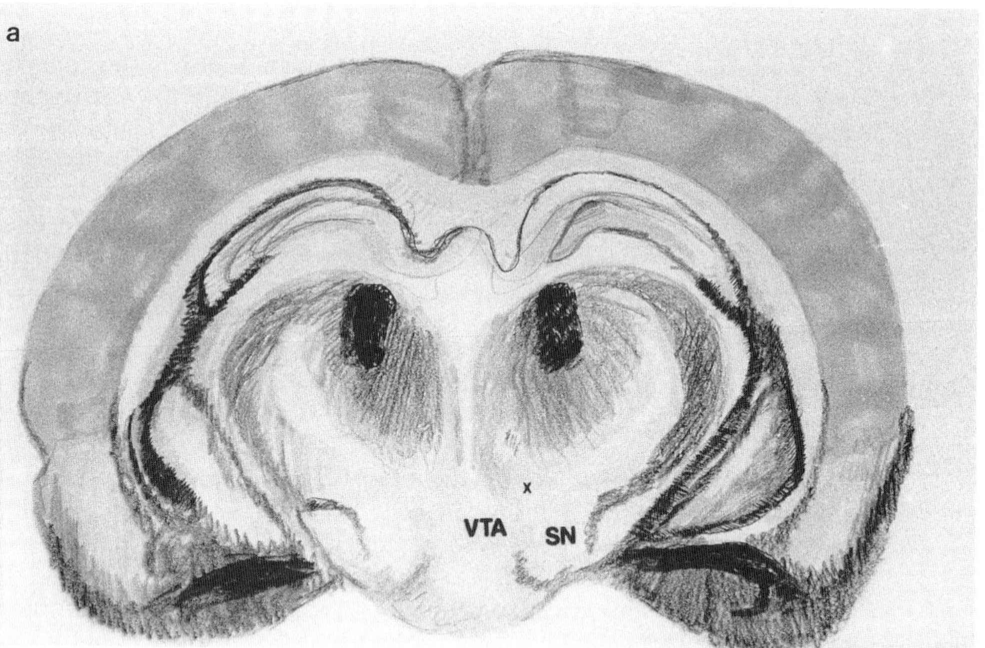

b

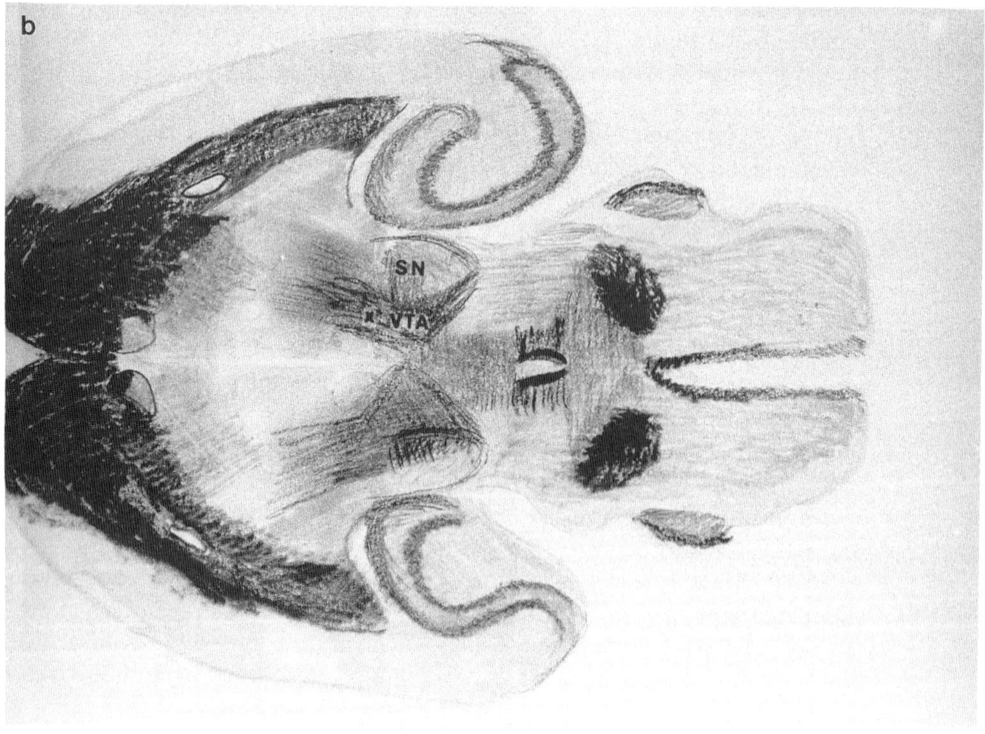

the solution. Diffusion distance is increased and therefore distributed more broadly and evenly to our target cell population. Once we worked out this problem, we achieved a 70% success rate. The 85–90% success rate we now realize came when we empirically established coordinates with each animal batch as described previously.

We inject 8 μg of 6-OHDA-HBr in a 4-μl 0.02% citrate solution. In the hours and early days following surgery, placing the animal on a surface and making noise can often reveal a contralateral (away from the lesion) spontaneous rotation indicative of an animal that will eventually rotate well in response to a drug challenge. We test the animals for contraversive rotation in response to 0.1 mg/kg apomorphine-HCl, delivered subcutaneously (sc) every 2 weeks for 6 weeks. We have observed that the rotation rates are stabilized by 6 weeks. Rotation rates can increase by as much as 60–70% in some animals between 4 and 6 weeks (groups average 20–25% increase in rotation rates during this time; see Fig. 4). If an experiment involves monitoring rotation rate as the dependent variable following an experimental manipulation, use of animals lesioned for less than 6 weeks is therefore not recommended. Using three baseline assessments also has the advantage of reducing the probability that apomorphine sensitization will affect the results.

Always verify lesions after an experiment. Perform DA assessment of the striatum or tyrosine hydroxylase stains of the mesencephalon. Dopamine assessment has the advantage of being readily quantified. In our laboratory, rotation rates of greater than 300/hr are generally associated with >99% depletion of DA in the striatum.

Injection of Cells into Brain Parenchyma

The injection of cells into the striatum of a 6-OHDA-lesioned rat is rapidly becoming a widely used tool to study transplant strategies for Parkinson's disease (PD). The injection of cells into the striatum employs the same basic

---

FIG. 3 Depiction of approximate location of the needle tip used to completely lesion the dopamine neurons in the mesencephalon, using 6-hydroxydopamine (6-OHDA). Note that the tip of the needle [*X* in (a) and (b)] is located slightly superior to, and between, the substantia nigra compacta (SN) and the ventral tegmental area (VTA) (a). Fiber bundles leaving the SN and VTA ascend slightly and merge at about this point. On a horizontal section, note that the needle tip is rostral to the SN and VTA (b). If a beveled needle is used, the flow should be directed caudally. Using this injection location allows the fiber bundles leaving the SN and VTA to disperse the 6-OHDA to all the cell bodies in the mesencephalon, thereby increasing the number of animals that reach rotational criterion (300 rotations/hr).

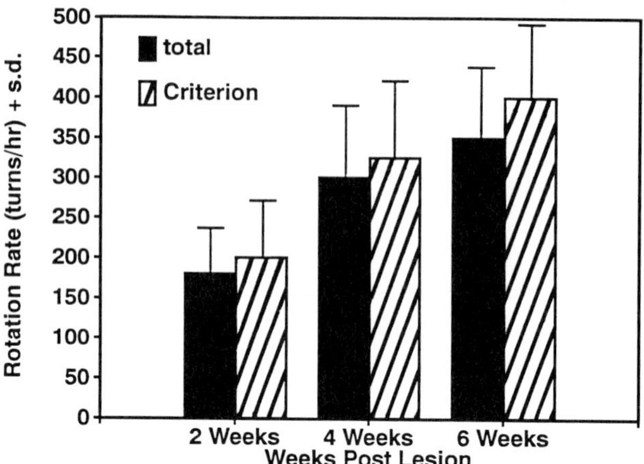

FIG. 4 Apomorphine (0.1 mg/kg of salt)-induced rotational rates (contralateral rotations/hr) in 120 male rats (94.5% of 127 animal batch) 2, 4, and 6 weeks following unilateral 6-OHDA lesion. Rotation rates increase gradually over 6 weeks and level out thereafter (no statistically significant change; data not shown). Note the dramatic increase in rate from 2 to 4 weeks as well as from 4 to 6 weeks. These increases in rotation rate occurred in all animals (total) as well as in those animals that went on to reach criterion (300 rotations/hr in this study; 89 of the 120 rotators). Because rotation rates statistically increase between 4 and 6 weeks, using animals that have been lesioned for only 4 weeks or less is not recommended.

strategies outlined above. The injection of cells does, however, pose an additional problem. When a solution is injected, it can, in most cases, simply diffuse away or is absorbed into surrounding tissue. When the injection needle is withdrawn, the suction created by that withdrawal therefore does not significantly affect the diffusion pattern provided the needle is left in place for several minutes after the injection. Cells cannot, however, diffuse away or be absorbed into surrounding tissue. We have found that even slow withdrawal of the injection needle creates a negative pressure that draws cells up the needle track. Even if a traditional guide cannula is used, cells are drawn up into the guide cannula. The result is that one does not really know how many cells were actually injected.

The suction created by withdrawing the injection needle can also distribute cells into the ventricular system. The ventricular system offers little resistance to the injection of any solution including cells. The injection of cells into the striatum to study tarnsplantation for PD usually crosses this area of low resistance. Even if a lateral approach is used, the lateral ventricle may not be apparent but is still present and will offer a region of low resistance. Thus, when the injection needle is withdrawn, the suction created by the withdrawal often distributes cells into the ventricular system (see Fig. 5a). A similar problem occurs at the junction between white matter tracts and gray matter (3). Because this reflux occurs frequently, numerous animals are wasted unless this phenomenon is appreciated.

We have modified our technique to adapt to this particular problem. For injection of cells into brain parenchyma, our laboratory uses a 10-μl Hamilton syringe with a guide cannula. We have found that for injections of cells into brain parenchyma, the use of a guide cannula helps to prevent some cellular reflux, but not all of it all of the time. We reasoned that to prevent this reflux completely, the suction created by needle withdrawal had to be dramatically reduced. Leaving an air pocket on top of the column of cells in the Hamilton syringe and then injecting that air into the brain on top of the cells did not prevent reflux, probably because the air was absorbed rapidly into the parenchyma. It appeared that the injection site must receive a flow of air during withdrawal to reduce suction and the associated cell reflux.

To accomplish this we used a guide cannula with an internal diameter significantly larger than the outside diameter of the Hamilton syringe. This design readily allowed air to enter the guide cannula while the needle was being withdrawn. This idea of depositing the transplant with minimal reflux by using an oversized guide cannula for the Hamilton syringe is similar to the current usage of a cannula within a cannula in human transplants performed in Sweden (4).

A 20-gauge needle, with a sharp tip and a 45–60° beveled tip, is currently used in our laboratory as a guide cannula. The Hamilton syringe fits loosely inside the cannula and extends 1 mm beyond the cannula tip when in place. The guide cannula was fashioned with a tight-fitting stylet similar to the design described previously. If a stylet is not present in the guide cannula while it is being inserted, a corridor of tissue will fill the cannula. Because we implant the guide cannula and inject the cells in one operation without a recovery period, insertion of the injection needle into a guide cannula that was implanted without a stylet left tissue between the external surface of the injection needle and the interior surface of the guide cannula. Air could not flow readily and cell reflux again occurred when the needle was withdrawn. Keeping the cannula clear of brain tissue by inserting it with a stylet present also prevented the Hamilton needle from becoming clogged on insertion into the cannula.

To begin the injection, the guide cannula, plugged with the snug-fitting stylet that is flush with the beveled tip of the cannula, is slowly lowered to the desired depth and left in place for 5 min. Prior to removing the stylet and inserting the Hamilton syringe into the guide cannula, the Hamilton syringe should be washed with water, saline, and then the same buffer in

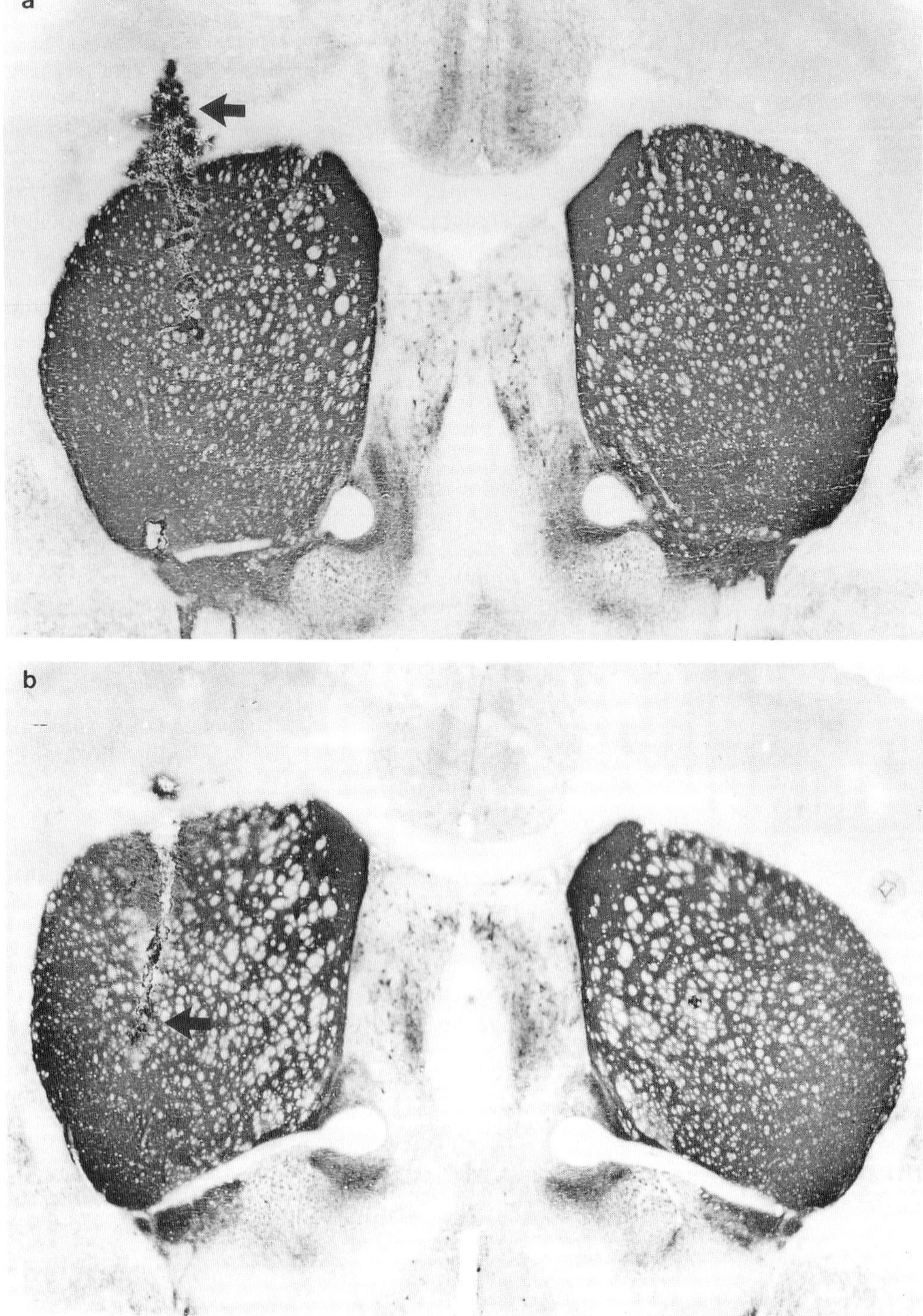

a
b

which the cells are bathed. After washing the Hamilton syringe, the cells to be infused, which are kept on ice, are gently stirred and then drawn up into the syringe. The needle is then slowly inserted into the guide cannula.

For the injection itself, three basic principles are followed: cells are injected slowly over time, in small volumes, and over short distances. These principles promote the implantation of a column of cells over any desired distance. Typically a small volume is deposited at the most inferior point of the target, 1 min is allowed to pass, and the cannula and syringe are withdrawn a short distance. This procedure is repeated as many times as is necessary to cover the target site. Injecting small volumes causes minimal tissue displacement, and when a small total volume is used, intracranial pressure is only minimally increased. The less intracranial pressure is raised, the less likely it is that the implanted cells will be forced into an area of less resistance, such as the ventricles or white matter tract and gray matter junctions. Finally, the deposition of only a small volume of cells at each point along the injection corridor increases the contact between the implanted cells and the cells in the vicinity. Creating a vertical corridor of tissue also increases the probability of adequate oxygenation and nutrient support for all of the implanted cells; this can become problematic if a large-diameter tissue bolus is injected.

When injecting rostral mesencephalic tegmental (RMT) cells into striatum, for example, we use the following strategy. The concentration of RMT cells is 100,000 cells/μl in a total volume of 3 μl. A 0.3-μl volume is injected in the inferior part of the center of the striatum, followed by a 1-min wait, and the stereotaxic arm is raised 0.3 mm. The procedure is repeated until the 3 μl is deposited over 3 mm. The entire injection takes 10 min. At the end of the last injection, the Hamilton syringe and guide cannula are left in place for 5 min. We assume that during this period the implanted cells settle down into the implant site, further minimizing reflux, especially into the ventricle. Both the Hamilton syringe and guide cannula are then withdrawn slowly so as not to create a vacuum. Using this procedure, we have minimal cell reflux up the cannula track or into the ventricles (Fig. 5b). When injection is complete, the cells remaining in the Hamilton syringe should be counted on a hemacytometer to verify that the cellular concentration thought to be injected was actually injected.

FIG. 5 Distribution of tyrosine hydroxylase-immunoreactive cells (PC-12) in the striatal region following injection with a syringe (a) and with a syringe that fits loosely into the guide cannula (b). In (a) note how the cells are concentrated in the superior region of the cannula tract and how many of the cells have dispersed throughout the ventricular system (arrow). In (b) note how the cells have been dispersed evenly through the cannula track within the heart of the striatum (arrow), ostensibly due to the lack of reflux associated with the loose-fitting guide cannula.

Acknowledgments

We would like to thank Michelle Einert and Dr. Jack Lipton for their help with the illustrations. Special thanks go to Dr. Jeff Kroin, who taught us most of what we know about this topic. This work was supported by a grant from the United Parkinson Foundation.

References

1. D. A. Perese, J. Ulman, J. Viola, S. E. Ewing, and K. S. Bankiewicz, *Brain Res.* **494,** 285 (1989).
2. G. Paxinos and C. Watson, "The Rat Brain in Stereotaxic Coordinates," 2nd ed. Academic Press, San Diego, 1986.
3. A. Bjorklund, U. Stenevi, R. H. Schmidt, S. B. Dunnett, and F. H. Gage, *Acta Physiol. Scand., Suppl.* **522,** 9 (1983).
4. O. Lindvall, S. Rehncrona, P. Brundin, B. Gustavii, B. Astedt, H. Widner, T. Lindholm, A. Björklund, K. Leenders, J. C. Rothwell, R. Frackowiak, C. D. Marsden, B. Johnels, G. Steg, R. Freedman, B. J. Hoffer, A. Seiger, M. Bygdeman, I. Stromberg, and L. Olson, *Arch. Neurol.* (*Chicago*) **46,** 615 (1989).

Section VI

Using Implanted Living Tissues within the Brain

[14] Factors Important in the Survival of Dopamine Neurons in Intracerebral Grafts of Embryonic Substantia Nigra

Roger Barker, Rosemary Fricker, and Stephen B. Dunnett

Introduction

A number of common human neurodegenerative conditions of the central nervous system (CNS) are currently under consideration as potential targets for neural transplantation therapy. These include Parkinson's disease (PD), Alzheimer's disease (AD), Huntington's chorea (HC), and amyotrophic lateral sclerosis (ALS). In each case, the pathology that lies at the core of the disease is relatively well described but the etiology remains largely unknown (1–4). Consequently, present approaches to treatment focus on pharmacological approaches to reversing neurochemical pathology rather than on halting the degeneration or replacing lost neurons. This approach has proved to be most successful in PD, with the use of dopaminergic agents to replace the degenerating nigrostriatal system, the loss of which constitutes the pathological hallmark of this condition (1, 5). By contrast, in other diseases such as ALS there is no effective agent currently available to substitute for the degenerating motor neurons (4, 6). However, even in the case of PD, pharmacological replacement therapy with drugs will always be limited in the absence of being able to halt or reverse the etiopathological process. As the disease progresses, undesirable and often intolerable side effects of the drugs increase. Thus, in PD, this is characterized by the "on–off" phenomena, wearing off effects, and dyskinesias associated with long-term 3-hydroxy-L-tyrosine (L-dopa) treatment (7).

New treatments are therefore required that circumvent these problems, most logically employing a delivery system that actually reverses or replaces the neuronal loss and more closely mimics the endogenous release of the missing transmitter or transmitters, in a fashion analogous to insulin replacement in young-onset diabetes mellitus (8). One obvious candidate for such a delivery system in PD is replacement by intracerebral transplantation of the lost dopaminergic nigral neurons themselves (1, 9). This approach not only replaces the missing transmitter in a more physiological way than can be achieved by extrinsic drug delivery systems, but also, if the disease is the result of an intrinsic defect in the patient's own dopaminergic nigral neurons (10), then replacement by transplantation has the potential to offer an actual cure.

Methods in Neurosciences, Volume 21

In this chapter we concentrate on PD and its treatment by intracerebral transplantation of embryonic nigral neurons, as this condition has been the one that has received the most attention and has now entered the first stages of clinical trials (11, 12). Other neurodegenerative conditions have been studied from a transplantation perspective and the same principles discussed for PD can also be applied to these conditions.

Nigral Grafts

Background

The first successful use of rat embryonic nigral grafts as a means of overcoming experimentally induced dopaminergic depletions of the nigrostriatal bundle was reported almost simultaneously by the groups of Perlow and of Björklund in the late 1970s. Both groups showed that the rotational asymmetry induced by unilateral 6-hydroxydopamine (6-OHDA) lesions of the nigrostriatal pathway in rats can be reversed by embryonic nigral grafts placed in that dopamine-deafferented striatum (13, 14). Subsequent studies demonstrated that these nigral grafts can survive for long periods of time when grafted into the CNS (14, 15), that the axonal outgrowth forms synapses with appropriate targets in the host neostriatum (16), and that the grafts themselves also receive a distinctive pattern of afferent synaptic inputs from the host brain (17, 18). Electrophysiologically, the grafted neurons retain spontaneous electrical activity (19), and the level of dopamine in the axonal terminal field in the adjacent striatum is elevated (15). This dopaminergic reinnervation probably accounts for the ability of these grafts to reduce and even reverse the rotational behavior induced by dopaminergic drug stimulation in the 6-OHDA-lesioned rat (20). Moreover, the exact location of the nigral graft within the striatum is important: after unilateral lesions, grafts in the dorsolateral striatum decrease deficits in rotational behavior and spontaneous motor asymmetry, whereas grafts in the ventrolateral striatum decrease deficits in sensorimotor neglect (20, 21). The recovery appears to be a specific response to the dopaminergic cell replacement rather than a nonspecific graft effect because control striatal or brainstem grafts devoid of dopamine neurons do not produce functional recovery (22), neurotoxic lesion of the dopaminergic neurons within nigral grafts immediately abolishes the recovery (22), and nigral grafts reduce the striatal dopaminergic receptor supersensitivity that follows effective lesioning (23, 24). However, only some and not all of the more complex behavioral deficits induced by forebrain dopamine lesions are reversed by nigral grafts. Thus, for example, although the grafts can ameliorate contralateral sensory neglect this does not extend to include independent limb use (25).

Subsequent work on primates has largely supported the principles first determined in rats (26), although the more complex anatomy of the striatum and the more complex behavioral repertoire of primates has emphasized several important points. First, nigral grafts do not usually have an immediate effect on deficit reversal. Rather, recovery can take several months to develop in primates in contrast to the 3–6 weeks required in rats, which corresponds to the longer time course required for fiber ingrowth from the grafted neurons and reinnervation of the host striatum. Furthermore, as in rats, not all the behavioral deficits of a nigrostriatal lesion are reversed by nigral grafts, and this problem is not resolved simply by using multiple placements throughout the denervated striatum (26, 27).

The relative success of fetal nigral grafts in experimental animals has led to the first trials of neural transplantation for clinical application in a limited number of patients with advanced PD (11, 12). Patients receiving nigral grafts from aborted human fetuses appear in general to show some improvement after grafting; the improvement is not initially dramatic but takes several months to become apparent, in agreement with earlier studies in primates with allografts and in rats with xenografts of human mesencephalic tissue (28). Demonstration of continuing graft viability and survival has been demonstrated most convincingly *in vivo* by positron emission tomography, using 6-L-[^{18}F]fluorodopa as a ligand for dopaminergic terminals (29).

In summary, embryonic nigral grafts appear to survive transplantation to the lesioned striatum, and reverse many of the deficits that result from dopamine deafferentation of this structure. The capacity of the grafts to reverse the behavioral deficits induced by dopamine denervation is not total, and depends to some extent on the exact location of the graft within the striatum. The selective profile of recovery, combined with its abolition when the dopamine cells within the grafts are killed, and the ability of the grafts to release dopamine and to form and receive synapses with the host brain, all suggest that fetal nigral grafts work by recreating a new dopaminergic innervation within the denervated neostriatum.

Limitations

As outlined above, although nigral grafts are effective in ameliorating many of the behavioral deficits induced by unilateral nigrostriatal lesions, they do not reverse all of them. This may in part be attributable to the ectopic placement of the grafts in the striatum, so that although they restore a striatal reinnervation they do not reconstruct the damaged nigrostriatal projection per se (25). A second factor that is almost certainly of importance is the fact that only a small portion (typically 1–10%) of the dopaminergic neurons included within the graft dissection survive transplantation in the long term (30). This raises several fundamental questions about the grafting process. First, is the preparation of the tissue prior to grafting optimal? If not, can the technique be improved, for example by modifications of the tissue-handling and preparation techniques or by supplementation with neurotrophic factors? Furthermore, can the functional capabilities of the grafts be improved by transplanting the ventromesencephalon (VM) tissue to a homotopic rather than an ectopic site, that is, into the host substantia nigra? Although this was originally unsuccessful when rat nigral cells were transplanted to the rat nigra, and attempts to bridge this gap in the rat by transplanting embryonic rat nigral neurons into the host nigra along with a substrate bridge have met with only limited success (31), human nigral cells have been shown to bridge the nigrostriatal gap in the 6-OHDA-lesioned rat (32). The success of the xenografts is striking in that the axons from the human neuroblasts target all the normal dopaminergic structures. This implies that the human nigral neuroblasts are either uniquely programmed to follow this developmental pattern or that they are immune to the inhibitory signals within the rat CNS that prevent rat axonal growth and instead are attracted to their normal target structures (32, 33). This opens up the possibility that xenografts may be more effective than homografts, which is not only of great theoretical interest but has enormous therapeutic implications.

Basic Procedure

The two basic transplantation procedures are those involving cell suspensions or solid pieces of tissue. The solid graft procedure involves implantation of pieces of donor tissue directly into the host brain, either being placed into the lateral ventricle against the medial surface of the neostriatum, on the dorsal or lateral surfaces of the striatum in a preformed cavity, or inserted as a tissue plug directly into the striatal parenchyma (for examples, see Refs. 13 and 34; Fig. 1). In this chapter, we are primarily concerned with the cell suspension grafts. This technique has several advantages: it permits multiple graft deposits to be positioned with stereotaxic accuracy into deep as well as superficial brain sites, and with remarkably little additional extraneous damage. The cell suspension method is the one on which our own more recent results are based and has the greater potential for clinical applications.

The basic method for preparing the embryonic nigral tissue for transplantation as a suspension graft was introduced by Björklund and colleagues in

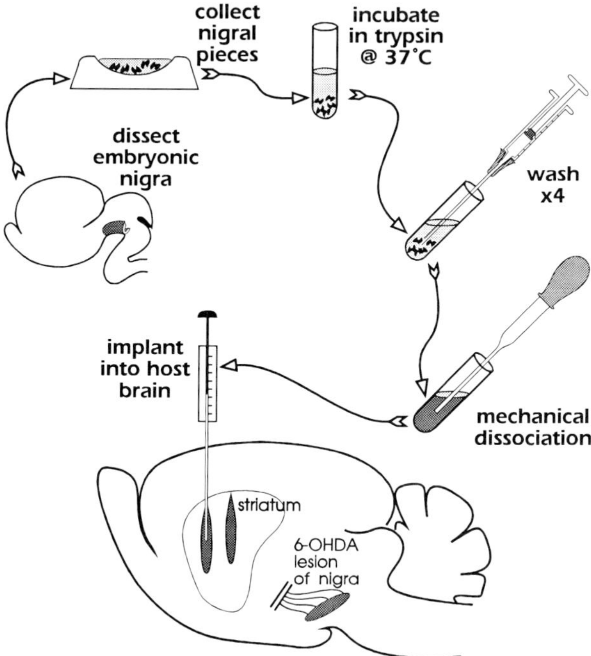

FIG. 1 Schematic illustration of the technique for preparing embryonic nigral tissue for grafting as a dissociated cell suspension into the striatum of unilaterally 6-OHDA-lesioned rats.

the early 1980s and has been described in detail (35). The procedure involves the removal of the embryo at a crown rump length of around 10–12 mm, which corresponds to a gestational age of E13–E14 days, with embryonic day E0 formally determined by the presence of a vaginal plug on the morning after an overnight mating. The embryo is removed from its chorion and amnion, and is then placed onto a small petri dish that can be viewed under a dissecting microscope. The ventral mesencephalon (VM), which contains the embryonic dopaminergic neurons, is then removed as a single piece of tissue (see Fig. 2) (35a). This single piece of VM is then placed into a solution of 0.9% saline and 0.6% glucose. The pieces of VM are stored in this solution until dissection is complete, following which they are placed into a Durham tube with 0.1% trypsin made up in the original saline–glucose solution. The Durham tube is then placed in a 1.5-ml Eppendorf tube containing 300–500 μl water to facilitate heat conduction, and the whole assembly incubated for 20 min at 37°C. At the end of this incubation the tissue pieces are lightly tapped to the bottom of the Durham tube, and the trypsin supernatant is

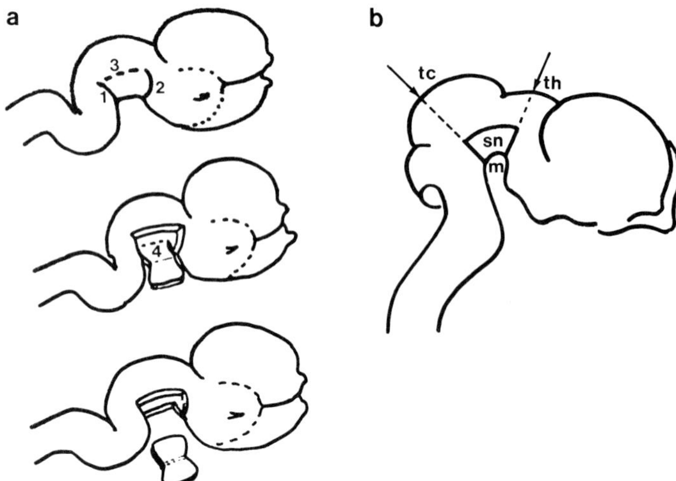

FIG. 2 Schematic figure demonstrating the procedure for dissection of the embryonic ventral mesencephalon in the rat. Abbreviations: m, mesencephalic flexure; sn, substantia nigra; tc, tectum, th, thalamus. 1–4 are the sequence of cuts required to remove the piece of ventral mesencephalon. [From Dunnett and Björklund (35a), with permission of Oxford University Press.]

removed by a fine 23-gauge needle and replaced and washed four times with 0.01% DNase made up in the original glucose–saline solution. At the end of the washes the final volume of DNase is added, to give a ratio of one VM to 6 μl of DNase. The VM is then triturated in this solution through a series of flame-polished Pasteur pipettes of diminishing diameter. The suspension is then allowed to settle and the viability and density of the suspension assessed using a vital dye (see Vital Dyes, below). The suspension is then aspirated into a 10-μl glass microsyringe and transplanted into the required site (typically the striatum) as a series of 2- to 3-μl deposits.

Strategies for Improvement

In the standard embryonic nigral graft only 1–10% of the transplanted dopaminergic neurons survive (30). The reason for this low yield is unclear but is probably a combination of factors including the preparation process, perioperatively when the graft site is edematous, ischemic and hypoxic, and finally postgrafting due either to programmed cell death or the loss of a neurotrophic input. Some of these factors are amenable to investigation, in particular the role of the different stages of the preparation procedure in the loss of dopaminergic neurons within the suspension.

Cell loss during preparation of dissociated cell suspensions can be a result of one of two factors. First, the cells may never enter the suspension and so are lost as solid pieces of VM, which implies that the proteolysis and trituration of the tissue are inadequate. Conversely, the cells may be lost as a result of chemical damage by the proteolytic enzymes or mechanical damage during the trituration procedure. Any method of preparation of the tissue involves striking a fine balance between getting the cells into suspension and not damaging them in the process. This particular aspect of the graft procedure is clearly of importance, and methodological improvements of this part of the grafting procedure would be of major therapeutic relevance and practice. This, coupled to the paucity of a clear neurotrophic factor for this neuronal population (36), has meant that this approach at present holds the greatest potential for improving dopaminergic cell survival within grafts.

Several factors in the preparation method of VM tissue for cell suspensions require analysis, including the developmental age/stage of the donor embryos, which (if any) proteolytic enzymes are used, the duration and concentrations of enzyme incubation, the presence or absence of DNase, and the trituration procedure itself. Although we have studied and will refer to results on all these factors, in view of limited space we here restrict a detailed discussion to the role of embryonic donor age.

The effects of different preparation protocols, including embryonic donor age, on dopaminergic cell survival in VM cell suspensions and grafts can be analyzed at three different levels.

Vital Dyes

Vital dyes can be used to stain cells in a dissociated suspension, revealing the number and density of viable cells within suspensions prepared in a variety of ways (37, 38). The vital dye technique is relatively easy to apply (see Use of Cell Suspensions and Vital Stains, below) and is useful in studying the behavior of dissociated cells immediately after preparation of the suspension. Its major limitation is that it does not differentiate between dopamine cells and other populations of neuronal and nonneuronal cells within the suspension. It is not known whether the dopaminergic neurons behave in a way similar to the other cells within the suspension, although there is some evidence to believe that this is the case (R. Barker, unpublished observation, 1994; 38).

In Vitro Cell Cultures

The use of *in vitro* cultures reveals the number of surviving dopaminergic neurons derived from VM suspensions after being grown for several days in culture. The culturing technique is relatively straightforward (39) and allows for an accurate description of the conditions under which the cells are grown. They therefore provide a powerful technique for assessing the role of different variables in the preparation of VM cell suspensions. The cultures can be maintained only for relatively short periods of time (typically 14–28 days) and so are more useful for studying the behavior of cells in the days immediately after suspension preparation rather than as factors involved in long-term viability. A second difficulty of the cell culture technique is that of generalization to the *in vivo* situation. In the most common culture techniques, the cells are plated onto a two-dimensional coverslip, with the nutritional requirements of the cells being met by the culture medium. This provides a cell environment quite different from that encountered following graft implantation, although the use of three-dimensional cultures may provide a somewhat closer approximation to the *in vivo* situation.

In Vivo Neural Grafts

The use of *in vivo* transplantation of the neuronal cell suspensions is necessary to reveal the functional capability of a graft and how this relates to its histological state in terms of the critical dopaminergic neurons. This is clearly the most direct means for assessing the effects of different variables on graft expression. However, these studies are complicated, time consuming, and intrinsically more variable than vital dye or culture techniques. First, they need to be carried out over relatively long periods of time. Second, the functional assessment of these animals needs to be qualified in terms of the tests employed. For example, the simplest and most widely used test for assessing unilateral dopamine lesions and nigral grafts relies on motor asymmetries induced by stimulant drugs in the 6-OHDA-lesioned rat. Whole body turning (''rotation'') is thought to reflect the differential release of dopamine in the striatum on the two sides. This asymmetry can be exaggerated by the use of drugs that provide a dopaminergic activation of the host striatum—apomorphine at the level of the postsynaptic receptor and amphetamine at the level of the presynaptic terminal (40). Thus the rotational behavioral response to these drugs in the lesioned animals and a restoration toward relative symmetry in grafted animals is believed to reflect a restoration of the level dopaminergic activation between the two sides of the brain (21). However, direct damage to the striatum on the lesioned side can itself influence rotational behavior, especially to apomorphine, and thus some of the effects of the graft may be mediated through potentially nonspecific mechanisms. Although this is probably not significant in embryonic nigral grafts, in particular when based on the use of amphetamine rather than apomorphine as the primary stimulant drug, it may be of greater significance with other grafts, especially adrenal medullary grafts (41, 42). Furthermore, the state of the graft at the time of histological analysis at the end of behavioral testing is the result of a multitude of variables, only some of which are associated with the preparation procedure. Thus, extrapolation on variables in suspension preparation and graft histology and effect are not straightforward. This can be circumvented to some extent by the use of acute studies designed to look at the grafts soon after transplantation, but this approach is fraught with technical problems, especially in terms of maintaining graft integrity. However, with substantial advances being made in the techniques for functional imaging of grafts *in vivo* using positron emission tomography (PET) scanners in animal studies as well as in patients (43, 44), this problem may soon be substantially overcome.

These three different approaches each have advantages and disadvantages, both theoretical and practical. They each monitor the behavior of nigral cells over different time periods and therefore the judicious use of all three approaches in combination can enable conclusions to be drawn on the crucial factors in cell survival with VM suspension grafts, which in turn have important therapeutic implications for the design of future experiments not only in rodents but also in other species, in particular humans.

Use of Cell Suspensions and Vital Stains

Vital stains are used to monitor the viability of cell suspensions both immediately after their preparation and during their use over several hours in the subsequent grafting procedure. Although several vital stains are available (37), the one that we routinely use is a 1 : 1 mixture of acridine orange and ethidium bromide. In this method viable cells accumulate acridine orange via an active uptake mechanism and show green nuclear fluorescence when viewed under incident ultraviolet illumination, whereas nonviable cells take up ethidium bromide passively through damaged membranes and are characterized by orange fluorescence when viewed under green illumination (45).

In the following study different gestational age embryos were dissected in sterile glucose–saline. Nigral cell suspensions were prepared by the procedure already described, but with the final washes being in 0.04% DNase in glucose–saline, leaving a final volume of one VM to 10 μl of solution. The cell suspensions were then stored at 4°C throughout the sampling period and measurements on cell viability made at various times after preparation by diluting an aliquot of the suspension 1 : 4 with a solution of acridine orange and ethidium bromide.

The results of this study are summarized in Fig. 3. There is a difference in viability at all time points between embryos of crown–rump length (CRL) 11–13 mm (E13–E14) and those of CRL greater than 13 mm (E15–E17). This difference is relatively small immediately after the preparation of the cell

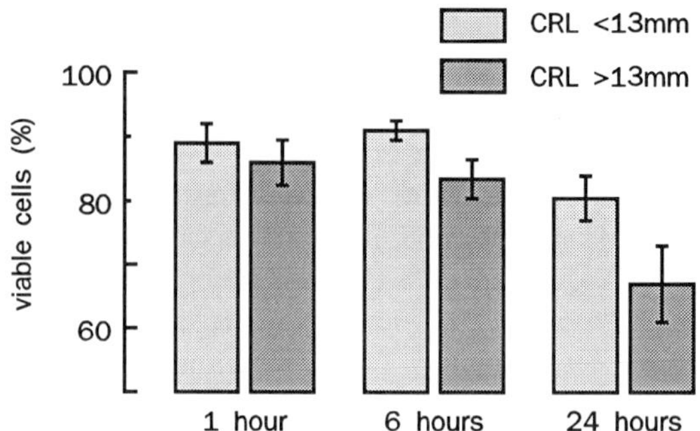

FIG. 3 The effect of donor embryo age on cell viability as assessed by the ethidium bromide–acridine orange method over time. CRL, Crown–rump length. (R. Fricker, unpublished data, 1994.)

suspension, but becomes more apparent with time and reaches statistical significance after 24 hr. This study therefore indicates that the age of the embryo is a factor influencing even the initial cell viability in suspensions, and not just long-term survival, although the effect becomes even more marked with time (see below). However, as previously stated, this method measures the total cell viability and one is unable to monitor the proportion of dopaminergic cells present and their fate relative to other cell types in the suspension. One way to try and evaluate the number of dopaminergic cells present in the suspension is to take a smear of it on a microscope slide and stain for one of the synthetic enzymes for dopamine, namely tyrosine hydroxylase. This can then be used to assess whether there are any changes in the proportion of dopaminergic neurons present in the suspension over time, by comparing it to the cell viability counts for the whole suspension.

Use of *in Vitro* Cultures

In vitro cultures are used to study the behavior of embryonic nigral neurons when grown in culture, usually on coverslips (two-dimensional cultures). Alternatively, the nigral neurons can be grown in three-dimensional culture systems, such as small porous tubes (46). This latter technique has the advantage that it resembles more accurately the situation within the graft and CNS, and can reveal aspects of cellular interactions that differ from those observed in the two-dimensional culture systems (47). The techniques used for culturing nigral neurons are variable (39). We have therefore used a technique that is similar in all essential respects to that used for intracerebral grafts (see below), although the final dilution per VM is much greater (~100 μl/VM). Once made, the suspension is then plated onto coverslips previously coated with 0.1% poly-D-lysine at a density of one VM per coverslip (approximately 750,000 cells). To this is added 0.3–0.4 ml of culture medium [80% (v/v) Dulbecco's modified Eagle's medium (DMEM), 20% (v/v) fetal calf serum (FCS), Fungizone (amphotericin B) streptomycin, and penicillin] and the coverslips are left in an incubator at 37°C for 2–3 hr to allow the cells to settle and adhere to the coverslips. After this 2 ml of the culture medium is added to each and the cultures incubated at 37°C in a 5% carbon dioxide environment. The cultures are then fixed in 4% paraformaldehyde and stained immunocytochemically for tyrosine hydroxylase after different lengths of time in culture. In general one set is fixed within 48 hr of plating and another at 7 days. The effects of the various manipulations in the preparation of the original cell suspension can then be assessed by counting the number of tyrosine hydroxylase (TH)-positive cells per coverslip. We have examined a multitude of factors in the preparation procedure (48) but here we focus only on the effect of embryonic age.

In this study embryos of different gestational ages were dissected in sterile Hanks' balanced salt solution. The age was determined by crown–rump length (35) and covered the range from 10 to 15 mm, corresponding to gestational age E13–E16. The dissected VM was then treated by 0.1% trypsin for 6 min at 37°C, followed by 0.01% DNase. The whole solution was then centrifuged at 100 *g* for 2 min, following which the supernatant was removed and triturating solution added. The tissue was then triturated through a flame-polished pasteur pipette (10–15 times). The suspension was then allowed to settle and cell viability and density assessed, following which it was plated out as described above.

The results are shown in Fig. 4. There was a clear effect of age on cell survival at both 1 and 7 days in culture. The embryos aged between E13

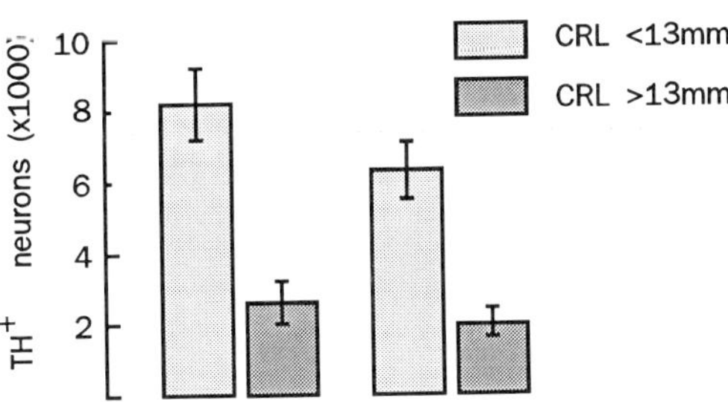

FIG. 4 The effect of donor embryo age on dopaminergic cell survival in culture. CRL, Crown–rump length. (R. Barker, unpublished data, 1994.)

and E15 (CRL 10–12 mm) give the highest yield at both time points. At older embryonic ages the yield is much lower, in agreement with other studies (see the next section). Thus the age of the embryo is probably one of the most important factors in influencing the survival of dopaminergic nigral cells in culture.

In Vivo Intracerebral Grafts

Intracerebral embryonic nigral grafts are now routinely done in several laboratories, although the vast majority of this work is in analyzing the functional capabilities of grafts in different locations within the CNS on a variety of behavioral tests (49). There has been relatively little attention given to the critical variables involved in the preparation and grafting of the cell suspension. Thus, the standard procedure devised by Björklund, Schmidt, and Stenevi (35a) generally provides the basis for techniques used elsewhere, and the minor modifications in each laboratory are based more on intuition than on any systematic evaluation of the factors influencing the survival of dopaminergic neurons within a graft. However, although systematic studies are designed to look at the preparation variables, only a few have considered individual variables, of which the most extensive are those designed to evaluate the effect of embryo donor age on survival. This has now been done not only in rats but in primate homografts (50) and in human xenografts (51). The study that best exemplifies the effect of age on graft survival in the rat is that by Brundin and colleagues (38, 52). In this study they examined cell survival at the time of preparation of the suspension from different-aged embryos and compared this to the results of grafts derived from similarly aged embryos. Their study involved unilateral 6-OHDA-lesioned rats of which the majority (22 of 31) received grafts prepared from CRL 13.5-mm embryos, whereas the remainder received grafts from 16-mm embryos. The suspension was then transplanted to the dorsal striatum at two sites and functional recovery monitored by amphetamine-induced rotation. Approximately 6 weeks after grafting the animals were sacrificed for histology. Cell viability was found to decline with increasing embryonic age regardless of the resuspension method, and this effect was seen in both the functional and histological findings in the grafted animals. At 5 weeks postgrafting none of the CRL 16-mm donor-grafted rats had a reduction in rotation but six of the younger donor group did. The animals that did show a reduction in rotation were characterized by having been grafted with suspensions of greater than 50% viability, and which had been stored for not more than 5.5 hr. However, in the older donor group there was no behavioral effect regardless of the viability scores *in vitro* of the suspensions used (36–86%), or their postdissociation storage times. This may relate to the fact that in these older donor animals few surviving dopaminergic cells were found in the graft site—none had more than 35 surviving dopaminergic neurons compared to up to 1300 in the younger donor group. This study therefore shows that age is critical in the survival of dopaminergic neurons in embryonic VM grafts. It also makes the point that the preparation of the tissue in terms of the time it is stored prior to grafting, regardless of its viability, is important (see also Fig. 3).

Thus the data on the importance of donor age on nigral graft success validate the vital stain and cell culturing techniques as a means of assessing dopaminergic cell behavior. It further illustrates that the importance of age is apparent shortly after the preparation of the cell suspension, and that this effect becomes increasingly more important with time.

Conclusions

In this chapter, discussion has been confined to experimental parkinsonism, which mimicks the essential neurodegenerative and functional features of human Parkinson's disease, and its treatment with intracerebral embryonic nigral grafts. The rationale behind this therapeutic approach relates to the fact that in the first instance the core of the symptomatology relates to the loss of a discrete population of dopaminergic neurons, and that the drug treatment of this deficit, although successful in the early stages of the disease, is frequently complicated by the development of profound side effects. The functional effectiveness of embryonic nigral grafts has been demonstrated in experimental parkinsonism, and they are now being considered for clinical application in humans. However, despite the basic feasibility of transplantation strategies to treatment, there still remain many fundamental questions, not least of which is why so few transplanted dopaminergic neurons survive. The reasons for such low yields of nigral dopaminergic neurons are unknown, but major contributory factors are the age of the donor embryos, the preparatory process for the suspension, and the environment of the graft within the CNS. These can be investigated by studying the behavior of nigral cells in response to systematic manipulations of the parameters for preparing the dissociated cell suspensions, using vital stains of cell viability in combination with the analysis of subsequent survival both in culture and in intracerebral grafts. The judicious use of these three approaches enables the critical factors influencing survival of embryonic nigral neurons to be defined. This not only has implications for developing improved techniques for intracerebral cell transplantation, but may also be important in revealing possible etiological mechanisms involved in the generation of PD itself.

Acknowledgments

The work presented in this chapter was funded by the Medical Research Council and the Wellcome Trust.

References

1. L. S. Forno, *in* "Parkinson's Disease" (G. Stern, ed.), p. 185. Chapman & Hall, London, 1990.
2. R. C. A. Pearson and T. P. S. Powell, *Rev. Neurosci.* **2,** 101 (1989).
3. J. B. Martin and J. F. Gusella, *N. Engl. J. Med.* **315,** 1267 (1986).
4. H. Mitsumoto, M. R. Hansen, and D. A. Chad, *Arch. Neurol.* (*Chicago*) **45,** 189 (1988).
5. J. E. Ahlskog, *Hosp. Formul.* **27,** 1 (1992).
6. Editorial, *Lancet* **336,** 1033 (1990).
7. C. G. Clough, *Lancet* **337,** 1324 (1991).
8. J. N. MacPherson and J. Freely, *Br. Med. J.* **300,** 731 (1990).
9. Y. Agid, P. Cervera, E. Hirsch, F. Javoy-Agid, S. Lehericy, R. Raisman, and M. Ruberg, *Movement Dis.* **4,** Suppl., S126 (1989).
10. P. Riederer and K. W. Lange, *Curr. Opin. Neurol. Neurosurg.* **5,** 295 (1992).
11. W. J. Freed, *Restor. Neurol. Neurosci.* **3,** 109 (1991).
12. S. Fahn, *N. Engl. J. Med.* **327,** 1589 (1992).
13. M. J. Perlow, W. J. Freed, B. J. Hoffer, A. Seiger, L. Olson, and R. J. Wyatt, *Science* **204,** 643 (1979).
14. A. Björklund and U. Stenevi, *Brain Res.* **177,** 555 (1979).
15. W. J. Freed, M. J. Perlow, F. Karoum, A. Seiger, L. Olson, B. J. Hoffer, and R. J. Wyatt, *Ann. Neurol.* **8,** 510 (1980).
16. R. F. Freund, J. P. Bolam, A. Björklund, U. Stenevi, S. B. Dunnett, J. F. Powell, and A. D. Smith, *J. Neurosci.* **5,** 603 (1985).
17. J. P. Bolam, T. F. Freund, A. Björklund, S. B. Dunnett, and A. D. Smith, *Exp. Brain Res.* **68,** 131 (1987).
18. G. Doucet, T. Murata, P. Brundin, O. Boster, N. Mons, M. Geffard, C. C. Ouimet, and A. Björklund, *Exp. Neurol.* **106,** 1 (1989).
19. S. M. Wuerthele, W. J. Freed, L. Olson, J. Morihisa, L. Spoor, R. J. Wyatt, and B. J. Hoffer, *Brain Res.* **244,** 1 (1981).
20. A. Björklund, S. B. Dunnett, U. Stenevi, M. E. Lewis, and S. D. Iversen, *Brain Res.* **199,** 307 (1980).
21. S. B. Dunnett, A. Björklund, U. Stenevi, and S. D. Iversen, *Brain Res.* **229,** 209 (1981).
22. S. B. Dunnett, T. D. Hernandez, A. Summerfield, G. H. Jones, and G. Arbuthnott, *Exp. Brain Res.* **71,** 411 (1988).
23. T. M. Dawson, V. L. Dawson, F. H. Gage, L. J. Fisher, M. A. Hunt, and J. K. Warmsley, *Exp. Neurol.* **111,** 282 (1991).

24. L. Rioux, D. P. Gaudin, C. Gagnon, T. DiPaolo, and P. J. Bedard, *Neuroscience* **44,** 75 (1991).
25. S. B. Dunnett, I. Q. Whishaw, D. C. Rogers, and G. H. Jones, *Brain Res.* **415,** 63 (1987).
26. S. B. Dunnett and L. E. Annett, *in* "Intracerebral Transplantation in Movement Disorders" (O. Lindvall, A. Björklund, and H. Widner, eds.), Vol. 4, p. 27. Elsevier, Amsterdam, 1991.
27. R. M. Ridley and H. F. Baker, *Trends Neurosci.* **14,** 366 (1991).
28. P. Brundin, R. E. Strecker, H. Widner, D. J. Clarke, O. G. Nilsson, B. Åstedt, O. Lindvall, and A. Björklund, *Exp. Brain Res.* **70,** 192 (1988).
29. G. V. Sawle, P. M. Bloomfield, A. Björklund, D. J. Brooks, P. Brundin, K. L. Leenders, O. Lindvall, C. D. Marsden, S. Rehncrona, H. Widner, and R. S. J. Frackowiak, *Ann. Neurol.* **31,** 166 (1992).
30. A. Björklund, *Curr. Opin. Neurobiol.* **2,** 683 (1992).
31. S. B. Dunnett, D. C. Rogers, and S.-J. Richards, *Exp. Brain Res.* **75,** 523 (1989).
32. K. Wictorin, P. Brundin, H. Sauer, O. Lindvall, and A. Björklund, *J. Comp. Neurol.* **323,** 475 (1992).
33. J. W. Fawcett, *Trends Neurosci.* **15,** 5 (1992).
34. I. Strömberg, C. Van Horne, M. Bygdeman, N. Weiner, and G. A. Gerhardt, *Exp. Neurol.* **112,** 140 (1991).
35. A. Björklund and S. B. Dunnett, *in* "Neural Transplantation: A Practical Approach" (S. B. Dunnett and A. Björklund, eds.), p. 57. IRL Press, Oxford, 1992.
35a. S. B. Dunnett and A. Björklund, *in* "Neural Transplantation: A Practical Approach" (S. B. Dunnett and A. Björklund, eds.), p. 1. IRL Press, Oxford, 1992.
36. R. A. Barker, S. B. Dunnett, and J. W. Fawcett, *Semin. Neurosci.* **5,** 431 (1993).
37. B. B. Mishell and S. M. Shiigi, "Selected Methods in Cellular Immunology." Freeman, San Francisco, 1980.
38. P. Brundin, O. Isacson, and A. Björklund, *Brain Res.* **331,** 251 (1985).
39. R. Barker and A. Johnson, *in* "Nerve Cell Culture. Volume I: A Practical Approach" (J. Cohen and G. Wilkin, eds.), IRL Press, Oxford (in press).
40. J. B. Becker, E. J. Curran, and W. J. Feed, *Can. J. Psychol.* **44,** 293 (1990).
41. J. B. Becker and E. J. Curran, *Restor. Neurol. Neurosci.* **4,** 172 (1992).
42. R. A. Barker and S. B. Dunnett, *Restor. Neurol. Neurosci.* **4,** 158 (1992).
43. P. Hantraye, A. L. Brownell, D. Elmalah, R. D. Spealman, U. Wüllner, G. L. Brownell, B. K. Madras, and O. Isacson, *NeuroReport* **3,** 265 (1993).
44. G. V. Sawle and R. Myers, *Trends Neurosci.* **16,** 172 (1993).
45. R. H. Schmidt, A. Björklund, U. Stenevi, and S. B. Dunnett, *in* "Nerve, Organ and Tissue Regeneration: Research Perspectives" (F. J. Seil, ed.), p. 325. Academic Press, New York, 1983.
46. J. W. Fawcett, E. Housden, L. Smith-Thomas, and R. L. Meyer, *Dev. Biol.* **135,** 449 (1989).
47. J. W. Fawcett, J. Rokos, and I. Bakst, *J. Cell Sci.* **92,** 93 (1989).
48. R. A. Barker, R. A. Fricker, J. W. Fawcett, and S. B. Dunnett, *Cell Transplant.* (submitted).
49. S. D. Iversen and S. B. Dunnett, *Psychopharmacol. Biol. Psychiatry* **13,** 453 (1989).

50. L. E. Annett, S. B. Dunnett, E. M. Torres, D. J. Clarke, R. M. Ridley, and H. F. Baker, *Restor. Neurol. Neurosci.* **4,** 185 (1992).
51. T. B. Freeman, E. M. Nauert, C. W. Olanow, and J. H. Kordower, *Restor. Neurol. Neurosci.* **4,** 180 (1992).
52. P. Brundin, G. Barbin, R. E. Strecker, O. Isacson, A. Prochiantz, and A. Björklund, *Dev. Brain Res.* **39,** 233 (1988).

[15] Techniques in Adrenal Medullary Transplantation for Experimental Nonhuman Primate Parkinsonism

Massimo S. Fiandaca and Jeffrey H. Kordower

Nonhuman primates have become important experimental animals in the study of various transplantation strategies in the treatment of Parkinson's disease (PD), Alzheimer's disease (AD), and Huntington's disease (HD). Indeed, monkeys have been used extensively in grafting studies for Parkinson's disease since the discovery that injections of *n*-methyl-4-phenyl-1,2,3,6-tetrahydropyridine (MPTP) cause extensive degeneration of the substantia nigra and induce a parkinsonian syndrome in these animals (1). Many different types of dopaminergic donor tissues have been employed in nonhuman primates. One such donor tissue, adrenal medullary cells, was originally grafted with success in rodents. This was followed by studies in nonhuman primates and human PD patients (2). Chromaffin tissue was proposed to replete the dopamine-depleted striatum under PD conditions with catecholamines, including dopamine, although grafts of adrenal medullary tissue can induce other effects as well (3). The addition of growth factors, such as nerve growth factor (NGF), or growth factor-producing tissues, such as sural nerve or intercostal nerve, enhances the survival and neural phenotypic expression of the chromaffin cells, making them a better graft material.

The authors have almost two decades of combined experience in experimental nonhuman primate surgery; this chapter attempts to convey their technical expertise to investigators interested in learning new transplantation techniques for use in nonhuman primates. The chapter is necessarily technical in nature, because it describes surgical methods and procedures that are not always straightforward or simple, and reading this chapter does not replace hands-on experience in the laboratory or operating room. Indeed, variability between animals can, and has, often led to difficulties even for experienced neurosurgeons. Because nonhuman primate experiments should not be undertaken lightly, investigators interested in using this species and the techniques described in this chapter should be experienced surgeons. Many of the surgical techniques utilized are similar, if not identical, to those used in human transplantation surgery. This chapter, therefore, describes the nonhuman primate operative procedures involved in the treatment of experimental PD with striatal grafting of adrenal medullary tissue, or cograft-

Methods in Neurosciences, Volume 21

ing of adrenal medullary tissue with peripheral nerve. However, it should be noted that the transplant approaches described in this chapter can also be used for other donor tissues as well.

Adrenalectomy in Nonhuman Primate

Nonhuman primates, like humans, normally have bilateral adrenal glands capping their kidneys in the retroperitoneal space. Safe and effective surgical resection of one of these glands can be readily performed, making chromaffin tissue available for autografting in the same animal. From the surgical perspective, there are two major approaches (retroperitoneal and transabdominal) to consider in performing a unilateral adrenalectomy. As in other surgical interventions, the general surgical principles of meticulous technique, hemostasis, and asepsis must be rigorously adhered to for success and animal safety in this type of surgery. Each technique is described in detail below, with comments made regarding advantages and disadvantages of each.

Retroperitoneal Approach

It has been our preference to perform adrenalectomies in nonhuman primates via a left retroperitoneal approach. This approach can be used with the animal positioned in a standad stereotactic apparatus, allowing the adrenalectomy and transplant procedure to be carried out simultaneously. The left gland is chosen because it is usually the larger of the two (at least in humans), and is the furthest from the vena cava, making isolation of its vascular pedicle easier (see below). In humans and nonhuman primates, the flank incision is also less painful postoperatively than the abdominal incision. Less stress is placed along the suture line with breathing or coughing, thereby reducing postoperative pain, increasing deep breathing and coughing, thereby reducing postoperative atelectasis or pneumonia. In addition, the flank incision and retroperitoneal approach do not routinely cause a postoperative ileus (gastrointestinal hypomotility) in the animal. At least a transient ileus is the norm following a transabdominal procedure and can occasionally impede postoperative nutrition and slow overall recovery from surgery.

After placing a small roll under the left chest to rotate the left flank up slightly, a longitudinal incision is placed along the lateral border of the left paraspinous muscles at the costophrenic angle. The superior limb of the incision is extended slightly above the lowest rib. Once the superficial muscles have been traversed, staying below the lowest rib and lateral to the paraspinous muscle bundle, the incision is carried deeper, reaching the quadratus lumborum muscle. This muscle spans between the lowest rib and the iliac crest, stabilizing the origins of the diaphragm during inspiration. Spreading or cutting through this muscle brings one to the retroperitoneal compartment, denoted by yellow fat. Finger palpation medially allows the surgeon to feel the kidney and aorta, which serve as important landmarks for the position of the adrenal gland. Palpation between the upper pole of the kidney and the aorta should allow the surgeon to feel the semilunar-shaped adrenal gland. Once this area is palpated, dissection through the fatty tissues will allow direct inspection of the upper pole of the left kidney and adrenal gland (Fig. 1) (4). Using vascular forceps, gentle dissection of a thin fibroareolar capsule off the adrenal gland and kidney allows easy distinction between the two organs. The kidney has the familiar reddish-brown color, while the adrenal is more yellow-tan in color. Attention should now be paid to the medial border of the adrenal, where the hilum and vascular pedicle are found. Being adjacent to the aorta, the left adrenal gland has a short arterial vessel supplying it and a longer vein or veins draining it to the vena cava. It is always more difficult to dissect the venous structures of the pedicle than the arterial, but longer veins are much easier to isolate and clip ligate

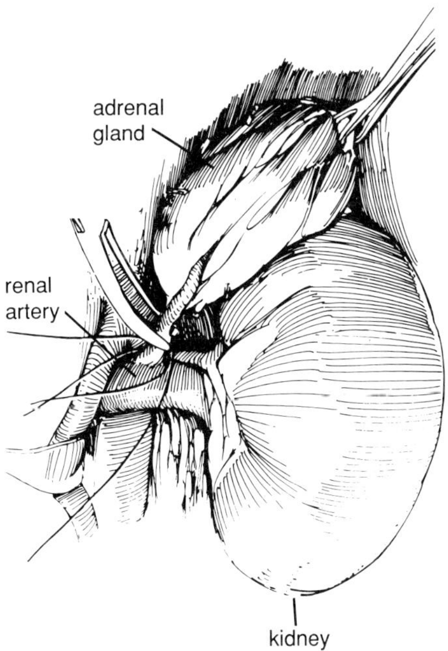

FIG. 1 Schematic illustration of the surgical exposure of the left adrenal gland, using the retroperitoneal approach. [Reprinted from Hinman (4), with permission.]

(using small or medium Weck vascular clips) than shorter ones. A single Weck clip is placed on the vascular pedicle adjacent to the gland, whereas double Weck clips are placed toward the aorta and vena cava, lessening the chance of hemorrhage once the pedicle is sectioned between the sets of clips. At this point the gland should be ready to be removed from the retroperitoneal compartment. The surgical bed is irrigated with warm saline and hemostasis is achieved by the use of bipolar cautery. With the vascular pedicle secured and the adrenal bed dry, routine closure is carried out using simple interrupted 3-0 Vicryl sutures on the muscle layers and simple interrupted 4-0 Dermilon on the skin. Interrupted sutures are used on the skin to prevent inadvertent wound dehiscence due to the animal picking at the wound edge. The animal can also be kept in a primate jacket to prevent it from scratching the incision site.

Transabdominal Approach

Either a midline or transverse abdominal incision can be utilized, but the animal is usually in the supine position for this procedure. This approach is less favored because the animal in a standard stereotactic apparatus is in the prone position, preventing easy access to the anterior abdomen. Therefore, the transplant procedure using this approach involves repositioning the animal in the prone position for the stereotactic procedure after the completion of supine transabdominal adrenalectomy. This adds potential morbidity from placing the animal on its fresh abdominal incision and significantly lengthens the time of the operation. The authors' preference when using this approach is to use a midline incision, extending from the xyphoid to just below the umbilicus, with the animal supine. For the added exposure necessary to properly visualize the retroperitoneal compartment via this approach, the length of the incision is necessarily longer than that used with the retroperitoneal approach. The left adrenal gland is targeted because the right gland is located behind the liver and immediately adjacent to the vena cava, making dissection and removal of the latter much more difficult.

The skin incision is carried down the midline of the abdomen, along the linea alba, and between the rectus muscle sheaths bilaterally. The peritoneal cavity is entered without cutting through muscle, after going through the deep fascia of the rectus aponeurosis. This approach minimizes muscle trauma and postoperative pain. Attention at this point must be paid to minimizing handling of the visceral organs of the abdominal cavity, reducing operative morbidity. With the abdominal incision fully opened, the omentum is elevated from below the stomach, exposing the small intestine and transverse colon. The small intestine is retracted out of the abdominal cavity and toward the right side of the animal, and wrapped in a warm, moist laparotomy pad. This mobilization of the small intestine on its mesentery is essential for visualization of the retroperitoneal space. Working on the left side of the abdomen, the left kidney is palpated in the retroperitoneal space, behind the stomach. The stomach is retracted to the right of the abdominal cavity by carefully dissecting between its greater curvature and the spleen. The transverse colon is retracted inferiorly on its mesentery, allowing visualization of the proximal intraabdominal aorta and the superomedial pole of the left kidney, which is capped by the left adrenal gland (Fig. 2). Crossing the midportion of the left kidney is the glandular-appearing tail of the pancreas. Attention is now given to the left adrenal, which is dissected free from the kidney and surrounding connective tissue. The vascular pedicle of the adrenal is visualized, isolated, and dissected, allowing clamping of arteries and veins with vascular clips (Weck clips) proximal and distal to the adrenal. Once the blood supply is interrupted the pedicle is divided between the clips and the gland delivered from the abdominal cavity. Attention is now given to making sure that the vascular pedicles are secured and that the adrenal bed is dry. Warm saline irrigation is now used to bathe the adrenal bed. Bipolar cautery is useful in obtaining hemostasis prior to closure.

At this point the intraabdominal organs are replaced in their original positions by reversing the steps used in exposing the left adrenal. The peritoneum

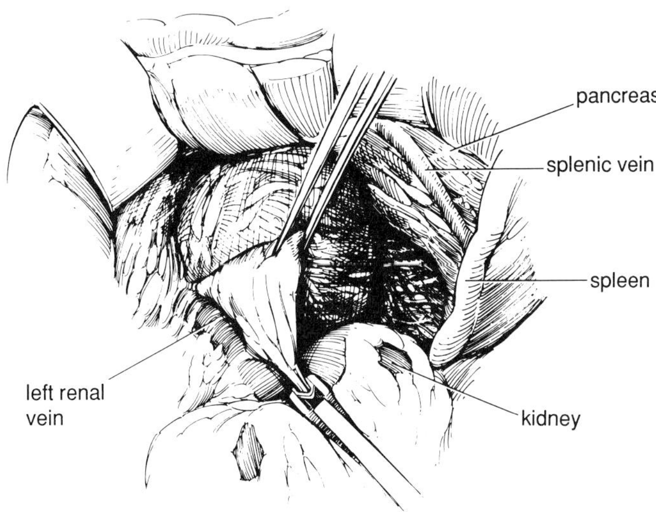

FIG. 2 Schematic illustration of the surgical exposure of the left adrenal gland, using the transabdominal approach. [Reprinted from Hinman (4), with permission.]

is closed with a running 4-0 chromic suture. The midline fascia is closed with a running 2-0 Vicryl suture, in two layers. The subcutaneous tissue is closed with interrupted 3-0 Vicryl suture. The skin is closed with interrupted 4-0 Dermalon suture. The abdominal incision must be covered with a sterile dressing and the animal placed in a primate jacket to prevent it from picking at the suture line.

Adrenal Medulla: Cell Preparation

Once the adrenal gland is removed, it is placed in a petri dish containing ice-cold Ringer's solution with 50% autologous serum. Using a dissecting microscope, a series of coronal cuts is made through the adrenal gland. The resulting coronal sections allow the adrenal medulla to be visualized along with its circumferential investment of adrenal cortex. Using a No. 11 scalpel blade, the medullary core is dissected away from the cortical zona reticulata and placed in a separate petri dish. At higher magnification, the remaining adherent cortical pieces can be separated from the medullary fragments. It is interesting to note that the adrenal cortex is far more interdigitated with the adrenal medulla in humans relative to monkeys. In nonhuman primates, large amounts of pure adrenal medulla can be dissected from the adrenal cortex, whereas this is often not true with the human gland. At this point, the medulla can be dissected into small, 1-mm^3 pieces for solid implants. Alternatively, the cells can be prepared for delivery in suspension. For the latter procedure, the adrenal medullary pieces are placed in a 0.1% trypsin solution at 37°C for 20 min. Then the suspension is centrifuged, decanted, and the pellet resuspended in buffer. The cells are triturated multiple times with a fire-polished Pasteur pipette to disperse them into a more homogeneous suspension. The cells can then be drawn up into a Hamilton syringe (26 gauge) for transplantation.

Isolation of Adrenal Chromaffin Cells

Implants of adrenal chromaffin cells can have complex effects on the host organisms. In this regard, grafts of adrenal medulla have been demonstrated to induce a host-derived TH-immunoreactive sprouting in rodents, nonhuman primates, and patients with Parkinson's disease (2). This response is particularly robust in MPTP-treated nonhuman primates, where the models employed often provide residual dopaminergic neurons within the ventral mesencephalon to manifest this response, a characteristic that appears necessary for a sprouting response to occur (2). The survival of adrenal chromaffin cells within the striatum without trophic factor supplementation has been poor in rats, monkeys, and humans (2). The prevailing hypothesis has been that these cells survived poorly owing to the absence of NGF-like trophic support. This hypothesis has been supported by the fact that infusion of NGF into adrenal graft sites (5) or cografting adrenal medulla with trophic factor-secreting cells (6), augments the viability of the graft and in some cases potentiates functional recovery. However, the fact that trophic factors such as NGF enhance graft viability does not mean that the lack of trophic support mediates the demise of these cells. We have demonstrated that large numbers of chromaffin cells can survive in rodents when the chromaffin cells are isolated from the fibroblasts and endothelial cells contained within the adrenal medulla (7). Using this isolation technique, we have observed that large numbers of chromaffin cells can survive following grafting into MPTP-treated monkeys (Fig. 3). Therefore, if the goal of an experiment is to induce large numbers of chromaffin cells to survive the grafting procedure, the chromaffin cells need to be isolated from the nonchromaffin cell constituents of the adrenal medulla.

The chromaffin cell isolation procedure was established by Sagen and co-workers for use in their studies examining the ability of chromaffin cells to decrease sensitivity to noxious stimuli (8). The methodology established by Sagen and colleagues is illustrated in Fig. 4. Usually, bovine or calf adrenal glands are utilized as donor material. These species of cells are excellent for study because a significant number of chromaffin cells is lost during the isolation procedure and the bovine or calf adrenal gland provides for a large initial population of cells. The glands are first trimmed of their fat and perfused with a calcium- and magnesium-free Locke's solution [1.5 *M* KCl, 0.04 *M* $NaHCO_3$, 0.06 *M* glucose, 0.05 *M* *N*-hydroxyethylpiperazine-*N*′-2-ethane-sulfonic acid (HEPES) at pH 7.2, 37°C] containing antibiotics [penicillin/streptomycin (100 U/ml) and kanamycin (25 mg/ml)] and antifungal agents [Fungizone (amphotericin B; 0.125 mg/ml)]. For 30 min, the glands are incubated in the Locke's solution and then perfused for another 30 min with a 0.1% (v/v) collagenase solution (Boehringer Mannheim, Indianapolis, IN), 0.05% (w/v) bovine serum albumin (BSA; Sigma, St. Louis, MO), and 0.01% (v/v) trypsin inhibitor (Sigma). The medullay tissue is then dissected from the surrounding cortex, minced, filtered through a fine nylon mesh, and washed several times with the Locke's solution. Then the chromaffin cells are suspended in a Percoll buoyancy gradient (45 ml of Percoll, 5 ml of 10× Locke's solution at pH 7.4) and spun at 12,000 rpm for 25 min in a refrigerated centrifuge (IEC B20, 4°C). This produces several bands with dense cell types (e.g., erythrocytes) on the bottom, viable cell types (adrenal medullary cells) in the middle, and lysed cell fragments layering the top. The band containing the adrenal chromaffin cells is removed and washed with Locke's solution.

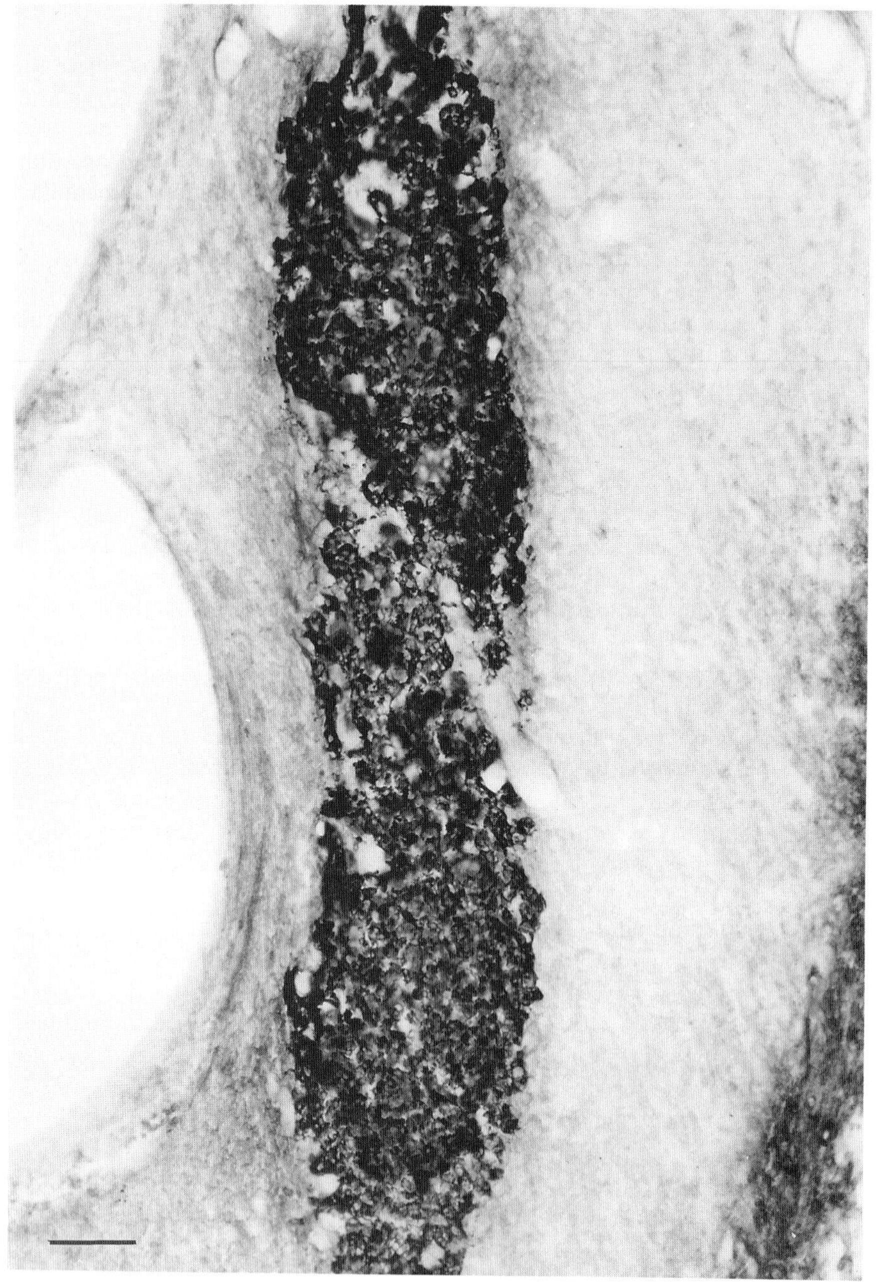

FIG. 3 Tyrosine hydroxylase immunohistochemistry through the striatum of an MPTP-treated rhesus monkey, illustrating the robust survival of healthy adrenal chromaffin cells once the cells are isolated from the nonchomaffin cell types (fibroblast and endothelial cells) of the adrenal medulla. Bar: 100 μm.

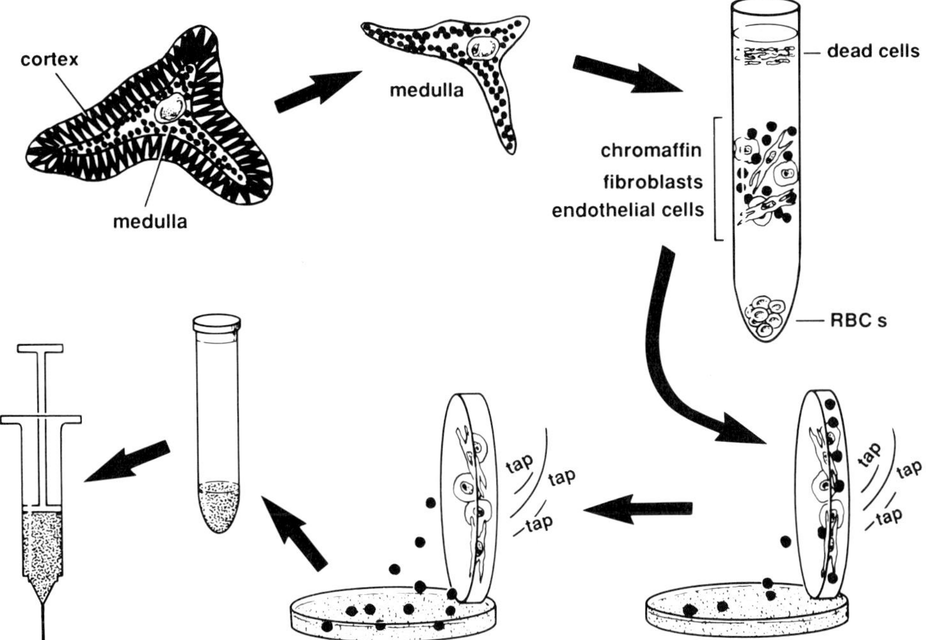

FIG. 4 Schematic illustration of the method used for the isolation of chromaffin cells. See text for details. [Reprinted from Schueler *et al.* (7), with permission.]

The cells are then plated on 100-mm tissue culture plates with DMEM : F12 medium (1 : 1) containing 5% (v/v) fetal bovine serum and antibiotics [penicillin/streptomycin (100 U/ml) and gentamicin (50 U/ml)]. The plates are incubated overnight (37°C, 5% CO_2) to allow the supporting cell types (endothelial cells and fibroblasts) to adhere to the culture plate. On the following day, the chromaffin cells are gently agitated from the plates and placed on a second Percoll gradient to further purify the chromaffin cell population. The viability of this cell preparation is usually in excess of 95% when tested for trypan blue exclusion. Supporting cells remaining on the plates are refed and can be allowed to grow for 3–5 days. These cells can then be removed from the plate and grafted alone or recombined with the isolated chromaffin cells to serve as control donor material.

Peripheral Nerve Harvesting in Nonhuman Primate

Peripheral nerve has been utilized to provide a living, long-lasting source of growth factors to enhance survival and transform phenotypic expression of adrenal chromaffin tissue grafted into the striatum of animals and humans suffering from experimental or clinical PD, respectively. Nerve growth factor, brain-derived neurotrophic factor, fibroblast growth factor, and ciliary neuronotrophic factor are all secreted by the Schwann cells ensheathing peripheral nerves following transection (2). We have used peripheral nerve grafts to provide a "trophic factor cocktail" to support the viability of chromaffin cells following grafting into MPTP-treated rhesus monkeys. These cografts greatly enhance the viability of adrenal autografts (6), induce phenotypic differentiation of some chromaffin cells (6), and can enhance functional recovery (9).

Investigators have utilized both intercostal nerves and sural nerves as readily available peripheral nerve graft sources. Intercostal nerves have been employed in the cograft procedure clinically, as these nerves are usually exposed during the adrenalectomy approach (10). Therefore, a second procedure for nerve harvesting is not required. Experimentally, we have preferred to use sural nerve. Painful intercostal nerve neuralgias are not uncommonly reported following human thoracic surgical procedures, during which the intercostal nerves are cut or otherwise traumatized. The sural nerve, however, is the most commonly sampled peripheral nerve in clinical medicine and usually does not have the same amount of associated morbidity with its resection. The surgical procedures for resecting each nerve type are described below.

Intercostal Nerve Resection

Intercostal nerves are composed of ventral rami of the thoracic roots and are mixed nerves, having motor and sensory components. The major intercostal nerves commonly run in a neurovascular bundle under the caudal edge of each rib and are commonly exposed during an adrenal medullary grafting procedure utilizing the costophrenic angle approach for the resection of the adrenal. It is not unusual to expose either the left T11 or, more commonly, the left T12 ventral ramus (subcostal nerve) as it traverses the surgical approach to the retroperitoneal space at the level of the quadratus lumborum muscle. A 4- to 6-cm length of intercostal nerve can commonly be isolated and resected at this time. Whenever possible, the proximal stump of the nerve should be buried within muscle to prevent the development of a painful subcutaneous neuroma. Despite this latter maneuver, a significant proportion of these proximal nerve stumps do develop symptomatic neuromas.

It has been our preference to immediately mince the segment of peripheral nerve under a dissecting microscope, using a razor blade or sharp scalpel, in a bath of 50% autologous serum–saline solution on ice. The peripheral nerve tissue is kept in the iced saline solution until it is ready to be mixed with the adrenal medullary tissue.

Sural Nerve Resection

The sural nerve is a pure sensory nerve and runs from the popliteal space along the posterolateral aspect of the lower leg, following the course of the lesser saphenous vein. With the animal in the Kopf stereotaxic frame, the sural nerve can be harvested from one or both legs at the same time as the cranial and flank procedures are being carried out. The distal lower legs are shaved, prepared, and draped in a sterile manner, exposing the lateral malleolus of each ankle. The sural nerve invariably runs behind and inferior to the lateral malleolus of the ankle and can easily be located here and dissected back proximally into the leg for a distance of up to 10–15 cm. The proximal course of the nerve from the popliteal space follows the path of the lesser saphenous vein. The nerve is usually found deep to the vein and attention must be paid so as not to be misled into thinking that the collapsed vein is the nerve. The best way to avoid this mistake is to find the nerve proximal to the lateral malleolus. At this level, the nerve begins to branch into several terminal segments, but still has a fairly consistent caliber. Once the nerve has been isolated, it is resected and transferred to the dissecting dish for mincing. Closure of the wound involves using interrupted 3-0 Vicryl sutures in the subcutaneous tissues and interrupted 4-0 Dermalon in the skin.

Striatal Grafting and Cografting for Nonhuman Primate Parkinsonian Syndromes

The transplantation of tissues into the primate striatum for the treatment of experimental parkinsonian syndromes has been well developed during the last 10 years. The majority of investigators have utilized stereotaxic implantation techniques, using various types of frames and hardware. Stereotaxic implantations have depended on the mapping of stereotaxic coordinates for various brain structures in species-specific atlases. Many investigators, however, have found the various commercially available atlases wanting, due to animal size or species differences, and have done their own mapping in groups of their own experimental animals. The Kopf stereotaxic frame remains the main stereotaxic system used for nonhuman primate stereotaxic procedures in the United States. Other systems are certainly available and can be as reliable.

We have used both a standard and modified Kopf stereotaxic apparatus for most of our transplant procedures. This apparatus holds the head in a stable position and many different types of attachments (e.g., electrode holders, microdrives) can be purchased to facilitate the procedure. Besides the stereotaxic implantation technique, an open microsurgical approach can be utilized to implant adrenal medullary tissue (with or without peripheral nerve) into the head(s) of the caudate, paralleling the strategy of Madrazo and colleagues (11). This latter surgical approach is inherently more difficult and associated with more animal morbidity. It is presented primarily for historical perspective because most experimental and clinical transplantation paradigms now utilize stereotaxic approaches.

For all of our surgical procedures, animals are tranquilized with ketamine [10 mg/kg, intramuscularly (im)] and an intravenous line placed for administration of drugs and fluids (D5 lactated Ringer's). For our multipart transplantation procedures a transurethral urinary catheter (5F feeding tube) is placed to monitor urine output during the procedure. Continuous electrocardiogram (EKG) monitoring is utilized. For both stereotaxic and open microsurgical procedures, general anesthesia via orotracheal intubation and inhalation agents should be employed. We prefer isoflurane delivered via a veterinary anesthesia machine and monitored by a veterinary technician. Animals are mechanically ventilated throughout the procedures. Steroids are not routinely used and intravenous antibiotics are not routinely utilized.

Stereotaxic Implantation

In our initial primate experiments, we employed the standard Kopf primate stereotaxic frame and ascertained our stereotaxic coordinates using the Kopf stereotaxic zero bar. Unlike rats, however, we found that there is considerable variability in the brain structure of primates, depending on size and species, and standard atlases are often inadequate. Consistent localization of even large brain structures such as the caudate nucleus and putamen can be problematic as deviation by just a few millimeters can place the target into the internal or external capsules. Furthermore, behavioral recovery following grafting is thought to be site specific and significant variability even within one structure (e.g., dorsal versus ventral caudate nucleus) can create variability in behavioral data that is magnified by the relatively small numbers of subjects usually employed in nonhuman primate studies. Therefore, we now use magnetic resonance imaging (MRI) techniques for target localization in all our transplant studies utilizing a stereotaxic procedure. This requires that all parts of the stereotaxic frame be nonmagnetic. Such units can be made

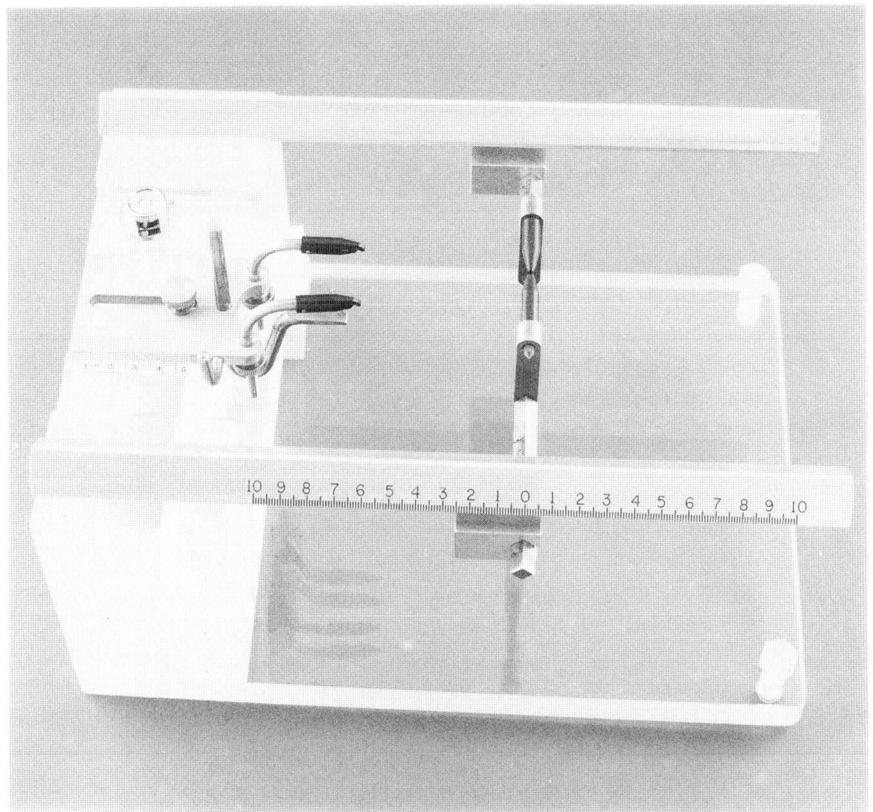

FIG. 5 MRI-compatible stereotaxic unit modeled after the Kopf stereotaxic frame.

from plastic or nonmetallic alloys (Fig. 5). Our MRI-compatible stereotaxic apparatus is based on the Kopf design and therefore can utilize the electrode holder and coordinate systems designed by this manufacturer. When we use MRI to scan our monkeys, they first receive an intramuscular injection of atropine (0.04 mg/kg). Then they are anesthetized with an intramuscular combination of ketamine (10 mg/kg) and xylazine (2 mg/kg). This allows for approximately 60–90 min of anesthesia. If the scan takes an unusually long time and the animal begins to awaken, the monkey is supplemented with one-quarter of the original dose. After the monkey is anesthetized, it is intubated, using the standard orotracheal method. They are then brought to the scanner and placed in the MRI-compatible stereotaxic apparatus. Because we do not scan our monkeys on the day of surgery, it is essential that the position of the head during the scan and subsequent operation be identical. Thus, we center the head of the animal with the coordinates on the ear bars. Then a needle bent at a 90° angle is mounted on a Kopf electrode holder (because the electrode holder is metallic this must be done outside the room with the scanner). The height of the needle when it contacts the lower edge of the animal's incisor teeth is then measured and recorded. The electrode holder is then removed and the animal is scanned in the stereotaxic unit on a 1.5-T General Electric MRI scanner, obtaining sequential scans in the coronal plane. The anterior–posterior (AP) zero is at the level at which the ear canals can be seen (Fig. 6A). The brain site of interest (e.g., caudate nucleus and putamen) can then be visualized on more rostral sections that are a known distance from the AP zero. The medial–lateral (ML) and dorsal–ventral (DV) coordinates can then be easily measured using standard software on the MRI scanner (Fig. 6B). The monkey is then removed from the scanner and stereotaxic unit. Prior to placing the monkey back in its home cage, the monkey receives tolazoline (2 mg/kg, im), which reverses the effect of the xylazine and facilitates recovery.

At the time of surgery, the monkey is tranquilized with ketamine (10 mg/kg, im), pretreated with atropine (0.04 mg/kg, im), and intubated via the orotracheal method. The head is shaved and the animal is replaced in the MRI-compatible stereotaxic apparatus. Then the height of its incisor teeth is measured as before, using the same electrode holder and bent needle. It is critical that this height be identical to that measured prior to the MRI scan or the stereotaxic coordinates will be incorrect. The head is then prepped with Betadine solution and draped, using sterile methods. A midsagittal scalp incision is placed from just behind the supraorbital ridge to the level of the interaural line. The right temporalis muscle is detached from the skull by cautery, exposing the right lateral frontal skull, bregma, and right coronal suture. Hemostasis of the scalp edges is obtained by bipolar cautery. The stereotaxic micromanipulator and injection cannula are then moved over the target as determined by the MRI coordinates. The injection needle is lowered to the skull surface, using the micromanipulator, to determine where to drill the entry hole for the injection cannula. Once the entry site is noted, the needle is rotated out of position and a burr hole is made with a high-speed drill. Once the inner table of the skull is penetrated, the dura is opened and the pia incised enough to allow entry of a 16- to 18-gauge Seldinger needle into the brain parenchyma without distortion. The Seldinger needle and its vertical bar holder is detached from the micromanipulator and brought to the microdissection area, where it is loaded for grafting. The number of pieces of adrenal medulla (and peripheral nerve) taken up into the needle is noted for future reference. With the Seldinger needle loaded with graft (or cograft material), it is reattached to the micromanipulator via its vertical

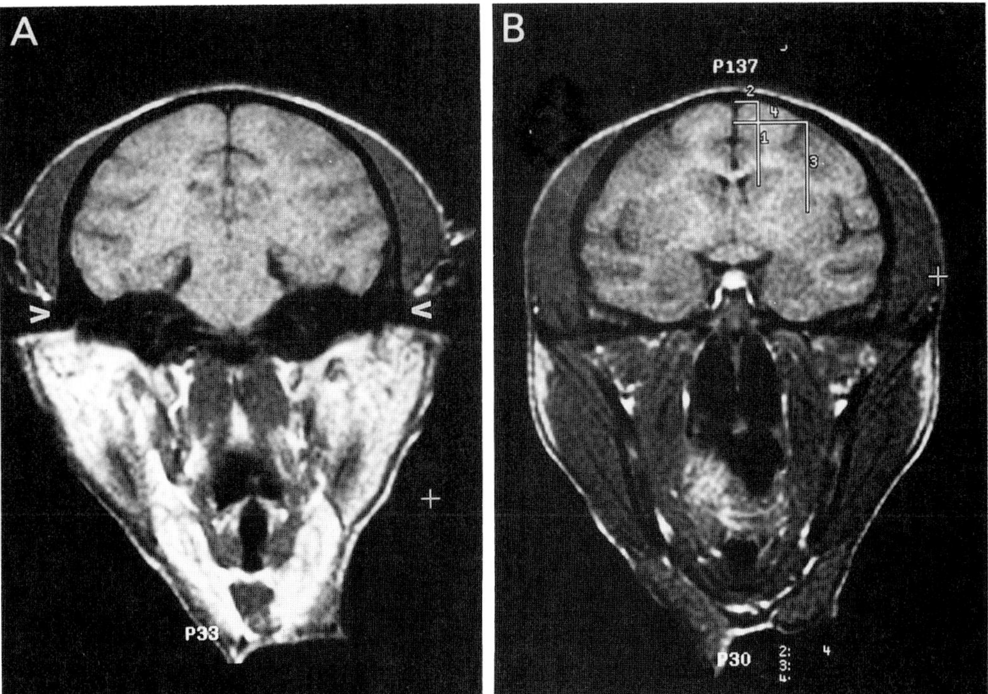

FIG. 6 MRI scans of a 4-kg cynomolagus monkey prior to transplantation. (A) This level of the brain serves as the AP zero, as the ear canals (arrowheads) can be clearly seen. (B) The stereotaxic coordinates for striatal implants are made on this scan, which is 14 mm rostral to the scan seen in Fig. (A). Numbers 1–4 denote the four measurements ascertained to provide mediolateral and dorsoventral stereotaxic coordinates for the caudate nucleus (1 and 2) and putamen (3 and 4).

bar, maintaining its position in reference to stereotaxic zero. With the micromanipulator already set to the AP and ML coordinates, the needle is then slowly lowered to the target on the basis of the MRI coordinates. The needle is left untouched for 2–3 min to allow it to equilibrate with the surrounding brain tissue. The contents of the Seldinger needle are injected slowly (3 min) via the stylet. After the final injection, the needle is left in position for an additional 2 min and then slowly removed. Occasionally (especially with cografts), a bit of graft material is often stuck to the tip on removal. The volume remaining on the needle tip is noted so that a determination of delivered graft volume can be made. This same procedure can be repeated at different sites.

On completion of the stereotaxic grafting, the burr hole is filled in with Gelfoam and the exposed skull irrigated with saline. The scalp wound is then closed with interrupted 3-0 Vicryl sutures in the galea aponeurotica, and interrupted 4-0 Dermilon sutures (or skin staples) in the skin. Animals recover quickly from this procedure and are ambulating in their cages within several hours after surgery.

Open Microsurgical Implantation

The animal again begins positioned in the Kopf head frame. Because this procedure does not use stereotaxic coordinates, either the standard or MRI-compatible apparatus can be employed. During this procedure it is not essential to have the head exactly centered as it was for the stereotaxic procedure, because we utilize the frame as a head holder rather than a localizing device. It is important, however, to position the head and neck in a way that would promote free venous drainage and not induce venous congestion. The head of the animal is shaved, prepared, and draped in a manner similar to the stereotaxic approach, but more of the scalp is exposed, allowing for the scalp flap. A U-shaped flap is cut using a No. 10 scalpel, with the pedicle based on the midline, astride the right coronal suture (Fig. 7). The dimensions of the flap are approximately 5 cm long by 3 cm wide. In some animals the medial temporalis muscle must then be dissected off the skull and retracted laterally. At this point the animal is given a bolus of intravenous mannitol solution [0.25–0.5 gm/kg, intravenously (iv)] to induce diuresis and decrease brain tension. The animal is moderately hyperventilated to a P_aCO_2 of approximately 30 mmHg. The exposed skull is then perforated with a high-speed drill, making four to six burr holes, the medial ones being on the midline. Great care must be used when drilling on the midline so as to avoid entering the superior sagittal sinus and causing a potentially lethal hemorrhage. Connecting cuts are then made between adjoining burr holes, so that a rectangular bone flap, measuring approximately 4 cm long and 2 cm wide, can be removed. On removal of the bone flap, bleeding from the area of the superior saggital sinus can be controlled with pieces of Gelfoam and Surgicel. Once good osmotic diuresis is obtained from the mannitol and the brain feels relatively slack, the dura can be safely opened.

The dura is then opened in a U-shaped flap based on the superior sagittal sinus, exposing the underlying parasagittal cortex. At this point the operating microscope is brought into the field and utilized for the remainder of the intracranial procedure. Under $\times 10$–$\times 16$ magnification, parasagittal bridging veins can be coagulated with bipolar cautery and cut, freeing the medial brain convexity for gentle lateral retraction. The medial brain convexity is covered with a sheet of Bicol and retracted laterally, using a self-retaining

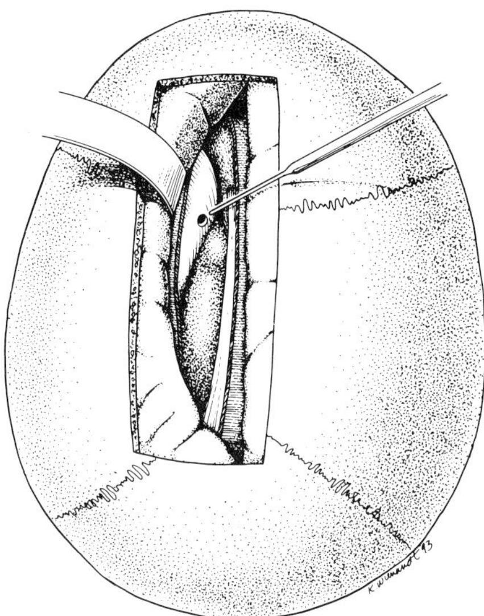

FIG. 7 Schematic illustration of the exposure obtained using the open microsurgical approach to the caudate nucleus.

brain retractor. A ball microdissector is used to open the arachnoid plane betwen the right hemisphere and the falx cerebri. At the level of the free edge of the falx, the arachnoidal adhesions between the cingulate gyri can be more difficult to dissect. Once opened, and the bilateral cingulate gyri separated, the ivory-colored corpus callosum is visualized. Running dorsal to the corpus callosum are the paired (or sometimes single) pericallosal arteries and veins. The veins may be coagulated if they are in the way of the approach to the callosum. The arteries are dissected to the left and right, exposing a relatively avascular midline.

Using the ball microdissector, a 2-cm incision is placed in the corpus callosum, deviating toward the right as the incision is carried deeper, allowing entry into the right lateral ventricle. Inspection of the ventricular landmarks (Fig. 7) allows the surgeon to become oriented and define the extent of the head of the caudate anterior to the foramen of Monro. After a piece of Gelfoam is placed over the ipsilateral foramen of Monro to prevent blood from draining into the third ventricle, a linear incision is made in the head of the caudate, using a No. 11 blade. Bleeding from this structure is guaranteed and bipolar cautery does not help, due to the friability of the tissue. We recommend that a pledget of Gelfoam be placed in the incision and left there for 3–5 min, with gentle suction applied through a cotton patty to obtain hemostasis. Once hemostasis is obtained, the incision in the head of the caudate is irrigated and the Gelfoam removed. At this point the transplant procedure can begin. Pieces of adrenal medulla (with or without peripheral nerve) can be placed within the incision under direct vision. Because of the texture of the tissue and the tissue pressure generated during grafting, the grafts must usually be held in place with a pledget of Gelfoam. Once the entire caudate incision is filled with graft material, surgeons have either stapled the grafts in place (11), made a Gelfoam net to hold the grafts in position (12), or left them alone after removing the Gelfoam. With hemostasis guaranteed via inspection and observation of the tumor bed during a Valsalva maneuver, closure of the wound can begin.

The microscope can be removed from the field and all retractors from within the brain and skull. The dura is now closed with running or interrupted 4-0 Vicryl, with an attempt made to make a watertight seal. A pledget of Gelfoam is then placed over the exposed dura. The bone flap is replaced using interrupted 4-0 Vicryl through predrilled holes in skull and bone flap. The wound is then copiously irrigated with saline. Finally, the scalp closure consists of interrupted 3-0 Vicryl sutures in the galea, and interrupted 4-0 Dermilon in the skin. The animal is then taken out of the Kopf frame and allowed to awaken from anesthesia while intubated. Once breathing well and beginning to cough, the orotracheal tube is removed and the animal placed in its cage under a heating lamp. The vast majority of animals undergoing this procedure will be ambulating in the cage within several hours.

Concluding Remarks

Grafting studies carried out in nonhuman primates are essential prior to initiating clinical trials. Because monkeys are expensive to purchase and maintain, and are an inherently valuable experimental resource, considerable care must be taken with their use. When used properly, they can be excellent predictors of results to be obtained following clinical transplantation. This turned out to be especially true in studies employing adrenal autografts for Parkinson's disease, in which extensive testing in nonhuman primates was not carried out prior to the initiation of clinical trials. Therefore, the clinical studies did not benefit from the knowledge gained later in monkey experiments demonstrating that without trophic factor support, adrenal medullary grafts survive poorly and a host-derived sprouting response may account for the modest benefit displayed by some patients (12, 13). For the most part, clinical trials employing the adrenal medulla as donor tissue have stopped. However, many of the procedures described herein can be employed in other grafting paradigms and their careful use in nonhuman primate models of neurodegenerative disease can provide critical information regarding their potential utility for clinical application.

Acknowledgments

The authors with to thank the many colleagues who have participated in the experiments, the methodologies for which are described herein.

References

1. S. Burns, C. C. Chieuh, S. Markey, H. Ebert, D. M. Jacobowitz, and I. J. Kopin, *Proc. Natl. Acad. Sci. U.S.A.* **80,** 4546 (1983).
2. J. H. Kordower, D. L. Felten, and D. M. Gash, *in* "Scientific Basis for Therapy in Parkinson's Disease" (C. W. Olanow and A. Lieberman, eds.), p. 175. Parthenon Press, Park Ridge, NJ, 1992.
3. M. S. Fiandaca, J. H. Kordower, J. T. Hansen, S.-S. Jiao, and D. M. Gash, Adrenal medullary autografts into the basal ganglia of cebus monkeys: Injury-induced regeneration. *Exp. Neurol.* **102,** 76 (1988).
4. F. Hinman, Jr., "Atlas of Urologic Surgery." Saunders, Philadelphia, 1989.
5. I. Strömberg, M. Herrera-Marschitz, U. Ungerstedt, T. Ebendal, and L. Olson, Chronic implants of chomaffin tissue into the dopamine-denervated striatum: Effects of NGF on graft survival, fiber growth and rotational behavior. *Exp. Brain Res.* **60,** 335 (1985).
6. J. H. Kordower, M. S. Fiandaca, M. F. D. Notter, J. T. Hansen, and D. M. Gash, NGF-like trophic support from peripheral nerve for grafted rhesus adrenal chromaffin cells. *J. Neurosurg.* **73,** 418 (1990).
7. S. B. Schueler, J. D. Ortega, J. Sagen, and J. H. Kordower, Robust survival of isolated bovine adrenal chromaffin cells following intrastriatal transplantation: A novel hypothesis of adrenal graft viability. *J. Neurosci.* **13,** 4496 (1993).
8. J. Sagen, G. D. Pappas, and J. D. Ortega, Host–graft relationships of isolated bovine chromaffin cells in rat periaqueductal gray. *J. Neurocytol.* **19,** 697 (1990).
9. R. A. E. Bakay, C. Herring, R. Watts, and L. Byrd, Delayed and acute stereotaxic cografting in the treatment of hemiparkinsonian monkeys. *Soc. Neurosci. Abstr.* **16,** 809 (1990).
10. R. L. Watts, A. Freeman, C. G. Goetz, S. Graham, G. O. Zakers, R. A. E. Bakay, G. T. Stebbins, and R. D. Penn, Autologous intrastriatal adrenal medulla/nerve cografts in Parkinson's disease: Early resultss. *Neurology* **A222** (1993).
11. I. Madrazo, T. Drucker-Colín, V. Daíz, J. Martinez-Mata, C. Torres, and J. J. Becerrel, Open microsurgical autograft of adrenal medulla to the right caudate nucleus in two patients with intractable Parkinson's disease. *N. Engl. J. Med.* **316,** 831 (1987).
12. G. S. Allen, R. S. Burns, N. B. Tulipan, and R. A. Parker, Adrenal medullary transplantation into the caudate nucleus in Parkinson's disease: Initial clinical results in 18 patients. *Arch. Neurol. (Chicago)* **46,** 487 (1989).
13. J. H. Kordower, E. Cochran, R. Penn, and C. G. Goetz, Putative chromaffin cell survival and enhanced host-derived TH-fiber innervation following a functional adrenal medulla autograft for Parkinson's disease. *Ann. Neurol.* **29,** 405 (1991).

[16] Technical Aspects of Transplantation of the Adrenal Medulla to the Caudate Nucleus as a Treatment for Parkinson's Disease

Stephen W. Carmichael, Susan L. Stoddard, and Patrick J. Kelly

Introduction

Parkinson's disease is characterized, in part, by a loss of dopaminergic cells in the pars compacta of the substantia nigra in the mesencephalon (6). A primary projection target of the axons from these cells is the neostriatum, that is, the putamen and caudate nucleus. Thus, in Parkinson's disease there is a notable decrease in the neurotransmitter dopamine within the striatum. It has been postulated that replacement of dopamine within this region of the brain may be of therapeutic benefit to patients with Parkinson's disease.

The chromaffin cells of the adrenal medulla synthesize dopamine as a precursor to norepinephrine and epinephrine (Fig. 1). The enzymes that convert dopamine to norepinephrine (dopamine β-hydroxylase) and norepinephrine to epinephrine (phenylethanolamine *N*-methyltransferase) are made more active by steroids produced by adrenal cortical cells (14). Chromaffin cells that are isolated from the adrenal cortex do not convert dopamine to epinephrine as readily as in the normally situated adrenal medulla. Thus, the isolated adrenal medulla has the potential to be a producer of dopamine that could be grafted to the basal ganglia.

In a highly publicized article, Madrazo and colleagues (9) reported observations from two patients in whom adrenal medullary tissue had been autologously transplanted to the caudate nucleus as a treatment for Parkinson's disease. In these individuals the parkinsonian symptoms were notably improved. This report stimulated the initiation of similar surgical procedures at many institutions throughout the world. The following is a report on the technical aspects of this procedure as it was performed on eight patients at the Mayo Clinic between September 1987 and April 1988.

Overview of Procedure

Autologous transplantation of the adrenal medulla to the caudate nucleus was planned. The patient was placed in a supine position to accommodate

Methods in Neurosciences, Volume 21

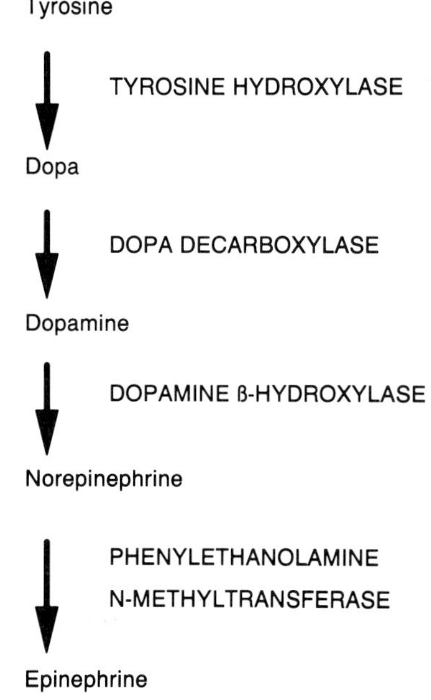

FIG. 1 Biosynthesis of catecholamines.

both the neurosurgical procedure and the laparotomy. The right adrenal gland was removed through a subcostal incision and a transperitoneal approach. The right gland was selected to avoid possible complications associated with left adrenalectomy (i.e., pancreatitis). The right adrenal gland was dissected free of all attachments before the adrenal vein was ligated; it was removed as an intact specimen. The adrenal medulla was dissected from the cortex and passed to the neurosurgeon for implantation.

Neurosurgical Procedure

Because patients undergoing adrenal medullary–caudate transplantation were debilitated, a minimally invasive surgical approach was developed that was a modification of previous approaches used for the resection of deep-seated brain neoplasms. The surgical approach was divided into three phases: database acquisition, treatment planning, and interactive surgical procedure, and is described briefly as follows.

Patients were fitted with a computed tomography (CT)-compatible stereotaxic head frame that attached to the skull at four points. The frame is relocatable by virtue of the osseous fixation and micrometer settings that allow the frame to be placed, removed, and reapplied in precisely the same location. Thus, database acquisition can be accomplished on one day and the surgical procedure on another.

The head of the caudate was selected from the stereotaxic CT images, displayed on a surgical planning computer. The computer calculated *X, Y,* and *Z* stereotaxic frame coordinates required to access the caudate. An arc-quadrant stereotaxic frame (COMPASS; Stereotactic Medical Systems, Inc., Rochester, MN) was used.

Stereotaxic craniotomy and transperitoneal right adrenalectomy were performed concomitantly while the patient was under general endotracheal anesthesia. For the craniotomy, a 7.6-cm incision made at the hairline of the skull was opened with a 3.8-cm diameter trephine and the dura mater was opened in a cruciate fashion. The sulcus between the superior and middle frontal convolutions was separated microsurgically and a 2-cm cylindrical retractor, which was held on the arc quadrant of the stereotaxic frame, was placed. The subcortical incision was deepened utilizing a carbon dioxide laser directed from a microslad mounted on the operating microscope. The subcortical white matter was incised with the laser and then dilated as the retractor was advanced over a special dilator. The right lateral ventricle was entered and the retractor advanced to the head of the caudate. An incision was made into the ependyma and a recipient site in the head of the right caudate nucleus prepared by removing a 7-mm diameter segment of the caudate head with a tumor biopsy forceps. This segment was assayed for catecholamines and receptor binding (4).

Within 1.5 to 19 min after adrenalectomy, multiple fragments of adrenal medulla were passed to the neurosurgical team for placement in the prepared bed within the caudate nucleus. The smaller fragments were placed deeper and the larger fragments were placed more superficially. The larger fragments were then clipped to the ependymal surface by means of small vascular clips. The stereotaxic retractor was removed as hemostasis was secured. The dura was closed, the bone replaced, and the scalp and abdominal incisions were closed. The patient was then removed from the stereotaxic frame and allowed to recover from the anesthesia.

Preparation of Adrenal Medulla

Weeks prior to the first surgical procedure, 24 unembalmed adrenal glands were obtained, with appropriate permission, from autopsied patients. Techniques for dissecting the medulla from the cortex were developed with three objectives in mind: obtaining as homogeneous a preparation of adrenal medulla as possible (purity), performing the dissection as quickly as possible (speed), and obtaining as many chromaffin cells from a single adrenal gland as possible (yield). The rationale for maximum purity was to isolate chromaffin cells from cortical cells, thereby minimizing the activating influence of cortical steroids on dopamine β-hydroxylase and phenylethanolamine N-methyltransferase, which in turn would maximize the amount of dopamine produced by the chromaffin cells. Speed was important because it is well known that adrenal chromaffin cells are metabolically active and are short lived when isolated. We increased the viability of the cells by performing the dissection on cold (4°C) sterile Teflon boards and holding the tissue, when not actually being dissected, in cold lactated Ringer's solution. There was no previously established rationale for maximizing yield, but we thought that it was logical to harvest as much of this limited tissue as possible for each patient.

The technique that was developed involved two people working simultaneously under ×12.5 binocular magnification. Person A received the gland from the surgeon in cold lactated Ringer's solution in an emesis basin. The gland was placed on a cooled Teflon board and sliced transversely with a new double-edged razor blade into 2- to 3-mm thick slices. The first slice containing medulla was passed to person B; person A continued to slice the gland. Medulla was apparent in the slice as a pearl-gray tissue, typically surrounded by a reddish-brown (or sometimes yellowish) cortex. The cortex was grasped with fine forceps (Dumont, No. 11254-20; Fine Science Tools) and the corticomedullary boundary was incised with Vannas scissors [straight, No. 1500-08 (Fine Science Tools) and angled up, No. OP-5587 (American V. Mueller)], separating the rim of cortex from the bulk of the medulla. The central vein was frequently noted to be surrounded by cortical tissue. Although this is not usually observed in the adrenal glands of most mammals, it was first described in the human adrenal gland by Kölliker in 1852 (8). In addition, islets of cortical tissue that varied in size were observed to be irregularly distributed within the medulla. As each slice was dissected, these islets, and the central vein and its associated cortical tissue, were removed. The first piece of medulla isolated by person B was passed to a pathologist, who confirmed the organ type from a frozen section. In our cases, 95–100% of the section was confirmed to be adrenal medulla.

Slices were stored in a small dish of cold lactated Ringer's solution, positioned between persons A and B. By the time person A finished slicing the gland (approximately 1 min), person B had isolated one or two pieces of medulla. Pieces of medulla were either passed to the neurosurgeon for implantation (as described above) or kept in another dish of lactated Ringer's until the neurosurgeon called for the tissue. The first piece of medulla was implanted about 90 sec after the adrenal gland was removed. At this point both persons A and B were dissecting medulla from each slice. Pieces of medulla that were too small for the neurosurgeon to implant were preserved for analyses and tissue culture. In our most protracted procedure, the last piece of medulla was implanted 19 min after the adrenal gland was removed. Twelve minutes of elapsed time was more typical.

Explants of transplanted adrenal medullary tissue were cultured to establish tissue viability. Cells were maintained in culture for over 2 weeks; electron microscopic examination of the chromaffin cells revealed essentially normal structure. Levels of catecholamines and several neuropeptides were measured in pieces of adrenal medulla too small for transplantation. Levels of all catecholamines were found to be significantly lower in tissue from parkinsonian patients than in control tissue (11). Similarly, levels of Met-enkephalin, neuropeptide Y, substance P, and vasoactive intestinal peptide were significantly decreased in adrenal medullary tissue from parkinsonian patients (12). Experiments with an animal model of Parkinson's disease have suggested that neurohormonal deficit observed in the adrenal medullas of parkinsonian patients is due to the disease, and not the chronic administration of antiparkinsonian medications (13).

The clinical outcome of these surgical procedures is described in detail elsewhere (3, 7). Briefly, one patient was categorized as moderately improved 1 year after transplantation; three patients were moderately improved, and four patients were unimproved. One patient died of an unrelated disease (myocardial infarction) about 2 years after the procedure and the neuropathological examination revealed no surviving chromaffin cells in the caudate. This is consistent with other autopsy findings (10).

Conclusions

We present here an effective technique for the autologous transplantation of adrenal medullary tissue to the caudate nucleus. The clinical outcome of this procedure was similar to that reported at several other centers (5); the limited improvement seen with this technique has not been sufficient to justify continuation of the risk and expense of the procedure (1, 2). We anticipate that new versions of this technique, perhaps including the application of trophic factors, may lead to a therapy for Parkinson's disease. A truly effective adrenal-to-brain transplantation procedure has yet to be clinically demonstrated.

References

1. J. E. Ahlskog, Parkinson's disease: New treatment strategies. *Compr. Ther.* **16,** 41 (1990).

2. J. E. Ahlskog, Cerebral transplantation for Parkinson's disease. *Mayo Clin. Proc.* **68,** 578 (1993).
3. J. E. Ahlskog, P. J. Kelly, J. A. van Heerden, S. L. Stoddard, G. M. Tyce, A. J. Windebank, P. A. Bailey, G. N. Bell, M. D. Blexrud, and S. W. Carmichael, Adrenal medullary transplantation into the brain for treatment of Parkinson's disease: Clinical outcome and neurochemical studies. *Mayo Clin. Proc.* **65,** 305 (1990).
4. J. E. Ahlskog, E. Richelson, A. Nelson, P. J. Kelly, H. Okazaki, G. M. Tyce, J. A. van Heerden, S. L. Stoddard, and S. W. Carmichael, Reduced D2-dopamine and muscarinic-cholinergic receptor densities in caudate biopsies of fluctuating Parkinson patients. *Ann. Neurol.* **30,** 185 (1991).
5. S. W. Carmichael and S. L. Stoddard, Chapter 16. Transplantation. *In* "The Adrenal Medulla, 1989–1991," pp. 401–429. CRC Press, Boca Raton, FL, 1993.
6. O. Hornykiewicz, Parkinson's disease: From brain homogenate to treatment. *Fed. Proc., Fed. Am. Soc. Exp. Biol.* **32,** 183 (1973).
7. P. J. Kelly, J. E. Ahlskog, J. A. van Heerden, S. W. Carmichael, S. L. Stoddard, and G. N. Bell, Adrenal medullary autograft transplantation into the striatum of patients with Parkinson's disease. *Mayo Clin. Proc.* **64,** 282 (1989).
8. A. Kölliker, *in* "Handbuch der Gewebelehre des Menschen" (W. Engelmann, ed.), p. 852. Leipzig, 1852.
9. I. Madrazo, R. Drucker-Colín, V. Díaz, J. Martínez-Mata, C. Torres, and J. J. Becerril, Open microsurgical autograft of adrenal medulla to the right caudate nucleus in two patients with intractable Parkinson's disease. *N. Engl. J. Med.* **316,** 831 (1987).
10. N. P. Quinn, The clinical application of cell grafting techniques in patients with Parkinson's disease. *Prog. Brain Res.* **78,** 619 (1990).
11. S. L. Stoddard, J. E. Ahlskog, P. J. Kelly, G. M. Tyce, J. A. van Heerden, A. R. Zinsmeister, and S. W. Carmichael, Decreased adrenal medullary catecholamines in adrenal transplanted parkinsonian patients compared to nephrectomy patients. *Exp. Neurol.* **104,** 218 (1989).
12. S. L. Stoddard, G. M. Tyce, J. E. Ahlskog, A. R. Zinsmeister, and S. W. Carmichael, Decreased levels of [Met]enkephalin, neuropeptide Y, substance P, and vasoactive intestinal peptide in parkinsonian adrenal medulla. *Exp. Neurol.* **114,** 23 (1991).
13. S. L. Stoddard, G. J. Merkel, J. A. Cook, A. R. Zinsmeister, and S. W. Carmichael, The adrenal medulla in Parkinson's disease. *Anat. Rec., Suppl.* **1,** 108 (1993).
14. R. J. Wurtman and J. Axelrod, Adrenaline synthesis: Control by the pituitary gland and adrenal glucocorticoids. *Science* **150,** 1464 (1965).

Section VII

Creating Cell Lines for Transplant Therapies

[17] Transplantation of Epidermal Growth Factor-Responsive Neural Stem Cell Progeny into the Murine Central Nervous System

Joseph P. Hammang, Brent A. Reynolds, Samuel Weiss, Albee Messing, and Ian D. Duncan

Introduction

Neurodegenerative disorders such as Alzheimer's, Parkinson's, and Huntington's disease, as well as demyelinating disorders such as multiple sclerosis (MS), are of serious concern in our society. Our understanding of the processes underlying these disorders is poor and treatments are few. Because of the wide array of central nervous system (CNS) disorders, possible therapeutic approaches are also diverse and include cell replacement via transplantation; neurotrophic factor delivery from implants of polymer-encapsulated or unencapsulated, genetically modified cell lines; and the systemic delivery of small, therapeutic molecules capable of traversing the blood–brain barrier. As each of these approaches has benefits and limitations, it may be necessary to combine some of them for successful therapeutic intervention.

Much attention is currently being directed toward the use of neurotrophic factors in the treatment of neurodegenerative disorders. The application of these factors to the CNS for therapeutic intervention has been delayed primarily by two obstacles. First, polypeptide growth factors are relatively large molecules and, in general, are unable to cross the blood–brain barrier. Second, it is unclear whether non-site-specific delivery will be effective in reversing the degenerative process that typically occurs in defined brain regions and whether nonspecific delivery will produce detrimental side effects. Although specific small molecules, capable of crossing the blood–brain barrier may be developed to overcome some of these problems, few options exist today for the delivery of neurotrophic factors to the CNS. One option is the use of a polymer encapsulation technology that provides a means for the delivery of neurotrophic factors and neurotransmitters to the site of disease within the nervous system (see Chapters [22]–[24], this volume). With this technology, one can safely encapsulate cell lines that have been genetically modified to secrete neurotrophic or other factors. The encapsu-

Methods in Neurosciences, Volume 21

lated device provides protection to the host from uncontrolled cell line growth while protecting the implanted cells from the host immune system.

A second approach in the treatment of neurodegenerative diseases is through cell replacement, by which unprotected cells are transplanted into the damaged or diseased nervous system. Potential cell therapy applications in humans include the replacement of oligodendrocytes in demyelinated MS lesions, replacement of dopaminergic neurons of the substantia nigra in Parkinson's disease, or the site-specific implantation of genetically modified, trophic factor-secreting cells to prevent or arrest neuronal loss. In experimental approaches for the treatment of demyelinating and inherited dysmyelinating disorders, progress has been made in animal models with the implantation of dissociated primary glial cells as well as a number of oligodendrocyte precursor cell lines. In these paradigms, oligodendrocytes or oligodendrocyte precursors have been shown to restore myelin in portions of the demyelinated or dysmyelinated nervous system (1–3). Progress has also been achieved with fetal cell transplants into patients with Parkinson's disease; however, the procedure has been largely dependent on the availability of fetal tissue, which is fraught with concerns of a moral and ethical nature as well as concerns over the uniformity, adequate supply, and the safety of the donor material (4, 5).

The lack of a reliable and safe supply of primary cells for human transplantation has resulted in the development of cell lines, specifically the oncogene-induced immortalization of CNS stem/progenitor cells (for reviews see Refs. 6 and 7). Although these cells have been extremely valuable in rodent transplant models, and in broadening our understanding of neural development and function, the use of oncogene-driven cells for human transplant therapy is questionable. Although the use of cell lines derived with temperature-sensitive or inducible oncogenes may be a logical alternative, their safety for transplantation into humans has not been addressed. An epidermal growth factor (EGF)-responsive neural stem cell culture system has been developed that may be an alternative to oncogene-generated cells (8–10). These growth factor-responsive, nontransformed neural stem cells can be continuously propagated in a cell line-like manner for indefinite periods in the presence of EGF. On removal of EGF, proliferation stops and the stem cell-generated progenitor cells can be differentiated *in vitro* into neurons, astrocytes, and oligodendrocytes.

In this chapter we describe aspects of this novel EGF-responsive stem cell culture system. The EGF-responsive cells can be isolated from embryonic and adult rat and mouse brain, and similar cells have been isolated from fetal human brain (B. Reynolds *et al.*, unpublished observations, 1994). In addition, we demonstrate that undifferentiated stem cell progeny are capable of forming oligodendrocytes when transplanted *in vivo*. Finally, we describe the development of genetically tagged, EGF-responsive stem cells derived from transgenic mice. These mice carry chimeric genes composed of mammalian cell-specific promoter elements that direct the expression of a reporter gene to either astrocytes or oligodendrocytes.

Production and *in Vitro* Characterization of Epidermal Growth Factor-Responsive Neural Stem Cells

Using sterile technique, the striata from litters of E14–15 Sprague-Dawley rats, or of BALB/cJ or CD1 mice, are dissected and separately pooled in L-15 dissection buffer (GIBCO, Grand Island, NY) and held on ice. The L-15 is removed and the dissected tissue is resuspended in a defined, DMEM: F12-based (GIBCO) serum-free medium containing glucose (0.6%), insulin (25 μg/ml), transferrin (100 μg/ml), progesterone (20 n*M*), putrescine (60 μM), selenium chloride (30 n*M*), glucose (0.6%), glutamine (2 m*M*), sodium bicarbonate (3 m*M*), *N*-2-hydroxyethylpiperazine-*N'*-2-ethanesulfonic acid (HEPES) buffer (5 m*M*) (all reagents from Sigma, St. Louis, MO), and EGF (20 ng/ml; Collaborative Research Incorporated, Waltham, MA) (subsequently referred to as complete EGF medium). The tissue is vigorously triturated 10–20 times with a fire-polished Pasteur pipette to achieve a single-cell suspension and the dissociated cells are plated at 100,000 cells/ml in T25 flasks and maintained in the complete EGF medium. Over the following 7–10 days, free-floating spheres of proliferating cells are formed. Without disturbing the attached cells, the spheres are removed, gently centrifuged at 800 rpm, and triturated with a fire-polished pipette to a single-cell suspension and plated at approximately 100,000 cells/ml in T25 flasks. By this method, the cells can be subcultured once per week (i.e., passaged) repeatedly, forming nonadherent spheres that float in suspension. The progeny can be identified by their immunoreactivity with antiserum to nestin, an intermediate filament protein expressed by undifferentiated neural stem/progenitor cells (11, 12). Under the appropriate differentiating conditions, the progeny of the EGF-generated cells lose their nestin immunoreactivity and differentiate into neurons, astrocytes, and oligodendrocytes. These EGF-responsive stem cells have now been routinely passaged more than 50 times over a period of 1 year and remain nestin immunopositive and multipotent.

Identification of Stem Cell Progeny and Their Differentiation Potential *in Vitro*

Differentiation and Immunolabeling Procedure

The EGF-generated cells can be induced to differentiate into oligodendrocytes, astrocytes, and neurons by altering the culture conditions (see Fig.

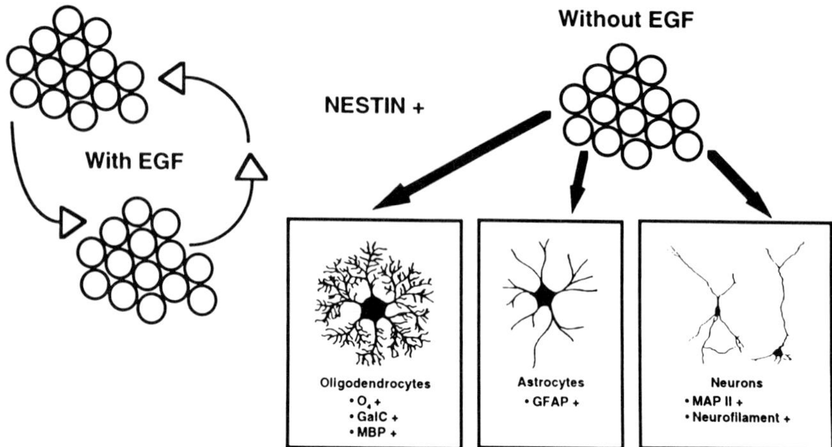

FIG. 1 Schematic representation of the EGF-responsive stem cell culture system. In the presence of EGF, and in a defined, serum-free medium, the stem cells can be propagated indefinitely. The stem cells grow as spheres (neurospheres) that are nestin positive. The stem cells can be influenced to differentiate by removing the EGF, and adding a small amount of serum to the defined medium. Under these conditions, the cells rapidly form the three major cell types in the CNS: neurons, astrocytes, and oligodendrocytes. The relative proportion of each differentiated cell type can be influenced using combinations of growth factors.

1). The free-floating, EGF-generated spheres are gently centrifuged, resuspended in the base medium (minus EGF) with 1% (v/v) fetal bovine serum, and plated on poly-L-ornithine-treated glass coverslips (10 μg/ml). The EGF-generated spheres attach firmly to the glass, and the cells slow or stop dividing and begin to differentiate. One to 14 days postplating, the cells on the coverslips are incubated unfixed, for 30 min at room temperature, with one of the following primary monoclonal antibodies; O1, O4 (13), galactocerebroside (GalC), or A2B5 (supernatants) (all provided by P. Wood, University of Miami) diluted in minimal essential medium with 5% (v/v) normal goat serum and 25 m*M* HEPES buffer, pH 7.3 (MEM–HEPES, NGS). Coverslips are gently washed five times in MEM–HEPES, and incubated for 30 min at room temperature in fluorescein- or rhodamine-conjugated secondary antibodies (Sigma) diluted in MEM–HEPES, NGS as recommended by the manufacturer. The coverslips are then washed five times in MEM–HEPES and fixed with acid alcohol (5% glacial acetic acid–95% ethanol) for 30 min to 1 hr at -20°C. Following this fixation, the coverslips are washed five times with MEM–HEPES, and either mounted and examined using fluorescence microscopy or immunoreacted with rabbit polyclonal antisera raised against glial fibrillary acidic protein (GFAP) (Dako, Carpinteria, CA), nestin (R. McKay, NIH), myelin basic protein (MBP) (Dako), or proteolipid protein

(PLP) (Serotec, Serotec Products, Harlan Bioproducts for Science, Inc., Indianapolis, IN). When subjected to a second round of immunolabeling, the coverslips are incubated first for 1 hr with 5% NGS in 0.1 *M* phosphate buffer with 0.9% (w/v) NaCl at pH 7.4 (PBS) followed by rabbit primary antibodies diluted in NGS for 1–2 hr at room temperature. Coverslips are washed three times with PBS, incubated with the appropriate secondary antibody conjugates diluted in NGS, washed with PBS, and then mounted on glass microscope slides with antifadent (Citifluor, Ltd., London, UK) mounting medium and examined using a fluorescence microscope. In cases in which samples are immunoreacted with antibodies raised against intracellular antigens and not immunolabeled live with the monoclonal antibody supernatants, the coverslips are fixed for 20 min with 4% paraformaldehyde in PBS (pH 7.4), washed with PBS, permeabilized with 100% ethanol, washed again with PBS, and incubated with 5% NGS in PBS for 1 hr. Primary antibodies and secondary antibody conjugates are applied as outlined above.

Formation of Mature Oligodendrocytes in Vitro from Epidermal Growth Factor-Responsive Stem Cell Progeny

To identify specific cell types 1 to 7 days after differentiation, cells on coverslips were immunolabeled with antibodies specific for oligodendrocyte precursors or mature oligodendrocytes. At 1 day postplating, the spheres attach to the substrate and many cells with a bipolar morphology migrate from the sphere. Most of the cells, especially flat cells at the base of the cluster, are immunoreactive for nestin. By 3 days, however, the nestin immunoreactivity in these flat cells diminishes whereas GFAP immunolabeling increases, consistent with the differentiation of astrocytes. During this same 3-day period, the bipolar cells, which are initially O4 positive, exhibit a decrease in O4 immunoreactivity and a concomitant increase in GalC immunolabeling by the third day postplating. Five to 7 days postplating, nestin and O4 immunoreactivity is significantly reduced in all cells and a fraction of the $O4^+/GalC^+$ oligodendrocyte precursors become immunoreactive to O1, MBP, or PLP. At this stage of differentiation in the culture system, these cells also possess a distinct oligodendrocyte morphology.

Formation of Myelinating Oligodendrocytes by Epidermal Growth Factor-Responsive Stem Cell Progeny when Transplanted *in Vivo*

Because the EGF-responsive stem cells are capable of generating oligodendrocyte precursors and oligodendrocytes *in vitro,* we examined whether these cells could respond to natural cues by differentiating into oligodendrocytes and myelinating CNS axons *in vivo*. The myelin-deficient rat (*md*) is an inherited dysmyelinating mutant and during their brief life span (approximately 25 days) the affected animals form virtually no myelin within the CNS. Prior to transplantation into the *md* rat, the EGF-responsive stem cells are maintained in EGF-containing medium for up to 35 passages. Nestin-positive cells (no mature oligodendrocytes) are collected and triturated into a single-cell suspension in the presence of 0.1% (w/v) bovine serum albumin (BSA). Epidermal growth factor-generated cells from different passages are used for injection into the mutant spinal cords. Myelin deficiency is an X-linked recessive trait and therefore only one-half of the male offspring born to carrier females are affected hemizygotes for the mutation. After laminectomy and exposure of the spinal cords, the mutants are readily identified at postnatal days 8–10 by the absence of myelin within the dorsal columns. At postnatal days 8–10, animals are anesthetized with halothane, a small longitudinal incision is made along the back, and a laminectomy performed, exposing the T13–L1 level of the spinal cord. A small incision is made in the dura mater to allow for the entry of the glass micropipette. To limit the number of animals, only the mutants are used for injection. Approximately 1.0–1.5 μl (50,000 cells/μl) of the stem cell progeny in Hanks' balanced salt solution (HBSS) is then injected into the dorsal columns just lateral to the midline. The site of injection is marked using sterile charcoal powder. Following the injection, the incision is sutured and the animals are gently warmed and allowed to recover from the halothane anesthesia. The animals are then returned to the dams and allowed to survive for approximately 2 weeks. Because the mutants usually die by approximately postnatal day 25, they are sacrificed at 21–24 days of age, using a pentobarbital overdose and aldehyde perfusion. Rats transplanted with the mouse stem cell progeny receive cyclosporin A (Sandoz, Switzerland) at a dose of 10 mg/kg intraperitoneal (ip), commencing on the day prior to cell injections. Spinal cords are removed and further postfixed in the same aldehyde fixatives for at least 24 hr, postfixed with osmium tetroxide, dehydrated, and processed for Epon embedding (1).

FIG. 2 The undifferentiated stem cells are capable of differentiating into myelinating oligodendrocytes when implanted into the myelin-deficient CNS. Photomicrographs of a section of the dorsal columns of an *md* rat spinal cord (T13–L1) 2 weeks postimplantation of undifferentiated mouse neurospheres. There is abundant normal myelin, especially along the midline in these sections. *Top:* At the edge of the photomicrograph, an apparent oligodendrocyte is seen that is in close contact to a cluster of myelinated fibers (arrow). One-micrometer Epon-embedded section stained with toluidine blue. Bar: 100 μm.

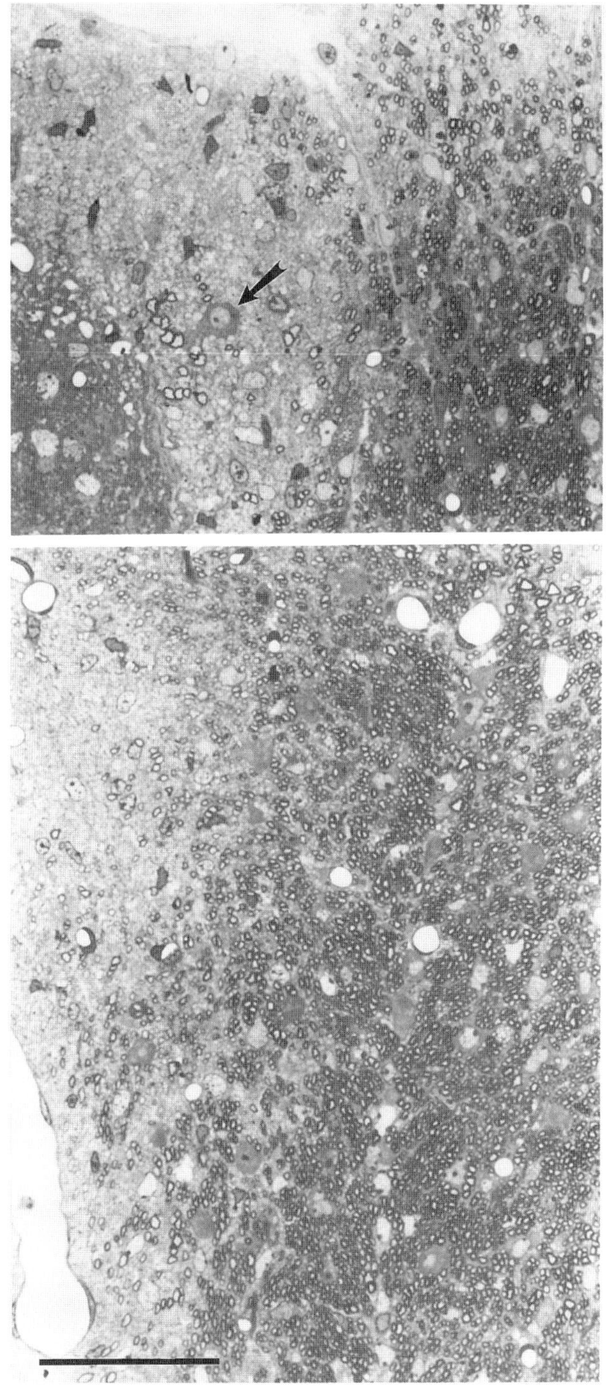

Histological analysis on toluidine blue-stained, 1-μm Epon sections was performed on the implanted spinal cords. Varying numbers of myelinating oligodendrocytes were seen in the implanted spinal cords with all myelin being confined to the dorsal columns (Fig. 2). Generally, within the core of the myelinated zones, the myelinated fibers were densely packed, and the myelin appeared to be of normal thickness, although this was not quantitated. At the edges of the zones, a number of myelinating oligodendrocytes were seen in contact with several axons. There was no obvious evidence of inflammation or abnormal cell death in any of the implant sites by light or electron microscopy.

In vitro, the majority of the EGF-responsive stem cell progeny form astrocytes under the standard differentiation protocol. Therefore, it was possible that astrogliosis would have been seen in the injected spinal cords. To determine whether the stem cell-derived astrocytes directly or indirectly caused any astrogliosis, we examined regions of the spinal cords that had received stem cell implants using immunocytochemistry for GFAP. For this analysis, we used 1-μm Epon sections that were essentially adjacent to those used in the analysis of the extent of myelination. None of the spinal cord sections containing the implanted stem cell progeny exhibited an increase in GFAP immunoreactivity relative to the spinal cords in the uninjected *md* rat. Furthermore, electron microscopy (EM) analysis of the grafted areas revealed no evidence of hypertrophied astrocyte fibers. Together, these experiments indicate that the injection of the stem cell progeny does not lead to glial scarring and that the implanted cells preferentially differentiate into oligodendrocytes in resopnse to the nonmyelinated CNS.

Although we have demonstrated a significant amount of myelin formation in the mutants, their short life span may limit the extent of myelination that is possible during this period. Because of the short interval between cell injection and sacrifice it is possible that some cells retained the potential to divide and myelinate at a later time. To address this issue, we performed [^{3}H]thymidine autoradiography on semithin sections to determine the extent of cell division in the injected and the uninjected mutants in the regions of myelination. [^{3}H]Thymidine labeling was seen within the myelinated patches in all animals examined. This is consistent with the development of stable, mature oligodendrocytes within the core of myelinated fibers, whereas in regions containing naked axons a few precursor cells remain with the capacity to divide. It is important to note that we observed no hyperplasia or hypercellularity as a result of the injections in any of the animals examined in this study. Although the number of labeled cells seen at the periphery of the myelinated zones in the injected animals appears to be significantly greater than that seen in the naive *md* rats, quantitation of labeling indices is required.

Differentiation and Survival of Epidermal Growth Factor-Responsive Stem Cells, Genetically Tagged with *Escherichia coli* β-Galactosidase Gene, When Implanted into Mouse Cerebral Cortex

We were interested in determining if the genetically tagged stem cell progeny would integrate into the developing CNS and if they would continue to express the reporter gene *in vivo*. Reports have demonstrated the negative regulation of retroviral long terminal repeats (LTRs) in transplanted cells, possibly through the actions of cytokines within the CNS (14). Proliferating,

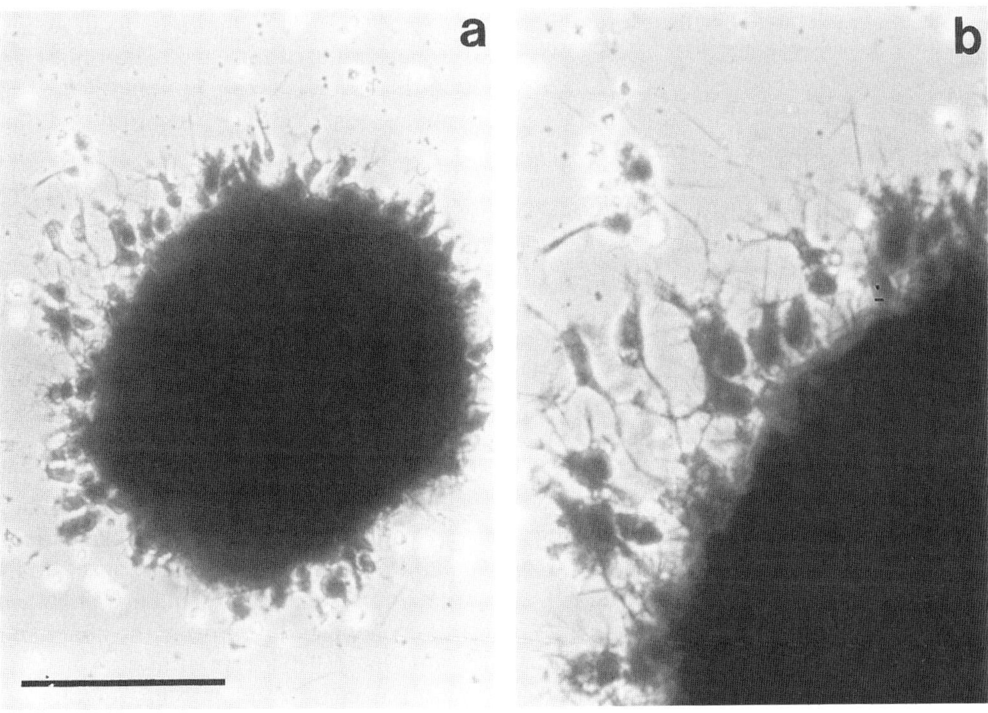

FIG. 3 Genetically modified EGF-responsive stem cells express the β-galactosidase reporter gene *in vitro*. A photomicrograph of genetically modified stem/precursor cells infected with a retrovirus containing the β-galactosidase gene (a). Cells containing the gene exhibit a characteristic blue reaction product after X-Gal histochemistry. (b) A higher magnification photomicrograph of (a), showing labeled cells migrating away from the sphere, extending processes, and taking on the morphology of differentiated CNS cells. Bar: 50 μm.

EGF-responsive cells are exposed to conditioned medium from the CRE BAG 2 packaging cell line (ATCC CRL 1858) for 1 day in the presence of Polybrene (8 μg/ml). Following this exposure, the cells are selected in Geneticin (400 μg/ml) (G418; GIBCO). Antibiotic-resistant spheres form within the first week and some of these spheres are expanded for several passages to produce sufficient cells for implantation (Fig. 3). One- to 3-day-old CD1 mice are anesthetized on ice. A small incision is made in the skin, a flap of bone is retracted, and a 2- to 3-mm^2 area of cortex is removed by aspiration. Undifferentiated mouse stem cell progeny are prepared for injection as described in the previous section. Approximately 50,000 cells are injected into each animal, using a micropipette. Three to 4 weeks later, the animals are deeply anesthetized with pentobarbital and perfused with 4% paraformaldehyde. The brains are removed, postfixed overnight in the same fixative, and cryoprotected in 25% sucrose and frozen in liquid nitrogen. The brains are cryosectioned (10–15 μm) and every fifth section is taken through the implantation region and processed for β-galactosidase activity, using the method of Vandaele *et al.* (15) with minor modifications. β-Galactosidase-labeled cells are seen in all of the animals (Fig. 4). These results demonstrate that transgenes inserted *in vitro* can be expressed *in vivo* following transplantation of the genetically modified, EGF-responsive stem cells.

Transgenic Mouse-Derived Neural Stem Cells: A Source of Marked Glial Cells for Central Nervous System Transplantation

In the section Formation of Myelinating Oligodendrocytes (above), we described the implantation of the EGF-responsive stem cell progeny into the dysmyelinated CNS. In this transplant paradigm, the presence of abundant myelin at the site of the implant clearly identified cells of donor origin. However, for the majority of transplant studies, the identification of donor cells or tissues after implantation remains a significant challenge. In some cases it is possible to identify cells of xenogeneic origin within the host using species-specific antibodies such as M6 (16, 17). Current strategies used to tag donor cells prior to implantation suffer from inherent problems of dilution, toxicity, and stability of gene expression over the long term. Furthermore, methods used to tag cells genetically *in vitro* with reporter genes generally suffer from low efficiency and the eventual identification of the cells *in vivo* is made more difficult if a majority of the implanted cells are never labeled in culture.

To provide a more stable and efficient method of cell labeling, we have used the promoter elements for the human glial fibrillary acidic protein (GFAP) gene (18) and the human myelin basic protein (MBP) gene (L. Wra-

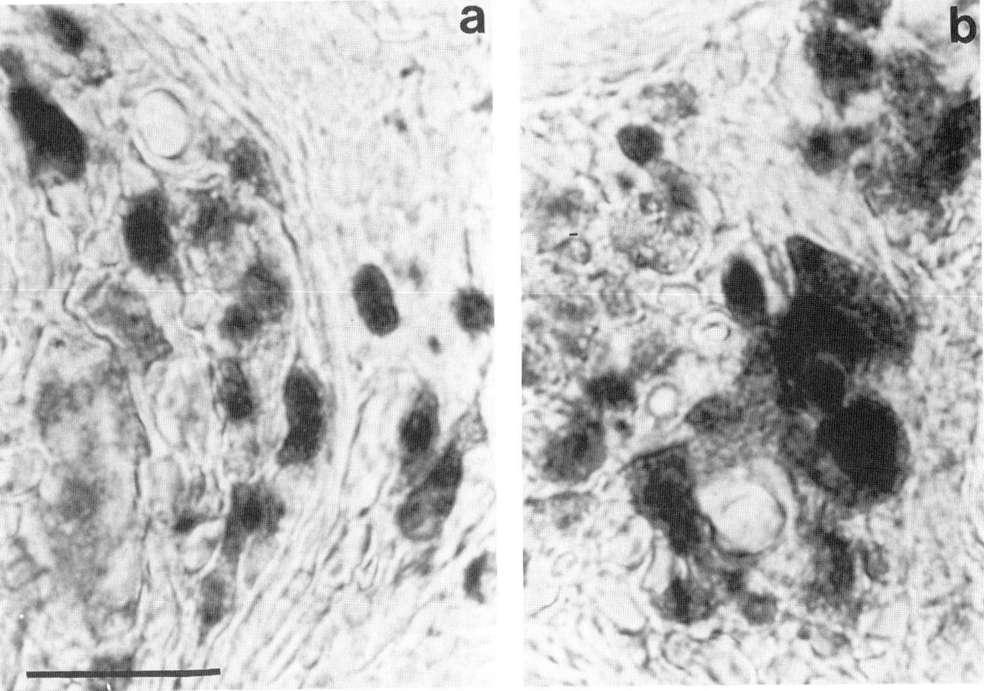

FIG. 4 EGF-responsive stem cells, genetically modified *in vitro,* survive transplantation. Photomicrographs of a section of cerebral cortex from a 4-week-old mouse that had been implanted with genetically modified cells on the day of birth (a and b). X-Galactosidase histochemistry was performed on free-floating, Vibratome sections. The large number of blue cells demonstrates that the genetically modified stem cell progeny can survive transplantation and express the transgene. Bar: 50 μm.

betz, personal communication) to direct the expression of the *Escherichia coli* β-galactosidase reporter gene in transgenic mice. Transgenic mice are produced using standard pronuclear injection of the MBP and GFAP constructs into fertilized F2 mouse eggs derived by crossing B6SJLF1 parents. Transgenic lines are maintained by back-crossing to B6SJLF1 mice. Epidermal growth factor-responsive stem cells have been prepared from individual fetuses from both of these transgenic mouse lines and propagated in the presence of EGF in serum-free, defined medium. *In vitro,* the stem cells derived from these transgenic animals appear to be identical to those derived from nontransgenic animals in their ability to proliferate and differentiate. When the stem cell progeny are allowed to differentiate, cell-specific expression of the reporter gene occurs in astrocytes (GFAP-*lacZ*) and in oligodendrocytes (MBP-*lacZ*) in a developmentally regulated manner. Identification of the β-galactosidase-positive cells is accomplished using double labeling with antibodies raised against GFAP (Dako) or MBP (Dako). The expression of the reporter genes is highly stable, as it is seen in thirtieth passage cultures and appears to be expressed in virtually 100% of the appropriate cells. We are currently investigating the expression of the reporter gene after transplantation in the rodent CNS. The use of mammalian promoter elements that are cell specific should eliminate the problems of inactivation or negative regulation seen with the use of retroviral LTRs. Transgenic mouse-derived neural stem cells represent a novel means of obtaining genetically tagged, stable populations of cells for transplantation.

Conclusions

Central nervous system stem cells represent a novel source of cell types for future transplant therapies, both for neuronal or glial cell replacement. Although the experiments that are presented here are of a preliminary nature, stem cells derived from humans could prove to be widely applicable in CNS transplantation. Studies are in progress to examine the feasibility of inducing differentiation of the stem cell progeny in culture prior to transplantation in the CNS in order to produce neural cells with specific phenotypes.

Acknowledgments

We wish to thank D. Rhode and D. Springman for assistance with the animal colony, Dr. D. Archer for his contributions to the *md* rat transplant experiments, and B. Dean for assistance with the stem cell cultures. We also thank our collaborators in the transgenic mouse studies (M. Brenner, L. Wrabetz, and J. Kamholz). I.D.D. was supported by grants from the NIH and The Myelin Project. A.M. was supported by a grant from the MS Society. S.W. was supported by grants from the MRC of Canada, Ciba-Gergy, and the NCE neural regeneration network.

References

1. I. D. Duncan, J. P. Hammang, K. F. Jackson, P. M. Wood, R. P. Bunge, and L. Langford, Transplantation of oligodendrocytes and Schwann cells into the spinal cord of the myelin-deficient rat. *J. Neurocytol.* **17,** 351–360 (1988).
2. A. K. Groves, S. C. Barnett, R. J. Franklin, A. J. Crang, M. Mayer, W. F. Blakemore, and M. Noble, Repair of demyelinated lesions by transplantation of purified O-2A progenitor cells. *Nature* (*London*) **352,** 453–455 (1993).

3. S. C. Barnett, R. J. Franklin, and W. F. Blakemore, *In vitro* and *in vivo* analysis of a rat bipotential O-2A progenitor cell line containing the temperature-sensitive mutant gene of the SV40 large T antigen. *Eur. J. Neurosci.* **5,** 1247–1260 (1993).
4. W. J. Freed, M. Poltorak, and J. B. Becker, Intracerebral adrenal medulla grafts: A review. *Exp. Neurol.* **110,** 139–166 (1990).
5. W. J. Freed, Substantia nigra grafts and Parkinson's disease: From animal experiments to human therapeutic trials. *Restor. Neurol. Neurosci.* **3,** 109–134 (1991).
6. E. Cattaneo and R. D. G. McKay, Identifying and manipulating neuronal stem cells. *Trends Neurosci.* **14**(8), 338–340 (1991).
7. E. E. Baetge, Neural stem cells for CNS transplantation. *Ann. N.Y. Acad. Sci.* **695,** 285–291 (1993).
8. B. A. Reynolds and S. Weiss, Generation of neurons and astrocytes from isolated cells of the adult mammalian central nervous system. *Science* **255,** 1707–1710 (1992).
9. B. A. Reynolds, W. Tetzlaff, and S. Weiss, A multipotent EGF-responsive striatal embryonic progenitor cell produces neurons and astrocytes. *J. Neurosci.* **12**(11), 4565–4574 (1992).
10. B. A. Reynolds and S. Weiss, EGF-responsive stem cells in the mammalian central nervous system. *in:* "Restorative Neurology and Neuroscience: Neuronal Death and Repair," (A. C. Cuello, ed.), Vol. 6, pp. 247–255. Elsevier, Amsterdam, 1993.
11. U. Lendahl, L. B. Zimmerman, and R. D. G. McKay, CNS stem cells express a new class of intermediate filament protein. *Cell* **60,** 585–595 (1990).
12. L. Zimmerman, U. Lendahl, M. Cunningham, R. McKay, B. Parr, B. Gavin, J. Mann, G. Vassileva, and A. McMahon, Independent regulatory elements in the nestin gene direct transgene expression to neural stem cells or muscle precursors. *Neuron* **12,** 11–24 (1994).
13. M. Schachner, S. U. Kim, and R. Zehnle, Developmental expression in central and peripheral nervous system of oligodendrocyte cell surface antigens (O antigens) recognized by monoclonal antibodies. *Dev. Biol.* **83,** 328–338 (1981).
14. M. Schinstine and F. H. Gage, *in:* "Molecular and Cellular Approaches for the Treatment of Neurologic Diseases," (S. G. Waxman, ed.), ch. 16. Raven Press, New York, 1993.
15. S. Vandaele, D. Nordquist, R. M. Feddersen, I. Tretjakoff, A. C. Peterson, and H. T. Orr, Purkinje cell protein-2 regulatory regions and transgene expression in cerebellar compartments. *Genes Dev.* **5,** 1136–1148 (1991).
16. R. D. Lund, M. B. Houston, C. F. Lagenaur, H. W. Kunz, and T. J. Gill, Cellular events associated with induced rejection of neural xenografts placed into neonatal rat brains. *Transplant. Proc.* **21,** 3174–3175 (1989).
17. C. Lagenaur, V. Kunemund, G. Fischer, S. Fushiki, and M. Schachner, Monoclonal M6 antibody interferes with neurite extension of cultured neurons. *J. Neurobiol.* **23,** 71–88 (1991).
18. M. Brenner, W. C. Kisseberth, Y. Su, F. Besnard, and A. Messing, GFAP promotor directs astrocyte-specific expression in transgenic mice. *J. Neurosci.* **14,** 1030–1037 (1994).

[18] Application of Astrocyte Transplants as a Therapeutic Intervention

J. Patrick Kesslak and Richard J. Bridges

Introduction

Although classically perceived only in terms of their structural contributions to the CNS, accumulating evidence indicates that glia, particularly astrocytes, have a critical role in the response of the central nervous system (CNS) to injury (1, 11). Astrocytes increase in both number and size in brain areas compromised by either traumatic or neurodegenerative damage. Studies demonstrating the ability of astrocytes to regulate the homeostasis of the extracellular environment, participate in neurotransmitter synthesis and metabolism, express receptors for transmitters and growth factors, and synthesize and secrete neurotrophic factors highlight the capacity of these cells to contribute to CNS function under both normal and pathological conditions (2, 17). Any number of these activities could foreseeably contribute to establishing conditions that would support neuroplastic processes. Thus it seems logical to target astrocytes as a possible cell type to implant in the brain as a therapeutic approach to improve CNS recovery and function. Consistent with such a strategy, a number of studies have demonstrated that the implantation of astrocytes can lead to increased behavioral recovery following selective lesions. In this chapter we focus on a discussion of the methodological aspects of astrocyte implantation. These approaches should prove useful in evaluating the ability of astrocytes to promote CNS recovery, as well as in studying more general aspects of astrocyte function.

Methodological Considerations for Implantation

As in neural transplantation studies, a large number of variables must be taken into consideration in the design of astrocyte transplant experiments. Although the guiding principles for a given study will, necessarily, be dependent on the objectives of the investigation (e.g., recovery of function, survival of host neurons, integration of transplanted neurons, or characterization of implanted astrocytes), there are a number of common variables, including (a) the time course of the lesion, implantation, and assessment, (b) culture conditions, and (c) implant density and form. Indeed, it is the ability to

Methods in Neurosciences, Volume 21

control these variables that makes the implantation of astrocytes such a flexible, interesting, and potentially useful approach.

When astrocyte implants are incorporated into studies of neural plasticity and behavioral recovery, timing of both the implant and the assessment of function is especially critical. To enhance neuron survival and promote neurite sprouting, previous studies concluded that the astrocytes should be implanted as close to the time of injury as possible. In this manner, a ready source of neurotrophic factors is available immediately preceding the neuronal damage. Alternatively, it is also possible to implant astrocytes by injection, prior to a surgical or chemical lesion. This permits the evaluation of potential prophylactic activity of the cells. As the time between the initial injury and glial implantation increases, endogenous responses of the host brain (e.g., astrocyte migration and proliferation) make it difficult to judge the relative effectiveness of the implanted cells. This is especially true if the implant serves only to enhance the rate of recovery, as opposed to promoting neuron survival that would not ordinarily have occurred. If this is the case, a time course for assessment must be chosen that can distinguish between spontaneous and implant-facilitated recovery.

Not surprisingly, the cellular characteristics of the astrocytes being implanted can be strongly influenced by both their original source and the conditions under which they are grown (3, 7, 8, 19, 20). Thus, primary astrocytes can be isolated from any number of specific brain regions simply by modifications of the microdissection procedure (see Culture Preparation, below). This should prove to be an important consideration in view of accumulating evidence that astrocytes exhibit anatomical heterogeneity. Furthermore, demonstrations that astrocytes can be purified from adult brain allow the developmental state of the astrocytes to be varied (23). Once isolated, *in vitro* culture conditions provide yet another level of variability. For example, numerous studies have demonstrated that culture conditions (e.g., defined media vs serum-supplemented media) can dramatically alter the morphology and biochemical properties of the astrocytes (8, 19, 20). Similarly, the length of time in culture, the extent of confluency reached by the cells, as well as any additional molecules they have been exposed to, could all potentially influence the physiological properties of the astrocytes. Fortunately, as an experimental system, *in vitro* tissue culture is amenable to following cellular growth, characterizing physiological properties, and controlling the extracellular environment of the astrocytes prior to their isolation for implantation.

Finally, the fact that astrocytes are cultured before implantation provides a significant amount of flexibility in the manner in which the cells are introduced into the host. Thus, the astrocytes can be injected as a cell suspension of known density, implanted as a solid plug of isolated cells, or introduced after they are grown on an implantable matrix. Embedding glia within such a matrix provides a strategy to reduce migration and ensure that the glia are not displaced. A number of studies have used Gelfoam as a biologically inert support system for implanting astrocytes (12, 13). Pieces of Gelfoam can be taken directly from the secondary culture wells and placed into the host brain. Astrocytes appear to adhere to surfaces and will distribute themselves over any vacant area. The density of astrocytes can be controlled to some extent by the length of time in culture, although exact quantitation of cell number appears limited. Short culture times limit the migration of astrocytes into the interior of a three-dimensional matrix of the Gelfoam, resulting in cells primarily covering the outer perimeter. Promising alternative mechanisms for isolation and implantation of transplants are currently being developed and are discussed elsewhere in this volume (Ch. 24).

Preparation and Implantation of Astrocytes into Brain

Culture Preparation

The preparation of astrocytes (18) for implantation studies can be divided into three basic phases: (a) microdissection of the brain area of interest, (b) primary culture of the astrocytes for the purpose of purification, and (c) secondary culture to provide sufficient cell numbers and set the type of implant (e.g., cell suspension, Gelfoam). In the following sections we describe the typical protocol used in our studies of the actions of implanted cortical astrocytes on behavioral recovery following lesion. It is important to remember, however, that each phase of the methodology holds the potential for modification, depending on the intended study. As previously mentioned, different brain regions could be used as the tissue source for the astrocytes to be implanted. Similarly, the astrocytes could be cultured under differing conditions, such as with or without medium including a serum supplement. These variations emphasize the versatility of this approach as well as highlight the number of interesting questions remaining to be addressed.

Dissection

Cortical tissue is collected from 4- to 6-day-old neonatal rats. The preparation is carried out using sterile technique in an appropriate tissue culture hood. After rinsing the head of the rat pup with 70% ethanol, it is rapidly decapitated into a petri dish containing 10 ml of Ca^{2+}/Mg^{2+}-free buffer [CMF: Hanks' balanced salt solution (GIBCO, Grand Island, NY) supplemented with 20 mM N-2-hydroxyethylpiperazine-N'-2-ethanesulfonic acid (HEPES), 4.2 mM sodium bicarbonate, 1 mM sodium pyruvate, bovine serum albumin (BSA; 3 mg/ml)]. While immobilized with a pair of fine dissecting forceps, a longitudinal incision is made from the neck to the nose and the skin covering the dorsal surface of the head is peeled away. The dorsal portion of the skull is removed in a similar fashion. The exposed brain is teased away from the remainder of the skull and allowed to fall into a second petri dish containing CMF. With the aid of a dissecting microscope, the meninges are carefully and thoroughly removed from the brain. This is easily accomplished by immobilizing the brain with one pair of forceps, and gently teasing away the meninges with a second, very fine pair. We have found it most efficient to remove the meninges first from the ventral surface and then from the dorsal surface of the brain. The brain is then divided into its two hemispheres. With the medial surface exposed, the midbrain and hippocampal tissues are removed using the fine forceps, leaving a thin, hollow shell of cortical tissue. The dissection is completed by carefully removing any obvious blood vessels (i.e., those containing erythrocytes). The cortical tissue is then transferred to a third petri dish containing 4 ml of CMF buffer. This procedure is repeated until all of the tissue required for the preparation has been collected.

Dissociation

The collected cortices and CMF buffer are transferred into a 15-ml capped test tube with a 10-ml disposable pipette. This same pipette is used to break up the hemispheres by triturating them slowly 10–12 times. The test tube is then capped and allowed to incubate in a shaking water bath for 10 min at 37°C. The tube is gently agitated about every 2 min. The tissue is then pelleted in the test tube, using a clinical centrifuge (3 min). The supernatant is removed and 2 ml of a mixture of Dulbecco's modified Eagle's medium and Ham's F-12 medium buffered with 25 mM HEPES and 14.3 mM $NaHCO_3$ (pH 7.4) and supplemented with 15% (v/v) fetal bovine serum (DMEM/F12 + 15% FBS) is added to the tissue. After first suspending the pellet by gentle trituration with a 2-ml disposable pipette, it is transferred to a second 15-ml tube. The tissue is furthered triturated with a flame-constricted siliconized Pasteur pipette (0.3- to 0.5-mm i.d.) to produce a homogeneous suspension. Care is taken to minimize the amount of foam produced during the trituration. Microscopic inspection of the suspension should show a majority of isolated single cells with very few cell clumps.

Primary Culture

An aliquot of cells can be removed at this point to determine the density of the suspension. As a general procedure, however, we typically divide the preparation at a ratio of one brain hemisphere per 75-cm^2 flask, each of which contains 10 ml of DMEM/F12 + 15% FBS. The flasks are gently shaken to dilute the aliquot, after which they are returned to the incubator (37°C, 5% CO_2, 95% humidity). Twenty-four hours after plating, the medium in the primary culture flasks is removed, the cells are rinsed three times with 4 ml of DMEM/F12 − FBS, and given 10 ml of medium containing 10% FBS. Medium is replaced every 3–5 days with DMEM/F12 + 10% FBS.

Purification

Oligodendrocytes, type II astrocytes, and microglia are removed from the primary cultures by agitation. After the cultures have reached approximately 80% confluence (about 8 days), fresh medium is added and the flasks are shaken on a rotary shaker (250 rpm) for 24 hr at 37°C. To maintain sterile conditions, the flasks are sealed in plastic bags. Immediately following the removal of the flasks from the shaker, the cultures are rinsed three times with 4 ml of DMEM/F12. It should be noted that the medium removed following the shaking procedure can be used in the preparation of other glial cultures (10, 18). The purified astrocytes are given 10 ml of DMEM/F12 + FBS and allowed to grow to confluence (about 12 days).

Secondary Culture

The confluent astrocytes are harvested from the primary culture flasks with trypsin. The cultures are rinsed and allowed to incubate with 10 ml of CMF buffer for about 1 min. The CMF medium is removed and 5 ml of a 0.25% (v/v) trypsin (in CMF buffer) is added to the flasks. The flask is tilted to ensure that all of the cells are exposed to the trypsin, after which it is returned to the incubator (37°C) for about 5 min. The flask is then checked every 2 min until a majority of the cells are observed to be lifting. The trypsin reaction is quenched by adding 7 ml of DMEM/F12 + 10% FBS and the suspension transferred to a sterile 50-ml capped tube. After all of the flasks have been harvested, the combined supernatants are centrifuged for 5 min in a clinical centrifuge. The supernatant is removed, after which the pellet is resuspended with a flame-constricted Pasteur pipette as described above. After determining the density of the suspension, the cells are replated either into a second set of 75-cm^2 flasks (1–3 $\times$ 10^6 cells/flask) or directly onto Gelfoam squares in a 24-well plate (see the next section). These secondary cultures are returned to the incubator and grown in a manner identical to the primary cultures. Once these secondary cultures have reached confluence, the cells are harvested by trypsinization and suspended by trituration for implantation.

Gelfoam

As an alternative to implanting the astrocytes as a cell suspension, the cells can be directly grown on an implantable piece of sterile Gelfoam (30–80 mm^3). The squares of Gelfoam are incubated in DMEM/F12 + 10% FBS overnight to ensure saturation. An aliquot of harvested cells ($1–2 \times 10^6$) is then directly pipetted onto pieces of Gelfoam placed in a 24-well culture plate. Two to 4 hr later, additional medium can be added to the wells (0.5 ml). The cells are maintained in an incubator at 37°C (5% CO_2 and 95% humidity) and given fresh DMEM/F12 + 10% FBS every 2–3 days as described above. Although this approach does raise some difficulties in quantifying the number of astrocytes that are actually implanted, it does provide a strategy to efficiently implant cells that have not been disrupted by a harvesting procedure.

Implantation Techniques

Cell Suspensions

The procedures for intracerebral injection of glial cell suspensions are similar to those used for implanting neurons. Animals are anesthetized, the scalp is shaved and swabbed with antiseptic, and placed into a stereotaxic instrument. An incision is made in the scalp to expose the skull over the region of interest and holes are drilled to expose the top of the brain. The glial cell suspension is then aspirated into a 1.0-mm o.d., thin-walled glass cannula, fitted to the arm of the stereotaxic instrument, and connected via Tygon tubing to a 25-μl Hamilton syringe. Cell density of the suspension can be determined and adjusted prior to injection. The injection system is filled with phosphate-buffered saline (PBS; pH 7.4). A small air bubble should separate the cell suspension and PBS to reduce dilution of cells and help monitor the rate of injection of cells. The cannula is lowered slowly into position, so as to reduce damage to overlying neural tissue. Approximately 10 μl of cell suspension or control solution is injected over a 10-min period at each implant site. The cannula is retracted over a 5-min period to reduce flow up the cannula tract. Sterile Gelfoam is placed into the wound cavity, the incision is closed, and the scalp swabbed with antiseptic. All animals are placed on a warm heating pad and monitored postoperatively until they have recovered from the anesthetic.

Astrocytes Cultured in Gelfoam Matrix

Astrocytes cultured in Gelfoam can be placed into brain as follows. Animals are anesthetized, the scalp is shaved and swabbed with antiseptic, and the head placed into a stereotaxic instrument. An incision is made in the scalp to expose the skull over the region of interest and holes are drilled to expose the top of the brain. After the meninges are cut, brain tissue is aspirated to form a cavity to receive the Gelfoam. Implants should be placed only after the bleeding has stopped. This will promote survival and facilitate proper placement. The cavity is cleared of debris so that the floor and sides of the area can be visualized. Cultured astrocytes in Gelfoam are then placed into the cavity, sterile Gelfoam is added to fill the remainder of the cavity, the incision is closed, and the scalp swabbed with antiseptic. To increase the number of astrocytes in the wound cavity a slurry of cells in suspension can be placed on the cavity floor before the astrocyte-containing Gelfoam is implanted. All animals are placed on a warm heating pad and monitored postoperatively until they have recovered from the anesthetic.

Characterization of Astrocyte Implants

Anatomical and Biochemical

After the astrocyte implants are placed into the host, the localization of cells is necessary to verify implant placement and determine any migration from the injection site. Standard immunohistological techniques can be used to identify astrocytes. For example, glial fibrillary acidic protein (GFAP) is typically used to provide an estimate of the density of reactive astrocytes at the implant site, although it may be difficult to differentiate between implanted and endogenous astrocytes (Fig. 1). Gelfoam implants can offer additional problems. The porous matrix may degrade after an extended time in the host and is prone to displacement from the lesion cavity. Furthermore, as the Gelfoam does not integrate with the host brain, extraction of the brain for histological analysis requires the surface of the brain to be clear of meninges and any connective tissue that may adhere to the implant. Particular attention must be given when removing the skull proximal to the implant site. Embedding of the brain will anchor the Gelfoam in the lesion cavity and make sectioning of the brain considerably easier. Injection of cell suspensions

---

FIG. 1 Astrocytes *in vitro* are easily identified with GFAP and show a flattened appearance with processes developing as the cells reach confluence (A). After implantation the astrocytes are not easily identified in sections stained with cresyl violet (B), but can be readily identified with GFAP (C). Higher magnification of the GFAP-positive astrocytes illustrates the characteristic stellate morphology (D).

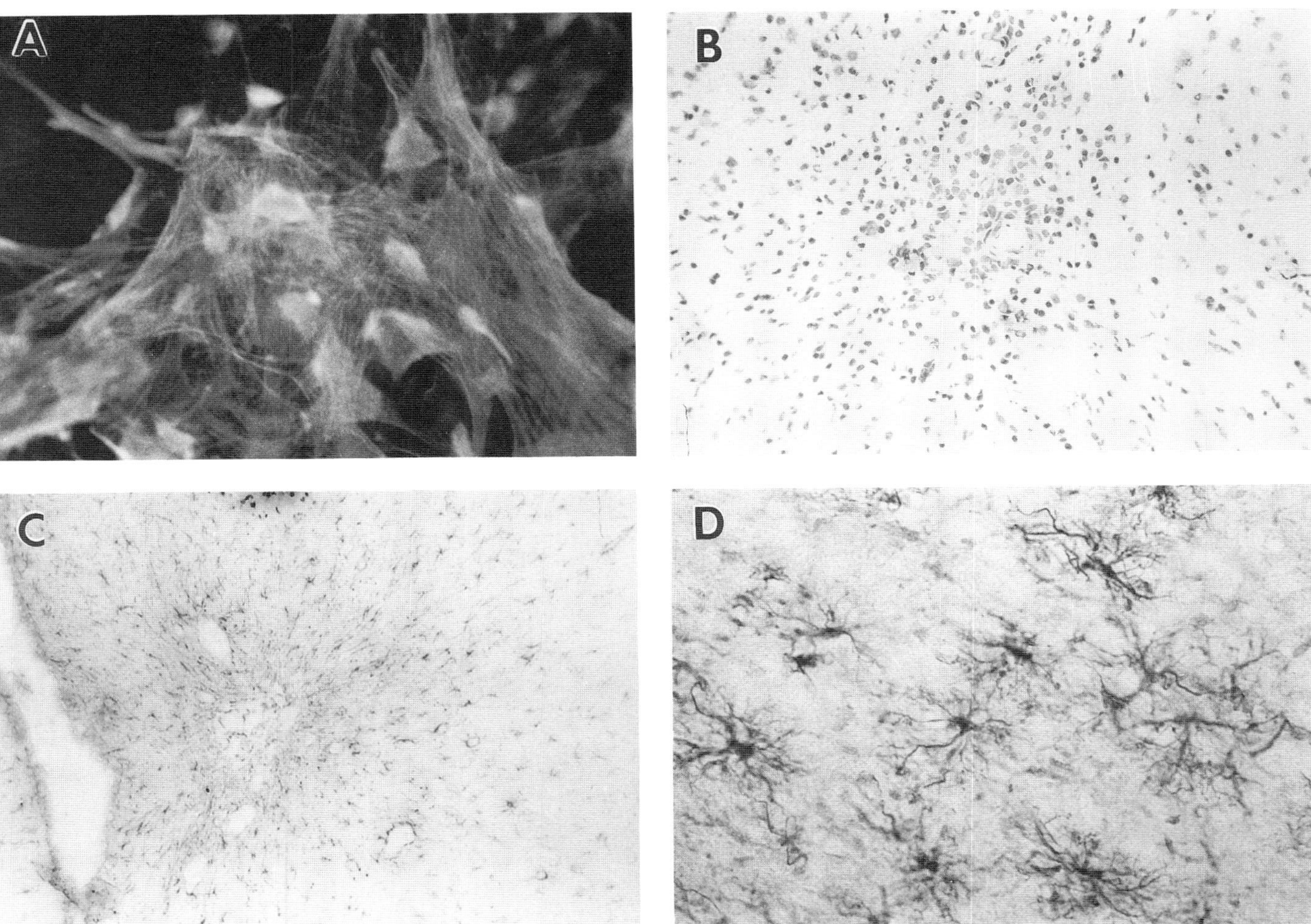
A
B
C
D

within the host tissue avoids many of the complications for tissue preparation and handling.

A number of approaches have been applied in an attempt to distinguish implanted cells from the endogenous astrocytes. Astrocytes prelabeled with [^{3}H]thymidine *in vitro* can be implanted into the host brain and localized by autoradiography (16). The [^{3}H]thymidine is incorporated into the DNA of the glia during the mitotic phase. An alternative method for identification of astrocyte implants relies on the use of the fluorescent dye Fast Blue, which has been shown to be effective in transplanted oligodendrocytes (9). Cells are incubated in culture medium containing Fast Blue and rinsed before implantation. The cells can also be labeled with *Phaseolus vulgaris* leukoagglutin (PHAL) while in culture. Double labeling of host brain for PHAL and GFAP can then be used to identify the implanted astrocytes and to monitor migration from the implant site (4). Studies have indicated that the astrocytes retain the lectin for up to 3 months after implantation. It is important to note, however, that there are potential drawbacks to these localization techniques. In the methods employing [^{3}H]thymidine the labeling must be timed to provide maximum incorporation. Studies with PHAL and Fast Blue must avoid allowing mitotic activity to dilute the label. In this respect, further mitotic activity after implantation would be expected to dilute the marker. It is also possible that implanted astrocytes will be phagocytized or that cell marker released from the implant is incorporated by the host as part of its normal response. The label incorporated by host cells would be expected to be less intense than transplanted cells, but a definitive differentiation between cells is not assured by these methods.

Xenographic implants can circumvent some of the problems associated with labeling homotypical cells *in vitro*. Species and stain-specific characteristics make it possible to localize implants by immunohistological identification of specific proteins. Species or subspecies-specific antibodies have been developed that recognize specific structural proteins that can be used for differentiation and localization of implanted cells. For example, donor astrocytes from mouse have been implanted into rat brain to examine cell migration (26). Xenographic implants can also be combined with the labeling techniques described above to monitor mitotic activity of the implanted cells. Decreased or absent labeling in immunopositive cells would suggest the transplants proliferate within the host brain. It should be noted, however, that these studies also warrant methodological considerations such as species differences and immunosuppression, each of which impact on astrocyte implant survival and activity. Astrocytes derived from different areas of the brain may also provide distinct characteristics, such as neurotransmitter transport (5), that may be useful for differentiation of implant and host cells.

Functional Characterization

The functional impact of astrocyte implants can cover a wide range of activities, from neural transmission to behavior. Glial cells can be applied to facilitate a recovery for a variety of dysfunctions, such as localized lesions in the brain, developmental deficits, demyelinating diseases, and spinal cord injury. In this section we focus on describing how astrocytes can be applied to facilitate functional recovery, and discuss variables that may affect implant activity. When a lesion occurs in the CNS there are a number of variables that impact on recovery from the insult, including lesion location, size, rate of growth, and developmental period (25). Behavioral assessments are also influenced by a number of variables, such as task complexity, time since injury, and exposure to the task prior to the damage. The fundamental mechanisms of functional recovery present a fascinating and complex issue that is beyond the scope of this chapter. It is clear however, that astrocytes can be an integral component of functional recovery.

Astrocyte implants have been shown to facilitate behavioral recovery after lesions in the frontal cortex (12, 13) and visual cortex (21), but not after selective neurotoxin lesions to the hippocampus (14). Success in enhancing behavioral recovery with astrocyte implants may depend on the extent of damage as well as on the neural circuit involved. Behavioral studies have shown that astrocyte implants can enhance the rate of recovery. Our studies have indicated that implants of astrocytes immediately after damage can accelerate the rate of recovery on a spatial learning task. Lesions of the frontal cortex produce a transient deficit on reinforced alternation in a T-maze that recovers within a 15-day period. Placement of astrocytes in the wound cavity immediately after the lesion promotes an accelerated rate of recovery. If astrocyte implants are delayed for 10 days postlesion they do not increase the rate of recovery of function on a spontaneous alternation task (J. P. Kesslak, unpublished observations, 1994). Thus, the success of astrocyte implants to facilitate recovery of function and promote neurotrophic activity suggests their natural response to injury is beneficial, and introduction of astrocyte implants in a timely manner may augment the natural response.

Timing of astrocyte implants should also be considered with regard to the developmental role that the cells can play in modification of the existing CNS circuitry. Immature astrocytes may be required for normal neural development, and introduction of these astrocytes at a later stage may promote neural rearrangements to compensate for developmental deficits. For example, Muller and Best (21) implanted immature astrocytes into the visual cortex of cats that had ocular dominance impairments due to restricted vision during the critical developmental period. After the astrocytes had been implanted into the visual cortex of adult cats, the impaired side exhibited normal ocular dominance. In this instance the neurons required for the ocular function were present but dysfunctional. Astrocytes may promote synaptic plasticity by providing neurotrophic factors and/or stimulating a growth response by the presence of the immature cells. Thus, astrocytes can modify existing neural arrangements to promote functional recovery.

The site and extent of damage in the CNS can play a critical role in the ability of astrocyte implants to facilitate recovery of function. When CNS damage produces a prolonged behavioral deficit, such as impaired spatial learning after lesion to the hippocampus, astrocyte implants may be insufficient to compensate for the damage. Kainic acid (KA) lesion of the CA3 pyramidal neurons produces a long-term deficit on spatial maze learning. Astrocytes implanted either 4 days before or 10 days after KA lesions did not facilitate recovery on a forced-choice alternation task (14). However, transplants of embryonic neurons after KA lesion of CA3 did promote recovery. The astrocytes implanted prior to the KA injection did not appear to reduce the neurotoxicity, possibly due to the potent action of KA and the observation that astrocytes are not involved in KA transport and metabolism. This dissociation between neural and nonneural transplants indicates there are limits to the application of glial implants. Neural transplants may function to augment the damaged neural circuit by providing new neural connections or supplementing the general availability of neurotransmitters. Although astrocytes may be able to provide trophic support and limited interactions with the neurotransmitter systems, it does not appear that astrocytes are sufficient for restoration of function in all cases.

Summary

The implantation of astrocytes into the CNS offers a means to develop well-defined studies to address a variety of anatomical, biochemcial, and behavioral issues. It is apparent that glial cells far exceed the limited structural and support functions historically assigned, and the actions of astrocytes can be either detrimental or beneficial. Invariably, astrocytes are present in neural transplants and can affect neuron survival and integration. Following damage, astrocytes can form a glial limitans or scar that can prohibit innervation by blocking neurite extension. The glial limitans, however, also reestablishes the blood–brain barrier to inhibit the influx of detrimental substances. The phagocytic activity of astrocytes also acts to maintain a homeostatic environment to support neural function. There is accumulating evidence from lesion and transplant studies that indicates that astrocytes or astrocyte-derived factors may actually facilitate mechanisms of neural plasticity. Survival of neural transplants and recovery of function are enhanced when the tissue is placed into the host brain after a period of delay (i.e., conditioning lesion) that allows the injury-induced neurotrophic response to reach a peak, approximately 15 days in adult rats (6, 22). This time course also corresponds to an increase in the density of astrocytes in the lesioned area, suggesting that these cells may contribute to the trophic response. Furthermore, Gelfoam that is present in the wound cavity during this conditioning time has been shown to promote neural survival *in vitro* and recovery of function *in vivo* (12, 13, 22). Analysis of the Gelfoam indicates that it not only contains soluble neurotrophic factors but also a high density of astrocytes. These observations suggest that the production of trophic factors by astrocytes may represent a mechanism to promote neural survival and growth following injury.

Consistent with a role in the neurotrophic response, astrocytes have been shown to be capable of synthesizing and secreting a wide range of factors, including nerve growth factor (NGF), basic fibroblast growth factor (bFGF), and ciliary neurotrophic factor (CNTF) (24). A glial-derived neurotrophic factor (GDNF) has been isolated from a cell line and demonstrated to promote survival and differentiation of dopaminergic neurons *in vitro* (15). The capacity of glia to produce trophic factors provides a mechanism to sustain neuron survival and promote neurite sprouting *in vivo*. In terms of behavioral and functional recovery, secretion of factors may be sufficient to promote the development of compensatory responses by the CNS either directly, by providing missing or insufficient components, or indirectly, by augmenting and sustaining existing neurons and glia.

As the role of astrocytes in the CNS becomes better defined, the potential applications of the manipulation of these cells dramatically increase. Characterization of the heterogeneous populations of astrocytes from different brain regions, developmental expression, and reactivity to aging, disease, and trauma promise to provide new insights into the activity of astrocytes and their contributions to normal CNS functions. In terms of therapeutic applications glia, modified glia, or derived factors may prove beneficial. It has already been illustrated that astrocyte implants can facilitate recovery from some traumatic and developmental deficits. There are certainly limitations to the application of implants, but new avenues are being developed. Developmental studies that apply astrocytes to examine migration and innervation appear promising. Manipulation of astrocytes and other glial cells also may have a pivotal role in the treatment of disorders characterized by demeylination, or provide a substrate for reinnervation of damaged neural circuits.

Genetic modification of transfected astrocytes, or other cell types, may provide a ready source of specific trophic factors and neurotransmitters directly to localized areas of the brain (see [20] in this volume). With the evolution of transplant technology and increased awareness of astrocyte function, it is evident that therapeutic applications can be developed to incorporate astrocytes or components of the cells to address basic experimental issues and develop effective therapeutic interventions.

References

1. M. Aschner and R. M. LoPachin, Jr., *J. Toxicol. Environ. Health* **38,** 329 (1993).
2. B. A. Barres, *Neuroscience* **11,** 3685 (1991).
3. B. A. Barres, L. L. Chun, and D. P. Corey, *J. Neurosci.* **9,** 3169 (1989).
4. J. J. Bernstein and W. J. Goldberg, *Brain Res.* **491,** 205 (1989).
5. R. J. Bridges, J. P. Kesslak, M. Nieto-Sampedro, J. T. Broderick, and C. W. Cotman, *Brain Res.* **415,** 163 (1987).
6. C. W. Cotman, and J. P. Kesslak, *Prog. Brain Res.* **78,** 311 (1988).
7. S. Drejer, O. M. Larsson, and A. Schoeusboe, *Exp. Brain Res.* **47,** 259 (1982).
8. P. S. Eriksson, E. Hansson, and L. Ronnback, *Neuropharmacology* **30,** 1233 (1991).
9. A. Espinosa de los Monteros, M. A. Zhang, M. Gordon, M. Aymie, and J. de Vellis, *Dev. Neurosci.* **14,** 98 (1992).
10. D. Giulian and T. J. Baker, *J. Neurosci.* **8,** 2163 (1986).
11. E. Hansson and L. Rönnback, *Cell. Mol. Biol.* **36,** 487 (1990).
12. J. P. Kesslak, M. Nieto-Sampedro, J. Globus, and C. W. Cotman, *Exp. Neurol.* **92,** 377 (1986).
13. J. P. Kesslak, L. Brown, C. Steichen, and C. W. Cotman, *Exp. Neurol.* **94,** 615 (1986).
14. J. P. Kesslak, A. Walencewicz, L. Calin, M. Nieto-Sampedro, and C. W. Cotman, *Brain Res.* **454,** 347 (1988).
15. L.-F. H. Lin, D. H. Doherty, J. D. Lile, S. Bektesh, and F. Collins, *Science* **260,** 1130 (1993).
16. R. M. Lindsay, C. Emmett, G. Raisman, and P. J. Seeley, *Ann. N.Y. Acad. Sci.* **495,** 35 (1987).
17. D. C. Martin, *Glia* **5,** 81 (1992).
18. K. D. McCarthy and J. de Vellis, *J. Cell. Biol.* **85,** 890 (1980).
19. A. Michler-Stake, S. R. Wolff, and S. E. Bottenstein, *Int. J. Dev. Neurosci.* **2,** 575 (1984).
20. S. Miller, R. S. Bridges, and C. W. Cotman, *Brain Res.* **618,** 175 (1993).
21. C. M. Muller and J. Best, *Nature* (*London*) **342,** 427 (1989).
22. M. Nieto-Sampedro, J. P. Kesslak, R. Gibbs, and C. W. Cotman, *Ann. N.Y. Acad. Sci.* **495,** 108 (1987).

23. J. A. Olson, K. T. Shiverick, S. Ogilvie, W. C. Buhi, and M.K. Raizada, *Endocrinology (Baltimore)* **129,** 1066 (1991).
24. A. J. Patel, J. Kiss, and C. Gray, *in* "Neurodegeneration" (A. J. Hunter and M. Clark, eds.), p. 59. Academic Press, San Diego, 1992.
25. D. G. Stein, S. Finger, and T. Hart, *Behav. Neural Biol.* **37,** 185 (1984).
26. H. F. Zhou and R. D. Lund, *J. Comp.Neurol.* **317,** 145 (1992).

[19] Development of Immortalized Cell Lines for Transplantation in Central Nervous System Injury and Degeneration Models

M. Giordano, H. Takashima, M. Poltorak, H. M. Geller, and W. J. Freed

Introduction

Neural transplantation in the mammalian central nervous system is a valuable methodology that has been used to increase our understanding of neural development and injury-induced plasticity. It also provides a technique to replace damaged tissue and thereby, in some cases, to restore function. Neural grafts have been shown to reafferent and to receive inputs from the host brain, and in several animal models can reverse functional and behavioral deficits. The source of tissue for neural grafts has traditionally been fetal tissue, both for its resilience and its capacity to grow and develop connections with the host nervous system. Fetal brain has thus proved to be the ideal tissue for transplantation in many respects. However, the use of fetal tissue complicates the understanding and identification of the factors involved in the functional efficacy of grafts. This is partly due to the variety of cellular populations that are present in fetal tissue, and to the difficulty in obtaining pure populations of cells with specific characteristics.

New techniques and developments in cellular and molecular biology have led to a number of possibilities for developing cell lines with defined properties. Transplantation of pure populations of cells may ultimately contribute to refined transplantation techniques through which the elements necessary for the functional effects of grafts may be identified. The characteristics and differences between cell lines can be well defined *in vitro*. The determination of which cell lines promote or do not promote functional recovery in a given animal model will aid in reducing the range of possible factors involved. A related aspect of the use of cell lines for neural transplantation is the possibility of designing cell lines to fulfill specific functions. Through the use of gene transfer techniques, cell lines that produce a certain neurotransmitter, possess a certain kind of adhesion molecule, or secrete a specific trophic factor can be produced.

Cell lines can be generated using several strategies (1–3). One is the culture and cloning of tumor cells, examples of which include the PC12 cell line

Methods in Neurosciences, Volume 21

derived from a pheochromocytoma (4), the B16/C3 line derived from a murine melanoma (5), the IMR-32 line derived from a human neuroblastoma (6), and the C6 cell line cloned from a rat glial tumor (7). Each of these lines has been used for studies of brain transplantation (8–11). Another is to produce hybrid cells from fusion of primary cells with tumor cells. Examples include two cell lines derived from rat and mouse embryonic mesencephalic cells and the murine neuroblastoma–glioma cell line N18TG2 (12, 13). Both cell lines are described as having neuronal properties not found in the N18TG2 cell line (12, 13). More recently described methods for generating cell lines from intact brain provide another possibility. One example is the HCN-1 human neuronal cell line (14). Another is the generation of neuronal stem cells from brain via "neurospheres" and other techniques, as have been described (15–17). One of the problems that may be associated with the use of certain cell lines is a potential for tumorogenicity, which limits their use in transplantation studies (1). More recent strategies include the use of genetically altered cells that carry a specific cDNA, for example, primary fibroblasts genetically modified to express tyrosine hydroxylase or nerve growth factor (NGF) (18–21), derivation of immortal cell lines from transgenic mice (22, 23), and immortalization of primary neural cells through incorporation of an immortalizing gene (24). Examples of these include olfactory bulb, cerebral and cerebellar cortical cell lines, and the A7 glial cell line (Fig. 1) immortalized using the *myc* vector, polyoma large T antigen, and simian virus 40 (SV40) large T antigens, respectively (25, 26). Immortalized hippocampal, raphe, mesencephalic, and striatal cell lines have also been developed using the *ts*A58 allele of SV40 large T antigen (27–31).

This chapter focuses on the methodology for one of the techniques using immortalizing genes to generate cell lines. Characterization and transplantation of these cell lines is also discussed.

General Guidelines

When generating an immortalized cell line one of the first steps is the selection of the brain region of interest and its optimal gestational age. The ability of the primary cells to divide is the key to successful immortalization, because integration of viral genes into the host genome requires that the host cell undergo at least one round of DNA synthesis (1). In the case of mouse striatal tissue the peak of cell division is on day 14 or 15, although neurogenesis occurs between day 12 of gestation and the first few days after birth (32). Another step is selection of the gene to be used for immortalization. The two genes that have been studied most extensively are v-*myc* and SV40 large T antigen. One factor to consider is the possibility of controlling the

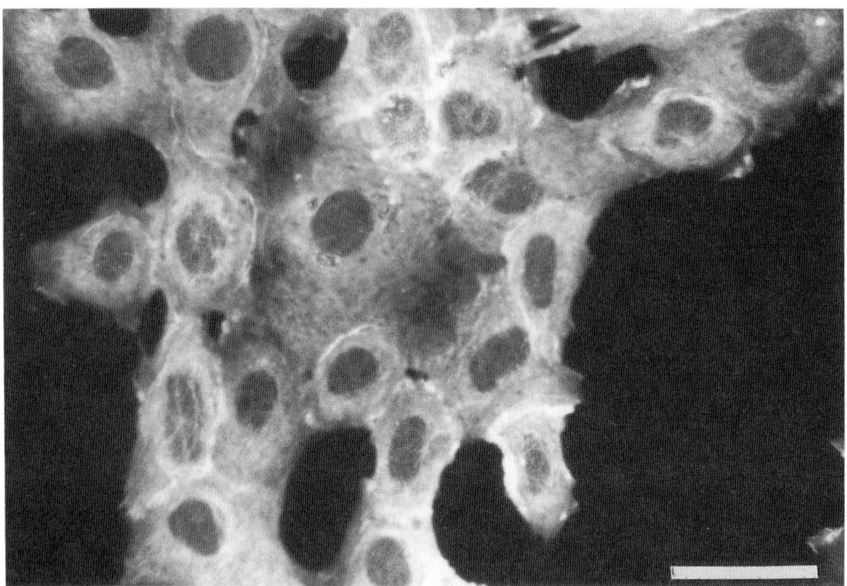

FIG. 1 A7 cells in culture processed for indirect immunofluorescence against anti-tubulin. Bar: 30 μm.

activity of the gene; temperature-sensitive mutants allow the gene to be active at the permissive temperature and inactive at the nonpermissive temperature, which may promote differentiation (1).

In the next section we outline the procedure we have used to generate immortalized cell lines from fetal rat ventral mesencephalic and striatal tissue (see Fig. 2).

Establishment of Immortalized Cell Line

In general, once the tissue has been dissected and infected, a primary cell culture is established (Figs. 3 and 4). The choice of medium depends on the type of cells that are to be immortalized. To promote the survival of cells of neuronal origin, we have used chemically defined or serum-free medium. The primary cultures are maintained for a variable period of time before separating immortalized cell lines from other cells. Usually the immortalizing vector carries a drug resistance gene, such as the neomycin resistance gene, which confers drug resistance to infected cells, and thereby allows for selection of the transformed population. Once normal cells have been killed by

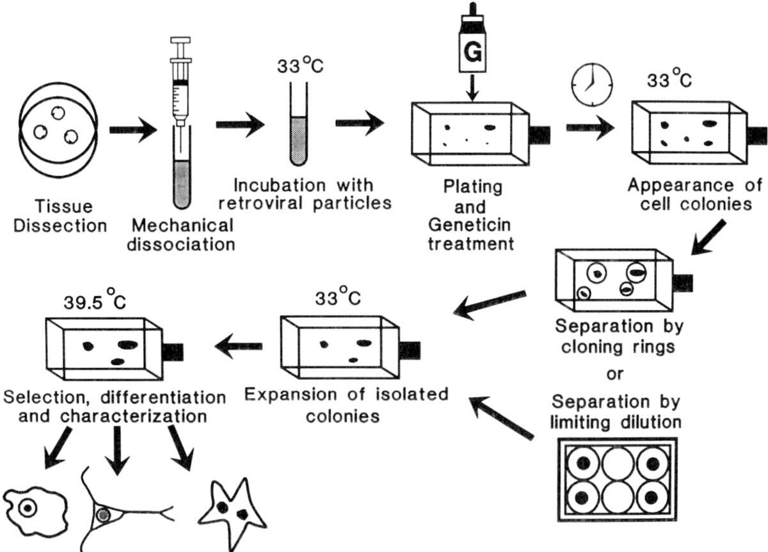

FIG. 2 General procedure for immortalization of primary cells using a temperature-sensitive allele of SV40 large T antigen.

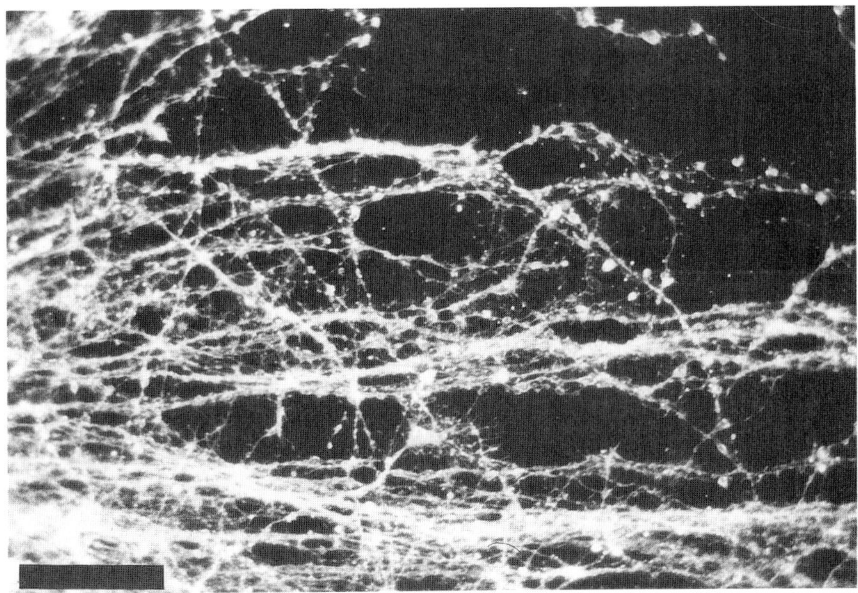

FIG. 3 Photomicrograph of a primary culture of striatal tissue (E14) in serum-free medium processed for indirect immunofluorescence against growth-associated protein 43. Bar: 100 μm.

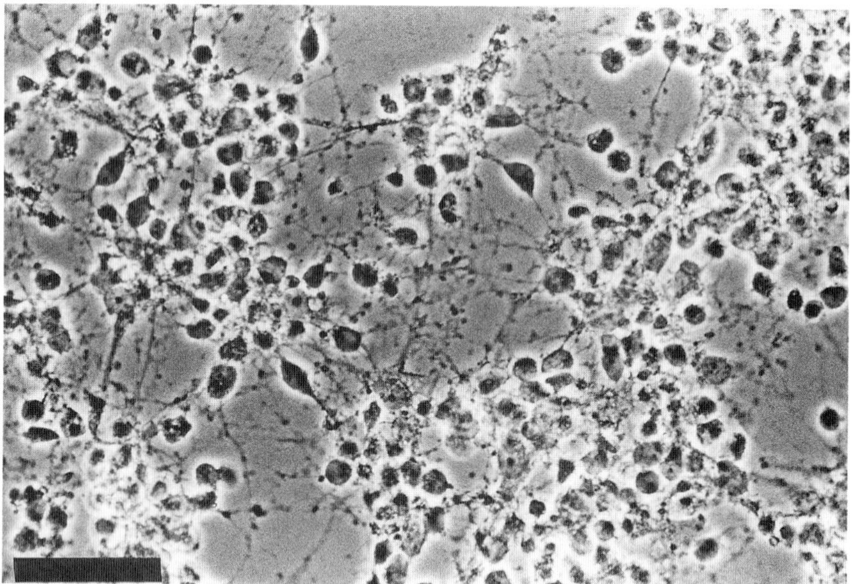

FIG. 4 Photomicrograph of a primary culture of striatal tissue (E14) in serum-free medium. Bar: 50 μm.

neomycin and only immortalized cells are present in the culture, the immortalized cell colonies can be separated and cloned. To clone the transformed cell lines one can screen a mixed population of immortalized cells for a particular characteristic, for example, the expression of a certain protein or a distinct morphology. Then clones can be separated by using the limiting dilution method (33), expanded, and characterized again. Other approaches include separating colonies using cloning rings (33), and cutting the dish on which cells are plated and dropping the pieces into culture flasks (J. W. Fawcett, Cambridge University, unpublished observations, 1993). These latter methods are possible only when the colonies are separate enough and there is no risk of contamination from one clone with another.

To obtain immortalized cell lines from mesencephalic and striatal cells we use the temperature-sensitive A58 allele of the SV40 large T antigen (*ts*A58). A Ψ2 cell line producing a defective recombinant retrovirus that contains the neomycin resistance and SV40 large T genes (34), provided by Cepko (35), is the source of the vector. Fetal striatal [embryonic day 14 (E14)] and mesencephalic (E12) tissue from Sprague-Dawley rats is dissected under sterile conditions and collected in oxygenated Dulbecco's modified Eagle's medium/Ham's F-12 nutrient mixture (DMEM/F12, 1 : 1) and 10% (v/v) fetal calf serum (FCS; GIBCO, Grand Island, NY). The tissue is washed and resuspended in 3 ml of filtered Ψ2-conditioned medium (syringe filter, 0.45-μm pore size; Gelman Sciences, Ann Arbor, MI) and mechanically dissociated with a 19-gauge needle in the presence of Polybrene (4 μg/ml). The tissue is incubated at 33°C for 4–12 hr, then resuspended, washed, mechanically dissociated in fresh 10% FCS, and plated on a 25-cm^2 flask previously coated with poly-D-lysine (20 μg/ml). The following day the medium is changed to a chemically defined medium (DM) consisting of DMEM/F12 (1 : 1), glucose (3.15 g/liter), 15 m*M* *N*-2-hydroxyethylpiperazine-*N'*-2-ethanesulfonic acid (HEPES), 4 m*M* glutamine (2 m*M* for striatal tissue), penicillin G (100 U/ml), streptomycin (100 μg/ml), transferrin (100 μg/ml), insulin (25 μg/ml), 60 μ*M* putrescine, 20 n*M* progesterone, 30 n*M* triiodothyronine (T_3), and 30 n*M* selenium. The medium is replaced every 2 days. After a minimum of 1 week and a maximum of 4 weeks, the cultures are treated with Geneticin (200 μg/ml) in 10% FCS for 10 days. After Geneticin treatment, all flasks are screened for the presence of cell colonies for up to 1 week. Once a colony is detected, it is allowed to expand and maintained at 33°C in 10% FCS. When a colony reaches a size of approximately 100 cells, it is separated with cloning rings, further expanded, and characterized. If several colonies are close together the cells are dissociated with a nonenzymatic dissociation solution (Sigma Chemical Co., St. Louis, MO). A portion of the cell suspension is frozen in 10% (v/v) dimethyl sulfoxide (DMSO) and another portion is plated at high dilution (10 cells/ml) in 96-well plates (Costar, Cambridge, MA). Each well contains 0.1 ml, so that the average well will contain one cell. These 96-well plates are screened for cells, and when colonies are found they are replated, expanded, and characterized. The selection of colonies is made on the basis of morphology alone.

Selection and Characterization

About 80 striatal cell lines and 30 mesencephalic cell lines were generated using the methods described above. Selection of ventral mesencephalic cell lines was made on the basis of staining for tyrosine hydroxylase and SV40 large T antigen. For the striatal cells, in view of their greater heterogeneity, a preliminary screening process included indirect immunofluorescence staining for the intermediate filament protein vimentin and for SV40 large T antigen. Those cell lines that were positive for vimentin were excluded from further characterization. This protein is found in cells of nonneuronal origin and our goal was to limit ourselves to the study of cell lines with potential neuronal phenotypes. Using immunocytochemical markers such as this, it is possible to screen large numbers of cell lines.

Another approach that can be used for selection of cell lines is the production of neurotransmitters or trophic factors. In this case, the cell culture supernatants are screened for the presence of the relevant factors. Alternatively conditioned medium effects on a second preparation can be evaluated. For example, Engele *et al.* (36) evaluated the effect of media conditioned by several glial cell lines on cell cultures of rat mesencephalon. Finally, the fastest approach is to screen cells by phase-contrast microscopy and select cells for further characterization according to their morphology. However, selection on the basis of morphological criteria is often difficult, because cells will express altered morphologies depending on the particular cell culture conditions, and the morphologies of many different cell lines are similar, even though they differ in key properties.

With regard to techniques for immunostaining of cells in culture, there are various methods. Peroxidase–anti-peroxidase- or streptavidin–biotin-based detection systems are sensitive methods, but have the disadvantage of producing higher background, which can lead to false positive results. In contrast, indirect immunofluorescence is less sensitive and requires a higher concentration of primary antibody, but is a rapid and reliable method for staining cell cultures, especially when staining for cell surface antigens. For indirect immunofluorescence commercially available primary antibodies are generally used at dilutions of 1 : 25 to 1 : 200. The method described herein is derived from Schachner (37).

Characterization of cell cultures is easily done using commercially available (Lab-Tek, Nunc Inc., Naperville, IL) chamber slides with two, four, or eight chambers per slide. The chambers have removable walls attached to plastic or glass slides. The use of chambers requires less time as compared to the staining of cell cultures on coverslips. The cells in each chamber can be stained separately for a specific antigen. Chamber walls may then be removed, the stained cells are coverslipped, and the slide is ready for observation. The slides can be coated with poly-D-lysine, poly-L-lysine, collagen, fibronectin, lamininin, or any other substrate, depending on the relative strength of attachment of the cell line. This is particularly important for glass slides. Photographs of cell cultures plated onto glass slides are of better quality than those of cell cultures on plastic slides. The advantage of plastic slides is that no coating is necessary.

The first step before staining is to determine whether the antigen of interest is located on the cell surface or in the intracellular compartment. In the latter case, permeabilization of the cell surface is required, and a different labeling protocol is to be used. For visualization of surface antigens, cultures are washed in Hank's balanced salt solution (HBSS), phosphate-buffered saline (PBS), or Dulbecco's phosphate-buffered saline (DPBS). The medium should be gently aspirated, because the cells are alive. Cells are then incubated with the primary antibody in a blocking buffer [e.g., washing medium plus 10% (v/v) goat or horse serum and 2% (w/v) bovine serum albumin] for 20 min at room temperature. The cultures are washed and fixed for 5 min in 4%

(w/v) phosphate-buffered paraformaldehyde, washed again, and then immersed for 10 min in blocking buffer. The blocking buffer is removed and the appropriate secondary antibodies are added for a 30- to 60-min incubation period. Affinity-purified anti-immunoglobulin antibodies conjugated with fluorescein isothiocyanate or tetramethylrhodamine isothiocyanate are recommended over bulk labeled antiserum. Secondary antibodies are usually used at 1 : 50–1 : 200 dilutions. After washing repeatedly, the chamber walls are removed and the cell cultures are mounted in glycerol–phosphate-buffered saline containing sodium azide (250 mg/50 ml) or another commercially available "fade retarding" medium.

For visualization of intracellular antigens, cultures are first fixed in 4% phosphate-buffered formalin for 5 min, then washed three times. Cell surfaces are then permeabilized in 5% acetic acid in ethanol for 2–5 min or in acetone for 30–60 sec at −20°C. The cells are repeatedly washed and then incbuated with the blocking buffer. Finally, they are stained with primary antibodies followed by the appropriate secondary antibodies.

Double immunolabeling with two primary antibodies of different origin can usually be done using either of two procedures: (a) primary antibodies are added together, and the culture is then rinsed and secondary antibodies are also added together, or (b) antibodies are applied successively, that is, the first antigen is reacted with the first antibody and an appropriately labeled secondary antibody, then the second antigen is reacted followed by the appropriately labeled secondary antibody.

Differentiation

Differentiation of cell lines is clearly the most important aspect of the generation of immortalized cell lines, for two reasons. First, if these cell lines are to be used to replace damaged tissue, they must possess the characteristics of the tissue to be replaced. Second, it is precisely the phenomenon of differentiation that is of interest when working with these pure cell populations. To promote differentiation, culture medium containing FCS is replaced by chemically defined medium and then a variety of substances such as growth factors, hormones, and enzymes may be added to the medium. In the case of cell lines immortalized using a temperature-sensitive allele, the change from the permissive to the nonpermissive temperature may be the first signal for differentiation to start.

The selection of the particular factors to be used depends on the target cell population, its availability, and on the results of past experiments. Examples of factors that have been used to promote differentiation include dibutyryl cAMP, nerve growth factor (NGF), basic fibroblast growth factor (bFGF), and retinoic acid, among others. Ronnett *et al.* (14) and Poltorak *et al.* (38) used a combination of NGF (25 ng/ml), dibutyryl cAMP (0.5 m*M*), and 3-isobutyl-1-methylxanthine (IBMX) (0.5 m*M*) to induce differentiation of the HCN-1 cell line. These factors appeared to induce the elongation of processes from the residue of retracted cytoplasmic membranes. If the factors were removed, the cells lost these processes and reverted to their original shape (38). It has become feasible to use reverse transcriptase-polymerase chain reaction (RT-PCR) to determine the spectrum of growth factor receptors present on a cell line, and then evaluate the effects of the agonists on cell division and differentiation (39). Mehler *et al.* (40) described the effects of cytokines for differentiation of immortalized hippocampal cells. The cytokines included interleukins 5, 7, 9, and 11, added to the culture medium, alone or in combination with bFGF, and transforming growth factor α (TGF-α) (40). The results of these and other studies indicate that each particular cell line may need to be sequentially exposed to a series of factors to differentiate. Indeed, this situation probably reflects more accurately what happens during *in vivo* neural development.

Cell Labeling

Whether the goal is to deliver a specific factor to the brain, replace damaged tissue, or test the ability of the cell line to differentiate, the final test is transplantation *in vivo*. Cells to be transplanted first must be marked so that they can be distinguished from host cells. There are several alternatives. One is to mark the clone by retroviral infection with a retrovirus carrying the gene for a marker such as a β-galactosidase (1) or alkaline phosphatase (41). Other methods include using an anti-gene antibody or preloading the cells with a fluorescent dye (9). The advantage of marking the cells with a marker such as β-galactosidase is that the marker is located in the cell cytoplasm, so that the morphology of the cells can be clearly visualized and examined for any changes, that is, elongation of processes.

The methodology to infect the cells with a second retrovirus is essentially the same as described for the initial infection. Cells are incubated at the permissive temperature with the filtered producer cell conditioned medium with (8 μg/ml) or without Polybrene. The cells are then seeded, grown, colonies are separated, and histochemically or immunohistochemically stained. The clones that have been successfully infected are then expanded and cryopreserved for future use. In the case of β-galactosidase staining, some researchers have found that repeated infections with the LacZ-encoding retrovirus may be needed to increase the percentage of β-galactosidase-positive cells (27, 42). It is not essential to isolate clones of labeled cells, as it may be sufficient to obtain a population in which a known percentage of the cells are labeled. A new retroviral vector, DAP, which encodes the human placental enzyme alkaline phosphatase, appears to result in more intense staining around cell bodies and processes than does β-galactosidase staining, and may provide better morphological definition (40).

There are a variety of intracellular markers that have been used to label cells for transplantation. One marker used is bisbenzimide (Hoechst 3342), a fluorescent vital dye that labels cell nuclei (43). To label the cells with bisbenzimide, the cells are dislodged from the culture dish or flask after incubation with trypsin–ethylenediaminetetraacetic acid (EDTA) or the non-enzymatic cell dissociation solution (Sigma Chemical Co.). After washing, the cells are incubated in serum containing medium with 5 μM bisbenzimide (Calbiochem, La Jolla, CA) for 30 min, washed, resuspended in serum-free medium, and gently dissociated by passing the cells through a 21-gauge metal needle (9). Cells can then be tested for viability by trypan blue exclusion and the density of the cell suspension is adjusted by adding fresh medium.

Similar procedures were used by Renfranz *et al.* (27) to label the hippocampal HiB5 cell line with tritiated thymidine, 1,1′-dioctadecyl-3,3,3′,3′-tetramethylindocarbocyanine perchlorate [DiI-C18-(3)], and green fluorescent latex microspheres to show the cell morphology and ascertain their origin. Other markers include rhodamine latex microspheres (0.1%, w/v) (Lumafluor, Inc., NJ), rhodamine-dextranamine (10%, w/v) (Molecular Probes, Eugene, OR), carboxy-fluorescein ester (5 *M*) (Molecular Probes), and Cascade Blue latex beads (0.1%, w/v) (Molecular Probes) (44). The most intense initial labeling was observed with the rhodamine compounds, and the highest selectivity for live cells occurred with the rhodamine-dextranamine and carboxy-fluorescein ester (44). After testing a variety of fluorescent dyes and other markers *in vitro,* Onifer *et al.* (42) found that only DiI was retained by proliferating or differentiating RN33B cells (an immortalized cell line from the raphe nucleus). The other markers weakly labeled cells or were not retained after some time *in vitro,* whereas others were toxic (42). An advantage of DiI over other fluorescent nuclear markers is that it labels cell membranes, revealing the morphology of the cell.

It appears that retroviral-mediated markers, such as galactosidase and alkaline phosphatase, generally have advantages over fluorescent dyes or microspheres. One advantage is that, at least in the case of the *lacZ* gene, the marker gene is constitutively expressed and passed on to all daughter cells in equal dose (42). These markers allow for visualization of somata and neurites, and allow for identification of infected cells *in vivo* (41, 42). A problem, however, is that expression of the histochemical marker, in the case of the *lacZ* gene, decreases with increasing number of passages, probably as a result of downregulation of inserted vector sequences driven from the retroviral long terminal repeat (LTR) (42, 45). Similar downregulation of the LTR appears to occur after transplantation into brain (46). Several possible solutions to the decrease in expression from the viral LTR have been suggested (46).

Transplantation

Cell lines are transplanted into the brain using ordinary stereotaxic techniques, involving injection of cell suspensions through metal or glass cannulas. Several aspects of the methodology are important, including steps that are needed to prevent the cells from being damaged by turbulence of shearing forces and steps to ensure that the cells are in fact ejected from the needle lumen.

Generally, cells are grown to confluence or near confluence in large 75-cm^2 flasks, in a medium such as DMEM or DMEM/F12 containing 10% fetal calf serum. Appropriate modifications should be made if the cells are grown in larger or smaller flasks. After aspirating the medium from the flask, cells are detached by incubating them in 2–3 ml of nonenzymatic cell dissociation solution (Sigma Chemical Co.). The cells will detach faster if the solution is at the same temperature as the cells. In this condition the cells are usually detached after 5 min. If using trypsin–EDTA IX (Sigma Chemical Co.) the cells detach faster and it is important to observe the cells through the microscope to stop the enzymatic reaction as soon as the cells start to detach from the flask. Trypsin is inactivated by adding medium with serum to the cells. The cells are transferred to a centrifuge tube and spun at approximately 600 *g* for 1 min. After this, the pellet should be visible. The medium is removed, replaced with serum-free medium, and resuspended by trituration. At this point cells can be incubated with intracellular markers as previously discussed. Once labeled, cell lines are implanted as cell suspensions of varying densities, for example, 1.5×10^5 cells/μl (42), 7.5×10^4 cells/μl (27), 1×10^4 cells/μl (45), and 5×10^3 cells/μl (47), suspended in phosphate-buffered saline or serum-free culture medium. The cells are mechanically dissociated and kept on ice until implantation. After incubation, cells are counted with a hemacytometer and the proportion of viable cells can be determined by the trypan blue dye exclusion test. For transplantation, cells may be kept for at least 1 hr in suspension while several animals receive cell transplants. It is necessary to agitate the cells periodically to prevent clumping.

Host animals are prepared for stereotaxic surgery using standard methods. The cells are aspirated into relatively large-bore needles to prevent damage of the cells and slow infusions are employed, of less than 1 μl/min. Cells are aspirated into metal or glass needles fitted to a glass Hamilton syringe, attached to a stereotaxic frame, or connected via polyethylene tubing to a syringe driven by a syringe pump (9). If using metal needles, the lumen should be smoothly polished. Alternatively, a glass capillary tube, about 1 mm in diameter, beveled and fire polished, can be glued onto a metal needle (64 mm × 0.025 in i.d.) using a cyanoacrylate adhesive, and then fitted onto the glass syringe (48). The advantage of using a glass needle is that the cells are visible and it is easy to assess if the appropriate volume was transplanted. In any case, the ability of cells to withstand ejection through various types of cannulas can be tested by ejecting the cells into a culture dish.

To transplant 100,000 cells into a region of the brain parenchyma, in a volume of 2 μl, cells should be suspended in medium in the appropriate volume. A volume of cells larger than that to be transplanted is aspirated into the infusion cannula. The cannula is lowered to the appropriate site in the brain, and the 2 μl of cells implanted slowly. The cannula should be left in place for at least 2 min and preferably longer. The cannula is then withdrawn and the remaining material ejected onto a glass slide to allow examination of the cells for viability.

An alternative method is to suspend the cells in a semisolid medium, such as Matrigel (Collaborative Research, Inc., Bedford, Massachusetts) (49), in order to provide support for the cells. In our laboratory we have successfully transplanted cell lines after reaggregation in a plasma clot following the method described by Lindsay *et al.* (50). Cells are washed and resuspended in 2–3 ml of citrated bovine plasma (GIBCO-Bethesda Research Laboratories, Gaithersburg, MD), mixed, and pelleted. The supernatant plasma is discarded and 100 μl of fresh plasma is added. Aliquots (10 μl) of plasma, containing the cells, are placed on a tissue culture dish and 8–12 μl of thrombin (bovine plasma thrombin; Sigma Chemical Co.) is added. After about 10 min at room temperature, a plasma clot is formed. These plasma clots can be injected into the brain of a host (50) or they can be placed on the surface of the exposed cortex.

It is also possible to simplify the transplantation technique, depending on the hardiness of the cells and the degree to which they can withstand manipulation. For example, PC-12 cells seems to be fairly fragile and must be treated carefully. B16 melanoma cells or mouse 3T3 cells, on the other hand, are quite hardy and can be transplanted into the brains of mice by simple freehand injection through burr holes, using 100-μl Hamilton syringes (gas-tight syringes work best). It is possible to transplant cells reliably into large targets (lateral ventricles or striatum) by this method. To transplant cells freehand, several animals are anesthetized, their scalps are cleaned with Betadine and alcohol, and incisions and burr holes are made in locations determined with reference to bregma. The syringe is loaded with medium, and approximately 3 μl of cell suspension is aspirated into the syringe. The syringe is inserted into the appropriate location and 2 μl of cells is slowly injected into the brain (over 1 min). The syringe is then left in place for approximately 30 sec, withdrawn, and the remaining cells are discarded. Several animals may be rapidly injected in succession in this way (2, 9).

For this method to be successful, there are several important considerations. Deflected point needles are much better than ordinary needles, because they do not become plugged by tissue when inserted into the brain. This allows the cells to be more easily ejected from the needle and may reduce damage to the transplanted cells. It may require some experience to perform this type of procedure successfully, as the cannulas must be held quite steady and the cells must be injected slowly to avoid displacing them into areas other than the target sites.

Following a predetermined interval, the hosts are sacrificed and the brain tissue is processed for histochemistry and immunohistochemistry. In the case of cells labeled with the *lacZ* gene, the tissue can be processed for X-Gal (5-bromo-4-chloro-3-indolyl-β-D-galactopyranoside) (27, 45) or immunohistochemistry (42). For cells labeled with alkaline phosphatase the tissue is processed for enzyme histochemistry as detailed in Fields-Berry *et al.* (41). In our laboratory we routinely use fresh frozen tissue sectioned at 12–16 μm and stained using indirect immunofluorescence (47). For detection of intracellular antigens, such as neurofilaments or glial fibrillary acidic protein (GFAP), sections are dried, washed in Tris-buffered saline, and incubated in primary antibody for 20 min at room temperature. Then cells are washed, fixed in 4% phosphate-buffered paraformaldehyde for 10 min, washed and incubated for 10 min in Tris-buffered 1.5% (w/v) saline containing 10% (v/v) horse serum, then incubated with anti-immunoglobulin antibodies conjugated to fluorescein isothiocynate or tetramethylrhodamine isothiocynate for 30 min. Finally, sections are mounted in glycerophosphate-buffered saline containing 0.05% (w/v) sodium azide (47). For visualization of bisbenzimide fluorescence, sections are dried, mounted, and examined with a fluorescence microscope equipped with filters for ultraviolet radiation. To aid in the anatomical localization of the graft, alternating sections can be stained using routine staining such as cresyl violet or hematoxylin–eosin. Finally, when sections are ready to be visualized under light microscopy, transplanted cells can be examined for expression of desired markers, for example, neurofilament and cell adhesion molecules. Effects of transplanted cells on the host brain, including the presence of an astroglial reaction and macrophages, also should be examined when determining the suitability of a cell line for transplantation.

Conclusions

The ability to use cell lines in place of primary neurons is a frequently stated goal of studies of neural transplantation. The potential advantages of cell lines are obvious. Problems of tissue uniformity would be reduced or eliminated, and experiments could be controlled in ways that are not possible when using primary cells. For human application, cell lines may ultimately obviate the problems associated with procurement of fetal tissue at appropriate developmental stages and testing for contamination, and various ethical and legal problems. These difficulties can be overcome for small numbers of patients on an experimental basis, but would be difficult to apply on a large scale, even if efficacious therapeutic techniques are developed. As an illustration, a study of fetal tissue transplantation in a patient with Parkinson's disease employed four fetuses (51). Although such large amounts of tissue may not ultimately be needed, at least for this particular application, it emphasizes the potential logistical problems that can be associated with the use of primary cells.

There are, however, some potential obstacles associated with the use of cell lines. It may be that an ideal cell line would have to substitute entirely for fetal tissue grafts. If this is the case, such a cell line would be required to perform a considerable number of functions such as extension of neurites, establishing appropriate postsynaptic contacts, forming synapses, and releasing neurotransmitters into the synapses at rates modulated in response to appropriate inputs. These functions require expression of a large number of proteins, each of which must be modulated appropriately. It is not clear whether cells that can accomplish these functions can be found or generated using current technology. On the other hand, cells that can perform a limited set of these functions (such as neurotransmitter release) may be partially or even entirely effective. In animal models of Parkinson's disease it has been observed that some of the behavioral deficits following substantia nigra lesions can be reversed by diffuse, nonsynaptic delivery of catecholamines (52). Thus, cell lines that simply release dopamine into the extracellular space may prove to be useful for transplantation.

The earliest approach to obtaining cell lines has involved the use of tumor cells. A number of tumor cell lines that produce neuroactive substances are available. Notably, the PC-12 pheochromocytoma cell line has been used for intracerebral transplantation in Parkinson's disease models (53, 54); however, because the cells are tumor cells, for long-term studies it has been necessary to encapsulate the cells to control their growth (53, 54). Other approaches to controlling growth of tumor cells may include further genetic alterations (7), or the use of chemical treatments to render the cells amitotic

(10). Because the use of tumor cells depends on the relatively haphazard availability of cells from spontaneous tumors, many groups have begun to consider the possibility of intentionally altering cells so that properties useful for neural transplantation are expressed.

There are essentially two routes by which new cell lines might be produced through genetic manipulation. One is that cells with the appropriate growth characteristics (e.g., astrocytes) might be altered genetically (55) so that they express the appropriate neuronal properties. Cells of a variety of types, such as fibroblasts, have already been altered to express tyrosine hydroxylase activity, nerve growth factor (56), or glutamic acid decarboxylase (57). Although such cells may be useful for the delivery of neurotransmitters or growth factors, it is not likely that they could be altered to form functional synapses with target neurons. For one thing, this would require a large number of genetic alterations, and other properties of the cells would be likely to interfere with the establishment of functional synapses. Finally, it is unclear which would be the ideal cell line for such applications, because cells that can be grown readily in culture may overgrow when transplanted into brain.

The contrasting approach is the immortalization of primary cells, the approach that has been emphasized in the present chapter. This approach has considerable potential advantages. If primary neurons could be immortalized at the final cell division stage, they would be committed to expressing the desired functional properties. In theory, therefore, it would be necessary only to alter primary cells to have the ability to grow under the appropriate tissue conditions.

There are, of course, difficulties. A fundamental difficulty is that primary neural cells must be altered to grow in culture, while at the same time the cells must stop growing after transplantation to prevent tumor formation. Approaches to controlling cell growth include the use of temperature-sensitive genes (1). There is also evidence that the LTR promoter is downregulated in cells that have been transplanted intracerebrally (46), which may help to control cell growth. A fundamental problem is that altering cells so that they can be grown in culture tends to alter other properties of the cells as well. Cells that are dividing tend to become locked in an undifferentiated state. Current methods for immortalization of cells tend to generate immature cells, which lack differentiated neuronal properties. There does not, however, appear to be a theoretical obstacle to generation of cells by immortalization techniques that cannot eventually be overcome. Indeed, some data support the concept that the brain provides appropriate differentiating factors for immortalized neuronal cells to become mature neurons (cf. 27, 45).

In the near future, it is envisioned that an increasing number of tumor cell lines, genetically altered cell lines, cells generated from normal brain, and immortalized cells will become available that can be employed for basic studies of neuronal transplantation. Cell lines will permit numerous studies that are not presently feasible. It may be possible, for example, to employ experimental designs in which the cells implanted in the control and experimental groups differ only in expression of a single protein. In the long term, cell lines may be developed that are able to perform the functions of primary cells to an increasing degree. Although intracerebral transplantation of cell lines for therapeutic purposes is a more distant possibility, it is already a realistic goal.

References

1. C. L. Cepko, *Annu. Rev. Neurosci.* **12,** 47 (1989).
2. W. J. Freed, H. M. Geller, M. Poltorak, H. E. Cannon-Spoor, S. L. Cottingham, M. E. LaMarca, M. Schultzberg, M. Rehavi, S. Paul, and E. I. Ginns, *Prog. Brain Res.* **82,** 10 (1990).
3. H. M. Geller, V. Quiñones-Jenab, M. Poltorak, and W. J. Freed, *J. Cell. Biochem.* **45,** 279 (1991).
4. L. A. Greene and A. S. Tischler, *Proc. Natl. Acad. Sci. U.S.A.* **73,** 2424 (1976).
5. F. Hu and P. F. Lesney, *Cancer Res.* **24,** 1634 (1964).
6. J. J. Tumilowicz, W. W. Nichols, J. J. Cholon, and A. E. Greene, *Cancer Res.* **30,** 2110 (1970).
7. P. Benda, J. Lightbody, G. Sato, L. Levine, and W. Sweet, *Science* **161,** 370 (1968).
8. O. Okuda, J. Bressler, L. Chang, and M. Brightman, *Exp. Neurol.* **113,** 330 (1991).
9. W. J. Freed, A. M. Adinolfi, J. D. Laskin, and H. M. Geller, *Brain Res.* **485,** 349 (1989).
10. D. M. Gash, M. F. D. Notter, S. H. Okawara, A. L. Kraus, and R. J. Joynt, *Science* **233,** 1420 (1986).
11. G. Bing, M. F. D. Notter, J. T. Hansen, C. Kellogg, J. H. Kordower, and D. M. Gash, *Neuroscience* **34,** 687 (1990).
12. G. D. Crawford, Jr., W. Le, R. G. Smith, W. Xie, E. Stefani, and S. H. Appel, *J. Neurosci.* **12,** 3392 (1992).
13. H. K. Choi, L. A. Won, P. J. Kontur, D. N. Hammond, A. P. Fox, B. H. Wainer, P. C. Hoffmann, and A. Heller, *Brain Res.* **552,** 67 (1991).
14. G. V. Ronnett, L. D. Hester, J. S. Nye, K. Connors, and S. H. Snyder, *Science* **248,** 603 (1990).
15. B. A. Reynolds and S. Weiss, *Science* **255,** 1707 (1992).
16. L. J. Richards, T. J. Kilpatrick, and P. F. Bartlett, *Proc. Natl. Acad. Sci. U.S.A.* **89,** 8591 (1992).
17. B. E. Wojcik, F. Nothias, M. Lazar, H. Jouin, J. F. Nicolas, and M. Peschanski, *Proc. Natl. Acad. Sci. U.S.A.* **90,** 1305 (1993).

18. L. J. Fisher, H. A. Jinnah, L. C. Kale, G. A. Higgins, and F. H. Gage, *Neuron* **6,** 371 (1991).
19. P. Horellou, P. Brundin, P. Kalen, J. Mallen, and A. Björklund, *Neuron* **5,** 393 (1990).
20. M. B. Rosenberg, T. Friedman, R. C. Robertson, M. Tsuzynski, J. A. Wolff, X. O. Breakfield, and F. H. Gage, *Science* **242,** 1575 (1988).
21. P. Ernfors, T. Ebendal, L. Olson, P. Moulton, I. Stromberg, and H. Persson, *Proc. Natl. Acad. Sci. U.S.A.* **86,** 4756 (1989).
22. P. S. Jat, M. D. Noble, P. Ataliotis, Y. Tanaka, N. Yannoutsos, L. Larsen, and D. Kioussis, *Proc. Natl. Acad. Sci. U.S.A.* **88,** 5096 (1991).
23. P. L. Mellon, J. J. Windle, P. C. Goldsmith, C. A. Padula, J. L. Roberts and R. I. Winer, *Neuron* **5,** 1 (1990).
24. C. L. Cepko, *Trends Neurosci.* **11,** 6 (1988).
25. E. F. Ryder, E. Y. Snyder, and C. L. Cepko, *J. Neurobiol.* **21,** 356 (1990).
26. H. M. Geller and M. Dubois-Dalcq, *J. Cell Biol.* **107,** 1977 (1988).
27. P. J. Renfranz, M. G. Cunningham, and R. D. G. McKay, *Cell (Cambridge, Mass.)* **66,** 713 (1991).
28. H. Takashima, M. Marone, H. M. Geller, and J. W. Freed, *Soc. Neurosci. Abstr.* **18,** 413 (1992).
29. M. Giordano, H. Takashima, A. Herranz, M. Poltorak, H. M. Geller, M. Marone, and W. J. Freed, *Exp. Neurol.* **124,** 395–400 (1993).
30. D. E. Bredsen, K. Hisanaga, and F. K. Sharp, *Ann. Neurol.* **27,** 205 (1990).
31. L. A. White and S. R. Whittemore, *J. Chem. Neuroanat.* **5,** 327 (1992).
32. C. Fentress, B. B. Stanfield, and W. M. Cowan, *Anat. Embryol.* **163,** 275 (1981).
33. R. I. Freshney, "Culture of Animal Cells: A Manual of Basic Technique." Wiley-Liss, New York, 1987.
34. P. S. Jat, C. L. Cepko, R. C. Mulligan, and P. A. Sharp, *Mol. Cell. Biol.* **6,** 1204 (1986).
35. C. L. Cepko, B. E. Roberts, and R. C. Mullilgan, *Cell (Cambridge, Mass.)* **37,** 1053 (1984).
36. J. Engele, D. Schubert, and M. C. Bohn, *J. Neurosci. Res.* **30,** 359 (1991).
37. M. Schachner, *in* "Immunohistochemistry" (A. Cuello, ed.), p. 399. Wiley, New York, 1983.
38. M. Poltorak, M. Isono, W. J. Freed, G. V. Ronnett, and S. H. Snyder, *Cell Transplant.* **1,** 3 (1992).
39. K. Shimoda, K. Inoue, T. Kitagawa, N. Kuno, K. Takahashi, and J. W. Commissiong, *Soc. Neurosci. Abstr.* **19,** 32 (1993).
40. M. F. Mehler, R. Rozental, M. Dougherty, D. C. Spray, and J. A. Kessler, *Nature (London)* **362,** 62 (1993).
41. S. C. Fields-Berry, A. L. Halliday, and C. L. Cepko, *Proc. Natl. Acad. Sci. U.S.A.* **89,** 693 (1992).
42. S. M. Onifer, L. A. White, S. R. Whittemore, and V. R. Holets, *Cell Transplant.* **2,** 131 (1993).
43. H. G. J. M. Kuypers, M. Bentivoglio, C. E. Catsman-Berrevoets, and A. T. Bharos, *Exp. Brain Res.* **40,** 383 (1980).
44. G. K. Pyapali, D. A. Turner, and R. D. Madison, *Exp. Neurol.* **116,** 133 (1992).

45. E. Y. Snyder, D. L. Deitcher, C. Walsh, S. Arnold-Aldea, E. A. Hartweig, and C. L. Cepko, *Cell (Cambridge, Mass.)* **68,** 33 (1992).
46. M. Schinstine and F. H. Gage, *Res. Publ.—Assoc. Res. Nerv. Ment. Dis.* **71,** 311 (1993).
47. M. Isono, H. M. Geller, M. Poltorak, and W. J. Freed, *Res. Neurol. Neurosci.* **4,** 301 (1991).
48. M. Giordano, S. H. Hagenmeyer-Houser, and P. R. Sanberg, *Brain Res.* **446,** 183 (1988).
49. S. R. Whittemore, V. R. Holets, R. W. Keane, D. J. Levy, and R. D. G. McKay, *J. Neurosci. Res.* **28,** 156 (1991).
50. R. M. Lindsay, G. Raisman, and P. J. Seeley, *Neuroscience* **21,** 685 (1987).
51. O. Lindvall, P. Brundin, H. Widner, S. Rehncrona, B. Gustavii, R. Frackowiak, K. L. Leenders, G. Sawle, J. C. Rothwell, C. D. Marsden, and A. Björklund, *Science* **247,** 574 (1990).
52. W. J. Freed, M. Poltorak, H. Takashima, M. E. LaMarca, and E. I. Ginns, *J. Cell. Biochem.* **45,** 261 (1991).
53. S. R. Winn, P. A. Tresco, B. Zielinski, L. A. Greene, C. B. Jaeger, and P. Aebischer, *Exp. Neurol.* **113,** 322 (1991).
54. D. F. Emerich, B. R. Frydel, T. R. Flanagan, M. Palmatier, S. R. Winn, and L. Christenson, *Cell Transplant.* **2,** 241 (1993).
55. E. F. La Gamma, G. Weisinger, N. J. Lenn, and R. E. Strecker, *Cell Transplant.* **2,** 207 (1993).
56. F. H. Gage, M. D. Kawaja, and L. J. Fisher, *Trends Neurosci.* **14,** 328 (1991).
57. F. C. Zhou, C. Cheng, and S. Bledsoe, *Cell Transplant.* **2,** 193 (1993).

Section VIII

Using Implanted Living Cells within the Central Nervous System

[20] Use of Genetically Modified Cells to Deliver Neurotrophic Factors and Neurotransmitters to the Brain

Lisa J. Fisher, Gordon R. Chalmers, and Fred H. Gage

Introduction

The strategy of using living cells as "vehicles" for delivering compounds to the central nervous system (CNS) has been pursued with great interest since the demonstrations in 1979 that fetal substantia nigra neurons grafted into the rat brain could functionally replace the neurotransmitter dopamine (2, 27). Although fetal tissues have been explored in most detail in this strategy, such heterogeneous tissues have the disadvantages that they do not produce some factors in sufficient quantities (i.e., neurotrophic factors) or purity (i.e., a single neurotransmitter) to assess the effectiveness of a discrete compound within the brain. Some of these limitations may be circumvented by using established cell lines, producing specific neuroactive substances, as donor material for grafting (see [19]). We have pursued an alternative strategy of using gene transfer techniques to create a population of cells that expresses a new genetic program that enables them to produce a specific compound of interest. These modified cells are then implanted into the brain to achieve localized delivery of the compounds to the CNS (14; see Fig. 1).

In considering applications to the CNS, we have genetically modified cells to produce a variety of neurotrophic factors, such as nerve growth factor (NGF), brain-derived neurotrophic factor (BDNF), and basic fibroblast growth factor (bFGF), and the synthetic enzymes necessary for producing neurotransmitters, such as dopamine (tyrosine hydroxylase; TH), γ-aminobutyric acid (glutamic acid decarboxylase), and acetylcholine (choline acetyltransferase; ChAT). These modified cells have been placed into both the developing and adult nervous systems to explore the role of the engineered product in the CNS (i.e., 20). In addition, genetically modified cells have been used in animal models of neurodegenerative disease, both as an approach for intervening in the disease process and as a method for replacing lost function (13).

This chapter describes some of the techniques involved in creating, characterizing, and using genetically modified cells as a method for delivering compounds to the CNS. Two representative model systems illustrate some

Methods in Neurosciences, Volume 21

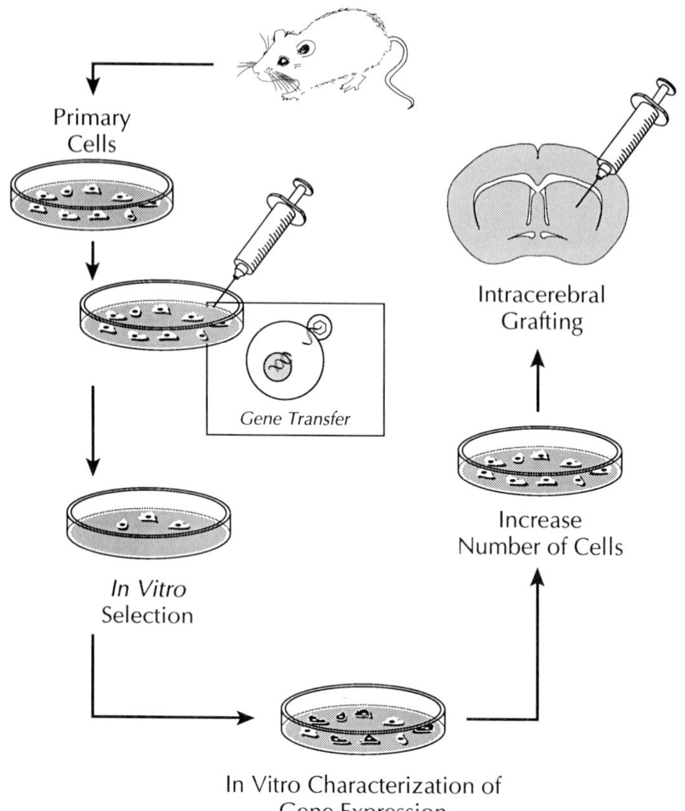

FIG. 1 Schematic of the gene transfer/intracerebral grafting strategy. Primary cells are obtained from a donor and placed in culture. A gene encoding a product of interest is inserted into the target cells, using the retroviral infection technique, and those cells that successfully incorporate the transgene are characterized *in vitro*. The transgene-containing cells are grown to sufficient numbers for grafting and then implanted into the CNS. Continued functioning of the engineered cells *in vivo* is assessed by a variety of anatomical, chemical, and behavioral techniques. [Figure modified from Gage *et al.* (13).]

of the techniques we use to assess the *in vivo* functioning of cells engineered to produce either a neurotrophic factor (NGF) or neurotransmitters (acetylcholine, dopamine). Although this strategy may be pursued with a variety of cell types, we have focused on the use of primary cells (fibroblasts), rather than established cell lines, for genetic modification because the power of the technique can be fully realized only with a cell type that will survive noninvasively for prolonged periods in the CNS [e.g., 5, 18, 21].

In Vitro Development and Characterization of Engineered Cells

Fibroblast Preparation

The method used for isolating primary skin fibroblasts from rats was modified from a procedure described by Sly and Grubb (30). Although any species of rat may be used for this procedure, the use of an inbred strain of rat (such as the Fischer 344) as both fibroblast donor and graft recipient minimizes problems with immunological rejection of the transplanted cells. The rat is anesthetized with a mixture of ketamine (75 mg/kg), rompun (4.0 mg/kg), and acepromazine (5.6 mg/kg) and its abdomen is shaved and cleansed with alcohol. A piece of skin approximately 1 cm^2 is removed, cut into small fragments (1–2 mm^2), and then placed into a 60-mm culture dish containing Dulbecco's minimal essential medium (DMEM) supplemented with 10% (v/v) fetal bovine serum and 0.1% (v/v) glutamine. Cultures are maintained at 37°C in a humidified incubator with a 10% CO_2 atmosphere and the medium is replaced once or twice per week. Fibroblasts grow out of the explant pieces within a few days and are passaged with 0.05% (v/v) trypsin and 1 m*M* ethylenediaminetetraacetic acid (EDTA) in phosphate-buffered saline (PBS) when approximately 90% confluent. Cells are replated in a T75 flask and the feeding schedule is increased to two or three times per week as the fibroblasts expand. Fibroblast cultures typically contain cells of varying shapes, ranging from thin and elongated to a flat, fried egg appearance. These differences in cellular morphologies reflect the health and age of the cells (1). Prior to gene transfer, some of the cells are passaged into a new T75 flask at low density and the remaining fibroblasts are frozen at −70°C in medium containing 10% (v/v) dimethyl sulfoxide (DMSO).

Gene Transfer

A variety of gene transfer techniques can be used to introduce new genetic material into cells. We primarily use the retroviral infection method (7) for the primary fibroblasts because this procedure is easy and more efficient than many other techniques (19). Briefly, the internal components of the retrovirus are removed and replaced with the gene of interest under the control of the viral 5′ long terminal repeat (LTR). An internal promoter is also typically inserted downstream of the gene of interest to drive the expression of a selectable marker gene such as that encoding for neomycin resistance. This second gene provides a method for screening cells after the infection procedure for those that have successfully incorporated the new genetic material. Because the internal components of the retrovirus have been replaced with other genes, the virus is incapable of producing infectious particles. The retroviral vector must therefore be inserted into a "helper" cell line, such as ψ2 producer cells, to generate the virus that will be used for gene transfer. For optimal infection efficiency using the retroviral technique, target cells should be replicating throughout the entire infection procedure. Primary fibroblasts are plated in a T75 flask such that they are 20–30% confluent. Five milliliters of virus-containing medium is collected from the ψ2 cells and mixed with Polybrene (4 μg/ml), a charged compound that promotes viral adherence to the cell surface, and added to the fibroblast cultures. On each of the following 2 days, the virus-containing medium is removed from the fibroblasts and the infection procedure repeated. On the fourth day, the medium is removed from the fibroblast cultures and replaced with fresh medium (DMEM with 10% fetal bovine serum) supplemented with 400 μg/ml of the neomycin analog G418 (GIBCO, Grand Island, NY) or an alternative drug that is appropriate for the selectable marker within the retroviral vector. Cells that were not successfully infected die in the G418 medium during a 1- to 2-week period, leaving a population of cells that have randomly incorporated the viral vector. These engineered cells will express the inserted gene ("transgene") at varying levels, perhaps reflecting the genomic insertion site or the state of the cell. Although the genetically modified fibroblasts may be subcloned to isolate a population that expresses the transgene at relatively uniform and/or high levels, the subcloning procedure (increased cellular doublings) may compromise the health of the cells. We typically use a bulk population of infected fibroblasts for grafting.

Verification of Transgene Function

Genetically modified fibroblasts are characterized *in vitro* prior to grafting to ensure that the selected cells express the transgene at discernible levels. For simplicity, the techniques that are used most frequently to obtain rapid assessments of transgene activity are described. In general, we rely on biochemical assays for determining the production of NGF or ChAT within modified cells, whereas we primarily employ histological techniques for identifying engineered cells that express TH or the *Escherichia coli* β-galactosidase (B-Gal) transgene. Fibroblasts expressing the B-Gal transgene, which has no therapeutic application in the CNS, are typically used in the grafting paradigms for control comparisons.

Nerve Growth Factor ELISA

Mouse NGF production by genetically modified fibroblasts is determined by a two-site enzyme immunoassay using commercially available reagents and a modification of the manufacturer protocol (Boehringer Mannheim, Indianapolis, IN). The primary antibody, anti-mouse NGF (Boehringer, Mannheim), is diluted in plate-coating buffer [$Na_2CO_3/NaHCO_3$, 50 mmol/liter; sodium azide, 0.1% (w/v); pH 9.6] by adding 100 μl of the stock antibody (at 30 μg/ml) to 6.5 ml of the coating buffer. Each well of a 96-well plate (Nunc-Immuno plate Maxi Sorp; Nunc, Inc., Naperville, IL) is filled with 100 μl of the dilute antibody solution and the plates are incubated for 2 hr at 37°C. It is important that the plate material have a high protein-binding capacity such as that found in the plate specified above. During the incubation period the standards are made and the samples diluted. To make standards, mouse NGF stock (Boehringer Mannheim) is added to the sample conjugate buffer (SCB) {50 ml of 10× (0.5 *M* Tris-HCl, pH 7.0); 100 ml of 25× (1 *M* NaCl); 10 ml of 50× (0.5 *M* $CaCl_2$); 5 ml of 100× 10% (v/v) Triton X-100], 5 g of bovine serum albumin (BSA); and 330 ml of H_2O} to produce standards of 1280, 320, 160, 80, 20, 10, 5, and 0 pg/ml. The samples may be diluted 1 : 10 to 1 : 20, depending on the concentration of NGF expected, so that the resulting measurement is below the 160-pg/ml point in the calibration curve. This permits the two highest standards to be excluded from the calibration curve so the curve is more accurate at the lower levels. Each well is then washed three times with wash buffer {50 ml of 10× (0.5 *M* Tris-HCl, pH 7.0); 100 ml of 25× (1 *M* NaCl), 10 ml of 50× (0.5 *M* $CaCl_2$), 5 ml of 100× [10% (v/v) Triton X-100], 5 ml of 100× [5% (w/v) NaN_3]; and 330 ml H_2O} and 50 μl of sample or standard is added per well, with each measurement being done in triplicate. Note that the volume placed in the well is far less than the volume of the coating solution, to avoid contact of the former with any uncoated surfaces. Plates are incubated at 4°C overnight and then washed three times with 150 μl of wash buffer per well. The stock secondary antibody, mouse anti-mouse NGF conjugated with β-galactosidase (4 U/ml activity; Boehringer Mannheim) is diluted in SCB, 150 μl of antibody to 3 ml of buffer (final activity, 0.2 U/ml), 50 μl is aliquoted per well, and plates are incubated for 4 hr at 37°C. For increased sensitivity the secondary antibody may be diluted half as much, for a final concentration of 0.4 U/ml. During the incubation, the substrate for the final reaction step is prepared by adding 24.5 mg of *O*-nitrophenyl-β-D-galactopyranoside (ONPG) to 7 ml of substrate buffer {50 ml of 10× [1 *M* *N*-2-hydroxyethylpiperazine-*N'*-2-ethanesulfonic acid (HEPES)], 75 ml of 25× (1 *M* NaCl), 5 ml of 100× (0.2 *M* $MgCl_2$), 10 ml of 100× [5% (w/v) NaN_3], 5 g of BSA; and 360 ml H_2O}. Each well is then washed three times with 150 ml of wash buffer; 100 μl of the substrate is added, and plates are incubated in the dark at 37°C for 2 hr. The plates are then read on an enzyme-linked immunosorbent array (ELISA) meter with the test filter set to 410 nm. The average of the triplicate measures for each sample and standard is determined and a standard curve is drawn, permitting sample levels to be determined by linear regression. The detection limit for

NGF by this procedure is in the range of 5–10 pg/ml. The typical NGF secretion level from low-passage fibroblasts containing the β-NGF transgene is approximately 170 pg of NGF/hr/10^5 cells (22).

Choline Acetyltransferase Assay

The technique used to determine ChAT activity within the engineered fibroblasts is modified from a method described by Fonnum (11). Fibroblasts in log-phase growth are removed from tissue cultures plates with trypsin and washed several times with sterile PBS. Cells suspended in the final PBS wash are transferred to a 1.5-ml Eppendorf tube and sonicated three times for 10 sec each. A 10-μl aliquot of the homogenate is placed in another Eppendorf tube and incubated with 10 μl of a solution containing 0.2 m*M* [^{14}C]acetyl-CoA, BSA (1 mg/mg), 18 m*M* EDTA, 0.6 m*M* NaCl, and 0.1 m*M* NaH_2PO_4 for 5 min at 37°C. The reaction is stopped by adding 100 μl of ice-cold distilled water. Samples are extracted with 1 ml of extraction buffer (15 g of sodium tetraphenylboron in 850 ml of toluene and 150 ml of acetonitrile) and 0.65 ml of the organic phase is removed to 5 ml of scintillation cocktail (National Diagnostics, Atlanta, GA) for a 10-min count. Activity is corrected for protein as determined by a Coomassie protein assay. Bulk populations of primary fibroblasts expressing the *Drosophila* form of ChAT show variable levels of expression that typically range from 250 to 1000 nmol of acetylcholine per hour per milligram of protein (10).

In Vitro Histochemistry and Immunocytochemistry

The expression of the *lacZ* transgene within engineered fibroblasts can be detected by the histochemical demonstration of the B-Gal enzyme. Typically this is done on fibroblasts plated on two-, four-, or eight-well Lab-Tek chamber slides (Nunc, Inc.) to minimize the amount of reagent needed. Plastic slides are superior to glass because the cells adhere better during the culture and histochemical procedures. Cells are rinsed (all rinses with PBS), fixed in 4% paraformaldehyde in 0.1 *M* PBS for 30 min, and then rinsed twice more. The reaction solution is prepared from 40 μl of 0.5 *M* potassium ferrocyanide, 40 μl of 0.5 *M* potassium ferricyanide, 4 μl of 1.0 *M* $MgCl_2$, 40 μl of X-Gal stock [40 mg of 5-bromo-4-chloro-3-indoly-β-D-galactopyranoside (X-Gal; Sigma, St. Louis, MO) dissolved in 1 ml of DMSO] and 3.9 ml of PBS. The X-Gal stock solution should be stored in the dark at 4°C and may be used as long as it remains colorless. Cells are incubated in this solution for 6–18 hr at 37°C and then rinsed twice. Plastic slides cannot be run through a dehydration series of alcohols and xylene because they melt and bend, therefore, after removing the wells the slides are coverslipped with a PBS and 10% (v/v) glycerol mixture and sealed with nail polish.

Immunocytochemistry is used for the detection of a transgene product for which no histochemical reaction exists, such as TH. Cells expressing the transgene are plated onto plastic slides, rinsed twice with PBS, and fixed as described above. Fixed cells are rinsed twice with Tris-buffered saline (TBS) and then placed in a blocking solution containing 5% (v/v) normal horse serum and 0.3% (v/v) Triton X-100 in TBS for 1 hr (this solution is used to dilute all antibodies). A primary antibody (e.g., Boehringer Mannheim mouse anti-TH IgG used at a 1 : 200 dilution) is applied for an overnight incubation at room temperature. Control wells are incubated in solution without primary antibody to determine the specificity of the subsequent steps. There is a risk, however, of incubation medium leaking from one well to another on the slides because the wells are often not sealed adequately from each other. Accordingly, it is important to run controls lacking a component of the normal procedure on a separate slide. The next day, cells are rinsed three times for 10 min each with the blocking solution and then incubated in the appropriate secondary antibody (e.g., biotinylated horse anti-mouse IgG, 6 μl/ml; Vector Laboratories, Burlingame, CA) for 1 hr at room temperature. An avidin–biotin complex mixture is made 30 min before use (AB Elite, 9 μl of avidin plus 9 μl of biotin in 1 ml of TBS; Vector Laboratories), as the cells are rinsed three times in TBS for 10 min each. Cells are incubated in the AB Elite mixture for 1 hr and then rinsed three times in TBS for 5 min each. The antibody is visualized by reaction in a 0.025% (v/v) diaminobenzidine tetrahydrochloride (DAB) solution containing 0.5% (v/v) nickel chloride and 0.018% (v/v) hydrogen peroxide, and the reaction is stopped by rinsing the wells with TBS when cells contain visible reaction product. Depending on the level of expression exhibited by the cells, the DAB incubation may last as long as 10 min. In a typical confluent chamber well containing a bulk population of primary fibroblasts expressing TH from the retroviral LTR promoter, over 80% of the cells show positive TH immunoreactivity. Rinsed slides are coverslipped as described above.

In Vivo Characterizations of Engineered Cells

Septohippocampal System

Cells within the medial septal nucleus send projections, 50% of which are cholinergic (34), through the fimbria–fornix (FF) to the hippocampus to terminate immediately above and below the pyramidal cells of the regio inferior, in the hilus of the dentate gyrus, and in the supragranular region of the dentate gyrus (24). Lesions of the FF axotomize the cholinergic septohippocampal fibers and result in the degeneration, then death, of 50% of the cholinergic neurons in the medial septum. Further, there is a marked downregulation of cholinergic markers (acetylcholinesterase histochemistry, ChAT activity, and NGF receptor immunohistochemistry) in 25–30% of the surviving septal cholinergic cells following transection (8, 12, 16). The loss of acetylcholine (ACh) from the hippocampus that follows septal cholinergic deterioration has been associated with learning and memory deficits in animals and is considered to play a role in the cognitive deterioration that occurs in Alzheimer's disease (4, 6).

Selection of Transgene

The degeneration of septal cholinergic neurons and the concomitant loss of ACh from the hippocampus that occurs after FF lesions provide a model system to assess the ability of intracerebral grafts of genetically modified cells to intervene in the cholinergic changes. Cholinergic neurons within the septum may be rescued after axotomy by the exogenous provision of NGF to replace the endogenous NGF previously transported from the hippocampus (12, 16, 23). Thus, one method for intervening in the cholinergic changes following axotomy is to use genetically modified cells that have been engineered to produce NGF as a localized source of the trophic factor for damaged septal neurons. Alternatively, loss of ACh within the hippocampus may be reversed by implanting cells engineered to produce ACh directly into regions of cholinergic denervation. Techniques for assessing the effectiveness of genetically modified cells in both of these strategies are discussed in the following section. For the representative methods discussed, retroviral vectors were constructed as described above (see Gene Transfer, above) with the cDNA for either mouse β-NGF or *Drosophila* ChAT inserted under the control of the 5′ LTR promoter. An internal Rous sarcoma virus (RSV) promoter is used to drive the expression of a neomycin-resistance gene. Transgene expression is verified *in vitro* as described above prior to implanting the cells into the brain.

Septohippocampal System: Neurotrophic Factor Delivery

Preparation of Collagen-Embedded Fibroblast Grafts (Plugs)

Nerve growth factor-producing fibroblasts embedded in a collagen matrix may serve both as a source of trophic factor, to promote survival of septal cholinergic axons axotomized by the FF lesion, and as a bridging material providing a substrate for regrowth of regenerating cholinergic axons. Genetically modified fibroblasts are generated and maintained as described above and prepared for implantation as collagen matrix bridging grafts as follows. Confluent, low-passage fibroblasts are washed with PBS and detached with trypsin, and the number of cells is determined with a hemacytometer. To embed fibroblasts within a collagen matrix, 2.5 million cells are suspended in 3.5 ml of DMEM and then mixed with 1.75 ml of 0.15% (w/v) type 1 collagen in 0.1 *M* acetic acid. Sodium hydroxide (0.1 ml) is added to neutralize the pH, and the plugs are allowed to set overnight at 37°C. Before surgery, medium samples are taken from the collagen gels containing transfected fibroblasts so that levels of transgene production can be tested using an ELISA as described above.

Fimbria–Fornix Lesion and Implantation of Fibroblast Plugs

Adult female Fischer 344 rats (200–250 g), housed in standard laboratory cages, are used. For grafting, rats are anesthetized as described above; the heads of the rats are shaved and cleansed with Betadine and the animals are placed in a Kopf stereotaxic frame. A hole is drilled immediately lateral and caudal of bregma and a unilateral aspiration lesion through the overlying cingulate cortex into the right FF pathway is performed under a dissecting microscope. We utilize an aspirative lesion rather than a knife cut of the FF so that a cavity will be produced into which the bridging matrix can be placed. In rats receiving a FF lesion bridging graft containing NGF-producing or control fibroblasts, a 1 × 2 mm piece of the fibroblast-embedded collagen plug is placed in the lesion cavity and held in place with Gelfoam. Additional rats receive only FF lesions or no treatment. Following grafting, the wound is dusted with antibiotic powder and closed with wound clips, and the rats are returned to cages that do not contain nonanesthetized animals. The rats are monitored closely for 1 week after surgery, then periodically through the course of the experiment.

Histological Processing

Rats are deeply anesthetized and perfused through the heart with cold saline followed by 4% (w/v) paraformaldehyde in 0.1 *M* phosphate buffer. Brains are postfixed overnight in the fixative and then placed in 30% (w/v) sucrose until saturated. The brains are cut in 40-μm sections on a freezing sliding microtome and collected into a cryoprotectant (glycerol–ethylene glycol–phosphate buffer) for storage at −20°C until processed. The choice of orientation for the brain sectioning depends on the view desired. Bilateral examination of the medial septum in a single section, which facilitates septal cell counting, is obtained with horizontal or coronal sections. Views showing the hippocampus and adjacent graft in the same section are best obtained with horizontal or sagittal sections.

Every sixth tissue section is processed for Nissl staining, using 0.5% (v/v) aqueous thionin and the next one-in-six series is reacted for acetylcholinesterase (AChE), using the method of Hedreen *et al.* (15). The remaining tissue sections are reacted for immunohistochemical detection of an antigen of interest. The procedure used is the same as described for *in vitro* immunocytochemistry, except that free-floating sections are incubated in 0.6% (v/v) hydrogen peroxide in TBS for 30 min before blocking. The primary antibodies typically used are mouse anti-NGF receptor (NGFr) IgG at 1 : 100 (3), Promega (Madison, WI) mouse anti-B-Gal IgG at 1 : 5000, or Boehringer Mannheim mouse anti-TH IgG at 1 : 200. The sections are mounted on gelatin-coated slides, allowed to dry overnight, dehydrated in a series of alcohols from 50 to 100%, cleared in xylene, and then coverslipped with Permount.

Examination of bridging grafts containing NGF-producing fibroblasts typically reveals a dense plexus of axons stained histochemically for AChE, whereas control grafts of B-Gal fibroblasts lack such staining (Fig. 2). In addition to reaching the NGF graft, regenerating AChE-positive septal axons are able to reinnervate the hippocampus, a phenomenon not observed in animals implanted with B-Gal-expressing fibrobasts.

Quantitation of Septal Cell Survival

Sections containing the medial septum that have been immunostained for either NGFr or ChAT can be used for quantitation of cholinergic cell number. The use of horizontal or coronal sections permits a clear distinction between septal cells ipsilateral and contralateral to the unilateral FF lesion. A portion of the medial septum is examined with $\times 10$ magnification and a 0.5×0.5 mm grid overlay. All immunoreactive cell bodies within the grid field are counted, and the process is repeated until the entire septal region in the tissue section is sampled. Approximately five tissue sections through the medial septum are similarly examined. Cell survival on the experimental side can then be expressed as a percentage of cells on the intact contralateral side. In a representative experiment, 62% of medial septal cells survived when an NGF-producing fibroblast graft was placed in the FF lesion cavity,

FIG. 2 Representative examples of bridging grafts containing NGF-producing (A) or control B-Gal (B) fibroblasts embedded within a collagen matrix and placed into a fimbria–fornix lesion cavity of an adult rat. Acetylcholinesterase staining reveals a dense cholinergic innervation of the NGF-producing grafts (A) and the extension of these processes into the adjacent hippocampus. In contrast, the B-Gal grafts are devoid of these features (B). Bar: 500 μm.

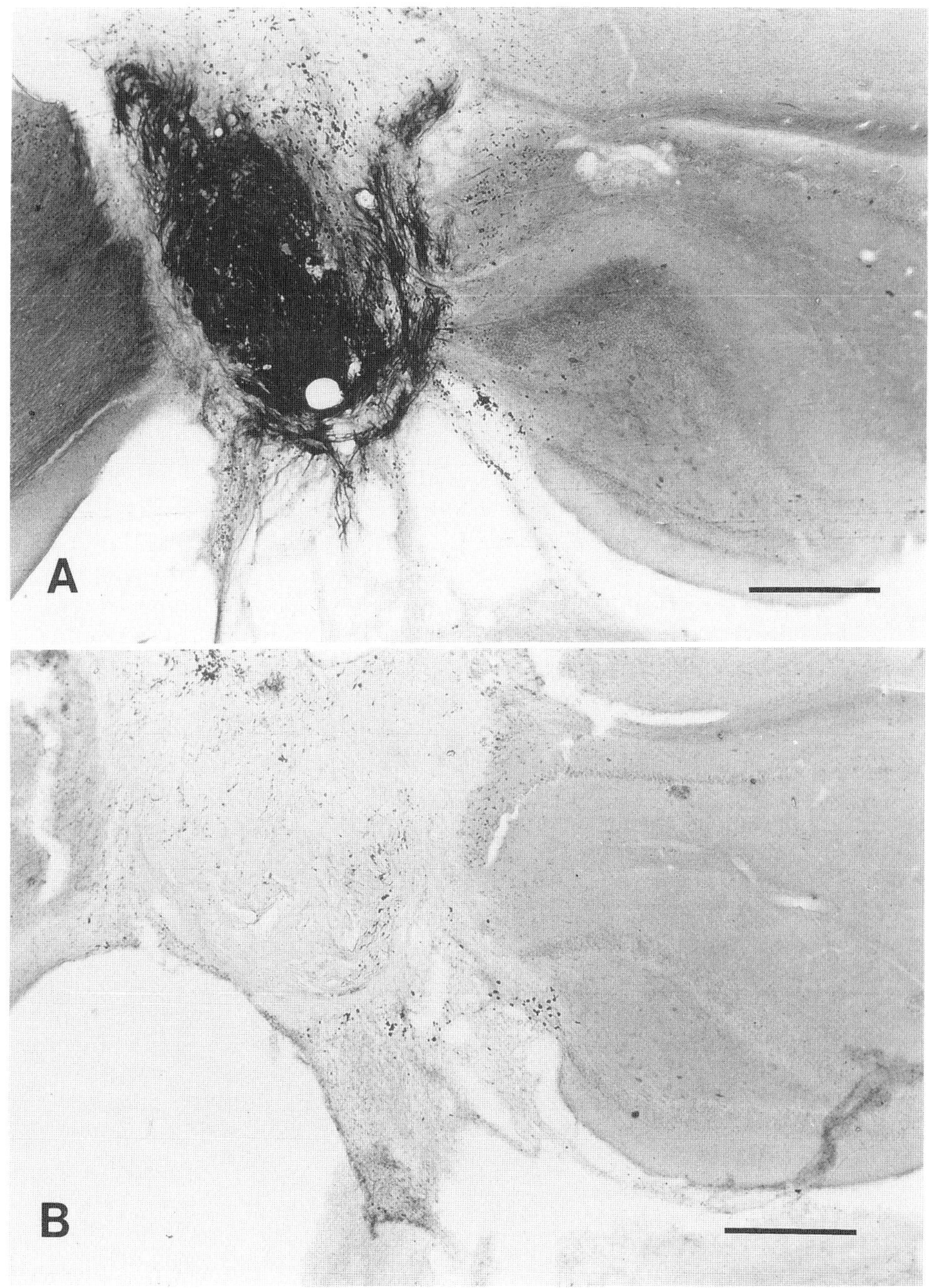
A
B

whereas only 47% survived when a B-Gal graft was similarly placed (22). Notably, an even greater saving of axotomized septal cells (75%) is achieved when a suspension graft of primary fibroblasts producing NGF is placed directly into the medial septum following FF lesion (22). Whereas increased cell savings are realized with more localized delivery of NGF to injured septal neurons, suspension grafts do not provide a physical substrate within the lesion cavity for regenerating axons. These combined results indicate that NGF-producing fibroblasts implanted into the brain continue to synthesize and release functionally active NGF that is able to support the survival of axotomized septal cholinergic neurons.

Septohippocampal System: Neurotransmitter Delivery

In Vivo Microdialysis

In addition to the use of engineered cells to deliver trophic factors to the CNS, genetically modified cells may be used to achieve site-specific supplementation of neurotransmitter levels within the brain. For this strategy, the technique of *in vivo* microdialysis provides a powerful method for assessing the extent to which genetically modified cells can continue to synthesize and release a neurotransmitter *in vivo*. The microdialysis method not only provides an on-line characterization of the functioning of the engineered cells within the brain, but also provides a localized route (through the indwelling probe) for manipulating the activity of the transgene in the grafted cells. The protocol is described for rats that have been implanted with ACh-producing fibroblasts in the septohippocampal system and should be modified as appropriate for the brain region of interest. The dialysis is performed one or more weeks after the implantation of fibroblasts into an aspiration cavity or into at least two adjacent sites in the hippocampus (AP, −3.0 mm; ML, 3.0 mm; DV, −3.5 mm; AP, −3.5 mm; ML, 3.0 mm; DV, −3.5 mm; incisor bar at +5 mm). For acute preparations, grafted rats are anesthetized and placed into a stereotaxic frame (incisor bar at +5 mm). The skull is exposed and a hole for the dialysis probe is drilled within 1 mm of the graft site(s). The dura is carefully removed and the cortical surface is rinsed with saline. A microdialysis probe (CMA/10; Bioanalytical Systems, West Lafayette, IN) with a 2- to 4-mm length membrane (depending on the vertical extension of the graft) is attached to a 1-ml Hamilton syringe filled with an artificial cerebrospinal fluid (CSF) solution (147 m*M* NaCl, 2.5 m*M* KCl, and 1.3 m*M* $CaCl_2$; pH 6.8) containing 15 μM neostigmine bromide. The high quantity of the AChE inhibitor in the CSF solution is included to improve resolution for detecting ACh release from the fibroblasts; lower amounts of neostigmine (1–10 μM) are more appropriate for measuring ACh overflow from neurons

(25). The pump is set to a flow rate of 1.5 μl/min and the probe is slowly lowered into the hippocampus to a depth of 4.0 mm. Samples are collected every 20–30 min for 90 min while the probe stabilizes. After the final sample collection, the infusion medium may be supplemented with additional compounds to determine if transgene activity can be modulated *in vivo*. For example, we have infused solutions containing 200 μ*M* choline chloride through indwelling probes positioned adjacent to the fibroblasts engineered to produce ACh (10). The new medium is perfused through the probe for at least 30 min and then thoroughly rinsed from the probe and tubing with the original CSF solution. Three or more 20-min samples are collected after the postcholine rinse. All dialysis samples are collected into Eppendorf tubes on ice and then transferred to a −70°C freezer until assessed by high-peformance liquid chromatography (HPLC, ESA, Inc., Bedford, MA) with electrochemical detection. Rats are kept on heating pads throughout the procedure and supplemented as necessary with anesthetic. The recovery rate of the microdialysis probes is always assessed *in vitro* prior to use and has been found to average 18% for the CMA/10 probes (from a 1 μ*M* solution of acetylcholine). Fibroblasts expressing the *Drosophila* form of ChAT have been found to produce an average of 20 pmol of ACh/30-μl sample *in vivo* (2 weeks postgrafting), which is readily discernible from the levels of ACh typically found within the intact (5 pmol/30-μl sample) or denervated (≤1 pmol/30-μl sample) hippocampus (10).

Nigrostriatal System

The striatum receives a dense innervation of dopaminergic fibers from the pigmented neurons within the substantia nigra pars compacta. In turn, the striatum sends projections containing the neurotransmitter γ-aminobutyric acid (GABA) back to the substantia nigra. This looped pathway is involved in normal sensory-motor functioning, as evidenced by the severe motor dysfunction that emerges in humans during the neurodegenerative deterioration of the substantia nigra (Parkinson's disease) or of the striatum (Huntington's disease). The loss of dopamine in the striatum that occurs in Parkinson's disease can be mimicked in the rat brain by destroying catecholamine neurons in the substantia nigra with 6-hydroxydopamine (6-OHDA). If this lesion is confined to one side of the brain, a distinctive set of behaviors linked to the dopamine depletion is induced (32, 33). Some of these behaviors can be reversed by supplying a localized source of dopamine within the striatum (2, 27) and thus the 6-OHDA-treated rat can be used as a "behavioral" assay to assess the success to which the genetically modified fibroblasts can effectively deliver and/or replace a neurotransmitter (dopamine) in the brain.

Selection of Transgene

The transgenes that are most appropriate for the dopamine-depleted rat model system are TH, the enzyme that converts tyrosine to L-dopa, and L-aromatic amino acid decarboxylase (AADC), the enzyme that converts L-dopa to the neurotransmitter dopamine. To date, most studies that have assessed the use of engineered cells as a method for delivering neurotransmitters to the brain have focused on the development of cells that express various forms of TH (9, 17, 18, 31, 35). Primary fibroblasts expressing TH must rely on the presence of endogenous cofactor (biopterin) and AADC within the brain to replace dopamine levels effectively. For our work, TH is inserted into a retroviral vector (as specified above) under the control of the 5′ LTR promoter and the neomycin resistance gene is placed downstream from an internal RSV promoter. Production of TH protein within the engineered fibroblasts is verified *in vitro* prior to implantation.

6-OHDA Lesion

Fischer 344 rats are anesthetized and placed in a stereotaxic frame (incisor bar at −3.3 mm). The skull is exposed and a small burr hole is drilled over the region of the medial forebrain bundle (AP, −4.4 mm; ML, 1.1 mm from bregma). The 6-OHDA (Sigma) is dissolved in saline supplemented with 0.1% (w/v) ascorbic acid at a concentration of 6 μg/μl. Because the 6-OHDA oxidizes readily in solution even in the presence of ascorbate, we typically weigh out a small quantity of the 6-OHDA into a clear Eppendorf tube and keep the powder on ice until it is suspended into solution immediately prior to use. The 6-OHDA is viable as long as it remains colorless. The solution is discarded as soon as there is any hint of a pink color change. Using a 5-μl Hamilton syringe with a 24-gauge (or smaller) needle, 1 μl of 6-OHDA solution is delivered at a depth of 7.3 mm below the dura and a second 1-μl deposit is made at 7.1 mm (injection speed, 1 μl/min). The syringe is raised 2 mm after the dorsal injection and left in place for at least 2 min to prevent the toxin from traveling up the needle track. The needle is then removed and the skin is sutured with metal wound clips.

Behavioral Testing of 6-OHDA-Treated Rats

Rats with good lesions display a marked asymmetric posture and walking pattern on waking from the 6-OHDA surgery. Although this spontaneous behavior will disappear within a few days, the circular walking pattern ("rotational behavior") can be reinstated by administering catecholamine drugs to the rats: amphetamine [5 mg/kg, subcutaneous (sc)] induces dopamine release from nigrostriatal fibers on the intact side of the brain and causes the rat to rotate toward (ipsilateral to) the side of the lesion, whereas apomorphine (0.1 mg/kg, sc) is a dopamine receptor agonist that stimulates upregulated dopamine receptors on the lesion side and causes the rat to rotate away from (contralateral to) the side of the lesion (32,33). Rats are allowed to recover for at least 1 week postsurgery to allow the system to stabilize prior to testing. The rotational testing is conducted using an automated system (San Diego Instruments, San Diego, CA), although the number of turns can also be manually counted by watching the rats. Drug-induced rotations are collected onto a Macintosh computer every 10 min for a 60-min period. Rats that display $\geq$7 net ipsilateral rotations/min to amphetamine over a 90-min period have been shown to have a greater than 95% loss of dopamine within the striatum (29). For apomorphine testing, we have found that Fischer 344 rats that display $\geq$4 rotations/min have virtually no TH immunoreactivity within the striatum on the lesion side. The drug testing is kept to a minimum because repeated exposure to catecholamine agonists increases the rotational behavior of the rats. Typically, we screen the rats only once with apomorphine to select those with good lesions and then test the rats with apomorphine every 2 weeks after fibroblasts are implanted into the brain. Behavioral testing with rats implanted with engineered cells is usually conducted for an 8-week period, after which the rats are sacrificed and the brains are histologically processed as described above.

Preparation of Fibroblast Suspensions

Fibroblasts are removed from tissue culture plates with trypsin and washed several times in PBS. An aliquot of the suspension is counted using a Coulter (Hialeah, FL) counter and the cells are centrifuged to remove the PBS. The fibroblasts are then resuspended in PBS supplemented with 1 μg of $MgCl_2$, 1 μg of $CaCl_2$, and 0.1% (w/v) glucose at a concentration of 5×10^4–1×10^5 cells/μl and kept at room temperature during the grafting procedure. Suspensions are used for approximately 2 hr and then a fresh batch is prepared if the grafting is not completed. Cell viability, as assessed with trypan blue exclusion, should remain at $\geq$80% throughout the procedure for optimal graft survival.

Grafting of Fibroblast Suspensions

The behaviorally characterized 6-OHDA-treated rats are anesthetized and placed in a stereotaxic frame. The skull is reexposed and two new burr holes are drilled over the striatum (AP, 0.2 mm; ML, 2.2 mm; and AP, 1.2 mm; ML, 2.0 mm from bregma; toothbar set at -3.3 mm). The rats are separated into at least two groups, with the experimental group receiving grafts of TH-expressing cells and the control group receiving implants of B-Gal-expressing fibroblasts (a third, nongrafted group is often included). The fibroblasts are injected into the brain using a 5-μl Hamilton syringe equipped with a 26-gauge (or smaller) beveled needle. Avoid the use of syringes that have plungers that extend through the length of the needle because the plungers may cause a disruptive shearing of the cells during injection and because the coating on the plungers has been observed to shed into the cell suspension and deposit in the grafts. The suspension is gently thumped a few times immediately prior to drawing the cells up into the syringe to distribute the fibroblasts evenly and reduce clumping. To minimize damage to the cells and avoid air bubbles in the suspension, the cells are slowly drawn into the syringe once. If air bubbles are evident in the suspension, the cells are gently ejected back into the Eppendorf and the air is removed by rinsing the syringe with saline and/or alcohol. Bubbles are never removed by repeated trituration of the suspension with the Hamilton syringe. At each of the two sites, a total of 1.5 μl of the suspension is injected in a series of three 0.5-μl deposits over a 1-mm span (DV: 4.5, 4.0, and 3.5 mm below the dura). The cells are injected at a rate of 1 μl/min, with a 1-min wait between each of the 0.5-μl deposits. After the most dorsal injection, the syringe is raised 1 mm and left in place for at least 2 min before the needle is slowly withdrawn from the brain and the skin is sutured closed with metal wound clips. Rats are returned to home cages and allowed to recover for at least 2 weeks before behavioral testing (described above) is initiated. However, active functioning of the implanted TH fibroblasts is indicated earlier by observing spontaneous contralateral rotational behavior of the rats immediately on waking from the surgery.

Histological Processing

Coronal sections through suspension grafts generally reveal elongated grafts with fibroblasts scattered throughout the implanted tissue (Fig. 3A). If the grafts are viewed periodically over an extended survival period, it is common to observe a reduction in both fibroblast number and graft volume through the first month after the cells are implanted into the brain. Thereafter, cell survival and volume usually stabilize and remain constant for periods of at least 6 months (21). Enhancing early fibroblast survival within the brain is achieved by varying the density of cells in the suspension (kept $\leq 10^5/\mu l$) and/or the total number of cells injected (kept $\leq$150,000 cells/site). Cell-free regions within the grafts are typical and primarily consist of collagen, a product that is normally secreted by, and supports the survival of, fibroblasts.

Immunohistochemical staining of the graft demonstrates active transgene expression within the implanted cells (Fig. 3B and C). It is typical for the cells to show variable levels of staining *in vivo,* a pattern that reflects the different intensities of labeling that characterize a bulk-infected population of cells *in vitro*. With increased time after grafting, there is often a decrease in the number of cells that show strong labeling of the transgene product.

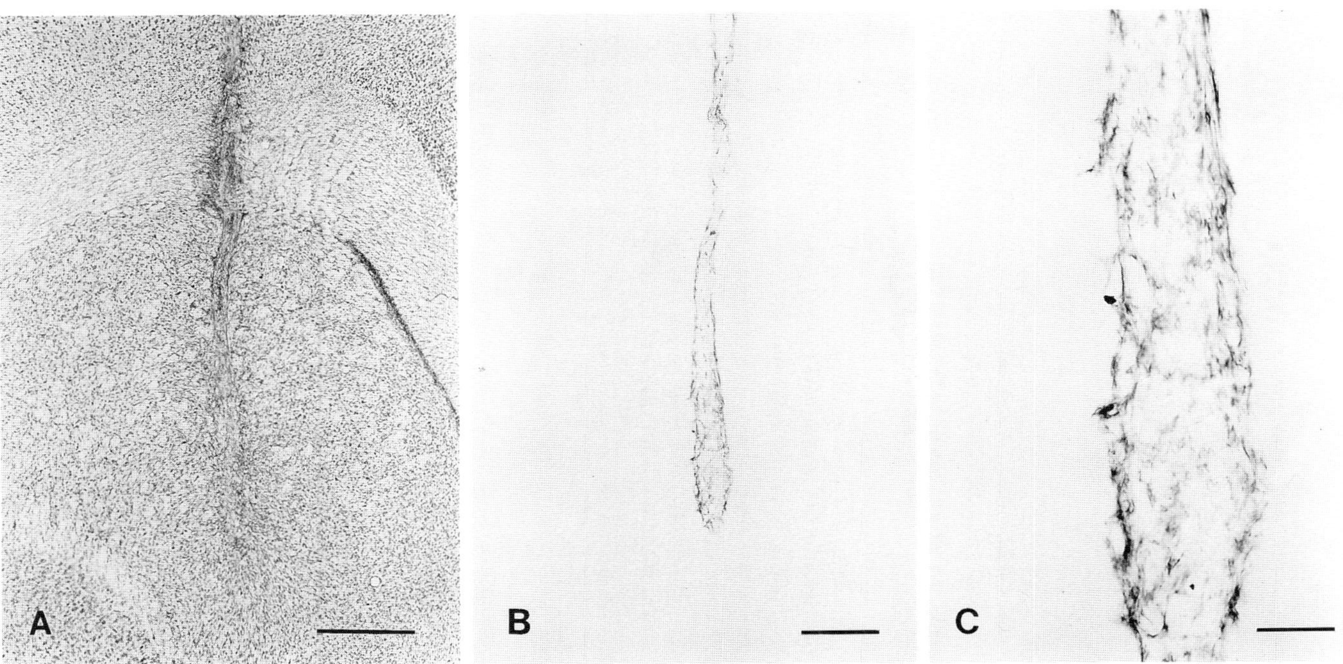

FIG. 3 Representative example of a suspension graft of primary fibroblasts expressing a B-Gal transgene placed into the 6-OHDA-treated striatum of rats. Surviving fibroblasts, demonstrated by thionin staining (A), are scattered throughout the grafts. Immunohistochemical labeling of the grafts reveals strong expression of the B-Gal transgene within the grafted cells (B). Higher power view of the B-Gal-labeled graft shown in (B) reveals the different intensities of cellular labeling that is typical of bulk-infected populations of cells (C). Bars: (A and B) 500 μm; (C) 100 μm.

Some of the changes in staining patterns that occur postimplantation reflect cell loss. In addition, however, it also appears that the retroviral promoters are subjected to regulatory influences within the host system (26, 28). Our approaches for increasing the stability of transgene expression within primary cells involve constructing alternative vector systems that allow the transgenes to be intentionally regulated with exogenous factors and/or to be preferentially influenced by cell-specific factors.

Summary

Work with genetically modified cells has demonstrated that engineered cells provide an effective vehicle for delivering both neurotrophic factors and neurotransmitters to the CNS. Although several types of cells have been used to transport engineered products into the brain, the use of primary cells for gene transfer and grafting generally assures that the cells will survive noninvasively for prolonged periods within the CNS. The particular advantage of using fibroblasts in this strategy is the ability to exploit the potent secretory nature of the cells to achieve a biological minipump administration of the compound of interest. The continued development of the gene transfer/grafting technique will lead to the increased use of this strategy for exploring the development, function, and repair of the CNS.

Acknowledgments

We would like to thank K. L. Eagle for providing the AChE-labeled sections and M. L. Gage for help in the preparation of the manuscript. Some of the work described was supported by grants from the NIH (AG10435) and the Broad Foundation.

References

1. K. Bayreuther, P. I. Francz, J. Gogol, C. Hapke, M. Maier, and H.-G. Meinrath, *Mutat. Res.* **256,** 233 (1991).
2. A. Björklund and U. Stenevi, *Brain Res.* **177,** 555 (1979).
3. C. E. Chandler, L. M. Parsons, M. Hosang, and E. M. Shooter, *J. Biol. Chem.* **259,** 6882 (1984).
4. J. T. Coyle, D. L. Price, and M. R. DeLong, *Science* **219,** 1184 (1983).
5. L. A. Cunningham, J. T. Hansen, M. P. Short, and M. C. Bohn, *Brain Res.* **561,** 192 (1991).
6. P. Davies and A. J. F. Maloney, *Lancet* **2,** 1403 (1976).
7. M. A. Eglitis and W. F. Anderson, *BioTechniques* **6,** 608 (1988).

8. W. Fischer and A. Björklund, *Exp. Neurol.* **113,** 93 (1991).
9. L. J. Fisher, H. A. Jinnah, L. C. Kale, G. A. Higgins, and F. H. Gage, *Neuron* **6,** 371 (1991).
10. L. J. Fisher, M. Schinstine, P. Salvaterra, A. J. Dekker, L. Thal, and F. H. Gage. *J. Neurochem.* **61,** 1323 (1993).
11. F. Fonnum, *J. Neurochem.* **24,** 407 (1975).
12. F. H. Gage, D. M. Armstrong, L. R. Williams, and S. Varon, *J. Comp. Neurol.* **269,**147 (1988).
13. F. H. Gage, M. D. Kawaja, and L. J. Fisher, *Trends Neurosci.* **8,** 328 (1991).
14. F. H. Gage, J. A. Wolff, M. B. Rosenberg, L. Xu, J. E. Yee, C. Shults, and T. Friedmann, *Neuroscience* **23,** 795 (1987).
15. J. C. Hedreen, S. J. Bacon, and D. L. Price, *J. Histochem. Cytochem.* **33,** 134 (1985).
16. F. Hefti, *J. Neurosci.* **6,** 2155 (1986).
17. P. Horellou, L. Marlier, A. Privat, and J. Mallet, *Eur. J. Neurosci.* **2,** 116 (1990).
18. S. Jiao, V. Gurevich, and J. A. Wolff, *Nature (London)* **362,** 450 (1993).
19. M. D. Kawaja, L. J. Fisher, M. Schinstine, H. A. Jinnah, J. Ray, L. S. Chen, and F. H. Gage, *in* "Neural Transplantation: A Practical Approach" (S. B. Dunnett and A. Björklund, eds.), p. 21. Oxford Univ. Press, Oxford, 1992.
20. M. D. Kawaja and F. H. Gage, *Neuron* **7,** 1019 (1991).
21. M. D. Kawaja and F. H. Gage, *J. Comp. Neurol.* **317,** 102 (1992).
22. M. D. Kawaja, M. B. Rosenberg, K. Yoshida, and F. H. Gage, *J. Neurosci.* **12,** 2849 (1992).
23. L. F. Kromer, *Science* **235,** 214 (1987).
24. S. Mosko, G. Lynch, and C. W. Cotman, *J. Comp. Neurol.* **152,** 163 (1973).
25. O. G. Nilsson, P. Kalen, E. Rosenberg, and A. Björklund, *Neuroscience* **36,** 325 (1990).
26. T. D. Palmer, G. J. Rosman, W. R. A. Osborne, and A. D. Miller, *Proc. Natl. Acad. Sci. U.S.A.* **88,** 1330 (1991).
27. M. J. Perlow, W. J. Freed, B. J. Hoffer, A. Seiger, L. Olson, and R. J. Wyatt, *Science* **204,** 643 (1979).
28. M. Schinstine, M. B. Rosenberg, C. Routledge-Ward, T. Friedmann, and F. H. Gage, *J. Neurochem.* **58,** 2019 (1992).
29. R. H. Schmidt, M. Ingvar, O. Lindvall, U. Stenevi, and A. Björklund, *J. Neurochem.* **38,** 737 (1982).
30. W. S. Sly and J. Grubb, *in* "Methods in Enzymology" (W. Jakoby and I. Pastan, eds.), vol. 58, p. 444. Academic Press, New York, 1979.
31. K. Uchida, K. Takamatsu, N. Kaneda, S. Toya, Y. Tsukada, Y. Kurosawa, K. Fujita, T. Nagatsu, and S. Kohsaka, *J. Neurochem.* **53,** 728 (1989).
32. U. Ungerstedt, *Acta Physiol. Scand., Suppl.* **367,** 49 (1971).
33. U. Ungerstedt, *Acta Physiol. Scand., Suppl.* **367,** 69 (1971).
34. B. H. Wainer, A. I. Levey, D. B. Rye, M. M. Mesulam, and E. J. Mufson, *Neurosci. Lett.* **54,** 45 (1985).
35. J. A. Wolff, L. J. Fisher, L. Xu, H. A. Jinnah, P. J. Langlais, P. M. Iuvone, K. L. O'Malley, M. B. Rosenberg, S. Shimohama, T. Friedmann, and F. H. Gage, *Proc. Natl. Acad. Sci. U.S.A.* **86,** 9011 (1989).

[21] Neuropeptide and Catecholamine Delivery to Central Nervous System by Implanted Chromaffin Cells

Jacqueline Sagen, John D. Ortega, and George D. Pappas

Introduction

The potential for neural transplants to serve as a means for restoring deficits resulting from injury or disease in the central nervous system (CNS) has been a subject of intense research for the past several years (cf. 1, 2). Much of this work has been focused on the ability of these transplants to function in a restorative capacity for the repair or replacement of damaged neuronal circuitries. It is possible that the full restoration of neural function will depend on the ability of such transplants to reproduce appropriate synaptic connections, and requires a specific pattern of host–graft integration. However, an alternative, and less demanding, role for neural grafts is that of providing a source of neuroactive agents to local regions of the CNS. This approach would be particularly useful in the restoration of neurochemical deficits or as an adjunct to traditional pharmacotherapies, and would not necessarily depend on extensive host–graft integration. In other words, cells transplanted to the CNS can act as living "pumps," providing a continually renewable source of needed neuroactive substances, and reducing the need for repeated exogenous administration of pharmacologic agents. In addition to providing a living, renewable source of pharmacological agents, this approach allows for the use of naturally derived neuroactive substances whose biological half-lives are too short to be delivered by any other means.

Work in our laboratory over the past several years has suggested at least two potential applications that are amenable to the use of transplanted cells as delivery agents for neuroactive substances: chronic pain (3–6) and depression (7–9). For these studies, adrenal medullary chromaffin cells have proved useful as graft sources, as they synthesize and secrete high levels of catecholamines as well as several pharmacologically active neuropeptides (10–13). When transplanted into the spinal subarachnoid space or the midbrain periaqueductal gray, these cells can provide a therapeutic source of opioid peptides and catecholamines for the reduction of pain (14). In addition, the development of tolerance to agents released from the transplanted cells is apparently limited (15), probably due to the synergistic coactivation of opioid

Methods in Neurosciences, Volume 21

and α-adrenergic receptors with low levels of exposure to subeffective levels of both families of agonists (16–19). Chromaffin cell transplants in the frontal neocortex can also be effective in alleviating behavioral deficits indicative of depression, most likely by providing a source of catecholamines for the restoration of monoaminergic imbalances (7–9, 20).

For the purpose of providing local CNS access to catecholamines and neuropeptides for therapeutic application, both allogeneic (between individuals of the same species) and xenogeneic (between donor and host of different species) sources have been used. Allogeneic sources are particularly important as this mimicks the most likely scenario for initial clinical application. In fact, preliminary clinical trials for alleviation of chronic pain in terminal cancer patients utilized adrenal medullary tissue from human organ donors (21). However, although human adrenal medullary allografts are the most likely sources for initial clinical studies, their limited availability and nonuniformity reduce their feasibility for widespread use. Xenogeneic donors are a potential alternative, and largely untapped, source of chromaffin cells for transplantation. For example, bovine adrenal glands are readily available, and large quantities of a relatively pure population of chromaffin cells can be easily isolated (22–24). This chapter describes the preparation and use of both adrenal medullary allografts and xenografts as an implantable local delivery source of catecholamines and opioid peptides to the CNS.

Graft Preparations

Adrenal Medullary Allografts

Allogeneic tissue for transplantation is obtained from adult rats (Sprague-Dawley; Sasco, Inc., Madison, WI). Donors are killed by cervical dislocation, and their adrenal glands removed aseptically and placed in ice-cold Hanks' buffer for dissection procedures. Adrenal cortical tissue is carefully removed from medullary tissue under a dissecting microscope and discarded. The medullary tissue is then cut into small pieces (0.5–1.0 mm^3 for spinal subarachnoid implantation or 0.25–0.5 mm^3 for intraparenchymal implantation) and kept in cold Hanks' buffer until transplanted (within 30 min).

Chromaffin Cell Xenografts

Bovine chromaffin cells are isolated as described by Ortega *et al.* (23). Bovine adrenal glands are purchased from a local abbatoir, trimmed of their fat, and immediately perfused with Ca^{2+}- and Mg^{2+}-free Locke's solution [1.5 *M*

NaCl, 0.05 *M* KCl, 0.04 *M* $NaHCO_3$, 0.06 *M* glucose, 0.05 *M* *N*-2-hydroxyethylpiperazine-*N*′-2-ethanesulfonic acid (HEPES) at pH 7.2, 37°C] containing antibiotics [penicillin/streptomycin (100 U/ml), kanamycin (25 μg/ml)] and antifungal agents [Fungizone] (amphotericin B, 0.125 μg/ml)]. Following a 30-min incubation in Locke's solution, the glands are perfused with a 0.1% collagenase solution [Boehringer Mannheim, Indianapolis, IN): 0.05% (w/v) bovine serum albumin (BSA; Sigma, St. Louis, MO) and 0.01% (w/v) trypsin inhibitor (Sigma)] for 30 min. After this perfusion, the medullary tissue is dissected from the surrounding cortex, minced, filtered through a fine nylon mesh, and washed several times with Locke's solution before purifying the cell population with a Percoll gradient. The washed cells are placed on a self-generating, buoyant density gradient (45 ml of Percoll, 5 ml of 10× Locke's solution at pH 7.4) and spun at 12,000 rpm for 20 min in a refrigerated centrifuge (IEC B20, Needhamitts, MA, 4°C). The band containing healthy chromaffin cells, as defined by morphological analysis, is removed from the gradient, washed several times with Locke's solution, and plated on 100-mm tissue culture dishes in medium [Dulbecco's modified Eagle's medium (DMEM) and Ham's F-12 (1 : 1 DMEM : F12)] supplemented with 5% (v/v) fetal bovine serum (FBS), antibiotics (penicillin/streptomycin, 100 U/ml; gentamicin, 50 μg/ml), and antifungal agents (Fungizone, 0.125 μg/ml). The plates are placed in an incubator overnight (37°C, 5% CO_2) to allow for differential adherence of unwanted cell types such as fibroblasts and endothelial cells. The next day chromaffin cells are removed from their plates by gentle agitation, and once again placed on a Percoll gradient to further enhance the purity and viability of the final chromaffin cell population. Trypan blue exclusion generally places the viability of all chromaffin cell preparations in excess of 95%.

Spinal Subarachnoid Grafts

Implantation into Spinal Subarachnoid Space

Both adrenal medullary tissues and cell suspensions are implanted into the rat spinal subarachnoid space via laminectomy. All surgical procedures are performed using aseptic technique and adequate anesthesia [pentobarbital, 30 mg/kg, intraperitoneal (ip), supplemented as necessary). A 3- to 4-mm segment of the spinal cord at the level of the lumbar enlargement is exposed, and a small slit in the dura and arachnoid membranes made with a needle tip under a dissecting microscope. Solid adrenal medullary tissue pieces are introduced via the slit and gently pushed away from the opening with a stylet. In general, medullary tissue from two adrenal glands are transplanted, as this amount has been shown to reliably reduce pain in rodent pain models

(3, 6, 14, 25). Equal volumes of striated muscle tissue, heat-killed adrenal medullary tissue, or Gelfoam can be used as controls.

To implant bovine chromaffin cell suspension, chromaffin cells are removed from their plates following a 2-day stabilization period by gentle agitation and washed in Hanks' buffered salt solution. Chromaffin cells are introduced into the subarachnoid space by insertion of polyethylene tubing (PE-10) into the subarachnoid space 2–3 mm past an incision made in the dural membrane. Two microliters of the cell suspension (50,000 cells/μl) is generally injected, as this reliably reduces nociception in animal models (14, 26). After 2 min, the tubing is withdrawn slowly to prevent backflow of cells. Animals receiving xenografts are immunosuppressed [cyclosporin A (Sandoz, East Hanover, NJ), 10 mg/kg ip daily] beginning the day of implantation. Studies in our laboratory suggest that it may be possible to discontinue this immunosuppression after several weeks, allowing for repair of the blood–brain barrier (22). For controls, equal volumes of vehicle (Hanks' buffer) or lysed chromaffin cells can be used.

Following all intraspinal surgical procedures, the overlying muscle is sutured with 3-0 silk, and the skin closed with wound clips.

Analysis of Neuropeptide and Catecholamine Delivery into Spinal Subarachnoid Space

The ability of intraspinal implants of either adrenal medullary allografts or bovine chromaffin cell xenografts to reduce pain has been demonstrated by acute analgesiometric assays (25, 26), as well as models for chronic arthritic and neuropathic pain (3, 6). Indirect pharmacological evidence suggests that this analgesia is due, at least in part, to the corelease of opioid peptides and catecholamines from the implanted chromaffin cells, because it can be attenuated using either opioid or α-adrenergic antagonists. More direct evidence for the delivery of neuroactive agents to the host spinal cord comes from neurochemical assays of the spinal fluid of implanted animals. To collect spinal cerebrospinal fluid (CSF) from animals with adrenal medullary implants, a spinal cord superfusion technique can be used (4, 5). Animals are anesthetized with urethane (1200 mg/kg), fitted with a tracheal tube, and placed in a stereotaxic frame with the head angled downward. An intrathecal catheter made of PE-10 tubing is threaded down the intrathecal space via a small slit in the atlantooccipital membrane so that the caudal tip of the catheter lays at the lumbar enlargement where the transplant had previously been placed. The rostral end of the catheter is connected to the infusion end of a push-pull pump, and artificial CSF is infused at a constant rate of 0.1 ml/min. Outflow is collected via PE-50 tubing placed over the opening in the dura. This tubing is connected to the withdrawal syringe of the push-pull pump, with intervening collection tubes kept on ice. A three-way stopcock arrangement is used to allow outflow to be directed to one of two collection tubes sequentially without interruption of the flow of artificial CSF. Following a 30- to 45-min stabilization period to allow for stabilization, samples can be collected sequentially for at least 4 hr.

Samples collected in this fashion can be analyzed for release of neuroactive substances, using standard assay procedures. In addition, pharmacological responsiveness, for example, response to stimulation of chromaffin cell surface receptors by nicotine, can also be measured using this procedure.

Neuropeptide Assays

All samples for measurement of peptide content are collected in the presence of a protease inhibitor (bacitracin, 5 μg/ml) and BSA (1 mg/ml) to minimize nonspecific binding of peptides. Samples are lyophilized and frozen (-30°C) until assayed. As an example, Met-enkephalin levels can be determined using standard radioimmunoassay procedures. The ^{125}I-labeled peptide and the Met-enkephalin antisera are purchased commercially (Incstar, Stillwater, MN). This antibody has been shown to cross-react 2.8% with Leu-enkephalin, 0.1% with α-endorphin, and <0.002% with substance P, β-endorphin, dynorphin$_{1-13}$, and α-neoendorphin. Prior to assay, samples are reconstituted in 0.2 *N* HCl and extracted on Sep-Pak preparatory cartridges (Waters, Milford, MA) to remove salts. Peptides are eluted from the columns with 60% (v/v) acetonitrile in 0.1% (v/v) trifluoracetic acid, and lyophilized. Lyophilized samples are reconstituted in 100 μl of assay buffer [Na_2HPO_4 (0.067 g/ml), NaCl (0.04 g/ml), BSA (0.01%, w/v) at pH 7.4]. Equal volumes of tracer (10,000 cpm/100 μl) and antibody (1 : 6000 final dilution) are added, the tubes vortexed, and incubated overnight at 4°C. The next day, 500 μl of IgGSorb [10%, diluted 1 : 40; The Enzyme Center] is added to precipitate the previously added Met-enkephalin antibody. After a 15-min incubation period (25°C) the tubes are centrifuged [Centra-R (IEC), 15 min at 2500 rpm, 4°C], the supernatant decanted, and the remaining pellet measured for radioactive decay using a Micromedic Systems γ counter. Met-enkephalin concentrations are calculated from a standard curve generated from 3.5–250 pg of cold Met-enkephalin. The recovery of authentic Met-enkephalin is 95–100%, and the sensitivity limit of this assay is 0.5 pg.

An example of Met-enkephalin release from animals with either adrenal medullary allografts or control striated muscle transplants is shown in Fig. 1. The mean basal Met-enkephalin release in control animals was 7.6 $\pm$ 2.4 pg in 5 min (Fig. 1A). This level of release remained essentially stable throughout the experiment. The injection of nicotine [0.1 mg/kg, subcutane-

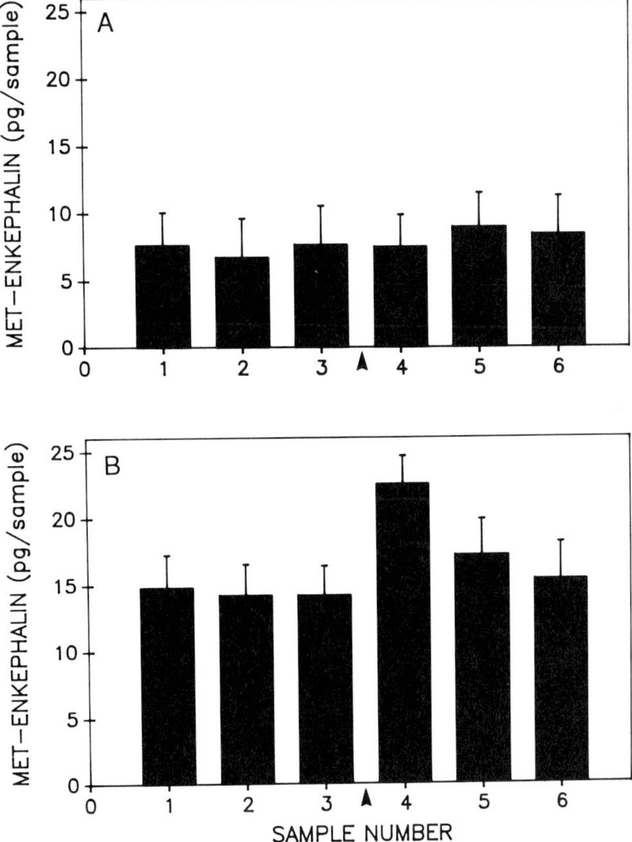

FIG. 1 Release of Met-enkephalin-like immunoreactivity into spinal cord superfusates in animals with (A) control striated muscle (n = 9 animals) or (B) adrenal medullary (n = 8 animals) transplants in the spinal cord subarachnoid space. Six 5-min CSF samples were collected: samples 1–3 to determine basal release, and samples 4–6 to determine release following the injection of nicotine (0.1 mg/kg, sc, at arrowhead). The ordinate is the mean ± SEM. Met-enkephalin levels per 5-min sample. [From Sagen and Kemmler (4).]

ous (sc)] following collection of the third sample did not alter the level of release in control animals. In animals with adrenal medullary implants, the basal levels of Met-enkephalin release were approximately doubled, to 14.8 ± 2.5 pg in 5 min (Fig. 1B). The injection of nicotine further increased the release of Met-enkephalin in these animals. When compared on an individual basis with changes in pain sensitivity, levels of Met-enkephalin release produced by the adrenal medullary transplants were found to be correlated with reductions in pain scores (Fig. 2).

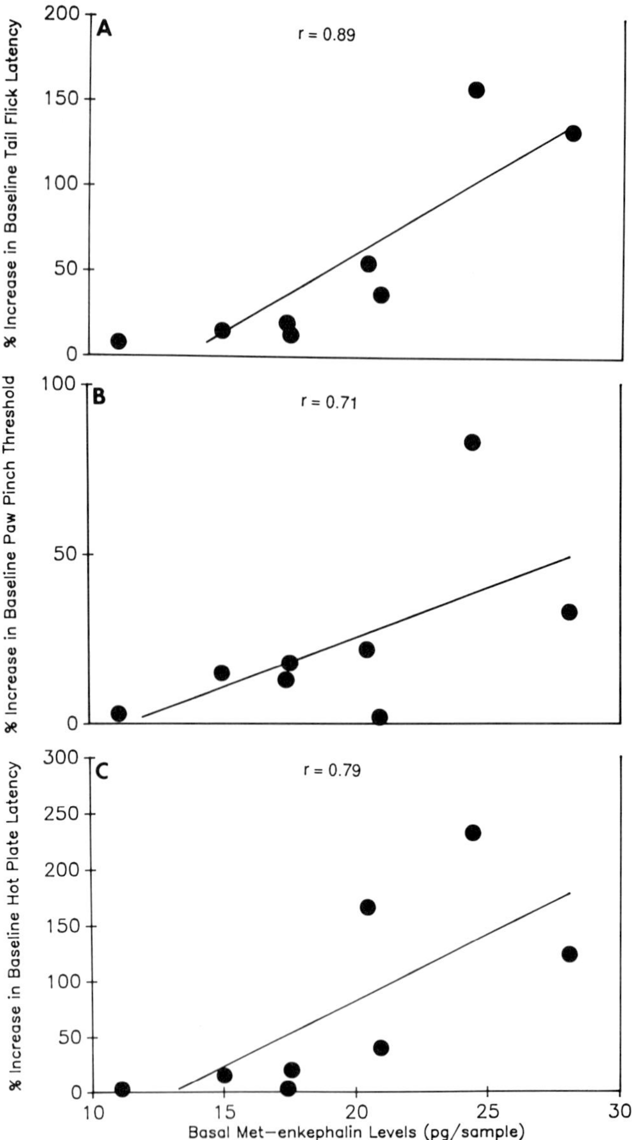

FIG. 2 Correlation between changes in baseline pain sensitivity following adrenal medullary implants in the spinal cord with basal levels of Met-enkephalin release. The ordinate indicates the percent increase in pain threshold from preimplantation levels following adrenal medullary implants as assessed by the tail flick (A), paw pinch (B), and hot plate (C) tests. The abscissa records the basal levels of Met-enkephalin release in 5-min superfusion samples from these animals. [From Sagen and Kemmler (4).]

Catecholamine Assays

All samples for catecholamine analysis are collected in tubes containing antioxidants [ethylenediaminetetraacetic acid (EDTA; 4 mg/ml), sodium *m*-bisulfite (0.5 mg/ml), and L-cysteine (2.5 mg/ml)]. Norepinephrine (NE), epinephrine (E), and dopamine (DA) levels are determined using modified alumina extraction and high-performance liquid chromatography (HPLC) (27, 28). Samples are incubated in 0.4 *N* perchloric acid, added to 20 mg of acid-washed alumina, and following pH adjustment to 8.6 they are vortexed, centrifuged, and the supernatant aspirated. Standards containing authentic amines are processed along with CSF samples. After three washes with distilled water, the amines are eluted from the alumina with 0.1 *N* perchloric acid. Catecholamines are quantitated by reversed phase HPLC and electrochemical detection over a 15-cm Waters Resolve C_{18} μBondapak column at a flow rate of 1.0 ml/min. The mobile phase contains 0.07 *M* Na_2HPO_4, 0.2 m*M* octyl sodium sulfate, 0.1 m*M* EDTA, and 2% (v/v) methanol at a pH of 4.8. The electrochemical detector is set at +0.6 mV versus an Ag-AgCl reference electrode. All sample concentrations are calculated using a Waters Baseline 810 system by comparison of relative peak areas with generated standard curves. Calculated concentrations are corrected for recovery, which is generally 75–85%. The lower detection limits for this assay are 5–10 pg.

Examples of catecholamine release in the CSF of animals with adrenal medullary transplants are shown in Fig. 3. Basal catecholamine levels shown are averages of three 5-min basal release samples. The mean basal norepinephrine level released into the CSF of control rats was 101.8 ± 13.8 pg in 5 min, whereas both epinephrine and dopamine levels were barely detectable (8.6 ± 6.4 and 7.3 ± 6.1 pg, respectively, at the lower limit of assay sensitivity). Both norepinephrine and epinephrine levels were markedly higher in the CSF of adrenal medullary-transplanted animals, with norepinephrine increased approximately 3-fold, and epinephrine increased over 100-fold. Dopamine levels were not appreciably altered. In addition, reductions in pain sensitivity could also be correlated with CSF catecholamine levels in animals with adrenal medullary transplants (Fig. 4).

Morphological Analysis

The viability and host–graft relationships following adrenal medullary tissue or cell implantation into the spinal cord subarachnoid space can be visualized by morphological analysis. Typically both immunocytochemistry and ultrastructural procedures are done. Figure 5 shows the appearance of an adrenal

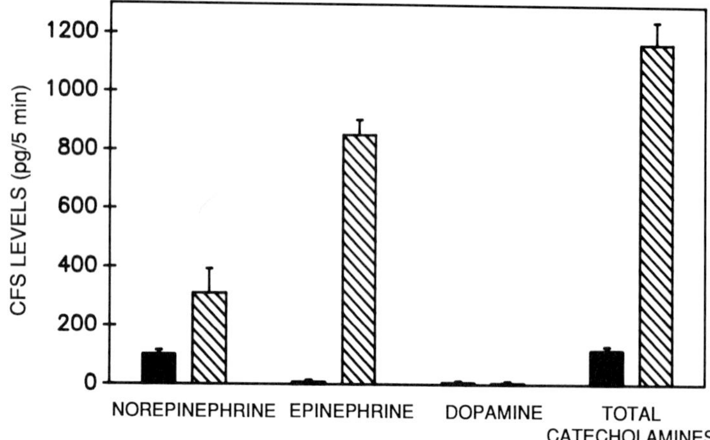

FIG. 3 Basal catecholamine release into spinal cord superfusates of animals with control striated muscle transplants (filled bars, $n = 8$) or adrenal medullary transplants (stripped bars, $n = 9$) in the spinal cord subarachnoid space. Bars represent mean ± SEM levels of norepinephrine, epinephrine, dopamine, and total catecholamine released per 5-min sample collection interval. [From Sagen *et al.* (5).]

medullary allograft in the rat spinal subarachnoid space 6 months following implantation. Using a tyrosine hydroxylase antibody, catecholamine-producing cells are readily identified. The adrenal medullary tissue typically remains in the subarachnoid space at the dorsal surface of the host spinal cord, surrounded by spinal roots, and does not integrate noticeably with the host parenchyma. A light micrograph of a toluidine blue-stained semithin section of bovine chromaffin cells grafted into the rat spinal subarachnoid space is shown in Fig. 6B. The graft is highly vascular, and there is a cellular and collagenous barrier between the grafted cells and the host spinal tissue. Chromaffin cells in both allografts and xenografts generally appear to retain their *in situ* cuboidal morphology. In contrast to intraparenchymally placed grafts, synaptic contacts between host and chromaffin cells grafted in the subarachnoid space are not apparent. These findings suggest that the ability of such grafts to reduce pain is due to the release of neuroactive substances into the CSF or extracellular spaces and diffusion to host spinal receptors, that is, via a "pump" mechanism, rather than via direct host–graft synaptic integration. An appreciation for this mechanism can be gained by Fig. 7, which shows a chromaffin cell in an adrenal medullary implant in the spinal subarachnoid space. This cell appears to release granular contents into the extracellular spaces of the graft.

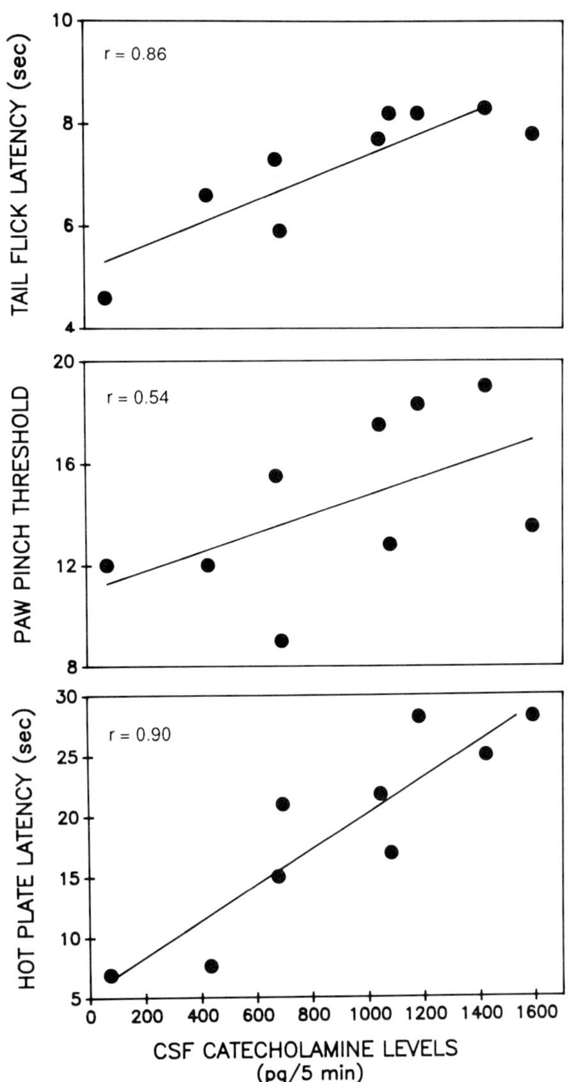

FIG. 4 Correlations between alterations in pain sensitivity following nicotine administration (0.1 mg/kg, ip) and mean release of total catecholamines per 5-min interval in animals with adrenal medullary implants in the spinal cord. Both the analgesiometric testing and the superfusion procedures took place 6 months following surgical implantation. The ordinate indicates the nociceptive threshold as assessed by the tail flick (top), paw pinch (middle), and hot plate (bottom) tests. [From Sagen *et al.* (5).]

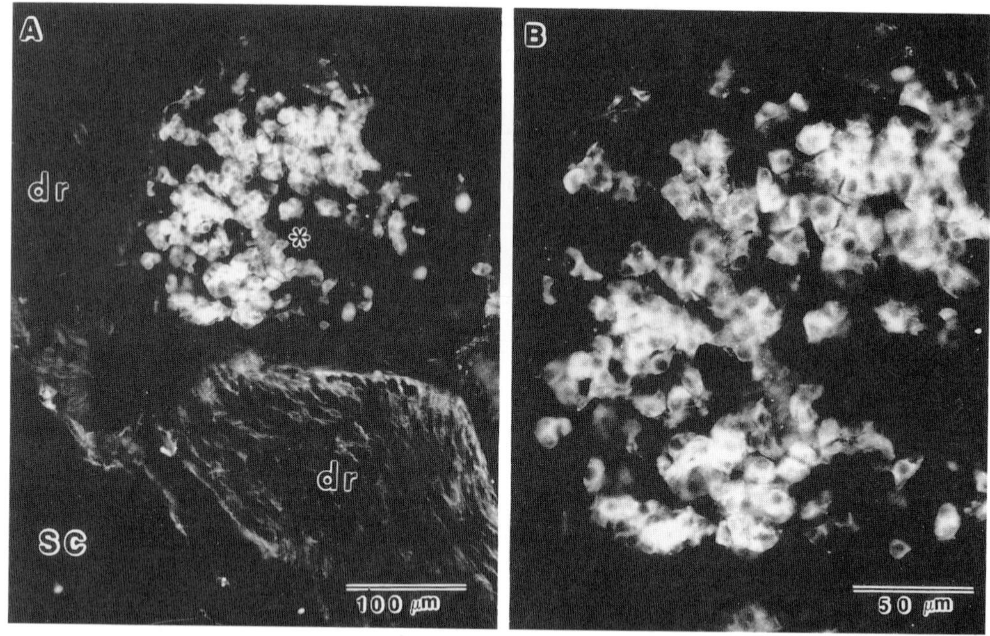

FIG. 5 (A) Appearance of a portion of an adrenal medullary transplant in the spinal cord subarachnoid space 6 months posttransplantation. Chromaffin cells in the transplant were immunocytochemically stained with an antibody to tyrosine hydroxylase, followed by a rhodamine-linked secondary antibody. The adrenal medullary tissue is marked by an asterisk, SC, Spinal cord; dr, dorsal root. (B) Higher magnification of the cluster of chromaffin cells in (A). Note that most of the chromaffin cells in the transplant retain their *in situ* cuboidal morphology. [From Sagen *et al.* (5).]

Intraparenchymal Grafts

Implantation into Periaqueductal Gray

Adrenal medullary allografts or chromaffin cell xenografts can also be placed in the parenchymal tissue of the brain for local delivery of neuroactive substances. The bulk of studies in our laboratory has focused on transplantation into the midbrain periaqueductal gray (PAG) because this is an important site of action of the analgesic effects of opiates (29, 30). However, when appropriate, these cells have been implanted successfully in other brain regions for local delivery of agents released by the chromaffin cells. For example, adrenal medullary allografts or bovine chromaffin cell xenografts can markedly reduce depressive symptoms in rat depression models when

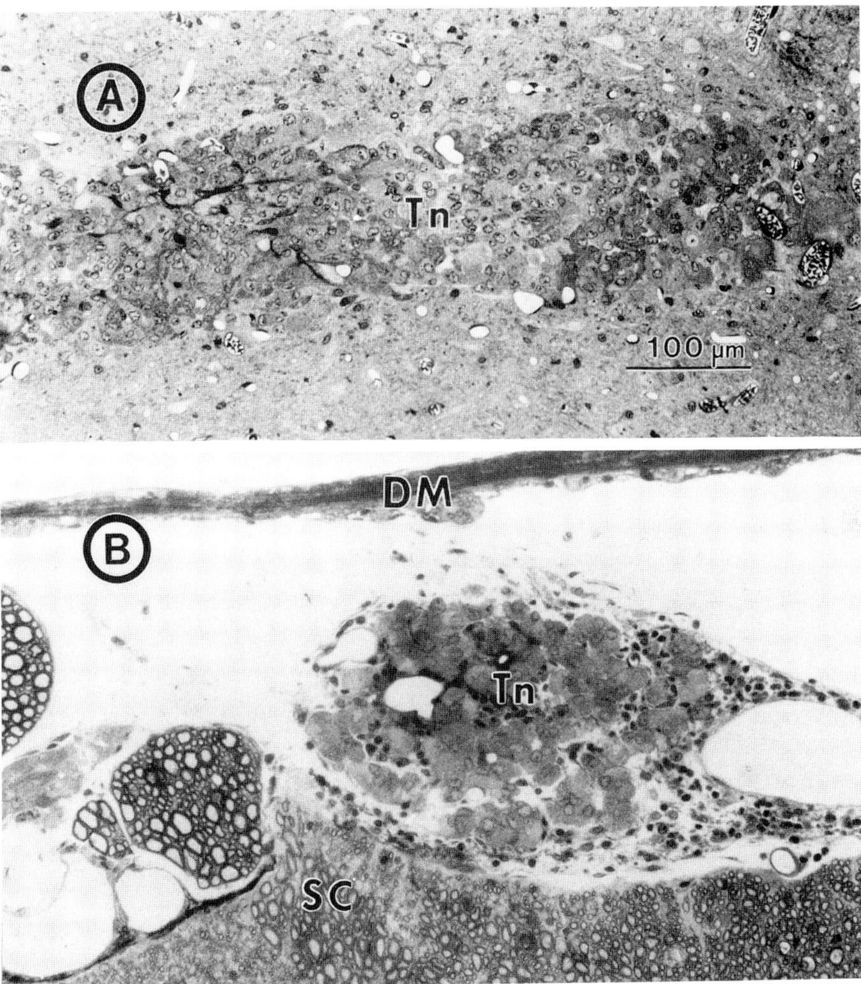

FIG. 6 Light micrographs of toluidine blue-stained semithin sections of bovine chromaffin cell suspensions implanted into the periaqueductal gray (A) and the subarachnoid space of the lumbar spinal cord (B). Note that the interface between the host and transplanted cells (Tn) in the periaqueductal gray is not well demarcated, suggesting good integration of grafted cells with host CNS tissue. In contrast, subarachnoid transplants [Tn in (B)] were not integrated with host tissue, but were separated by cellular and collagenous elements between the grafted cells and the spinal cord (SC). DM, Dural membrane. [From Ortega *et al.* (23).]

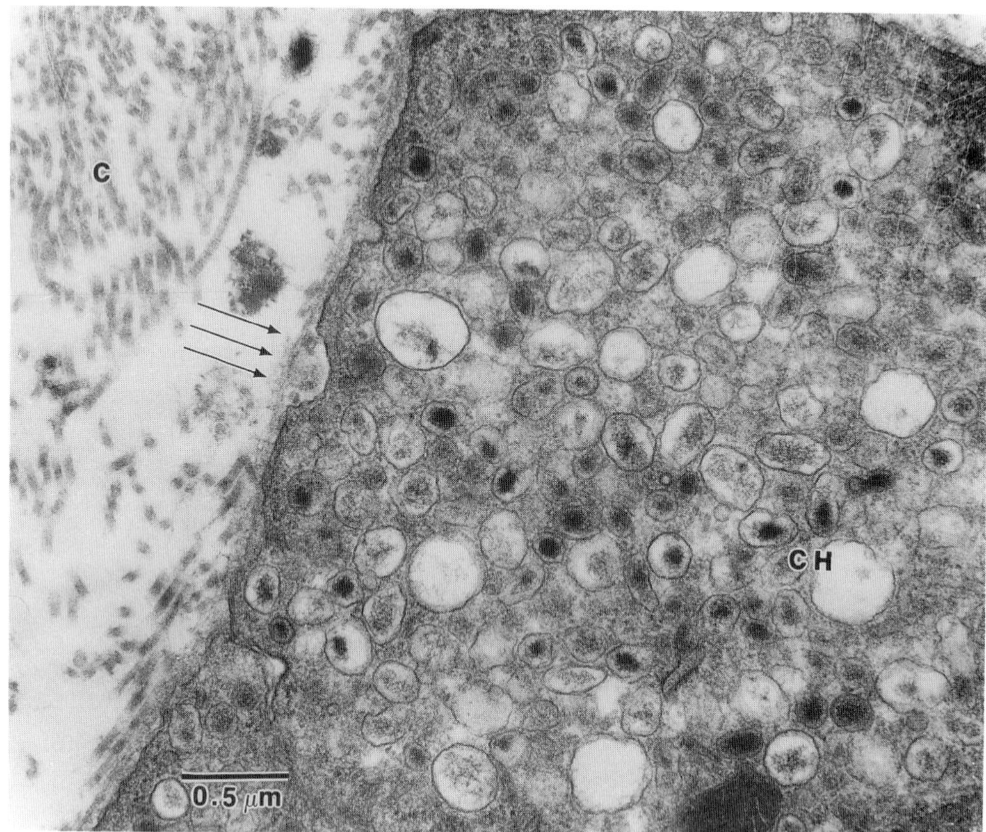

FIG. 7 Enlarged portion of a chromaffin cell (CH) in an adrenal medullary implant, giving the impression of releasing its granular contents into the extracellular spaces of the graft (at arrows). C, Collagen. [From Sagen and Kemmler (4).]

implanted into the frontal neocortex (7–9, 20). In addition, the survival of these cells is not limited to CNS regions rich in nerve growth factor, because they show robust survival in nerve growth factor-poor regions such as the striatum (23).

Both adrenal medullary allografts and bovine chromaffin cell xenografts are implanted stereotaxically in the rat parenchyma. Animals are anesthetized as above and placed in a stereotaxic frame. The scalp is shaved, and the surgical area prepared aseptically. An incision is made in the scalp, the skull cleaned, and a hole drilled at the appropriate region for implantation. For implantation of solid adrenal medullary tissue pieces, tissue from one adrenal medulla is loaded into a 25-gauge cannula, which is lowered to the desired coordinates. Tissue pieces are slowly extruded using a stylet, and left in place for 1 min prior to withdrawal of the injection cannula. For implantation of bovine chromaffin cell suspensions, the cells are allowed to settle at the bottom of a microfuge tube, and the concentrated suspensions of cells (50,000 cells/μl) are injected in 2-μl volumes into predetermined CNS areas. For example, the cell suspensions are injected stereotaxically via a 25-gauge needle into the PAG, using the following coordinates: A, +1.2 mm; L, −0.7 mm; H, +3.5 mm from the intraaural line; incisor bar, −2.5 mm (31). The injection is made over a 2-min period to minimize damage to brain tissue, after which the needle is slowly raised, and the scalp wound closed with wound clips.

Analysis of Neuropeptide and Catecholamine Delivery into Central Nervous System Parenchyma

Although the release of neuroactive agents from CNS sites can be accomplished by *in vivo* microdialysis, these methods are often not optimal because of technical difficulty and poor recovery. In particular, whereas monoamine recoveries can be 20–30%, the measurement of neuropeptides by this technique is a particularly difficult challenge, with recoveries often below 10%. We have presented an alternate method for measuring release of neuroactive substances, including neuropeptides, from cells transplanted into the CNS, using an *in vitro* slice preparation (32). As an additional advantage, the release of transmitters from the brain slices can be compared to that from bovine chromaffin cells maintained for similar periods of time in culture in order to assess the potential effects of the CNS environment on the function and pharmacological responsiveness of chromaffin cells.

A brain slice superfusion method was adapted from that used for electrophysiological studies (33). The use of superfusion chambers for the study of neural tissues has been described previously (34–36), but has not been used extensively in neural transplant studies. A brain slice chamber constructed for the biochemical and pharmacological study of intraparenchymal bovine chromaffin cell grafts is shown in Fig. 8. The brain slice chamber is made of a Plexiglas base (length, 10 cm; width, 10 cm; height, 2 cm) with a 10-mm diameter hole drilled exactly 0.5 cm into the top center of the platform. Another hole is drilled from the side to be fitted with polyethylene tubing for delivery of superfusion fluid. A smaller piece of Plexiglas (length, 3.5 cm; width, 3.5 cm; height, 0.5 cm) is drilled similarly, and fitted over the hole in the base, resulting in a chamber 1 cm in depth. This portion also contains a side port for attachment of polyethylene tubing (PE-160, 10 cm) to serve as an exit for the superfusate. A nylon netting is placed between

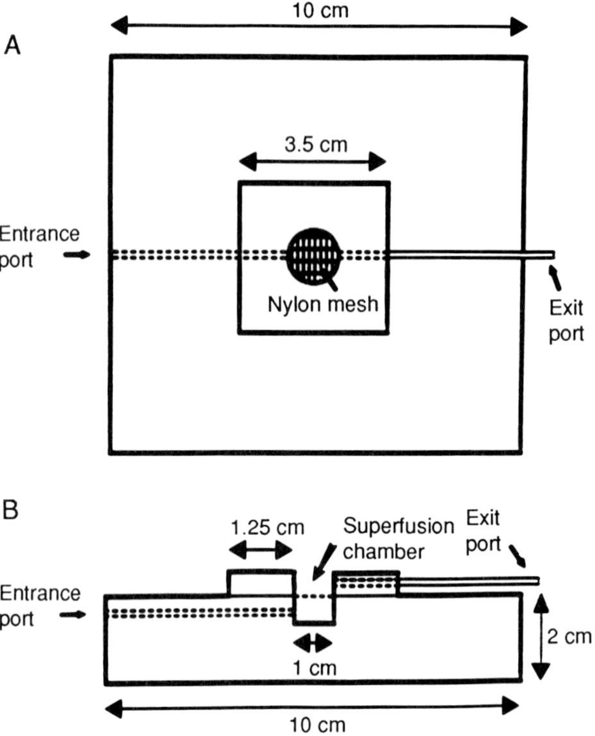

FIG. 8 A schematic diagram of the slice chamber. Top view (A) and side view (B). Superfusate enters the chamber from the entrance port and bathes the brain slice, resting on the nylon mesh, from below. The superfusate then exits from above the slice and can be collected from the exit port. [From Ortega and Sagen (32).]

the cylindrical holes, separating the chamber into upper and lower parts, and the Plexiglas pieces are secured with copper screws and water-tight sealant. The height of the exit hole is 0.3 cm above the level of the nylon mesh, assuring that brain slices are always submerged. This arrangement allows for the continuous flow of superfusate out of the chamber and into collection tubes.

To determine release of neuroactive agents from transplanted chromaffin cells, 5-mm^3 blocks containing the transplants are prepared from the brains of implanted rats, glued onto a chuck, and immediately placed into an Oxford Vibratome (Pelco, Redding, CA) trough filled with oxygenated artificial CSF (aCSF) cooled to 4°C. Brain slices (350 μm) containing the transplant are cut, placed in a slice chamber, and superfused continuously (2.0 ml/min by gravitational force, controlled by adjusting the height of the aCSF source) with oxygenated aCSF (maintained at 36.5°C by a heated water bath). This arrangement is shown in Fig. 9. A series of stopcocks placed immediately after the aCSF source allows for the introduction of pharmacological agents into the chamber containing the brain slice. Polyethylene tubing (PE-60) from the stopcocks to the entrance port of the chamber is immersed in a heated water bath to maintain superfusate temperature at 36.5°C. To assess recoveries from the slice bath, standards (e.g., authentic Met-enkephalin) can be collected from the slice chamber. Results from previous experience

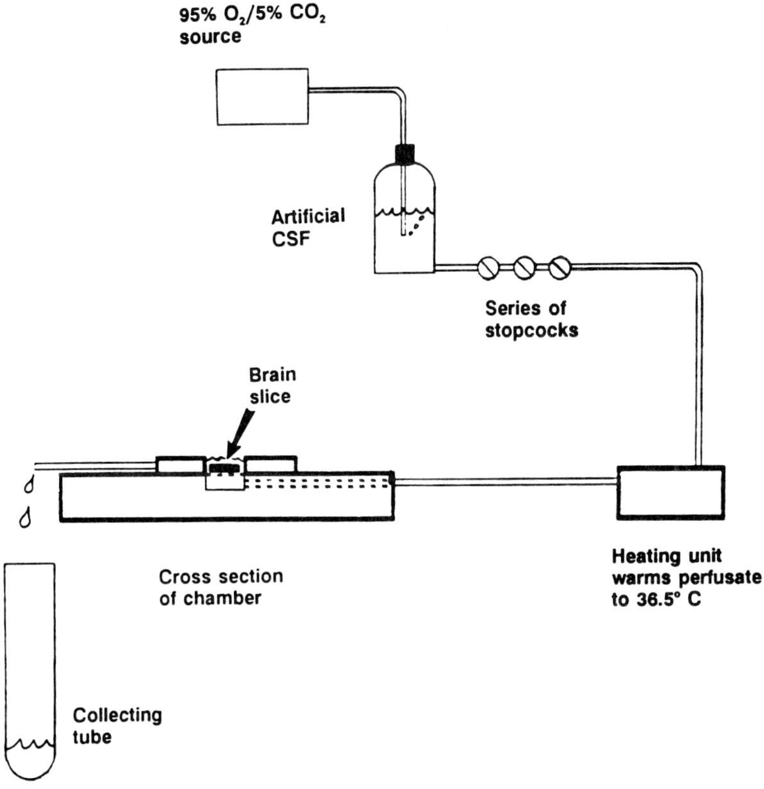

FIG. 9 Schematic diagram of the superfusion system used in these studies. O_2 source continuously oxygenates the artificial CSF (aCSF), which flows by gravitational force into the slice chamber containing the brain slice. The superfusate, which is maintained at 36.5°C by a heating unit, bathes the brain slice continuously. A series of stopcocks placed immediately after the aCSF source allows for the administration of pharmacological agents. All samples are collected as the superfusate exits the brain slice chamber. [From Ortega and Sagen (32).]

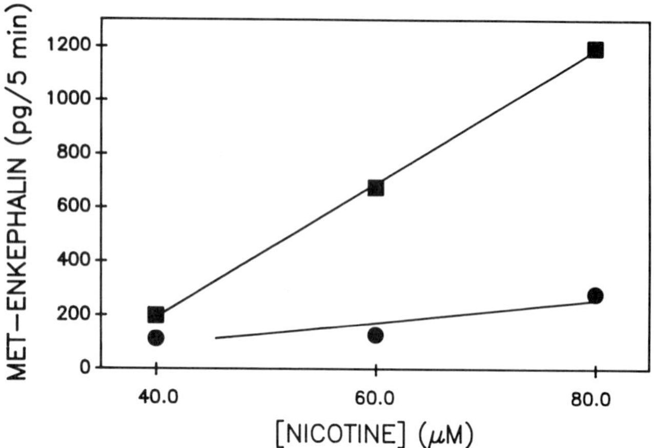

FIG. 10 Met-enkephalin content from superfusate samples collected from brain slices following stimulation with nicotine at concentrations ranging from 40 to 80 μM in nonimplanted animals (filled circles) or animals with bovine chromaffin cells implants (filled squares). Each stimulation period was followed by a 15-min washout period to confirm return to basal release. [From Ortega and Sagen (32).]

in our laboratory have indicated that approximately 65–75% of the standards are recovered within the first 5 min of application to the slice bath, and an additional 15–25% during the next 10 min. During a typical collection procedure, a 1-hr stabilization period is allowed, and superfusate samples are collected for 5-min periods. To assess pharmacological specificity, release in response to varying doses of nicotine can be evaluated. Each stimulation is followed by a 15-min washout phase and an additional 5-min collection period to confirm that release had returned to basal levels. All collected samples are frozen in liquid nitrogen, lyophilized, and stored at −30°C until assayed for neuropeptide or catecholamine content as described above.

FIG. 11 Electron micrographs of intraparenchymally transplanted chromaffin cells (Ch) infiltrated by neuritic processes of host origin. (A and C) Synaptic contacts can be observed on grafted chromaffin cells (arrowheads). These synaptic complexes are composed of adjoining pre- and postsynaptic densities (at arrowheads), frequently with many clusters of vesicles (V) in the presynaptic terminal. (D) Synaptic structures commonly seen at the host-graft border, but vesicle-containing neuronal processes (V) of host origin can often be found to intervene between clumps of grafted cells as well. (B) No clearly delineated synaptic structures are found in subarachnoid grafts, although occasional vesicle-filled processes (V) are observed. *, Extracellular material. [From Ortega *et al.* (23).]

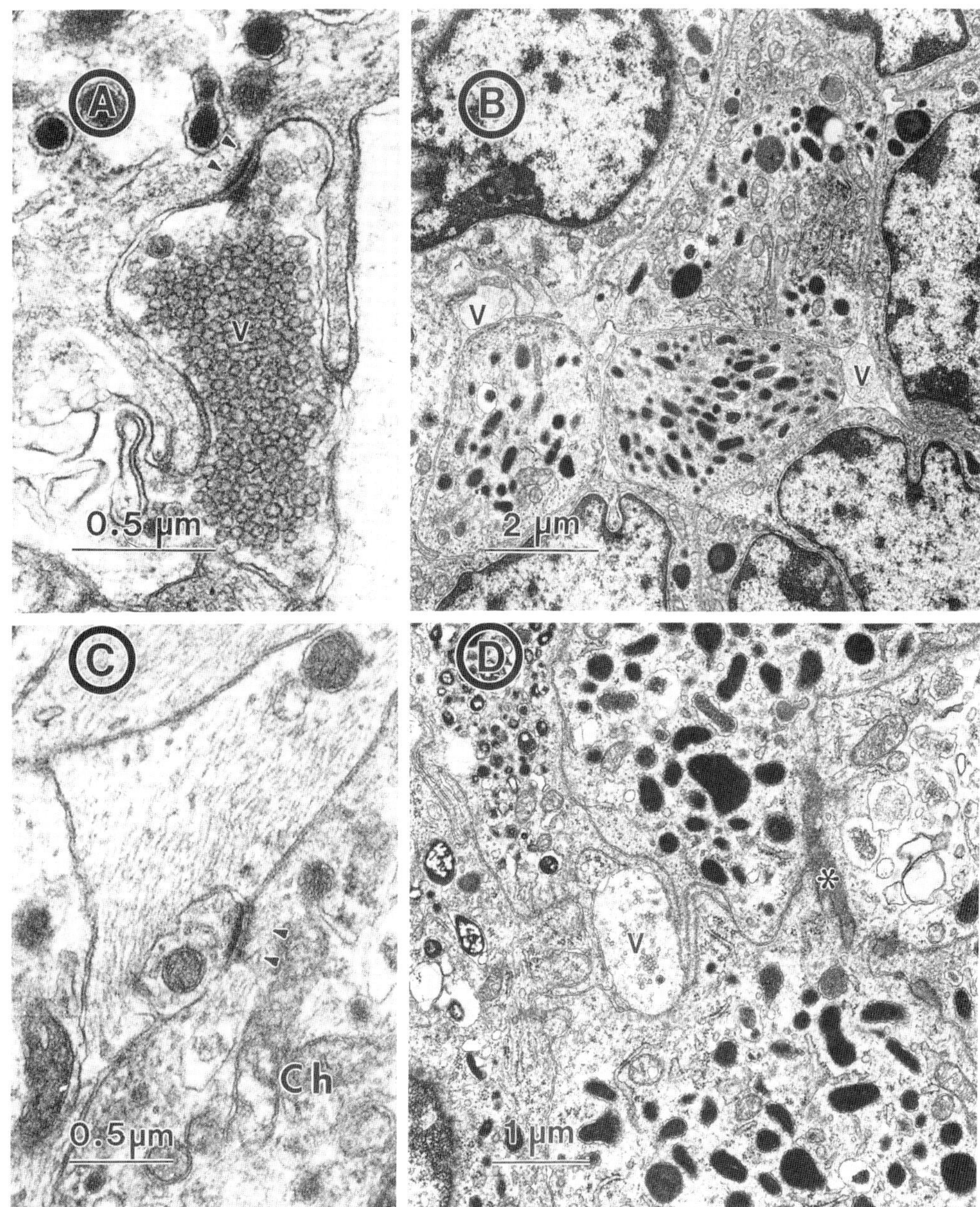
A
V
0.5 μm
B
V
V
2 μm
C
Ch
0.5μm
D
V
*
1 μm

An example of results obtained from these procedures is shown in Fig. 10, which shows the response of brain slices containing 8-week-old bovine chromaffin cell transplants in the rat periaqueductal gray to increasing concentration of nicotine. Results revealed a dose-related stimulation in Met-enkephalin release from the slices. Nicotine given in concentrations from 40 to 80 μM produced a sixfold increase in Met-enkephalin content in superfusate samples. During the 15-min washout phases Met-enkephalin release returned to prenicotine basal levels (60–115 pg/5 min). In addition, these levels showed no decrement over the time the slices were maintained in the bath (up to 6 hr), indicating good viability. For comparison, control brain slices from similar periaqueductal gray regions did not respond to these nicotine concentrations. Similar to implanted bovine chromaffin cells, cultured bovine chromaffin cells release increasing levels of Met-enkephalin in response to nicotinic stimulation. These studies provide further evidence suggesting that bovine chromaffin cells not only survive well in the rat CNS, but remain neurochemically active and pharmacologically responsive.

Morphological Analysis

Intraparenchymally placed grafts, like implants in the spinal subarachnoid space, are also evaluated using immunocytochemical or ultrastructural techniques. Figure 6A shows a toluidine blue-stained semithin section of a bovine chromaffin cell graft in the rat periaqueductal gray 8 weeks following transplantation. Note that, in contrast to the subarachnoid grafts, the chromaffin cells are tightly packed, with little intervening connective tissue. The grafted cells appear well integrated, with no apparent collagenous or gliotic scarring. Blood vessels are generally limited to the periphery of the graft, with only minimal vascularity deep within the graft itself, in contrast to extraparenchymally placed grafts, which tend to be highly vascular. Ultrastructural analysis of intraparenchymal grafts confirm that chromaffin cells integrate well with the host CNS tissue. A typical host–graft border reveals host neuropil in close apposition to grafted chromaffin cells. In addition, numerous neuritic processes of host origin can be found infiltrating the grafts and intervening between adjacent chromaffin cells. Frequent synaptic contacts are encountered on grafted chromaffin cells, when they are placed intraparenchymally, indicative of an increased level of integration not seen in the extraparenchymally placed spinal subarachnoid grafts (Fig. 11). These synaptic contacts can apparently form between immunologically disparate cells, as they result from presynaptic rat host CNS processes and implanted bovine chromaffin cells. In addition, there is rarely overt evidence of detrimental immunologic reactivity such as lymphocyte infiltration or perivascular cuffing in immunosuppressed animals.

Conclusions

Results from the methods presented in this chapter indicate that chromaffin cells can serve as a source of biologically active substances such as opioid peptides and catecholamines when transplanted into appropriate CNS sites. Both allogeneic and xenogeneic cells are potential candidates for donor material, and can survive and function when placed either intra- or extraparenchymally. This approach can be used for the local delivery of naturally produced neuroactive agents with short biological half-lives. In addition, the transplantation of living cells that continually synthesize these agents can overcome many of the inconveniences and potentially detrimental side effects of long-term or repeated exogenous drug administration.

Acknowledgment

This work was supported in part by NIH Grants NS25054 and NS28931.

References

1. E. C. Azmitia and A. Björklund, "Cell and Tissue Transplantation into the Adult Brain." N.Y. Acad. Sci., New York, 1987.
2. S. B. Dunnett and S.-J. Richards, "Neural Transplantation: From Molecular Basis to Clinical Applications." Elsevier, Amsterdam, 1990.
3. A. Hama and J. Sagen, *Pain* **52,** 223 (1993).
4. J. Sagen and J. E. Kemmler, *Brain Res.* **502,** 1 (1989).
5. J. Sagen, J. E. Kemmler, and H. Wang, *J. Neurochem.* **56,** 623 (1991).
6. J. Sagen, H. Wang, and G. D. Pappas, *Pain* **42,** 69 (1990).
7. J. Sagen, C. E. Sortwell, and G. D. Pappas, *Biol. Psychiatry* **28,** 1037 (1990).
8. C. E. Sortwell and J. Sagen, *Pharmacol. Biochem. Behav.* **46,** 225 (1993).
9. C. E. Sortwell, F. Petty, G. Kramer, M. Waddill, and J. Sagen, *Soc. Neurosci. Abstr.* **19,** 1319 (1993).
10. D. M. Gaumann and T. L. Yaksh, *Peptides (N.Y.)* **9,** 393 (1988).
11. H. Kondo, *Arch. Histol. Jpn.* **48,** 453 (1985).
12. B. G. Livett, D. M. Dean, L. G. Whelan, S. Udenfriend, and J. Rossier, *Nature (London)* **289,** 317 (1981).
13. S. P. Wilson, K.-J. Chang, and O. H. Viveros, *J. Neurosci.* **2,** 1150 (1982).

14. J. Sagen and G. D. Pappas, *in* "Cell and Tissue Transplantation into the Adult Brain" (E. C. Azmitia and A. Björklund, eds.), p. 306. N. Y. Acad. Sci., New York, 1987.
15. H. Wang and J. Sagen, *Soc. Neurosci. Abstr.* **15,** 1243 (1989).
16. K. Drasner and H. F. Fields, *Pain* **32,** 309 (1988).
17. S. E. Sherman, C. W. Loomis, B. Milne, and F. W. Cervenko, *Eur. J. Pharmacol.* **148,** 371 (1988).
18. G. L. Wilcox, K.-H. Carlsson, A. Jochim, and I. Jurna, *Brain Res.* **405,** 84 (1987).
19. T. L. Yaksh and S. V. Reddy, *Anesthesiology* **54,** 451 (1981).
20. D. D. Dougherty, C. E. Sortwell, and J. Sagen, *JAMA, J. Am. Med. Assoc.* **267,** 1268 (1992).
21. J. Sagen, G. D. Pappas, and A. P. Winnie, *Cell Transplant.* **2,** 259 (1993).
22. J. Ortega, J. Sagen, and G. D. Pappas, *Cell Transplant.* **1,** 33 (1992).
23. J. D. Ortega, J. Sagen, and G. D. Pappas, *J. Comp.Neurol.* **323,** 13 (1992).
24. J. Sagen, G. D. Pappas, and J. D. Ortega, *J. Neurocytol.* **19,** 697 (1990).
25. J. Sagen, G. D. Pappas, and M. J. Perlow, *Brain Res.* **384,** 189 (1986).
26. J. Sagen, G. D. Pappas, and H. B. Pollard, *Proc. Natl. Acad. Sci. U.S.A.* **83,** 7522 (1986).
27. R. E. Erny, M. W. Berezo, and R. L. Perlman, *J. Biol. Chem.* **256,** 1335 (1981).
28. L. J. Felice, J. D. Felice, and P. T. Kissinger, *J. Biol. Chem.* **31,** 1461 (1978).
29. V. A. Lewis and G. F. Gebhart, *Brain Res.* **124,** 283 (1976).
30. T. L. Yaksh and T. A. Rudy, *Pain* **24,** 229 (1978).
31. G. Paxinos and C. Watson, "The Rat Brain in Stereotaxic Coordinates." Academic Press, London, 1986.
32. J. D. Ortega and J. Sagen, *Exp. Brain Res.* **95,** 381 (1993).
33. B. E. Alger, S. Dhanjal, R. Dingledine, J. Garthweite, F. Henderson, G. L. King, P. Lipton, A. North, P. A. Schwartzkroin, T. A. Sears, M. Segal, T. S. Whittingham, and J. Williams, *in* "Brain Slices" (R. Dingledine, ed.), p. 381. Plenum, New York, 1984.
34. E. W. Black and J. M. Lakowski, *J. Pharmacol. Methods* **25,** 285 (1991).
35. H. L. Haas, B. Schaerer, and M. Vosmansky, *J. Neurosci. Methods* **1,** 323 (1979).
36. R. A. Nicoll and B. E. Alger, *J. Neurosci. Methods* **4,** 153 (1981).

Section IX

Using Implanted Encapsulated Cells within the Brain

[22] Microencapsulation of Cells in Thermoplastic Copolymer (Hydroxyethyl Methacrylate–Methyl Methacrylate)

M. V. Sefton, H. Uludag, J. Babensee, T. Roberts, V. Horvath, and U. De Boni

Introduction

Despite well-recognized limitations of L-dopa therapy, no viable alternative yet exists for the treatment of Parkinson's disease (PD). Tissue transplantation to replace striatal dopamine *in situ* has so far met with limited clinical success, and in the case of fetal tissue grafts is further hampered by lack of tissue and ethical concerns. As an alternative to naked tissue grafts, hollow fiber/cylindrical "macrocapsules" or spherical microcapsules have been used to separate cells from the host's immune system. Such immunoisolation units, or "hybrid artificial organs," are particularly interesting because they permit the use of xenogeneic cells or cell lines that, in the absence of a immunological or simple physical barrier, would not otherwise be considered. Whereas nutrients and products(s) freely diffuse across the membrane, the membrane prevents the immune system of the host from rejecting the donor tissue. Aebischer *et al.*, in conjunction with Cytotherapeutics, Inc., (Providence, RI) have used PAN/PVC "macrocapsules" with PC-12 cells, embryonic mesencephalon tissue, and adrenal chromaffin cells for dopamine delivery (1).

Rather than using preformed hollow fibers that are then filled with a cell suspension, we have used microencapsulation techniques to form a small spherical microcapsule that is, simultaneous with formation, filled with live cells. The capsule membrane constitutes a physical permeability barrier that restricts the survival of cell mass in a confined space but allows the release of cell-derived products. The fragile nature of the mammalian cells imposes severe restrictions on the process conditions of encapsulation as well as on the final properties of the resultant microcapsules. It is imperative that the exposure of mammalian cells to physical forces (such as shear, pressure, or osmotic) or toxic chemicals is minimized during this process. Once encapsulated, the cells rely on diffusion for maintenance of normal physiological activity and, therefore, it is important for the capsule wall to have high permeability for essential nutrients, growth regulatory factors, and end products of metabolism that might possess growth inhibitory action. In addition

Methods in Neurosciences, Volume 21

to the basic maintenance of viability, the encapsulated cells obviously must retain their functional or differentiated state (i.e., synthesize and secrete tissue-specific biomolecules). Additionally, the biocompatibility of the polymeric membrane becomes important for long-term success of transplantation by reducing the deleterious effects of tissue reaction against the microcapsule on the encapsulated cells and tissues.

A number of techniques based on the original work of Chang (2) have been reported for the microencapsulation of mammalian cells, with varying degrees of success. These include interfacial adsorption, commonly known as the poly(alginate)—poly(lysine) system (3, 4), polyelectrolyte complexation (5, 6), and interfacial polymerization (7). Alternatively, we have developed and subsequently modified an interfacial precipitation process to prepare polyacrylate microcapsules (8). A thermoplastic (i.e., non-cross-linked and hence soluble in an organic solvent) copolymer of hydroxyethyl methacrylate (HEMA) and methyl methacrylate (MMA) was chosen because of (a) demonstrated *in vivo* stability and biocompatibility of the parent homopolymers and (b) the feasibility of easy control over the physicochemical characteristics of copolymers (i.e., hence microcapsule properties). Using several mammalian cell types, we have demonstrated the retention of cell viability during the process of encapsulation and subsequent *in vitro* culture in microcapsules (9–11). The cells remained functional and expressed their tissue-specific functions.

Materials and Methods

Materials

An HEMA–MMA copolymer, nominally containing 75 mol% HEMA, is prepared by solution polymerization with azobisisobutyronitrile (0.001 mol/mol monomer) as initiator, as detailed elsewhere (12). The distilled water uptake (based on wet weight) is 31% and the value in phosphate-buffered saline (PBS) is not statistically different. For encapsulation, the copolymer is dissolved as 10% (w/v) in polyethylene glycol 200 (PEG 200; BDH Chemicals, Toronto, Ontario, Canada).

For encapsulation, individual cells (i.e., not tissue fragments or islets) are suspended in their normal tissue culture medium with serum at various concentrations from 1×10^5 to 1×10^7 cells/ml. For example, PC-12 cells [American Type Culture Collection (ATCC; Rockville, MD), CRL 1721, passage number unknown] are suspended in a medium consisting of RPMI-1640 with *N*-2-hydroxyethylpiperazine-*N*′-2-ethanesulfonic acid (HEPES) and L-glutamate (GIBCO Laboratories, Grand Island, NY), with 10% (v/v) donor horse serum (Hazleton Biologicals, Lenexa, KS), 5% (v/v) fetal bovine serum (Flow Laboratories, McLean, VA), and 100 μ/ml penicillin 100 ng/ml streptomycin (GIBCO). Before and after encapsulation, they are maintained at 37°C with 5% CO_2 and 95% air.

Capsule quality is improved by suspending cells in a more viscous medium, such as complete medium containing 20% (w/v) Ficoll 400 (Sigma Chemical Company, St. Louis, MO) (13). Anchorage-dependent cells such as HepG2 cells (ATCC) are suspended in Matrigel [1 : 1 (v/v) with complete tissue culture medium; Collaborative Research Incorporated, Bedford, MA]. Matrigel is prepared from a urea extract of Engelbreth–Holm–Swarm (EHS) tumors (14) and provides an extracellular matrix to which the cells attach and grow and which maximizes their expression of differentiated functions (e.g., plasma protein secretion by HepG2 cells).

Encapsulation Apparatus

Large-diameter microcapsules are prepared using the microencapsulation apparatus shown schematically in Fig. 1a, based primarily on the procedure defined by Crooks *et al.* (15). Two syringe pumps (model A-99; Razel Scientific Instruments, Inc., Stamford, CT) are used to pump the cell suspension and polymer solution to the double-barrelled extrusion needle (Fig. 1b). The coextrusion needle consists of a 16-gauge Luer-lok needle to which is added a side arm for the polymer solution and an inner 22-gauge disposable spinal needle (Becton Dickinson, Rutherford, NJ). A plastic pipette tip (Fisher Scientific, Don Mills, Ontario, Canada) is placed on the bottom of the 16-gauge needle to facilitate the shearing off of droplets. The pipette tip and the 22-gauge needle are blunt cut (Fig. 1b) and the needle is centered in the pipette tip opening, with it protruding ~100 μm past the end of the pipette tip. To facilitate the encapsulation of the Matrigel–cell suspension, gelatinous at room temperature, the polyethylene 50 (PE-50) tubing delivering this suspension is submerged in ice water. In this way an even distribution of the Matrigel–cell suspension among capsules is obtained (11).

Microcapsules are sheared from the coextrusion needle at the hexadecane–air interface as the needle is made to oscillate in the vertical plane by a motor and cam assembly. The frequency of oscillation is 30/min, with one droplet released each stroke. The capsules are collected in a 250-ml volumetric flask (Pyrex; Corning Co., Corning, NY) containing an aqueous precipitation solution that fills the flask, except for the top 7 cm in the neck, which is filled with a hexadecane (99% pure; Sigma) overlayer. The hexadecane prevents precipitation of the polymer solution on the needle tip and enables the formation of better capsules. A magnetic stirrer (8 mm diameter and 32

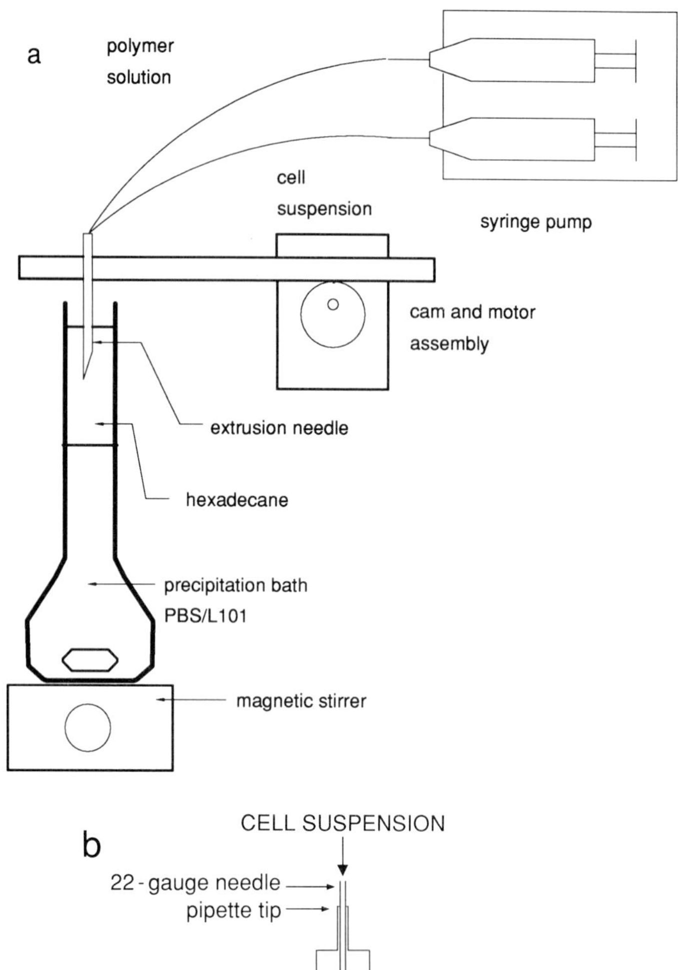

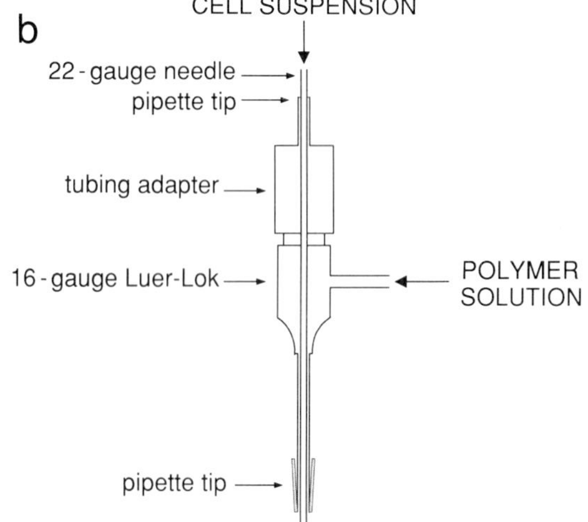

FIG. 1 Submerged jet microencapsulation apparatus: (a) Overall schematic; (b) detail of encapsulation needle. [(a) From Crooks *et al.* (15).] Copyright 1990, John Wiley & Sons, Inc.

mm long; Fisher Scientific) on low setting is employed to keep the capsules in suspension and prevent their agglomeration while they cure. Small-diameter capsules (as small as 400 μm) are made by a variation on this process, in which the needle is kept stationary and the hexadecane is pumped past the end of the needle (8).

The precipitation bath consists of PBS (0.14 *M* NaCl, 8.1 m*M* Na_2HPO_4, 0.98 m*M* KH_2PO_4, pH 7.4). Pluronic L101 surfactant (100 ppm; BASF Chemicals, Wyandotte, MI) is added to aid the passage of the microcapsules through the hexadecane–aqueous interface.

Encapsulation Procedure

All encapsulations are carried out in a laminar flow bench at room temperature (21–26°C). The cell suspension is pumped to the needle tip at a flow rate of ~0.02 ml/min and the ratio of polymer solution to cell flow rate varied from 1.5 : 1 to 2.67 : 1, depending on the cell suspension composition (viscosity) and the specific needle geometry. After 15 min of extrusion into a flask, the hexadecane is removed by pipette and then, after another 15 min of stirring at low speed, the original precipitant solution in each flask is decanted and replaced by fresh PBS without surfactant. The capsules are then allowed to stir for an additional 30 min for more complete curing of the polymer shell. Finally, capsules are recovered from the PBS and, if without cells, are stored in petri dishes in fresh PBS, or if they contain cells in complete tissue culture medium, at ambient conditions or in an incubator, respectively. Obviously defective or aggomerated capsules are removed by hand at this stage and again on day 1.

Capsules are opaque, and therefore it is not possible to see the capsule contents without destroying the capsule. As a routine check on capsule quality and encapsulation efficacy an aliquot of ~20 capsules is cut in half under a stereoscopic microscope for gross evaluation of capsule diameter and eccentricity. If care is taken not to lose the cells on cutting (easier with Matrigel capsules), encapsulated cells may also be stained (e.g., with MTT; see below Materials and Methods, MTT Assay). Encapsulation efficiency is routinely measured by determining the percentage of cells recovered in capsule core normalized by the calculated number of cells added to each capsule during extrusion. For this, the core contents are washed out from the cut-open capsules, and the cells are trypsinized (in the case of Matrigel, Dispase (Collaborative Research Incorporated, Bedford, MA) is also used to dissolve the gel) and counted in a hemacytometer. Viability is routinely assessed by trypan blue exclusion.

Scanning Electron Microscopy

To examine the wall structure microcapsules are rinsed in water, freeze-dried, and fractured using a razor blade. Ten to 15 capsule halves are mounted on an aluminum scanning electron microscopy (SEM) stud with double-sided tape, and coated with gold using a Polaron SEM coating system. Samples are examined at $\times 50$–$\times 10{,}000$ magnification with a Hitachi S520 SEM and photographed.

HEMA–MMA-microencapsulated cells are prepared for SEM examination by freeze cleavage of conductively stained specimens (10). This technique (and that used for light microscopy) avoids the use of conventional organic solvents such as ethanol or xylene, which would dissolve the capsule wall. Here the capsule wall remains intact and the cells are well preserved.

To preserve the microencapsulated cells during sample preparation, aqueous glycerol cryoprotection is necessary to prevent damage from ice crystals. Air drying is used as the drying method for SEM preparation. The negative impact of the surface tension effects associated with air drying must be tolerated because freeze-drying without cryoprotectant damages the cells. Osmium tetroxide staining is used, as this material is more conductive, diminishing charging effects during SEM analysis and requiring a thinner layer of gold, permitting better resolution of ultrastructural detail (Fig. 2).

Cell containing capsules are prepared for freeze-fracturing and SEM examination following the procedure of DeBoni (16), modified for this application (10). Briefly, microcapsules are fixed in a solution of 3.5% (v/v) glutaraldehyde (Polysciences, Warrington, PA) containing 2% (w/v) tannic acid (BDH Chemicals) in 0.1 *M* Sorenson's phosphate buffer (P-buffer). Prior to fixation, microcapsules are washed with PBS twice for 15 min each to remove serum proteins. Microcapsules are stored in fixative for at least 2 days at 4°C. To impart partial conductivity capsules are postfixed with osmium tetroxide (JBS, St. Laurent, Quebec, Canada) [1 hr, 1% (v/v) in P-buffer, prepared fresh from a 4% (w/v) aqueous solution] and exposed to 2% (w/v) aqueous tannic acid for 1 hr. The microcapsules are again postfixed with 1% (v/v) osmium tetroxide for 1 hr. Washings with P-buffer follow each step. The microcapsules are then cryoprotected with 7.5 and 15% (v/v) aqueous glycerol solutions, respectively, for 20 min each. Individual microcapsules are placed into liquid nitrogen and cleaved open by use of a microscalpel under a dissecting microscope. Because of the technical difficulty in cleanly fracturing a microcapsule, only half of the microcapsule pieces contain cells.

Following cleavage, microcapsules are transferred to a 15% (v/v) aqueous glycerol solution and then to a 7.5% (v/v) aqueous glycerol solution for 20 min and washed twice with distilled water for 15 min. They are then placed on dry Whatman (Clifton, NJ) 114 wet strength filter paper to air dry over-

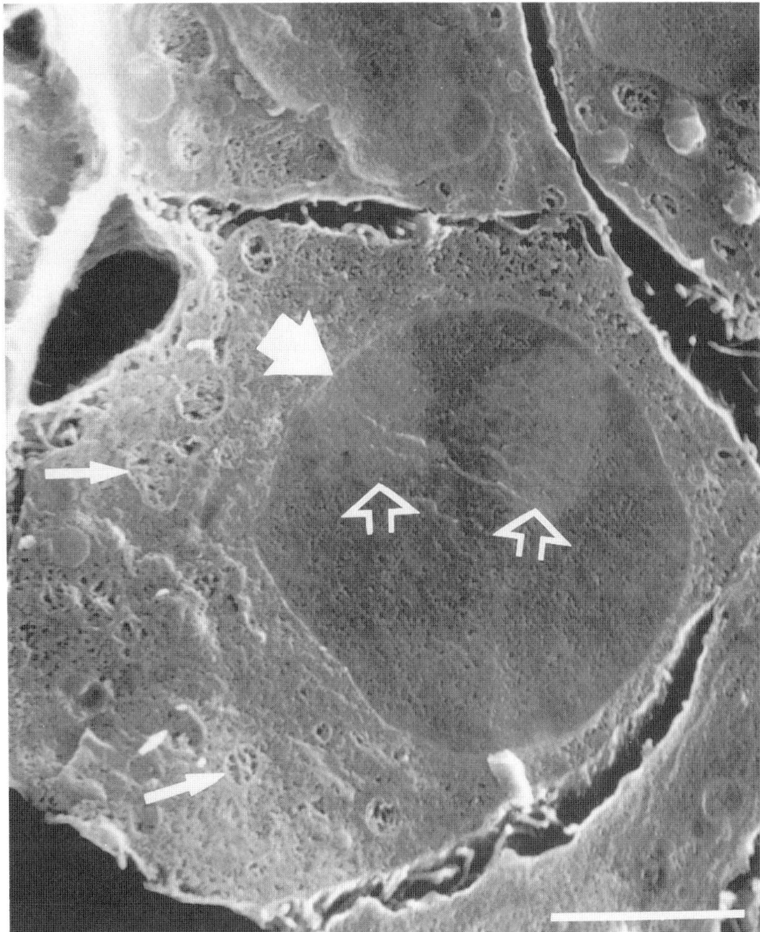

FIG. 2 Scanning electron micrograph of HepG2 cell within a Matrigel capsule, freeze-cleaved through the center of the cell. Note nucleus (solid white arrow) with two nucleoli (open arrows), and mitochondria (small solid arrows) with cristae. Bar: 4 μm. [From Babensee *et al.* (10).] Copyright 1992, John Wiley & Sons, Inc.

night, and then placed in a desiccator under vacuum, overnight. Aluminum stub-mounted samples are sputter coated with a thin layer of gold, in an argon atmosphere at 100 mtorr. The samples are examined using a Hitachi S-570 scanning electron microscope at an accelerating voltage of 20 kV and a working distance of 15 mm for low-magnification examination.

Light Microscopy

For light microscopy, aqueous toluidine blue staining of nucleic acids and some protein provides a rapid and easy method to localize cells and generally assess their morphology. Permount, a mounting medium that contains an organic solvent, may affect the polymer morphology but the capsule is retained on the slide, and the improved cellular resolution warrants its use.

Capsules are fixed and cryoprotected as described for SEM microscopy. A sample of 10–12 capsules is taken per postencapsulation time. The fixed microcapsules are washed twice with P-buffer for 15 min. Five or six capsules per plastic mold (Miles, Inc., Diagnostics Division, Elkhart, IN) are embedded in OCT compound [10.24% (w/w) polyvinyl alcohol, 4.26% (w/w) polyethylene glycol, 85.5% nonreactive ingredients; Miles Inc., Diagnostics Division], frozen, and stored on dry ice. Sections are cut using the Tissue-Tek microtome-cryostat (Ames Company, Elkhart, IN) at −20°C to a thickness of 10 μm and placed on gelatin–chrome alum [0.1% (w/v) gelatin, 0.01% (w/v) chromic potassium sulfate]-treated slides. The OCT embedding compound is dissolved in water and the sections stained with aqueous toluidine blue. Air-dried sections are mounted with Permount and observed with a light microscope.

MTT Assay

The MTT assay is used to determine the cellular viability or metabolic activity in microcapsules (17). It is based on the ability of metabolically active cells to transform a water-soluble dye[3-(4,5-dimethylthiazol-2-yl)-2,5-diphenyltetrazolium bromide] into an insoluble formazan. Quantitative determination of the amount of formazan gives an estimate of the number of cells in capsules. The simplicity and low cost of the assay make it a valuable tool with which to screen a large number of encapsulation parameters in a short period of time. It can be sensitive at a single capsule level, enabling one to look at capsule-to-capsule variations. Care should be taken in using formazan absorbance as a strict measure of cell number in capsules because changes in the metabolic state of the cells (i.e., metabolic deactivation or activation) will affect the results.

MTT solution (25 μl, 5 mg/ml) and 100 μl of fresh medium are added to each capsule (placed 1 per well in a 96-well plate) and incubated at 37°C for 5 hr, after which time the MTT–medium solution is removed by aspiration. Capsules are rinsed by a 10-minute incubation in distilled water followed by the addition of 100 μl of dimethyl sulfoxide (DMSO) and 12 μl of glycine buffer, pH 10.5. The capsules are allowed to dissolve for 30 min, with some manual agitation to aid in dissolution. The microplate is then read on an MR 700 microplate reader (Dynatech Laboratories, Inc., Chantilly, VA) at a wavelength of 570 nm, with the reference wavelength set at 630 nm. Blanks consisting of microcapsules with only culture medium as the core material are also assayed.

MTT is also used as a stain to obtain the overall arrangement of the cells in the capsule core. For this, the assay is carried out as described above but without the dissolution of formazan crystals. Investigation under a stereoscopic microscope (i.e., cells not forming the dye are not visible) will result in identification of the metabolically active cells.

Product Release

The therapeutic products of the encapsulated cell are assayed simply by incubating capsules in the appropriate release medium *in vitro*. The number of capsules per milliliter of medium and the incubation time are determined by the nature of the cell and the number of cells per capsule. For example, microcapsules containing PC-12 cells are incubated at 37°C in 1.5 ml of K^+/Ca^{2+} release medium [11.4 m*M* NaCl, 100 m*M* KCl, 1.3 m*M* $CaCl_2$, 1.0 *M* HEPES, 1.2 m*M* $MgSO_4$, 1.2 m*M* KH_2PO_4, 5.6 m*M* α-D(+)-glucose, 0.4 m*M* sodium ascorbate, and 0.05 m*M* L-tyrosine; pH 7.3] or RPMI-1640 for 15 min to 24 hr. Unencapsulated PC-12 cells are incubated in release medium or RPMI-1640 under similar circumstances as a control. The medium is stored at −70°C until analysis. Dopamine is measured by high-performance liquid chromatography (HPLC) (model 510; Waters Associates, Inc., Milford, MA) with an electrochemical detector (LC-40; Bioanalytical Systems, Inc., West Lafayette, IN) in the standard fashion (18).

Illustrative Results

Microcapsules

The present microencapsulation process results in microcapsules of ~700–900 μm diameter with a wall thickness of 50–150 μm. The wall interior is microporous, with a thin layer of dense skin on the outer and possibly the inner surface. A significant variation among capsule eccentricity was observed when tissue culture medium alone was employed as the cell-suspending medium. This heterogeneity was present within individual batches of capsules and was not just due to batch-to-batch differences. Supplementation of the cell suspending medium with density/viscosity enhancers [most effectively with 20% (w/v) Ficoll-400] resulted in better capsule morphology with reduced eccentricity (13) and a well-defined capsule core (Fig. 3). Reduction of the mixing of the polymer solution with the cell suspension as a result of increased viscosity of the inner core is presumed to give rise to the latter results. Encapsulation efficiency (viable cells recovered on day 1 as a percentage of the theoretical number of cells fed into each capsule during encapsulation) was found to be 65% with the Ficoll-400 supplementation of the cell suspension. The structure of the capsule wall and to a lesser extent the wall permeability can be varied by changing the preparation conditions (15).

The permeability of the HEMA–MMA microcapsules was measured by release experiments. A molecular weight cutoff of ~100 kD was observed (15), although the alcohol dehydrogenase (MW 150 kD) permeability was nonzero. This suggests that host antibodies could also reach the encapsulated

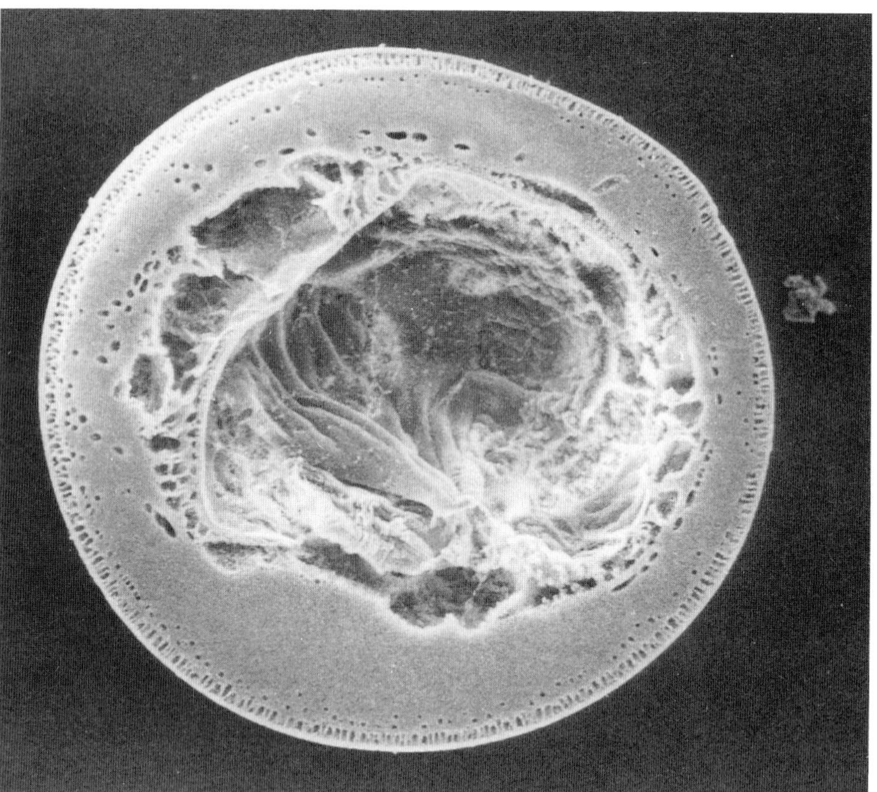

FIG. 3 Scanning electron micrograph of a typical ~900-μm HEMA–MMA capsule. [From Sefton and Stevenson (8).]

cells, although not necessarily in significant amounts. It is suspected that this low permeability to high molecular weight components is due to a subpopulation of relatively defective microcapsules. We have measured protein secretion from individual HepG2 capsules in order to gain further insight into the capsule-to-capsule variability in molecular weight cutoff (19).

Cell Viability

We have shown that a variety of cells survive encapsulation in HEMA–MMA and will grow or function for periods from 2 to >6 weeks *in vitro*. For example, they continued to secrete their particular products: insulin (rat or porcine pancreatic islets), dopamine (PC-12 cells/depolarization conditions), interleukin 2 (MLA 144 cells), epidermal growth factor (transfected FR3T3 cells), and various proteins [HepG2 cells (11)]. Encapsulated PC-12 cells secreted more dopamine per capsule as the time in culture increased (Fig. 4) and at a level that was comparable to unencapsulated cells, at least at

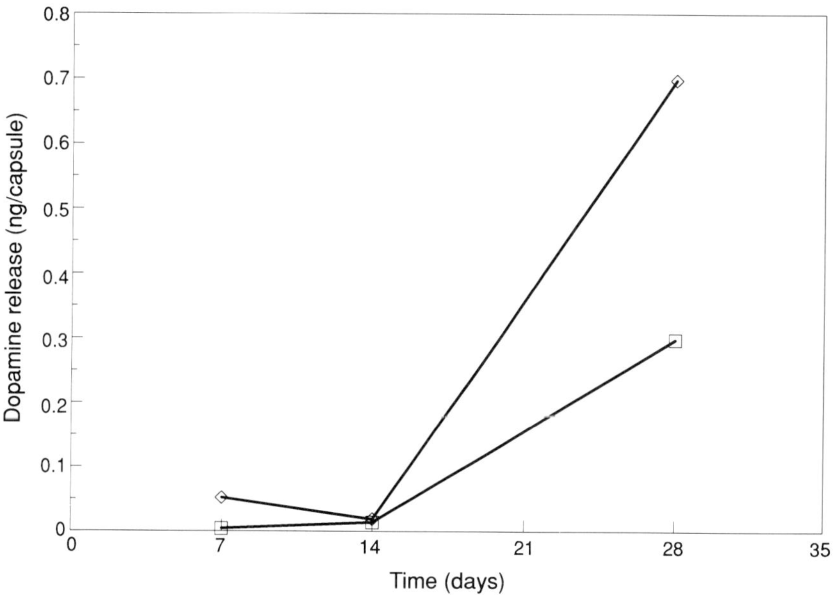

FIG. 4 Release of dopamine from microencapsulated PC-12 cells at various times after encapsulation during a 1-hr incubation in 101.2 m*M* K^+/0.05 m*M* tyrosine/1.3 m*M* Ca^{2+} at 37°C. Initial encapsulation density: (□) 4×10^5 cells/ml; (◇) 4×10^6 cells/ml.

comparable metabolic activities (MTT signal; Fig. 5). The time course of formazan production (MTT activity) for 4 weeks was followed to assess PC-12 survival and proliferation in microcapsules (Fig. 5) (20). Experiments were carried out using blank capsules and capsules for which the core solution cell concentrations (cells/ml) were 4×10^5 (low density) and 4×10^6 (high density) at the time of encapsulation. Similarly, HepG2 cells coencapsulated with Matrigel in large capsules released more protein 2 weeks after encapsulation (when there are more cells) than earlier (11). Interestingly, release of the larger protein (fibrinogen, 330 kDa) was not observed from the majority (~70%) of capsules, perhaps reflecting the influence of the capsule wall in restricting diffusion of large proteins.

Histological assays of large capsules have shown that, regardless of culture time (1–6 weeks) *in vitro* and even after brain implantation, a peripheral

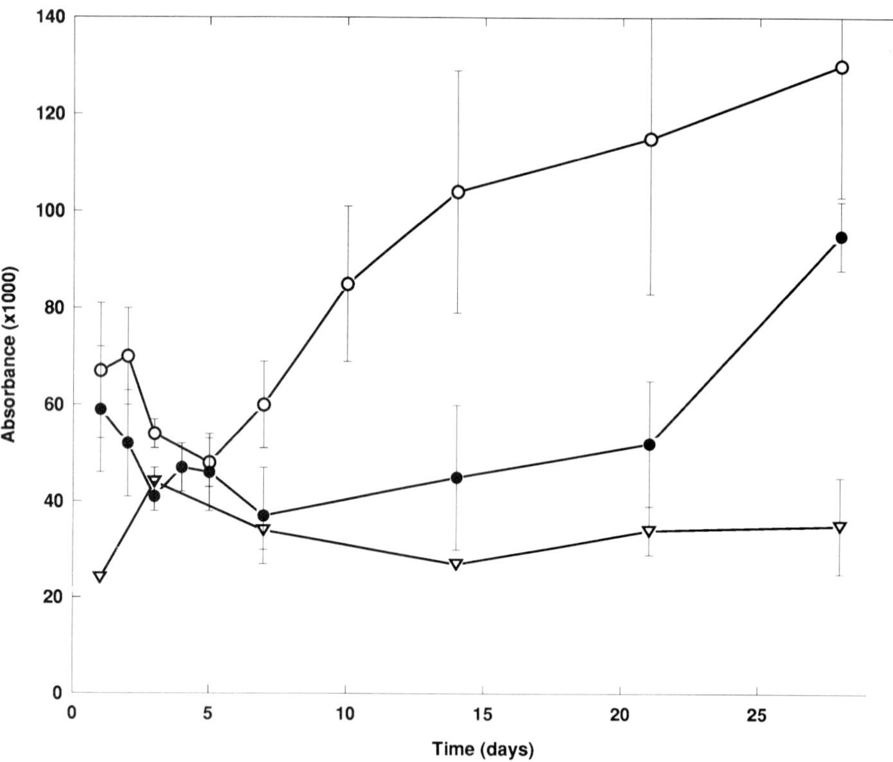

FIG. 5 Formazan absorbance (MTT signal) from (▽) blank, (●) low-density (4×10^5 cells/ml), and (○) high-density (4×10^6 cells/ml) PC-12 cell capsules (mean ± SD; $n = 3$ batchs). [From Sefton *et al.* (20).]

layer (~100 μm) of PC-12 cells intimately apposed to the interior aspect of the capsule appears viable and intact, as assessed by morphological criteria (Fig. 6) (40) similar to tumor spheroids (21). The cells comprising this layer are identical [by transmission electron microscopy (TEM); Fig. 7] to cells grown without encapsulation. In contrast, the cells closer to the center show distinct and progressive deterioration as a function of time *in vitro* and become necrotic. There is some increase in the thickness of the layer of viable, normal cells along the capsule periphery, presumably resulting from division of the most viable cells routinely found at this locus. It remains to be seen how long beyond 6 weeks such a "steady state" in viable cell behavior can be maintained. There was no evidence of cells breaching the

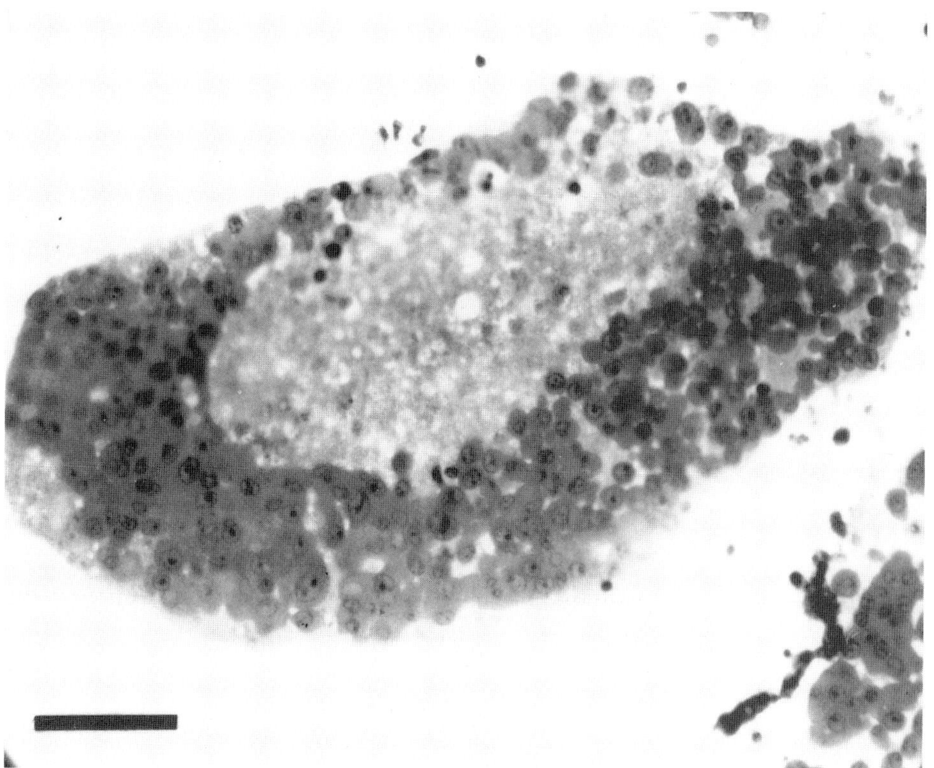

FIG. 6 Light micrograph of osmium tetroxide-stained encapsulated PC-12 cells 6 weeks after encapsulation in a large capsule (900-μm o.d.) at a density of 4×10^5 cells/ml, showing peripheral layer of viable cells under capsule wall (dissolved away) and central necrosis. Bar: 50 μm.

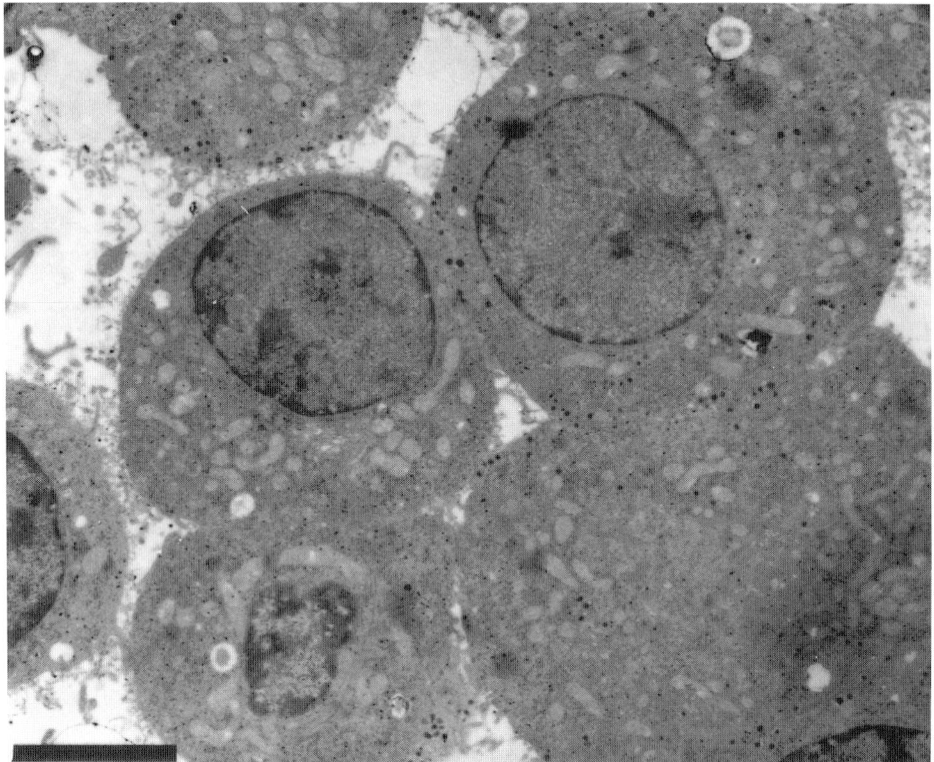

FIG. 7 Transmission electron micrograph of encapsulated PC-12 cells, 14 days after encapsulation. These cells were in the peripheral layer that surrounded the necrotic core. Bar: 4 μm.

capsule wall as a result of growth. Although a similar picture is seen for HepG2 cells in large capsules (10), early results from small (~400-μm o.d., 200-μm i.d.) capsules indicate that viable HepG2 cells fill the entire capsule interior without central necrosis. Because of the better use of internal volume we expect to concentrate our attention on these small capsules. Extrapolating from the tumor spheroid literature, we hypothesize that because of the physical restriction imposed by the capsule wall the rate of proliferation is less than it would be in unconfined (i.e., normal) culture with a corresponding increase in quiescent cells exhibiting functional differentiation leading to enhanced production of the target product (e.g., dopamine).

Conclusions

Microencapsulated cells hold considerable potential as controlled release devices for local or systemic delivery of bioactive molecules. The feasibility of encapsulating mammalian cells in polyacrylate membranes, using an interfacial precipitation process, has been demonstrated. The cells remained viable through the process of encapsulation as well as during subsequent long-term *in vitro* culture. A wide variety of cell phenotypes retained their differentiated functions in microcapsules, as determined morphologically and by secretion or tissue-specific bioactive molecules. Furthermore, secretion by the encapsulated cells was regulated in response to the appropriate physiological stimuli. Current research is focused on evaluating the performance of encapsulated cells *in vivo*.

Acknowledgments

Financial support was provided by the Natural Sciences and Engineering Research Council, the Medical Research Council, the Canadian Diabetes Association, and the Ontario Center for Material Research (OCMR).

References

1. D. F. Emerich, S. R. Winn, L. Christendon, M. A. Palmatier, F. T. Gentile, and P. R. Sanberg, A novel approach to neural transplantation in Parkinson's disease: Use of polymer encapsulated cell therapy. *Neurosci. Biobehav. Rev.* **16,** 437–447 (1992).
2. T. M. S. Chang, F. C. McIntosh, and S. G. Mason, Semipermeable aqueous microcapsules. I. Preparation and properties. *Can. J. Physiol. Pharmacol.* **44,** 115–128 (1966).
3. F. Lim and A. M. Sun, Microencapsulated islets as bioartificial endocrine pancreas. *Science* **210,** 908–910 (1980).
4. M. F. A. Goosen, G. M. O'Shea, H. Gharapetian, S. Chou, and A. M. Sun, Optimization of microencapsulation parameters: Semi-permeable capsules as a bioartificial pancreas. *Biotechnol. Bioeng.* **27,** 146–150 (1985).
5. T. Yoshioka, R. Hirano, T. Shioya, and M. Kaka, Encapsulation of mammalian cells with chitosan-CMC capsule. *Biotechnol. Bioeng.* **35,** 66–72 (1990).
6. S. Wen, Y. Xiaonan, and W. T. K. Stevenson, Microcapsules through polymer complexation. I. By complex coacervation of polymers containing a high charge density. *Biomaterials* **35,** 66–72 (1991).

7. B. Dupuy, H. Gin, C. Baquey, and D. Ducassou, In situ polymerization of a microencapsulating medium around living cells. *J. Biomed. Mater. Res.* **22,** 1061–1070 (1988).
8. M. V. Sefton and W. T. K. Stevenson, Microencapsulation of live animal cells using polyacrylates. *Adv. Polym. Sci.* **107,** 143–198 (1993).
9. H. Uludag and M. V. Sefton, Metabolic activity of CHO fibroblasts in HEMA-MMA microcapsules. *Biotechnol. Bioeng.* **39,** 672–678 (1992).
10. J. Babensee, U. De Boni, and M. V. Sefton, Morphological assessment of hepatoma cells (HepG2) microencapsulated in a HEMA-MMA copolymer with and without Matrigel®. *J. Biomed. Mater. Res.* **26,** 1401–1418 (1992).
11. H. Uludag and M. V. Sefton, Microencapsulated human hepatoma (HepG2) cells: In vitro growth and protein release. *J. Biomed. Mater. Res.* **27,** 1213–1224 (1993).
12. W. T. K. Stevenson, R. A. Evangelista, R. L. Broughton, and M. V. Sefton, Preparation and characterization of thermoplastic polymers from hydroxyethyl methacrylates. *J. Appl. Polym. Sci.* **34,** 65–83 (1987).
13. H. Uludag and M. V. Sefton, Metabolic activity and proliferation of CHO cells in hydroxyethyl methacrylate-methyl methacrylate (HEMA-MMA) microcapsules. *Cell Transplant.* **2,** 175–182 (1993).
14. H. K. Kleinman, M. L. McGarvey, J. R. Hassell, V. L. Star, F. B. Cannon, G. W. Laurie, and G. R. Martin, Basement membrane complexes with biological activity. *Biochemistry* **25,** 312–318 (1986).
15. C. A. Crooks, J. A. Douglas, R. L. Broughton, and M. V. Sefton, Microencapsulation of mammalian cells in a HEMA-MMA copolymer: Effect on capsule morphology and permeability. *J. Biomed. Mater. Res.* **24,** 1241–1262 (1990).
16. U. DeBoni, Chromatin and nuclear envelope of freeze-fractured, neuronal interphase nuclei, resolved by scanning microscopy. *Biol. Cell.* **63,** 1–8 (1988).
17. H. Uludag and M. V. Sefton, Colorimetric assay for cellular activity in microcapsules. *Biomaterials* **11,** 708–712 (1990).
18. I. N. Mefford, Application of high performance liquid chromatography with electrochemical detection to neurochemical analysis: Measurement of catecholamines, serotonin, and metabolites in the rat brain. *J. Neurol. Methods* **3,** 207–224 (1981).
19. H. Uludag and M. V. Sefton, unpublished observations, 1994.
20. M. V. Sefton, L. Kharlip, V. Howath, and T. Roberts, Controlled release using microencapsulated mammalian cells. *J. Controlled Release* **19,** 289–298 (1992).
21. R. M. Sutherland, Importance of critical metabolites and cellular interactions in the biology of microregions of tumors. *Cancer (Philadelphia)* **58,** 1668–1680 (1986).

[23] Hydrogel Applications for Encapsulated Cellular Transplants

Shelley R. Winn and Patrick A. Tresco

Introduction

Transplantation of polymer-encapsulated cells into discrete regions of the central nervous system (CNS) deficient in certain neuroactive compounds has successfully ameliorated experimental conditions modeling Parkinson's disease (1–3), Alzheimer's disease (4, 5), and pain syndromes (6). An encapsulated device typically consists of a polymer membrane (usually selectively permeable), cells/tissue that synthesize and secrete the desired compound(s), and in some cases an immobilization matrix. The cells encapsulated within the selectively permeable membrane are isolated from the host cellular and humoral immune factors. However, the pores or openings in the permeable membrane permit the bidirectional "passage" of neuroactive compounds by diffusion for functionality and low molecular weight solutes for maintenance of cell viability.

Hydrogel polymers can be broadly defined as materials, either synthetic or from natural sources, that swell in the presence of water and can be gelled by chemical interactions (7). Hydrogels represent a class of materials that may be useful as substitutes for soft tissues and offer potential in drug delivery technology (7). They have also been utilized as an immobilizing material within preformed thermoplastic hollow fibers or as a scaffold to which a semipermeable membrane can be attached, producing microcapsules by interfacial adsorption of polyelectrolytes (8). Our efforts have been focused on the application of biologically derived, water-soluble alginates in both micro- and macroencapsulation techniques. The polyelectrolyte-based microcapsules are transparent and offer an optimal geometry to facilitate diffusion (enhanced cell survival). They are, however, relatively fragile, difficult to retrieve, and may block the flow of cerebrospinal fluid when implanted within the ventricles (9). The thermoplastic macrocapsules, in contrast, are opaque, have less than optimal geometry for diffusion, but are mechanically more durable and easy to retrieve.

The use of an immobilizing matrix can serve several purposes. First, in cases of primary cells, for example, adult or neonatal-sourced tissues such as islets of Langerhans or adrenal chromaffin cells, the primary purpose of the matrices is to immobilize small tissue clusters and inhibit their reaggregation. In the absence of a matrix, considerable reaggregation of cell clusters has been observed, leading to the formation of larger clusters that develop central necrotic areas and a concomitant decrease in the production and release of neuroactive compound(s). Furthermore, the immobilization matrix can be used to prevent anchorage-dependent cells such as fibroblasts or endothelial cells colocalized with the aforementioned primary cell preparations, from overgrowing the device. In addition, immobilization matrices can be effective as a cellular scaffold for anchorage-dependent cells (10).

This chapter describes several methods in which hydrogels can be utilized in the fabrication of cell-loaded micro- and macrocapsules. Encapsulation methodology allows advantages that have previously been described (9, 11–13). In addition, however, site-specific transplantation of encapsulated cells has provided insights into the potential for humoral-mediated therapies in certain CNS disorders. Encapsulation has also provided a clean *in vitro* model system in which biochemical analyses, for example, catecholamine assays, can be carried out without the risk of contamination by aspirated cells during repeated manipulations.

Cellular Preparations

Cellular Isolation/Maintenance

Primary Cells

Adrenal chromaffin cells are isolated from either adult cows as described by Sagen *et al.* [21] in this volume) or adrenal glands of nonhuman primates (*Macaca fascicularis*) as described below. The adrenals are isolated from the circulatory system and perfused retrogradely *in vivo* with solutions of Ca^{2+}- and Mg^{2+}-free Hanks' balanced salt solution (CMF-HBSS; 4–8°C) for approximately 10 min. This solution is replaced with 50 ml of ambient HBSS containing 0.2% (v/v) collagenase (Worthington Biochemicals, Freehold, NJ) and 0.02% (v/v) DNase (Sigma, St. Louis, MO). Enzyme-perfused glands are incubated for approximately 12 min, washed with fresh CMF-HBSS, and the adrenal glands are excised. Following digestion, dissociated adrenal chromaffin cells are isolated as follows. The cortical tissue is removed after circumferentially cutting the glands, with the medullary portion from each gland pooled, and minced with a No.10 scalpel blade. Additional enzyme treatment, if necessary, is performed for 12–15 min. The cell suspension is spun through a density gradient and maintained as previously described (9). Chromaffin cell preparations are further purified by sequential plating techniques in Dulbecco's modified Eagle's medium (DMEM)–5% (v/v) fetal calf serum (FCS) to reduce the number of anchorage-dependent cells.

Cell Lines

PC-12 cells are cultivated either (a) on rat tail collagen-coated petri dishes in RPMI-1640 supplemented with 10% (v/v) heat-inactivated horse serum and 5% (v/v) fetal calf serum as previously described (14), or (b) in 500-ml spinner culture flasks at 80 rpm in a serum-free defined medium HL1 (Ventrex, Inc., Portland, ME). All cells are maintained at 37°C in a water-saturated, 5% CO_2 ambient air atmosphere.

For certain microcapsule experiments the fibroblast cell line rat1 N.8, genetically modified through infection with a retroviral vector containing the mouse nerve growth factor (NGF) cDNA, is used (15). The clonal line designated rat1 N.8-21 is maintained and prepared for encapsulation as previously described (9). [These cells were a generous gift from X. Breakefield and P. Short, Massachusetts General Hospital, Boston, MA).] The rat1 N.8-21 NGF-releasing clonal cell line was previously assayed by enzyme-linked immunosorbent assay (ELISA) and the measured release of NGF was 165 pg/10^5 cells/hr (9). The NGF released from rat1 N.8-21 cell-loaded microcapsules has been previously reported to be biologically active (9). More recently, a BHK cell line that secretes human NGF through a dihydrofolate reductase (DHFR)–metalloathionein I promoter has been used in encapsulation experiments whose levels of release are reported to be 100–300 times larger than the retrovirally mediated cell lines (5). This system maintains long-term expression for at least 25 passages *in vitro,* in the absence of continued methotrexate selection, and perhaps more significantly for 6 months *in vivo* (5).

Matrix Preparations

As an immobilization matrix two sources of alignate have been used (either KelcoGel LV and HV (Kelco, Clark, NJ) or UP alginate, Protan Biopolymer (Drammen, Norway)]. Powdered sodium alginates are brought to a 2.0% (w/v) solution by the addition of isotonic 0.85% (w/v) NaCl buffered to pH 7.3 with 5.0 m*M* *N*-2-hydroxyethylpiperazine-*N'*-2-ethanesulfonic acid (HEPES). Originally, the solutions were "sterilized" by a pasteurization process of ~80–90°C for 1 hr. The alginates can also be sterilized in Erlenmeyer flasks by an ethylene oxide gassing procedure and brought into sterile solution as described above.

For coseeding experiments, ready-to-use Matrigel (Collaborative Research, Lexington, MA), an extracellular matrix hydrogen containing predominantly laminin (7.0 mg/ml) and type IV collagen (0.25 mg/ml), is a liquid at 4–25°C and is utilized as a substratum for the anchorage-dependent fibroblasts. Matrigel is, however, known to contain various growth factors.

An alternative form of a temperature-responsive collagen, Vitrogen 100 (Celtrix Laboratories, Palo Alto, CA), is a purified, pepsin-solubilized bovine dermal collagen extract that is devoid of growth factors. Other possibilities include rat tail collagen extracts, gelatin shards, or porous gelatin microcarriers.

The hydrogels alginate and hyaluronic acid have also been utilized in the maintenance of two-dimensional cell cultures as coatings to inhibit attachment of anchorage-dependent cells and reaggregation of cellular clusters, respectively. Following standard polyornithine or polylysine (D- or L-form) treatment of tissue culture plates/flasks, a 0.5% alginate solution layered over the lysine is effective in preventing cell attachment and proliferation of fibroblasts and endothelial cells found in chromaffin cell preparations. Additionally, by including a 0.2% (w/v) hyaluronic acid solution within the tissue culture growth medium, one can effectively maintain a nominal aggregate size.

Microencapsulation Process

Adrenal chromaffin cells, independent of their source, are harvested by gentle trituration, followed by centrifugation at 100–200 *g*. If the size of the chromaffin cell clusters is generally between 40 and 100 μm, then centrifugation can be done between 50 and 80 *g*. If possible, try to avoid single cells, as they do not thrive in the encapsulation environment as well as do small cellular aggregates. The cells are resuspended in growth medium and counted with a hemacytometer after treatment with 1.0% (v/v) trypan blue to determine cell viability. [*Note:* If the cluster size impedes accurate cell counting, addition of a lysis solution, for example, 1.0% (v/v) Triton X, can be included prior to trypan blue exposure and a total nuclei count can be compared to percent viability.] One part of the cellular suspension is mixed with three parts of a 2.0% (w/v) solution of sodium alginate (KelcoGel HV; Kelco), resulting in desired densities ranging from 1 to 10 $\times$ 10^6 cells/ml. It is imperative that the volume of the pellet be accurately measured. Droplets of the cell/alginate suspension are formed by syringe-pump extrusion and gelled by immersion in a 1.0% (w/v) $CaCl_2$ [in 2.5 m*M* HEPES and 0.4% (w/v) NaCl, pH 7.4] solution. Syringe-pump extrusion (Fig. 1) utilizes a coaxial extrusion technique through an annular spinneret; the cell/matrix suspension at 0.5–2 ml/min flows through the center of the die (i.e., bore solution), while filtered nitrogen gas is passed through the outer tube, shearing off droplets from the spinneret assembly into a container of 1.0% $CaCl_2$. The filtered nitrogen stream is used in the range of 800–2000 ml/min. Sizes of the gelled beads can be controlled by altering the following: (a) the air

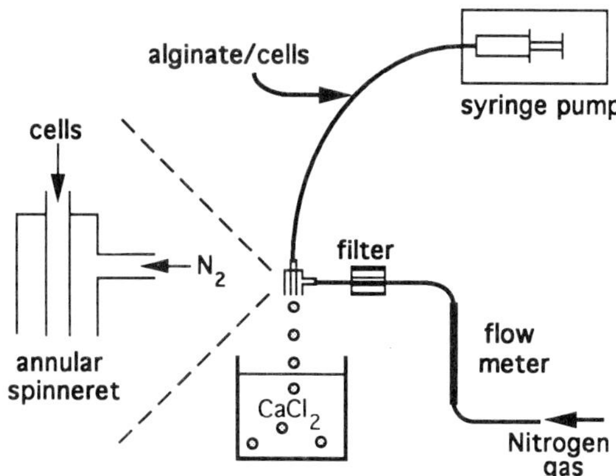

FIG. 1 Schematic illustration of the syringe pump extrusion technique. The alginate/cell suspension is extruded through the center of the annular spinneret at a desired flow rate while filtered nitrogen gas is passed through the outer tube, shearing off droplets from the spinneret assembly into a container of 1.0% $CaCl_2$.

flow rate, (b) the bore (cell/alginate) solution flow rate, (c) by manipulating the alginate viscosity, that is, by addition of multivalent cations, and (d) by changing the temperature of the bore solution (i.e., the cooling process causes an increase in alginate viscosity, thus smaller beads can be formed during fabrication).

Following a 4- to 7-minute gelation period, the cell-containing alginate beads are washed twice in 25 ml of 0.85% NaCl buffered to pH 7.4 with 2.5 m*M* HEPES, and once in 0.85% NaCl/HEPES, pH 7.8. A 0.05% (v/v) solution of poly-L-lysine in 0.85% NaCl, pH 7.8 (M_r 36,000; Sigma), is added to the gelled alginate beads and mixed for 6 min. Washes of 0.85% NaCl/HEPES, pH 7.0, are followed by immersion in 0.15% (w/v) sodium alginate in 0.85% NaCl/HEPES, pH 7.0, for 5 min. Following a wash in NaCl/HEPES, pH 7.4, the cell-containing microcapsules are additionally laminated, if desired, with the lysine/alginate solutions (see option designated by dashed lines in Fig. 2). The resulting cell-loaded microcapsules are washed in NaCl/HEPES, pH 7.4, prior to exposure of the beads to 25 ml of 50 m*M* sodium citrate for 5 min in order to reliquefy the entrapped alginate core. The reliquefication process can be eliminated if added rigidity of the hydrogel core is desired ("± citrate" in Fig. 2). The microencapsulated cell-containing beads are washed twice in 0.85% NaCl/HEPES, pH 7.4, and twice in the preferred maintenance medium before being placed in a water-saturated CO_2 incubator at 37°C. The entire procedure is outlined in Fig. 2. Approximately 100 cell-loaded microcapsules/well are transferred into a 24-multiwell tissue

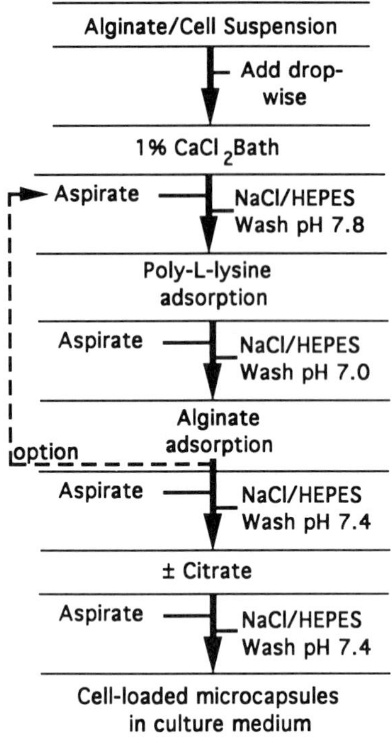

FIG. 2 Flow diagram outlining the microencapsulation process. The polyelectrolyes poly-L-lysine and alginate are sequentially adsorbed (interfacial adsorption) onto the alginate spheres following immersion in the 1.0% $CaCl_2$ bath. Details are outlined in text.

culture plate (Falcon 3047; Becton Dickinson, Paramus, NJ) for maintenance in culture medium and subsequent *in vitro* analysis.

Identical techniques have been utilized to form microcapsules containing the rodent-derived tumor cell line PC-12 (2). In this example, PC-12 cells are collected and mechanically broken up by passage through a glass-fired Pasteur pipette to ensure small cell clusters. The PC-12 cells are then seeded at densities between 5 and 50 × 10^6 cells/ml. The transparent nature of the microcapsules allows visual inspection and continual observation(s) after the microencapsulation process is complete (see Fig. 3A).

Coseeding

Under the coseeded conditions, 2 × 10^6 rat1 N.8-21 cells and 3 × 10^6 chromaffin cells mixed in 150 μl of Matrigel (Collaborative Research) are

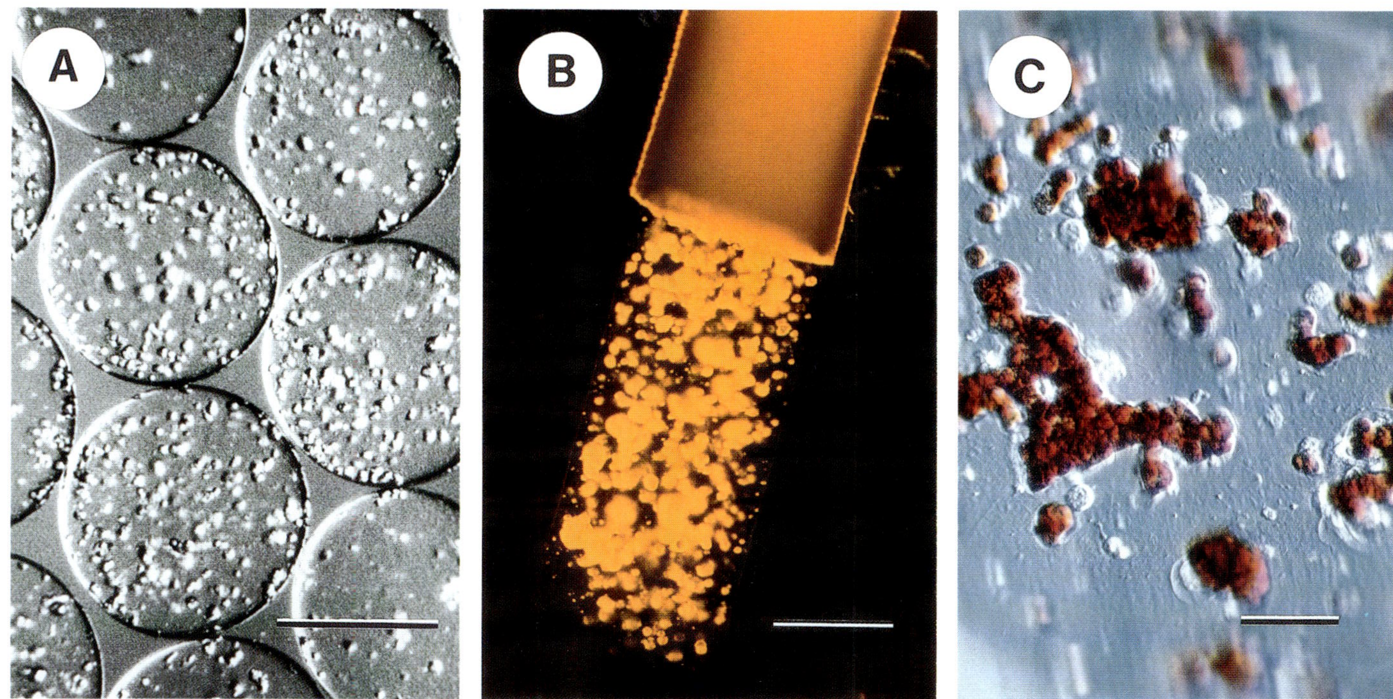

Fig. 3 Light micrographs of chromaffin cell-loaded capsules following the encapsulation procedure. (A) Phase-contrast microscopy of cell-loaded microcapsules shows the uniform size and cell distribution. (B) Phase-contrast microscopy of a cell-loaded macrocapsule in which the alginate core has been partially extruded to visualize the cellular distribution and viability. (C) A neutral red-stained microcapsule shows that the majority of encapsulated cells take up the stain. Bars: (A and B) 500 μm; (C) 50 μm.

suspended in 450 μl of 2% (w/v) isotonic sodium alginate. Matrigel is utilized as a substratum for the fibroblasts and gelation occurs with increasing temperature (e.g., 25–30°C); therefore, it is essential to maintain the temperature at or near 10–15°C. Anchorage-dependent cells, such as fibroblasts, astrocytes, and endothelium, do not survive well in the presence of alginate alone. The cell-loaded microcapsules are fabricated by syringe-pump extrusion as described above. As before, approximately 100 cell-loaded microcapsules are placed in individual wells of a 24-multiwell tissue culture plate.

Macroencapsulation

The following methodologies concerning macroencapsulation involve the use of sterile, preformed (i.e., prespun), hollow fibers fabricated by phase inversion using a dry-jet wet spinning technique (16). Cell-loaded macrocapsules are sealed by a heat pinch technique and subsequently the extremities can be dipped into a warm poly(acrylonitrile-co-vinyl chloride) (PAN–PVC) solution (in dimethyl sulfoxide).

Chromaffin cells are collected, pelleted by gentle centrifugation, and assessed for cell viability by counting with a hemacytometer after exposure to trypan blue. Once the cell number has been calculated, cells are again concentrated and the pellet suspended in the appropriate volume of 2.0% (w/v) physiological alginate to arrive at a desired concentration. The chromaffin cell/alginate suspension can be infused into sterile segments, for example, 8-cm long PAN–PVC preformed hollow fibers. The PAN–PVC hollow fibers in the present example are immunoisolatory, that is, they exclude the cytotoxic effect of antibody (IgG)-mediated complement lysis; see Cytotoxicity Assay (below).

Individual capsules 10 ($\pm$1) mm in length are fabricated containing chromaffin cells from a hollow fiber by a pinch and heat-sealing method. Approximately 50 μl of the cell suspension is drawn into an appropriately gauged intravenous (iv) catheter attached to a 100-μl Hamilton microsyringe. A tight friction fit can be made between the catheter tip and the PAN–PVC hollow fiber. Once the cell suspension has been infused into the fiber and approaches the distal end, a pinch is made with a pair of fine-tipped forceps perpendicular to the long axis of the hollow fiber, being careful not to allow the alginate/cell suspension to contact the washing bath. Approximately 2 mm from the point at which the forceps are in contact with the hollow fiber, heat is applied until the fiber bends at an angle 40–50° from its origin. At this point the fiber is pulled off of the catheter tip, pinched, and heat is applied on the opposite end as described. Be careful not to allow the fiber to dry during the pinch/heat seal process. After heat sealing both ends, the fiber is immersed in the same 1.0% $CaCl_2$ solution previously described for 4–5 min to form a gel.

Following the gelation period the cell-loaded fiber is maintained and washed in HBSS/HEPES between the steps of the cutting-down process. Measure the appropriate length and begin the cutting-down process by pinching and heating the fiber 10 mm from the original heat seal. After the 40–50° bend, immerse the fiber in HBSS, lift it out, and rotate the fiber 180°. Heat is applied to the other side of the forceps until the fiber bends again, reapproaching the original orientation of the fiber, that is, straight along the long axis. The heat-sealed portion should be transparent on visualization. Once visualized, the heat seal should be cut centrally with a pair of microscissors. For a secondary seal, and as a method for smoothing out the surface around the heat seal, the ends can be dipped into a warm polymer solution and rinsed in HBSS. Control capsules can be fabricated in an identical manner, with the exception of infusing matrix alone into the hollow fiber.

Coseeding

Cells of choice, for example, adrenal chromaffin and the nerve growth factor (NGF)-releasing fibroblast cell line rat1 N.8-21, or other cell lines secreting a growth/neurotrophic factor, can likewise be macroencapsulated; the mixing ratios are essentially as described in the microcapsule coseeding section and the procedure follows that outlined above for macrocapsule monoseeding.

Assessment

Several techniques are described that have been used to assess both the *in vitro* and *in vivo* performance of encapsulated cells for CNS implantation.

In Vitro Evaluation

Morphological

Immediately following the encapsulation process, visual inspection of the cellular density and distribution can be accomplished directly through the transparent microcapsules (Fig. 3A), and by extruding the alginate core from a macrocapsule (Fig. 3B). Included in this analysis can be a number of vital dyes; 0.2% (v/v) trypan blue for all cell types and, specifically for chromaffin cells, 1.0% (v/v) neutral red (Fig. 3C). Neutral red is a pH indicator that has an affinity for the highly acidic storage granules in adrenal chromaffin cells. In addition to viability, neutral red is also a predictor of chromaffin cell purity following adrenal medullary harvest, sequential platings, and subsequently encapsulation. Additionally, the combination of fluorescein diacetate and propidium iodide can be used to evaluate cells that are alive (green, fluorescein diacetate positive) and dead (red, propidium iodide-positive nuclei). Working solutions of the stains are prepared as previously described (17), the cellular preparations are exposed to the fluorescein diacetate–propidium iodide for 5–10 min, and viability is assessed by fluorescence microscopy. With cell-loaded macrocapsules, provided there is access to the alginate core, a method is available to reacquire the cellular suspension. Because gelation results from cross-linking by divalent Ca^{2+}, reliquefication can occur by the addition of a chelator, 50 m*M* sodium citrate. Use of this method requires a cell suspension for an accurate assessment of viability after the encapsulation procedure.

Other morphological methods employed in the analyses of cell-loaded capsules involve routine histochemical processes that employ dehydration, embedding, sectioning, and staining. These methods include paraffin embedding, the glycol methacrylate (GMA)-embedding technique (Fig. 4A) (1), and embedding in L. R. White or Spurr's low-viscosity resin (EMS, Fort Washington, PA) for ultrastructural observations (18). Limitations of the aforementioned techniques result from the considerable investment in time and resources and the fact that the resulting analyses is two dimensional; however, immunolabeling methods can be employed with paraffin and GMA. Ultrastructural observations are critical in deciphering cellular health, cell-to-cell and cell–matrix interactions, and the distribution of storage granules in secretory cells (Fig. 4B). When, instead of immobilizing cells, a matrix is utilized in macrocapsules to provide a scaffold for cells, the proper choice of techniques is essential. The techniques ultimately used should include a combination of acute and embedded morphological analyses.

Cytotoxicity Assay

Capsule integrity, that is, maintenance of immunoisolation, has been evaluated *in vitro* on PC-12 cell-loaded capsules, both in microcapsules as previously described (2) with guinea pig antiserum (19), and in macrocapsules by a cytotoxic challenge as follows. A paradigm/matrix was set up to assess the capability of the selectively permeable membrane to exclude the cytotoxic effect of antibody (IgG)-mediated complement lysis (see Table I). The antiserum against PC-12 cells was prepared in rabbits against the rat cell surface moiety Thy 1.1 (Accurate, Inc., Westbury, NY). Titers of the antiserum against unencapsulated PC-12 cells were determined and found to be cytolytic (in the presence of rabbit complement, 1 : 20; Pel Freez, Freez, Brown Deer, WI) in the range of 1 : 50–1 : 500. For the cytotoxic challenge, antiserum at 1 : 50 was left in multiwell plates under the various conditions (Table I) for 72 hr. Thereafter, a 2- to 3-hr incubation of fresh complement was added to

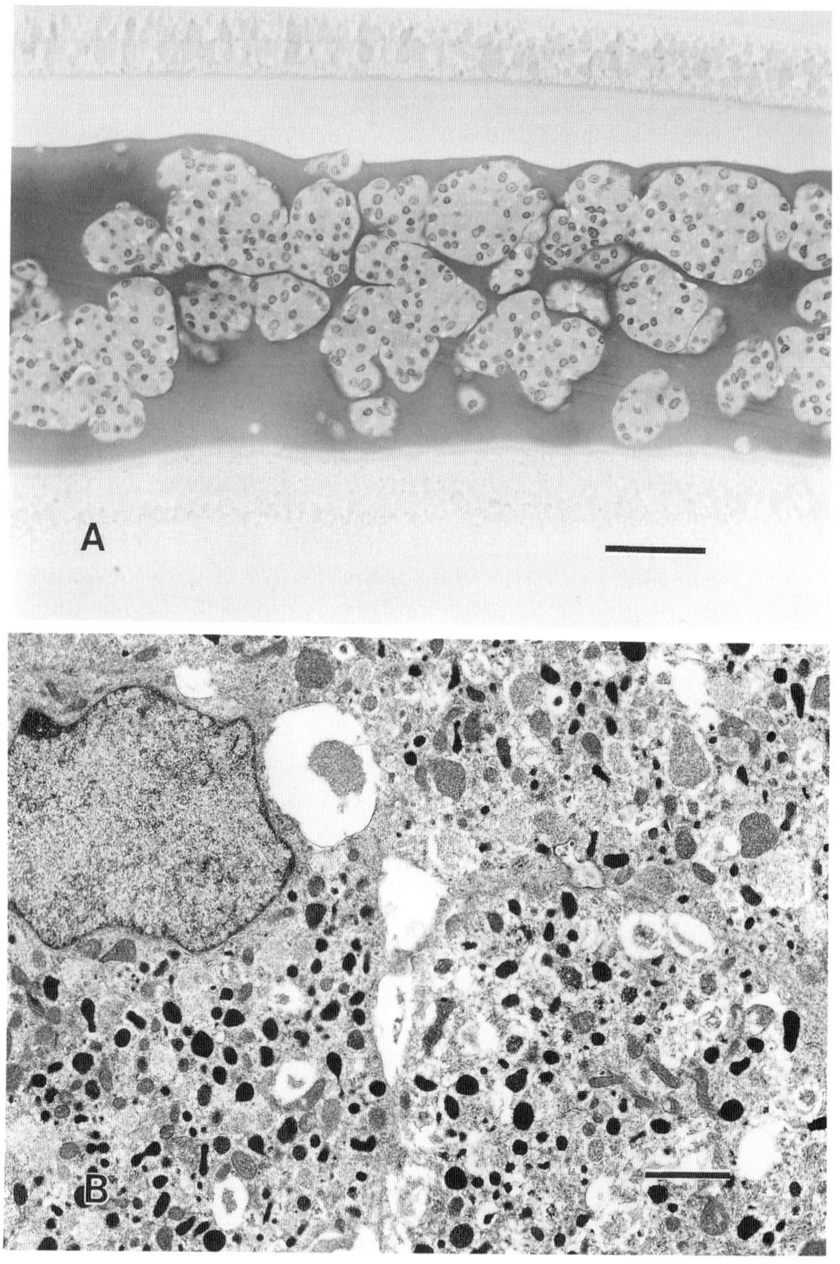

FIG. 4 Chromaffin cell-loaded macrocapsules processed for (A) GMA-embedded technique and stained with hematoxylin–eosin after 6 weeks in rat striatum, showing abundant viable cells. (B) A transmission electron micrograph shows the abundance of electron-dense secretory granules after 8 weeks *in vitro*. Bars: (A) 100 μm; (B) 2 μm.

TABLE I Antibody/Complement Screening Assay[a]

Condition	Cells	Antibody/medium	Complement/medium	Death (%)
Encapsulated	PC-12	Medium	Medium	<10
	PC-12	Antibody	Medium	<10
	PC-12	Medium	Complement	<10
	PC-12	Antibody	Complement	<10
Damaged capsules	PC-12	Antibody	Medium	<10
	PC-12	Antibody	Complement	100
Unencapsulated	PC-12	Medium	Complement	<10
	PC-12	Antibody	Medium	<10
	PC-12	Antibody	Complement	100

[a] n = at least three cell-loaded capsules/condition.

each well after washing, and the conditions were scored on the basis of percentage killed. The results were visualized by fluorescent microscopy, using the double-labeled fluorescein diacetate–propidium iodide technique as described above. As can be observed in Table I, in the presence of antibody and complement, the capsular membrane prevented antibody-mediated complement lysis, while complete killing (100%) was observed in cases of damaged capsules or with unencapsulated conditions.

Neurochemical

Acute lysates from 1×10^6 chromaffin cells are generally analyzed by high-performance liquid chromatography with electrochemical detection (LCEC) immediately after encapsulation by immersion in 1 ml of hypotonic 0.1 *N* perchloric acid to determine the cellular contents of catecholamines and their metabolites. Thus, by extrapolating the expected cellular content per capsule, and knowing what the expected percentage of release should be under potassium-evoked conditions, an estimation of catecholamine release can thus be predicted. Additionally, lysate samples can be collected for enkephalin analyses by immersion in hypotonic 1 *N* acetic acid.

Cell loaded capsules are routinely qualified by analysis of static constitutive and evoked release *in vitro* prior to implantation. Experience has proved this to be a good estimate as to the quantities of releasable neuroactive compounds. Constitutive release is measured for either 15 or 30 min in HBSS/HEPES, pH 7.3–7.4, with 10 μM free ascorbate [HBSS H1387 (Sigma) supplemented with 10 mM HEPES]. For eliciting an evokable response from chromaffin cells, the HBSS/HEPES can be spiked with the cholinergic agonist nicotine (20 μM tartrate (RBI, Natick, MA) or the potassium concentration can be elevated to 56 mM. For *in vitro* catecholamine analyses over time, the assay medium from individual capsules (or a group of microcapsules) was assayed by LCEC at selected times, for example, 3, 28, and 56 days postencapsulation (Fig. 5). Free-floating capsules were washed twice for 10 min with 1 ml of HBSS containing 10 μM free ascorbate to remove/wash out residual culture medium. Basal (constitutive release) samples were analyzed following a 15-min incubation in HBSS/HEPES, followed by a 15-min assay period in the HBSS/HEPES in which the potassium concentration has been elevated to 56 mM to evoke chemical depolarization. As an alternative to high potassium, a cholinergic receptor agonist such as nicotine at 20–63 μM can be utilized (11). Figure 5 reveals the concentrations of norepinephrine, epinephrine, and dopamine released from chromaffin cell-loaded devices maintained *in vitro* in the presence of HL1 medium after 3, 28, and 56 days. At selected times, a lysate of the capsule content can be performed in order to determine the relative percentage release under constitutive and evoked release compared to total catecholamine stores.

Additional *in vitro* analyses of chromaffin cell-loaded devices also have been characterized utilizing a perifusion apparatus (1). A specific number of microcapsules (e.g., 20) or a macrocapsule can be placed inside a chamber containing a 50- to 70-μl volume that is perfused at a constant flow rate. We typically have used a rate of 5 μl/min (Carnegie Medicin 100, Stockholm, Sweden) collected 50-μl perfusate volumes (i.e., 10 min) in 0.5-ml microfuge tubes containing 5 μl of 1.1 N perchloric acid on a fraction collector, and immediately assayed for catecholamines by LCEC. Following three or four constitutive fraction collections, the perfusate can be manipulated to contain a variety of secretagogues (e.g., 56 mM potassium, 20 μM nicotine, 50 μM acetylcholine, 50 μM veratridine). After an additional three or four fractions are collected, the perfusate can be returned to its original condition, collected, assayed for catecholamines, and the release characteristics plotted similar to that previously reported (1).

All samples for LCEC analyses were protected from oxidation by the rapid addition of a citrate-reducing acidified buffer, prepared and assayed according to Winn *et al.* (20) or Lavoie *et al.* (21). The concentrations of the catecholamines L-dopa, dopamine, norepinephrine, and epinephrine plus the dopamine metabolites DOPAC and HVA were quantified by comparing the peak heights of serially diluted standards run with each assay.

In Vivo Evaluation

Several animal model systems have been utilized to assess constitutive and secretagogue-induced release of neuroactive components from encapsulated cellular transplants. Table II outlines some of the model systems utilized in determining the potential efficacy associated with site-specific delivery of

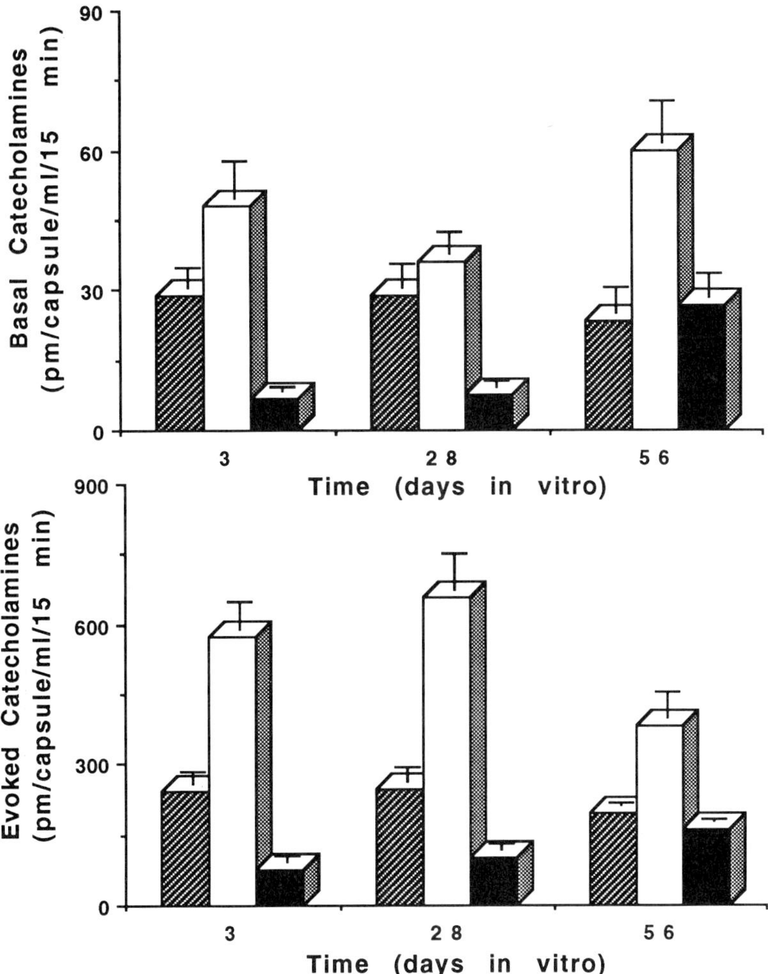

FIG. 5 Catecholamine release measured from static incubations over time of chromaffin cell-loaded macrocapsules maintained in serum-free HL1 medium *in vitro*. Basal catecholamines (constitutive release) are calculated and graphed (in pmol/capsule/15 min) over time from repeated analysis of the same capsules (top). Catecholamines evoked by chemical depolarization of 56 m*M* potassium in the sample medium are plotted over time (bottom). Striped bars, norepinephrine; open bars, epinephrine; black bars, dopamine.

TABLE II Encapsulation in Neurodegeneration[a]

Model system	Lesion type[b]	Animal	Ref.[c]
Parkinson's	6-OHDA	Rodent	1–3
	MPTP	NH primate	22
Alzheimer's	Aspirative	Rodent	4, 5
	Aspirative	NH primate	ip*
Huntington's	Excitotoxins	Rodent	ip
	Excitotoxins	NH primate	ip
Acute pain	NA	Rodent	6
Chronic pain	Ligation	Rodent	ip

[a] NH primate, nonhuman primate.
[b] 6-OHDA, 6-hydroxydopamine; MPTP, 1-methyl-4-phenyl-1,2,3,6-tetrahydropyridine.
[c] ip, Studies currently in progress.

neuroactive molecules produced by the encapsulated cells that diffuse through the membrane and into the surrounding host environment. Microcapsules loaded with bovine adrenal chromaffin cells (1) and PC-12 cells (2), as well as PC-12 cell-loaded macrocapsules (3), have been shown to be effective at alleviating drug-induced asymmetries associated with a unilateral dopamine deficiency in the striatum of rats following striatal transplantation. Similar observations have resulted after striatal implants of PC-12 cell-loaded devices in the unilateral MPTP-lesioned nonhuman primate model system (22).

Additional model systems in which the delivery of growth factors (e.g., NGF) (4, 5) has been assessed for efficacy include lesioned paradigms of Alzheimer's disease and Huntington's disease. Sagen and co-workers have also utilized xenografts of encapsulated chromaffin cells implanted in the subarachnoid space to reduce pain as assessed by acute pain models in rodents at 3 months (6) and up to 6 months (unpublished results, Sagen and Winn, 1993). Table II also indicates several studies that are ongoing as a means of evaluating encapsulated cell therapy in primate models. The ability to maintain long-term (i.e., at least 6-month) viable xenografts in the absence of host immunosuppression is an especially attractive feature of the encapsulated transplants.

Concluding Remarks

This chapter has described methods for the fabrication of cell-loaded micro- and macroencapsulation devices. Each encapsulation technique has advantages and disadvantages; nevertheless, each offers a means for evaluating therapies in chronic neurological disorders that may benefit from site-specific sustained release of neuroactive factors. Encapsulation also provides a useful *in vitro* model system in which neurochemical analyses can be performed without contamination by aspirated cells during repeated manipulations. Neural transplantation of encapsulated cells releasing growth factors may have enormous potential in certain chronic neurodegenerative states by reducing the rate of progression and/or stimulating regeneration of damaged nervous tissue. It is important to point out, however, that issues concerning safety and efficacy must be adequately addressed prior to large-scale human applications.

Acknowledgments

The authors thank their colleagues at CytoTherapeutics (CTI) and Brown University for input and assistance. Special thanks to Faith Kaplan at CTI for performing the cytotoxicity assay. Furthermore, much of this work would not have been possible without the guidance and support of Dr. Patrick Aebischer and CTI.

References

1. P. Aebischer, P. A. Tresco, J. Sagen, and S. R. Winn, *Brain Res.* **560,** 43 (1991).
2. S. R. Winn, P. A. Tresco, B. Zielinski, L. A. Greene, C. B. Jaeger, and P. Aebischer, *Exp. Neurol.* **113,** 322 (1991).
3. P. A. Tresco, S. R. Winn, S. Tan, C. B. Jaeger, L. A. Greene, and P. Aebischer, *Cell Transplant.* **1,** 255 (1992).
4. D. Hoffman, X. O. Breakefield, M. P. Short, and P. Aebischer, *Exp. Neurol.* **122,** 100 (1993).
5. S. R. Winn, J. P. Hammang, D. F. Emerich, A. Lee, R. D. Palmiter, and E. E. Baetge, *Proc. Natl. Acad. Sci. U.S.A.* **91,** 2324–2328 (1994).
6. J. Sagen, H. Wang, P. A. Tresco, and P. Aebischer, *J. Neurosci.* **13**(6), 2415 (1993).
7. N. A. Peppas, *in* "Hydrogels in Medicine and Pharmacy" (N. A. Peppas, ed.), Chapter 1. CRC Press, Boca Raton, FL, 1987.
8. F. Lim and A. M. Sun, *Science* **210,** 908 (1980).
9. P. Aebischer, M. Goddard, and P. A. Tresco, *in* "Fundamentals of Animal Cell Encapsulation and Immobilization" (M. F. A. Goosen, ed.), p. 197. CRC Press, Boca Raton, FL, 1993.
10. S. R. Winn, P. A. Tresco, B. Zielinski, J. Sagen, and P. Aebischer, *J. Neurol. Transplant. Plast.* **3**(2-3), 115 (1992).
11. P. A. Tresco, S. R. Winn, and P. Aebischer, *Trans. Am. Soc. Artif. Intern. Organs* **38,** 17 (1992).
12. D. F. Emerich, S. R. Winn, L. Christenson, M. A. Palmiter, F. T. Gentile, and P. R. Sanberg, *Neurosci. Biobehav. Rev.* **16,** 437 (1992).

13. L. Christenson, K. E. Dionne, and M. J. Lysaght, *in* "Fundamentals of Animal Cell Encapsulation and Immobilization" (M. F. A. Goosen, ed.), p. 7. CRC Press, Boca Raton, FL, 1993.
14. L. A. Greene and A. S. Tischler, *Proc. Natl. Acad. Sci. U.S.A.* **73,** 2424 (1976).
15. M. P. Short, M. B. Rosenberg, Z. D. Ezzedine, F. H. Gage, T. Friedmann, and X. O. Breakefield, *Dev. Neurosci.* **12,** 34 (1990).
16. I. Cabasso, *in* "Kirk-Othmer Encyclopedia of Chemical Technology" (M. Grayson and D. Eckroth, eds.), 3rd ed., Vol. 12, p. 492. Wiley, New York, 1980.
17. K. H. Jones and J. A. Senft, *J. Histochem. Cytochem.* **33,** 77 (1985).
18. S. R. Winn, P. Aebischer, and P. M. Galletti, *J. Biomed. Mater. Res.* **23,** 31 (1989).
19. V. H. Lee, L. A. Greene, and M. L. Shelanski, *Neuroscience* **5,** 1979 (1980).
20. S. R. Winn, L. Wahlberg, P. A. Tresco, and P. Aebischer, *Exp. Neurol.* **105,** 244 (1989).
21. M. Lavoie, M. Palmatier, F. T. Gentile, F. A. Kaplan, D. M. Fiore, T. F. Hazlett, W. J. Bell, and T. R. Flanagan, *Cell Transplant.* **2,** 163 (1993).
22. P. Aebischer, M. Goddard, R. Timpson, A. Signore, A. Beauregard-Young, and C. Rampone, *Soc. Neurosci. Abstr.* **16,** 963 (1990).

[24] Tests for Validating the Safety of Encapsulated Xenografts

T. R. Flanagan, B. Frydel, B. Tente, M. Lavoie, E. Doherty, D. Rein, D. F. Emerich, and S. R. Winn

Introduction

Xenografts are the most demanding form of cellular transplants because they directly confront the host immune system. At the same time there are clear advantages to working with cells from a well-characterized xenogeneic source, provided some method of immunoisolation or host immune modulation is available. This chapter provides suggestions for validating reproducible and safe devices for therapeutic applications of xenogeneic cells in polymer-encapsulated transplant studies.

Xenogeneic Cells in Transplants

Selecting a source of cells for a transplant study depends on the intended function of those cells. When clinical transplant strategies restrict cells to allogeneic sources (i.e., human donors), shortages can be expected. For example, it has been estimated that fetal catecholaminergic cell transplants for Parkinson's disease may require tissue from as many as 10 to 15 fetuses per treated patient (4). Provided an alternative cell source performed the intended transplant function, and survived once implanted for extended periods, xenogeneic cells are readily available from both established cell lines and primary cultures. Cell lines are typically well characterized and free of adventitious agents, but without effective immunoisolation they do not survive following cross-species transplantation. After encapsulation in an immunoisolatory device, identical lots of xenogeneic cells can be characterized in animal model systems leading to human applications.

This chapter describes our use of polyacrylonitrile–polyvinylchloride (PAN–PVC) thermoplastic hollow fiber immunoisolation devices [as described elsewhere; see Christenson *et al.* (7), Aebischer *et al.* (2), and [23] in this volume] with primary cultures of xenogeneic cells isolated from bovine sources or pheochromocytoma (PC-12) cells from a rat adrenomedullary tumor. Although immunosuppression (i.e., with cyclosporin A) may provide a measure of protection for transplanted xenogeneic cells (14, 24) our discussion is limited to the alternative strategy of immunoisolation.

Methods in Neurosciences, Volume 21

Tests for Uniformity of Immunoisolation Devices

Immunoisolation is critical for long-term xenograft survival. Key parameters for successful device performance include the ability to reliably reproduce (a) the membrane structure (i.e., physical dimensions), (b) the membrane characterizations (e.g., selective permeability and structural integrity), and (c) biological compatibility of the device within a specified implant site. Tests and representative results for each of these features are described below.

Membrane Structure

The physical characteristics of an immunoisolation device must permit the bidirectional diffusion of molecules necessary to support the survival of the encapsulated cells. These characteristics should be constant across the entire surface of the device, both radially and axially. One test to confirm uniformity in dimensions involves measuring the device with a calibrated ocular micrometer. Hollow fiber immunoisolation devices, for example, are easily transected with a razor blade, placed on a staging, illuminated with fiber optic lighting, and visually or electronically scanned. For documentation purposes, the use of video scanner systems is suggested [e.g., a compound microscope carrying a video camera and using Oracle video scalar software (Javelin Electronics) to display and to print the analysis]. The results of a video scanner analysis performed on a hollow fiber produced within our laboratories are shown in Fig. 1. Readily measureable physical features of the hollow fiber include the inner diameter, the wall thickness, the concentricity and the roundness of the fiber, the surface texture and color, and the constancy of all of these features along the length of the fiber. Morphological specifications will depend on the devices intended for use and require extensive testing to establish acceptable criteria.

A more detailed surface analysis can be obtained with scanning electron microscopy (SEM). Surface topography of an implanted device is an important variable for host tissue responses (19). Several hollow fiber surface morphologies are demonstrated in Fig. 2. Representative hollow fiber segments were trimmed with a razor blade, mounted on a sample stage with commercially available cyanoacrylate, and scanned with an AmRay SEM.

Membrane Characterizations

Characterization of hollow fiber immunoisolation devices should include data on the permselectivity of the barrier membrane. Measures of permselectivity

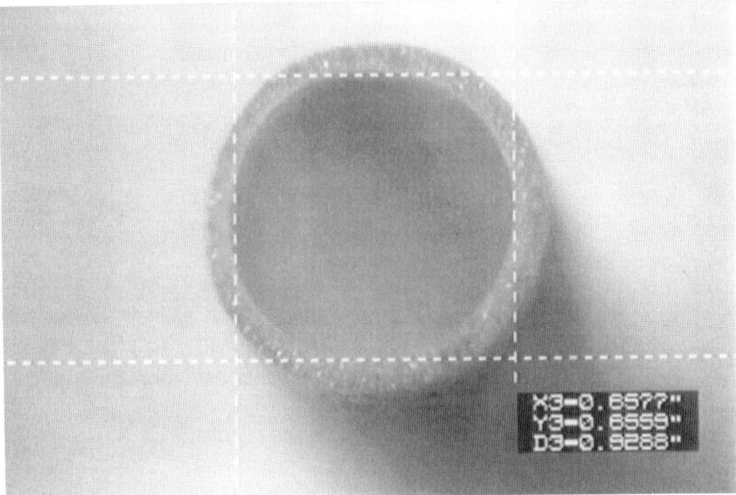

FIG. 1 Video scanner analysis of a representative hollow fiber. Inner diameter, outer diameter, and membrane thickness are all obtained by direct measurement. Concentricity is measured by comparing membrane thickness at four sites. The roundness of the hollow fiber may be measured by constructing a rectangle, each side of which is tangent to the inner surface of a fiber cross-section.

will provide information about the size of molecules that will pass the membrane and the rate that material can pass.

Diffusive tests are used to characterize the membrane molecular weight cutoff (MWCO). Hollow fiber segments mounted in a diffusion chamber can be loaded with solutions containing a known amount of material of a specified molecular weight. The diffusate is then periodically sampled, and the length of time required for molecules of differing size to reach equilibrium across the membrane can be determined. Detector systems include spectrophotometry (when a pure substance is being tested), size exclusion fast protein liquid chromatography with ultraviolet (UV) detection (when a mixture of substances is being tested), enzyme-linked immunosorbent assay (ELISA; when a single substance is being tested in the presence of many other substances), or radioimmunoassay (RIA). The rate of diffusive release of marker molecules from intact and from punctured membranes should be compared over time.

When characterizing membrane permeability with a mixture of molecular weight markers, uniform results can be achieved if dextrans are used in place of proteins. Dextran solutions are free from the intermolecular charges and hydrophobicity interactions that often complicate concentrated protein solu-

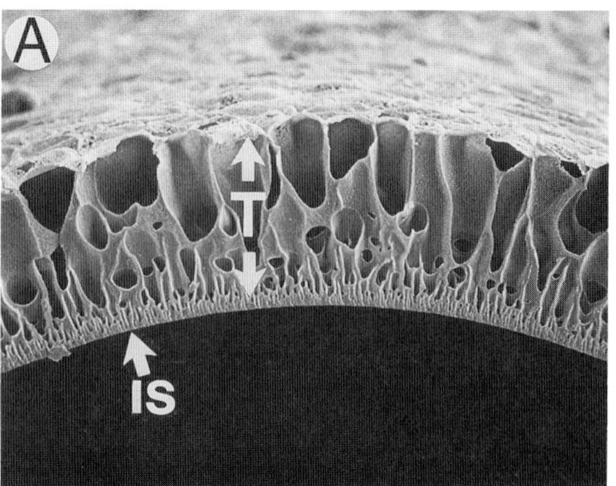
A
T
IS

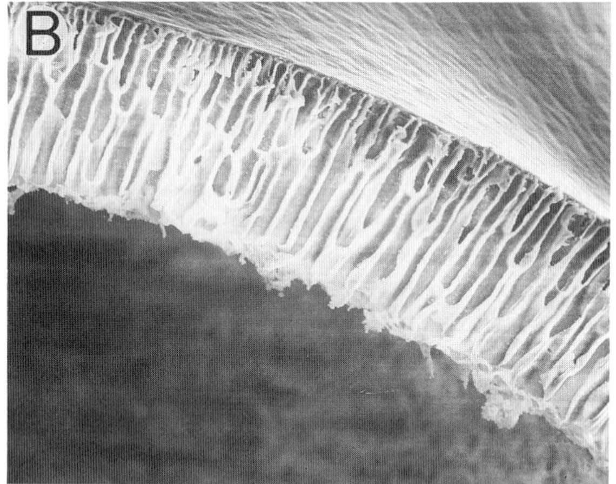
B

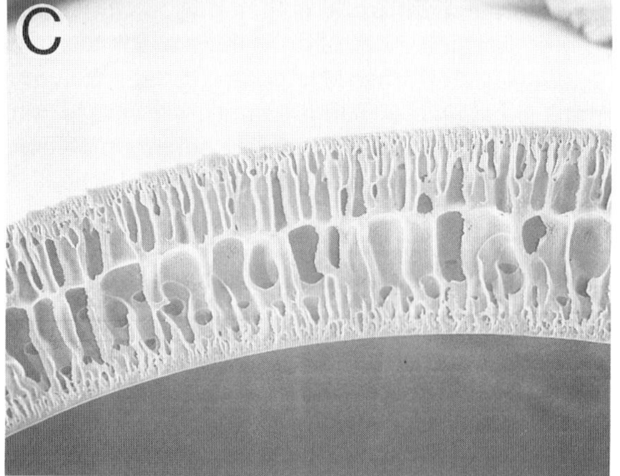
C

tions. Filtrate from a dilute dextran solution ultrafiltrated through fibers mounted in a chamber is periodically sampled and subjected to gel permeation chromatography (16). The membrane MWCO is defined as the molecular weight of the smallest dextran species that displays a log order reduction in transmembrane transport. Stated another way, if only 10% of the molecules of a given size class is able to pass through the membrane, then that membrane is designated as impermeable to that size molecule. Each dextran size class is assigned a rejection coefficient (unity minus the fractional portion of the test molecule solution that penetrates the membrane). A plot of the rejection coefficient against dextran size provides the molecular weight permselectivity of a membrane. Representative data are shown in Fig. 3. Note, however, that MWCO data obtained with dextran tracers will be shifted significantly toward higher masses relative to MWCO data obtained with protein standards.

The hydraulic permeability (HP) of the membrane is determined by the amount of water that is forced through a membrane under a defined set of convective conditions. Such measures are indicative of "porosity," or the density of molecular passages through the membrane. This measure should not be confused with MWCO, which is a measure of aggregate pore size that defines the permselectivity (see above). This HP parameter is expressed in terms of the total surface area of the membrane that was tested (ml of perfusate/min/mmHg pressure/m^2 of surface area tested). Although some membranes may have high MWCO and high HIP values (e.g., membranes with very large pores), other membranes may have low MWCO values and still have high HP values (e.g., membranes with many small pores).

Hollow fiber immunoisolation devices are sealed after cellular loading; and although the methods may vary, the seals should be validated with integrity tests both for effectiveness as an intact immunoisolating barrier and for mechanical strength. An ideal sealing procedure should produce seals that surpass the mechanical strength of the fiber itself.

FIG. 2 Three hollow fiber morphologies created under distinct extrusion conditions and viewed with SEM: coarse (A), dimpled (B), and smooth (C). These morphologies can accommodate a range of contact for host cells. Differences in the processes used to create these surface textures correlate with some structural features of the membrane trabecular space (T), but do not correlate with changes in the permselective properties of the inner membrane skin (IS).

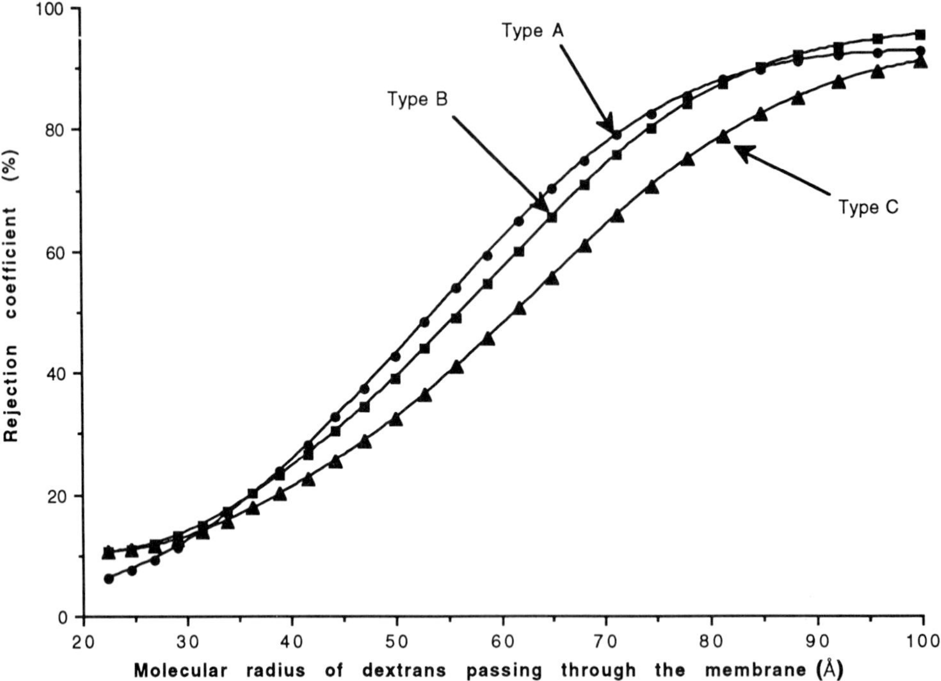

FIG. 3 Dextran rejection curves define the permselectivity range in a set of three fibers. The nominal MWCO of a fiber membrane is indicated here in terms of the size (molecular radius) of dextran molecules that are restricted from passing through the membrane (i.e., that display a 90% rejection coefficient). Note that fibers that display similar high molecular weight cutoff values (type A and type B) can concurrently display significantly different rates of passage for low molecular weight products.

Biological Compatibility of Devices

As applied in this chapter, the biological compatibility refers to a host tissue response to a PAN–PVC implanted device. Characterization of the response to an immunoisolatory device is performed by analyzing adjacent host morphology. Acceptable biocompatibility exists when host responses do not occlude the device and do not sustain host tissue perturbations over large distances (e.g., greater than 20 μm) from the device–tissue interface. The host cells that should be monitored will vary depending on the selected implant site; however, our discussion will concentrate on the central nervous system (CNS).

Adequate tissue preservation, that is, fixation, is essential for high-quality histological preparations. Best results can be expected when experimental animals are anesthetized, saline washed, and formaldehyde fixed through cardiac perfusion. A perfusion needle is inserted into the left ventricle and a large incision is made in the right atrium. A 0.9% (w/v) saline solution is then perfused for at least 1 min through the left ventricle, for example, at a rate of 60 ml/min (Masterflex peristaltic pump), after which the perfusion solution is changed to freshly prepared 4% (w/v) paraformaldehyde (4°C). Continue perfusing for 2 min, then reduce the perfusion speed to 20 ml/min and perfuse for an additional 30 min. Relevant tissues are then excised, postfixed in 4% paraformaldehyde, and are available for additional processing.

Histology

Histological analysis of CNS implant devices is accomplished with stains that differentiate between hematocytes, lymphocytes, and resident neuronal and glial cells. Hematoxylin–eosin (H–E) staining provides these distinctions. In addition, acidified 0.5% (w/v) cresyl violet (1 ml of acetic acid per 250 ml of stain) is a Nissl stain we routinely use to counterstain immunocytochemical preparations. Cryostat sections (20–30 μm thick) and plastic GMA (glycomethacrylate histo resin; Cat. No. 70-2218-500; Reichert-Jung) sections mounted on poly-L-lysine (Cat. No. P-8920; Sigma, St. Louis, MO)-coated slides are processed. Cryostat sections are first delipidated in ethanol–chloroform (1 : 1) overnight and are then processed like plastic sections. Plastic sections are hydrated, stained with hematoxylin, counterstained with eosin Y or cresyl violet, dehydrated (including clearing with methyl salicylate), transferred to xylene, and coverslipped. For Nissl staining, the sections are rinsed with tap water and treated with acidified ethanol to destain the sample. Destaining is monitored under a dissecting microscope until the background staining has been reduced to a desired level.

Examples from studies of the biocompatibility of CNS implant devices placed within the striatum are shown in Figs. 4 and 5. Representative coronal sections of a device fully implanted within the striatal parenchyma of a guinea pig at 4 weeks is shown in Fig. 4A. In this example, cellular interaction at the device–tissue interface is minimal. Figure 5A also shows representative staining of an implant device placed within the striatal parenchyma of a nonhuman primate for 8 weeks. In both cases, independent of host species, the relative absence of hematocytes and macrophages at 4 and 8 weeks is evidence of an acceptable (i.e., biocompatible) host response to the implant. Corresponding immurocytological staining of sections from this implant is discussed in the next ection.

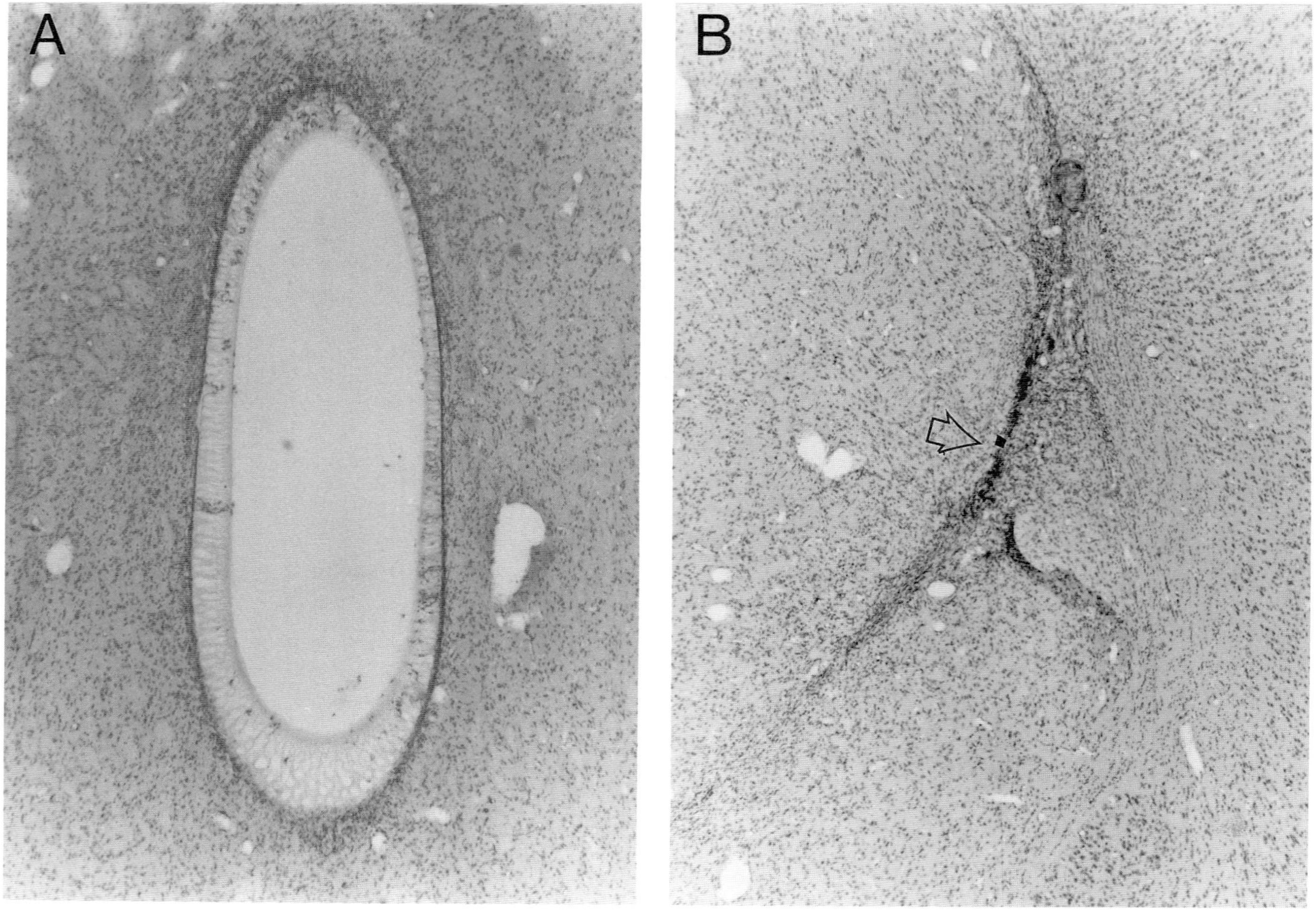

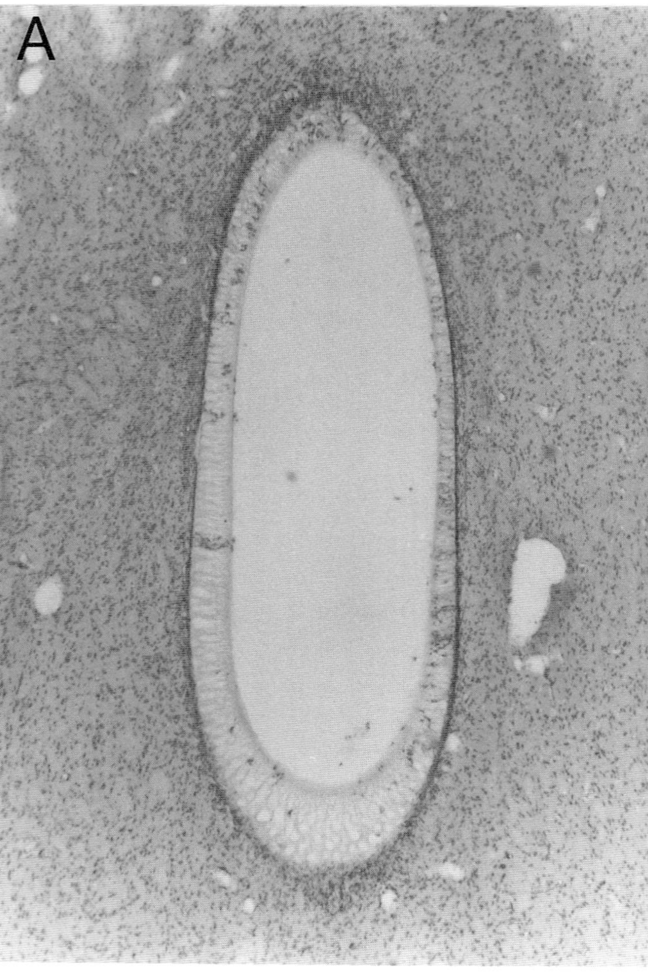
A

Immunocytology

Within the brain, astrocytes and microglia respond to intrusive brain trauma (20). Glial response is conveniently monitored immunocytologically with antisera directed against a glial-specific protein, glial fibrillary acidic protein (GFAP), and can also be directed against microglia. Tissue sections are mounted on poly-L lysine coated slides, hydrated into water, and preincubated for at least 1 hr in cold blocking solution. Sections are then processed according to Emerich *et al.* (9). As assessed by GFAP staining (Fig. 5B), the limited extent of astrocyte activation from a device implanted within the striatal parenchyma of a nonhuman primate striatum for 8 weeks is indicative of a biocompatible response. Fibronectin immunostaining reveals the limited extent of vascular damage caused by implantation of the device (Fig. 5C). Biologically relevant tests such as these can be evaluated against the host tissue responses to other neurological procedures (e.g., biopsies, resections, and indwelling shunts).

Qualitative Issues

Cell Selection

Xenogeneic cell sourcing for an encapsulated device begins with the desired function of the implant. For example, chromaffin cells are a known source of the opioid peptide enkephalin and norepinephrine (6, 8), and therefore have been utilized as a cellular delivery system to treat chronic, nonresponsive pain associated with extensive, disseminated cancer (25; also see [21] in this volume). Chromaffin cells are obtained as primary cultures enzymatically isolated from dairy cattle (15, 17). Chromaffin cells can be additionally purified by density gradients and differential plating methods. Tests for ensuring the safety, quality, and uniformity of these cells for xenogeneic transplants are described in the next section.

FIG. 4 Implantation studies to establish biological compatibility of devices in host brain tissue. Shown here is the relative absence of adverse cellular response in a histological sample of a hollow fiber device implanted for 8 weeks in guinea pig striatum (A). Implanted devices also were surgically removed after 8 weeks and the animals were held for an additional 4 weeks to assess the consequences of implant removal. Modest scar response (arrow) was observed in the guinea pig striatum following implant removal (B). Samples were stained with hematoxylin–eosin.

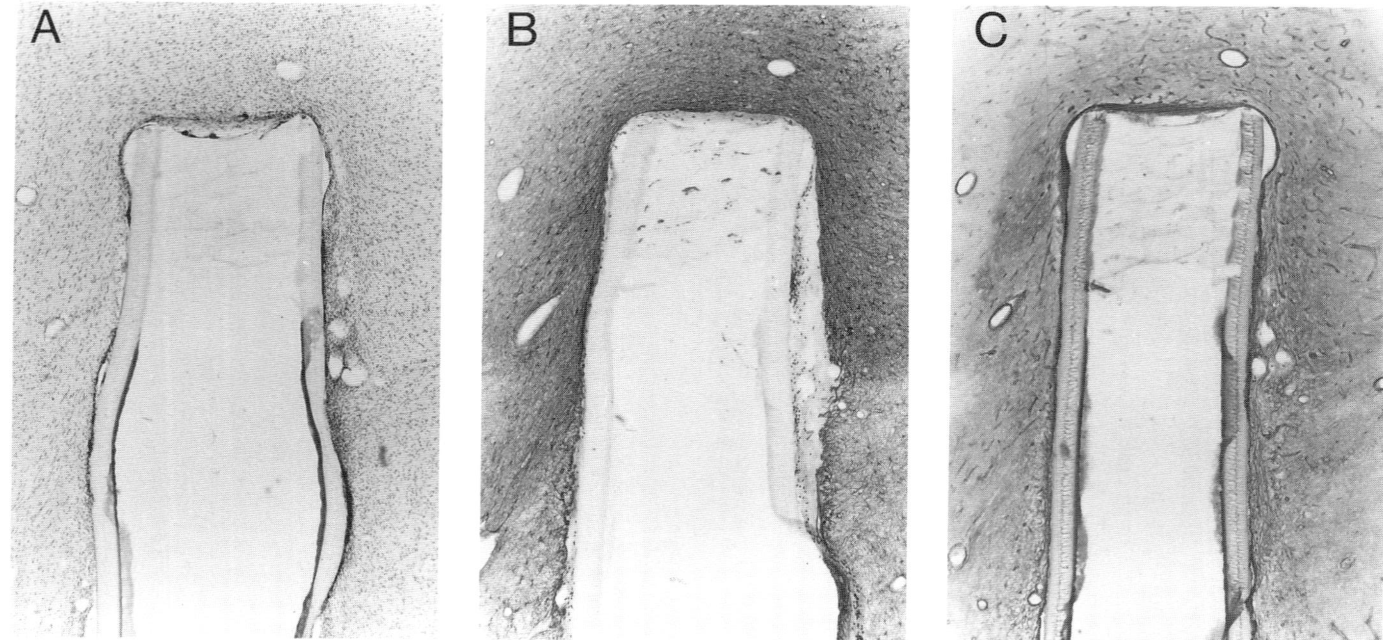

FIG. 5 Prototypes of implant devices tested in large animal models. A series of sections taken from a single hollow fiber implanted for 8 weeks in nonhuman primate striatum were stained with hematoxylin–eosin (A), and with antibodies to GFAP (B) and to fibronectin (C). The absence of immunological infiltration and the minimal glial response and fibronectin accumulation demonstrate favorable biological compatibility of the implanted cellular delivery device.

Safety of Transplantable Cell Sources

Cells for human implants must come from healthy donors or from stable, contaminant-free cell lines. This is particularly important for chronic implants, in which even slowly acting adventitious agents may compromise the outcome. Ensuring the health of a donor animal is best achieved through programs of immunization and daily health monitoring, the highest levels of which can be achieved in gnotobiotic herds. At the other end of the spectrum, within institutional animal care facilities, endemic health problems are generally detected by testing sentinel animals, and remedial actions are taken to treat the entire colony once an unhealthy sentinel is detected. To the extent that these colonies remain "clean" one may have confidence that cells from these donor animals are healthy. Within agricultural facilities, health surveillance can surpass those of the average insitutional animal care facility. Each animal in cattle herds on small dairy farms, for example, is individually monitored for health problems. This level of surveillance is possible because many dairy farms operate 24 hr/day, and thus workers are among the animals constantly and can detect a sick cow even before changes occur in milk production (a sensitive indicator of health).

The best means of ensuring the general health of donor animals and cell lines is through the participation of trained veterinarians and cell biologists, respectively. An animal caretaker can assess unusual behavior indicative of illness, and cell biologists can monitor cell growth and morphology of tissues being processed for cell isolations and cell lines. Lists of specific adventitious agents that will threaten the health of either the donor or the recipient will depend on the species involved (5, 12, 23).

To ensure a stringent level of quality control during isolations and cell culture, provided adequate on-site facilities are available, antibiotic-free conditions are recommended. This approach will detect breaches in sterility. However, even in the absence of obvious microbial contamination, slowly growing infectious agents within cell cultures will likely compromise the experimental study. In this context, xenogeneic cells, if adequately tested, can be safer than allogeneic transplant cells. With the long-standing use of bovine products in the dairy and meat industries, commercially available (and scientifically validated) tests exist for all common pathogens potentially transmittable from bovids to humans. One particularly rare pathogen, the noncultivable rickettsial agent *Coxiella burnetti* (the causative agent of Q fever), poses a potential health risk (18). Routine microbiological and virological culture methods will not detect this potentially infectious agent. Preventative health maintenance and proper housing of animals will significantly reduce the risk of this contaminant entering the cell isolation process. However, direct microscopic examination of isolated cells (i.e., by transmission electron microscopy directed to identify cytoplasmic rickettsial particles; or by fluorescent immunocytology directed to identify rickettsial antigens) will reliable detect extreme contaminations. Enhanced sensitivity for detecting these agents can be obtained through the use of customized polymerase chain reaction (PCR) assays. Informative manuals for handling cells and cell lines (e.g., 11) and affordable external services for screening common pathogens are available.

All cell sources carry some level of risk for microbial contamination (10, 21). The use of antibiotics (i.e., penicillin, streptomycin, and amphotericin B) (Cat. No. 600-5240PG; GIBCO, Grand Island, NY) to facilitate "sterile" isolations of primary cell cultures is a common practice. However, the use of such antibiotics in cell cultures destined for human use is not permitted because of the potentials for masking contaminants, altering cell physiology, and causing adverse reactions in transplant recipients. Thus, antibiotic use should be eliminated and a bioburden monitoring program substituted in its place. This program includes testing all organ transport fluids for total enumeration of aerobic bioburden by the membrane filtration technique (13). Additionally, a portion of the cell harvest is tested for sterility and endotoxins. Sterility tests require 2 weeks to complete and impede the rapid turn-around expected in most research applications. These tests are critical for validating sterile processes in routine transplant applications. In a production setting, such tests are mandatory components of implant product quality control and quality assurance programs (see Testing for Sterility and Endotoxins, below).

Quantitative Issues

Dosages of products released from implant devices can be predicted from pretransplant calculations by correlating cell number with metabolic or secretory measures. Where possible, nondestructive tests are preferred because they will allow individual characterization of each implant device before transplantation. Estimating cell number within an implant device is either direct or indirect: cells are recovered and counted or some form of cell-dependent activity is measured from which cell numbers are back-calculated. Metabolic activity is an indirect measure of cell number, and therefore need not be destructive. These tests fall into two general categories: measures of oxidative respiration, using an electron donor substance that becomes colorometrically and/or fluorometrically measurable once it has been reduced, or direct measures of nutrient flux within the culture medium.

Cell Counts

Measuring direct cell counts from encapsulated devices is both destructive and subject to counting errors. However limited, cell culture counting methods can be appropriate for this task if validated (e.g., trituration, enzymes, nuclei extraction, DNA content).

Metabolic Tracers

MTT (a tetrazolium salt) is converted to a formazan salt by mitochondrial dehydrogenases. When a population of cells contains equally active mitochondria, the MTT assay provides a sensitive measure of cell number; however, this assay is also destructive. Prior to transplanting, cohorts of implant capsules are incubated in medium containing reagent for several hours, during which time an insoluble formazan salt is produced. These capsules are cut open, the salt is subsequently solubilized with an alcohol solution during an overnight incubation, and analyzed thereafter.

Nutrient Flux

Lactate and dextrose are ubiquitous substances in the medium of cultured cells. Dextrose is consumed, and under fully nonoxidative conditions two molecules of lactate are produced for each molecule of dextrose. Rapid and sensitive tests for measuring lactate and dextrose have been developed that make use of enzymatic oxidations coupled with electrochemical measurement of derived peroxides. Self-calibrating instrumentation for lactate and dextrose analysis is available (e.g., YSI model 2700 Select; Yellow Springs Instruments, Inc., Yellow Springs, OH), with carousel sample-handling capacities for automation. Although this approach provides nondestructive measures without the addition of tracer materials to the implant device, nutrient flux from limited numbers of cells may require extended culture periods to generate measurable changes. Changes in dextrose levels are most reliably measured at later time points because most culture media contain high concentrations of dextrose. Monitoring trends in daily consumption of dextrose from encapsulated cells provides a rapid, safe, convenient, and reliable index of the number of metabolically active cells contained within an implant device (Fig. 6). Measures of glutamine consumption and/or alanine production parallel measures of dextrose use and lactate production in cell culture. Reversed-phase high-performance liquid chromatography with fluo-

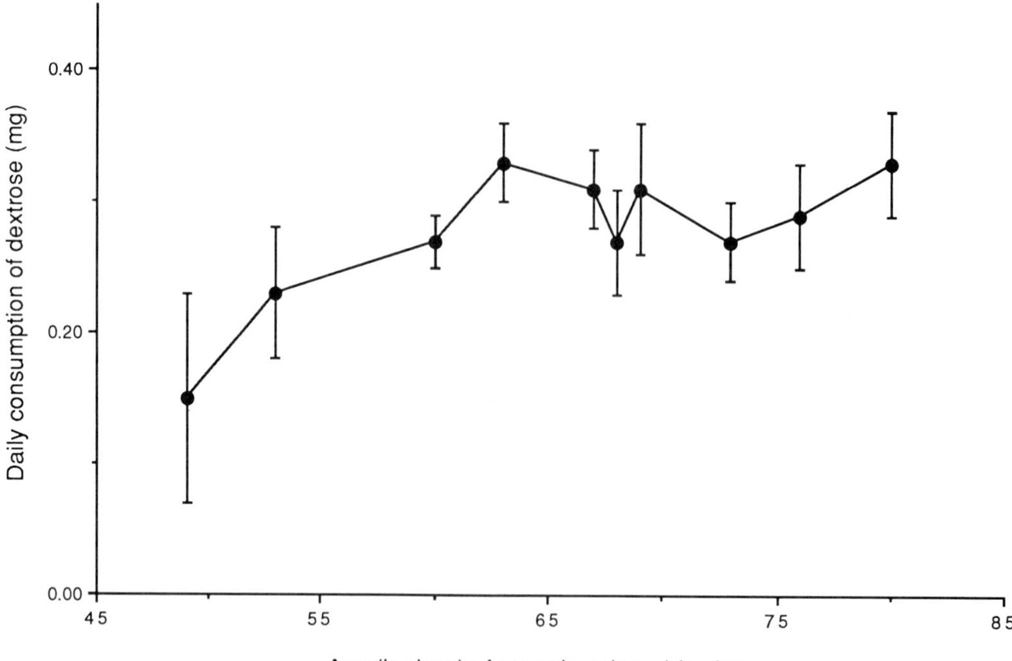

FIG. 6 Nutrient flux to monitor cell growth within implant devices. This graph shows a trend in the daily consumption of dextrose by fibroblasts within a set of implant devices cultured *in vitro* ($n = 4$; $x \pm$ SD). Cells were seeded into the devices at low densities and established stable and saturating nutrient utilization in approximately 2 months.

rometric detection has been used to measure *o*-phthaldehyde-derivitized amino acids from fresh and spent culture medium. An on-column derivitization protocol offers full automation of this assay (Waters Chromatography Division of the Millipore Corporation, Marlboro, MA).

Testing, Implanting, and Removing Devices

Testing for Sterility and Endotoxins

A bioburden assessment program has been implemented for all fluids, media, and device components (22). The program incorporates membrane filtration, conventional sterility tests, direct plating, component blending followed by membrane filtration, and environmental monitoring of air and surfaces by

RCS (Biotest) and RODAC testing for Class 10,000 and Class 100 aseptic processing areas. In a production environment bioburden assessment programs are an essential component of quality assurance. One approach to supplementing a higher degree of sterility assurance is to hold medium that has had device contact aerobically at 35–37°C. Most cell culture media and conditions will support the growth of a broad range of aerobic organisms, including skin contaminants (coagulase-negative staphylococci, diphtheroids, α-hemolytic streptococci, yeast, etc.). In addition, portions of the media may be added to a fluid thioglycolate medium (FTM) containing a reducing agent to allow for anaerobic outgrowth. Devices may be planted directly into FTM or Trypticase soy broth (TSB).

Implantable devices are also required to be essentially endotoxin free (pyrogenic material derived from gram-negative bacterial liposaccharides). The tests are verified by spiking the article with a known endotoxin standard amount [reported in endotoxin units (EU)]. Implants with cerebrospinal fluid (CSF) contact must have their chosen test method validated to at least the 0.06-EU/ml level. Endotoxins may be monitored using the *Limulus* amebocyte lysate (LAL) test by either the gel clot method (Associates of Cape Cod) or assayed quantitatively by a chromogenic end-point determination (BioWhittaker QCL-1000), using a multiwell plate reader at 405 nm (Molecular Devices). The chromogenic LAL method offers both ease of use and quantitative results. However, cell culture medium that undergoes a yellow color change with an acidic pH shift will often interfere with the chromogenic end-point determination. These methods are applied to all media, a percentage of final devices, and to all production baths that do not inhibit the tests. Capsules that either carry measurable endotoxin or have been exposed to biological contamination are excluded from further applications. In a production environment, any positive cultures are then submitted to more extensive screening so that their sources might be identified and steps taken to prevent future breaches in sterile processing.

Implantation Techniques

Techniques for the implantation of cell-loaded devices have been developed to utilize stereotaxic equipment for precise placement within the CNS. For example (see Fig. 7), rodent intrathecal implants are achieved by creating an incision from the back of the head to the base of the neck, dissecting the layers of fascia and muscle aside with forceps, and exposing the atlantooccipital region of the spinal cord. A cannula (e.g. 18 gauge) is loaded with a device, and a solid rod obturator is positioned behind the capsule. The tip of the cannula is inserted into a small incision in the spinal cord and gently

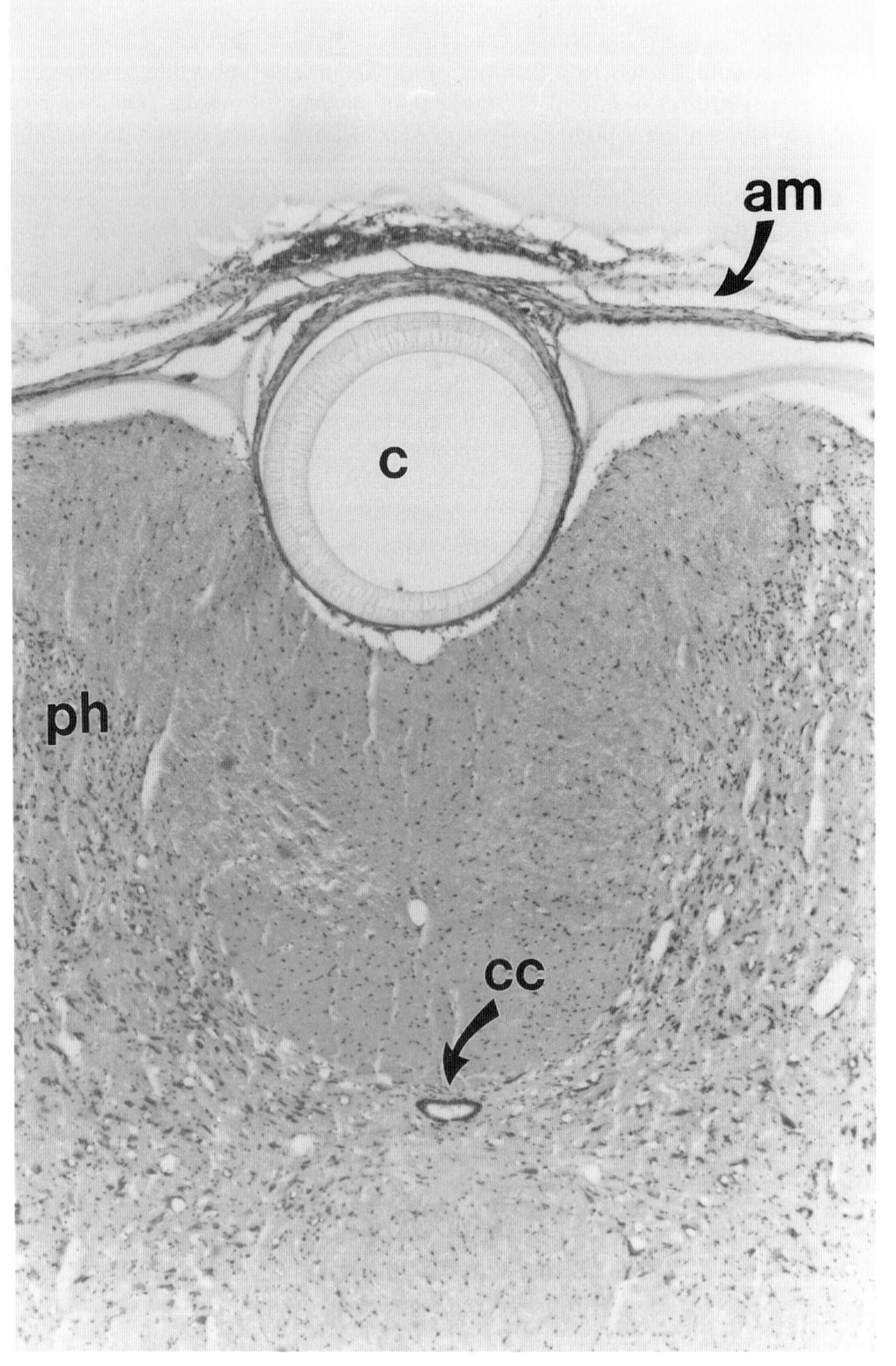
am
c
ph
cc

positioned into the cervical/thoracic region. The obturator is held in place while the cannula is withdrawn, leaving the capsule within the spinal cord; then the obturator is withdrawn and the incision is sutured. Animals are monitored for evidence of behavioral abnormalities. Cannula implantation approaches assure safe and precise placement, protect the device while guided to tissue target sites, and minimally perturb host tissue.

Host Tissue Response

As retrievability is an added benefit to encapsulated xenografts, the host tissue response to both implantation and device removal must be characterized, for example, from guinea pig striatum 4 weeks following implantation. As assessed morphologically, the striatum from animals housing devices for 8 weeks displayed only a trace level of wound reaction (Fig. 4A). Host tolerance may relate to the device occupying the cannula space (i.e., absence of a void), which, if occupied with host blood cells, could lead to significant scarring. Implants were surgically removed from a matched group of animals after 8 weeks; the animals recovered and survived for an additional 4 weeks, and were prepared for histological analysis. The host response to the withdrawn implant indicated a modest wound reaction along the space previously occupied by the device (Fig. 4B). Device removal likely produced a minimal amount of vascular disturbance contributing to a minimal level of wound response. Safe retrieval is a unique feature of encapsulated devices.

Device Response to Implant Procedures

Placement methods appropriate for recipients, that is, acceptable host biocompatibility, are also required so as not to influence the cell-loaded device negatively. Assessments are generally made at the conclusion of an *in vivo* test period by histo- and immunocytochemistry (see above). Cellular encapsulation facilitates identifying cells that have been implanted, as they are

FIG. 7 Stereotaxic approaches, such as cannula and obturator methods, for placing capsules into tissue target sites. Such methods improve confidence that transplanted cells are, and remain, positioned appropriately. Placement of experimental implant capsules into the subarachnoid space and onto the dorsal surface of the rodent spinal cord is confirmed histologically (arachnoid membrane, am; capsule, c; central canal, cc; posterior horn, ph).

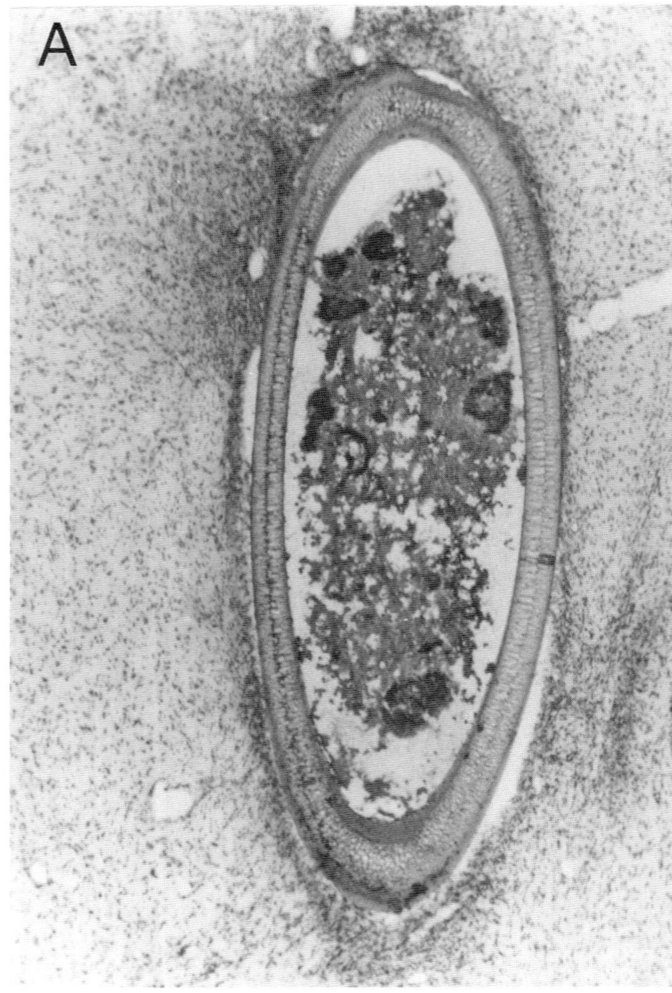
A

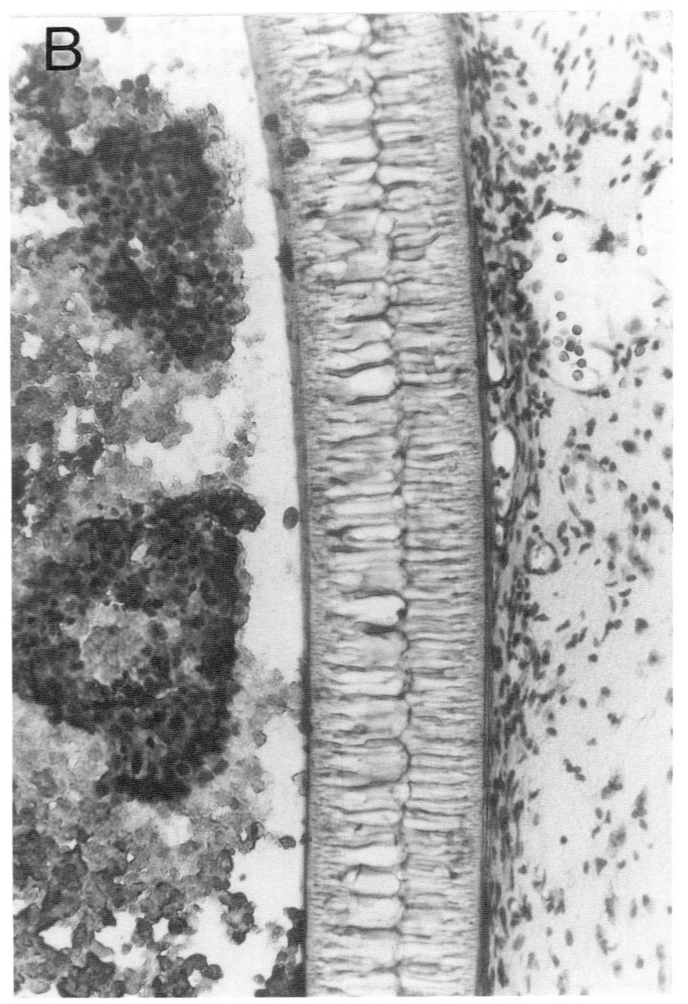
B

FIG. 8 The absence of host immune cell response to chronic xenografts (rat PC-12 cell-loaded device placed into guinea pig striatum) is taken as evidence of an appropriate combination of control over implant devices, encapsulated cells, and surgical placement. After 8 weeks within guinea pig striatum, capsules containing PC-12 cells showed only a modest GFAP-immunopositive response to the implant (A). (B) Higher magnification of the region indicated in the marked area of (A); healthy and abundant PC-12 cells immunopositive for tyrosine hydroxylase are evident with an adjacent acceptable host tissue response.

located within the boundaries of the device. A placement method that was not acceptable may damage the xenograft device during insertion, resulting in a host cellular immune response that rejects the cells within the device. With an appropriate combination of biocompatible device design, serum-free culture conditions, and appropriate placement methods, encapsulated xenografts are fully accepted by their hosts (Fig. 8). Encapsulated xenografts have been functioning without evidence of compromised performance in small animal hosts for periods of 3, 6, and 12 months [3 months in Aebischer *et al.* (3); 6- and 12-month data, unpublished, 1994).

Conclusion

Tests to validate the safety and reproducibility of encapsulated xenografts include evaluations of the device, cells, and host response. The tests discussed in this chapter are generally available to most researchers. Encapsulated chromaffin cell-loaded devices are currently under clinical evaluation in Switzerland for the management of intractable pain in terminal cancer patients (1). The tests described in this chapter are by no means complete, but nevertheless represent a program in support of clinical testing. These testing programs will be modified with the advent of validated, automated encapsulation processes. The field of cellular transplantation has been rapidly growing and as new applications arise parallel strategies to ensure the safety of this technology will be essential.

References

1. P. Aebischer, Is there a therapeutic future for tissue transplants to control pain? *Abst. World Congr. Pain, 7th,* Paris, France, *1993,* Abstr. No. 652 (1993).
2. P. Aebischer, S. R. Winn, P. A. Tresco, C. B. Jaeger, and L. A. Greene,

Transplantation of polymer encapsulated neurotransmitter secreting cells: Effect of the encapsulation technique. *J. Biomech. Eng.* **113,** 178–183 (1991).

3. P. Aebischer, P. A. Tresco, S. R. Winn, L. A. Greene, and C. B. Jaeger (1991). Long-term cross-species brain transplantation of a polymer-encapsulated dopamine-secreting cell line. *Exp. Neurol.* **111,** 269–275 (1991).
4. A. Björklund, Better cells for brain repair. *Nature (London)* **362,** 414–415 (1993).
5. A. Buxton and G. Fraser, "Animal Microbiology," Vol. 2. Blackwell, Oxford, 1989.
6. S. W. Carmichael and H. Winkler, The adrenal chromaffin cell. *Sci. Am.* **235,** 40–49 (1985).
7. L. Christenson, K. E. Dionne, and M. J. Lysaght, Biomedical application of immobilized cells. *In* "Fundamentals of Animal Cell Encapsulation and Immobilization" (M. F. A. Goosen, ed.), pp. 8–41. CRC Press, Boca Raton, FL, 1993.
8. R. E. Coupland, The natural history of the chromaffin cell—Twenty-five years on the beginning. *Arch. Histol. Cytol.* **52,** 331–341 (1989).
9. D. F. Emerich, P. McDermott, P. Krueger, M. Banks, J. Zhao, J. Marsalkowski, B. Frydel, S. Winn, and P. Sandberg, Locomotion of aged rats: Relationship to neurochemical but not morphological change in nigro striatal dopaminergic neurons. *Brain Res. Bull.* **32,** 477–486 (1993).
10. Food and Drug Administration, "Guideline on Validation of the *Limulus* Amebocyte Lysate Test as an End-Product Endotoxin Test for Human and Animal Parenteral Drugs, Biological Products, and Medical Devices, December." Division of Manufacturing and Product Quality (HFN-320), Office of Compliance, Center for Drug Evaluation and Research, 1987.
11. R. J. Hay, J. Caputo, and M. L. Macy, eds., "ATCC Quality Control Methods for Cell Lines," 2nd ed. American Type Culture Collection, Rockville, MD, 1992.
12. P. D. Hoeprich and M. C. Jordan, "Infectious Disease: A Modern Treatise of Infectious Processes," 4th ed., Lippincott, Philadelphia, 1991.
13. International Pharmaceutical Federation, Validation and environmental monitoring of aseptic processing, Committee on Microbial Purity. *J. Parenter. Sci. Technol.* **44** (No. 5) (1990).
14. B. D. Kahan, Immunosuppressive therapy. *Curr. Opin. Immunol.* **4,** 553–560 (1992).
15. D. L. Kilpatrick, F. H. Ledbetter, K. A. Carson, A. G. Kirshner, R. Slepetis, and N. Kirshner, Stability of bovine adrenal medulla cells in culture. *J. Neurochem.* **35,** 679–692 (1980).
16. J. K. Leypoldt, R. P. Frigon, K. W. DeVore, and L. W. Henderson, A rapid renal clearance methodology for dextran. *Kidney Int.* **31,** 855–860 (1987).
17. B. G. Livett, Adrenal medullary chromaffin cells in vitro. *Physiol. Rev.* **64,** 1103–1161 (1984).
18. T. J. Marrie, Epidemiology of Q fever. *In* "Q Fever" (T. J. Marrie, ed.), Vol. 1, pp. 50–66. CRC Press, Boca Raton, FL, 1990.
19. M. Mohanty, J. A. Hunt, P. J. Doherty, D. Annis, and D. F. Williams, Evaluations of soft tissue responses to a poly(urethane urea). *Biomaterials* **13,** 651–656 (1992).
20. M. K. Nicholas and B. G. W. Arnason, Immunological responses in central nervous system transplants. *Semin. Neurosci.* **4,** 273–283 (1992).

21. PDA Environmental Task Force, "Fundamentals of a Microbiological Environmental Monitoring Program," Tech. Rep. No. 13, *J. Parenter. Sci. Technol.*, Vol. 44, Suppl. PDA Environ. Task Force, 1990.
22. M. Pfeiffer, Testing medical disposables using the *Limulus* Amebocyte Lysate (LAL) test. *Med. Device Technol.*, May/June (1990).
23. J. A. Poiley, Methods for detection of adventitious viruses. *In* "Cell Cultures Used in the Production of Biotechnology Products in Large-Scale Mammalian Cell Culture Technology" (A. S. Lubiniecki, ed.). Dekker, New York, 1990.
24. J. Sagen and G. D. Pappas, Alleviation of chronic pain by adrenal medullary transplants. *Restor. Neurol. Neurosci.* **4,** 229 (1992).
25. J. Sagen, H. Wang, P. A. Tresco, and P. Aebischer, Transplants of immunologically isolated xenogeneic chromaffin cells provide a long-term source of pain-reducing neuroactive substances. *J. Neurosci.* **13,** 2415–2423 (1993).
26. G. Tkacik and S. Michaels, A rejection profile test for ultrafiltration membranes and devices. *Bio/Technology* **9,** 941–946 (1991).

Section X

Induced Gene Expression in Intrinsic Central Nervous System Cells with DNA Injected into the Brain

[25] Particle Bombardment for Gene Transfer into Nerve Cell Systems

Ning-Sun Yang, Shoushu Jiao, and Carolyn De Luna

Introduction

The development of gene transfer techniques has revolutionized molecular and cell biology, transforming many areas into genetic studies. In fact, gene transfer, in various forms, has become a necessary technology for virtually all biological disciplines. This is mainly due to recognition that the transgenic approach, in conjunction with gene cloning and sequencing, can provide powerful functional analyses of genes in homologous or heterologous biological systems. The application of gene transfer technologies has generated germ line-derived transgenic animal and plant systems, microbial genetic engineering systems, routine gene delivery systems for mammalian somatic cells in culture or *in vivo,* and, more recently, systems for human gene therapy.

Although several transgenic techniques have been effective in a wide spectrum of biological systems, their application to nerve cells has been comparatively limited and slow. This limitation may be due to the following difficulties in manipulating nervous tissue systems: (a) techniques for *ex vivo* manipulation of brain tissues and for establishing primary cultures from brain or other nerve cell types are not yet routinely applicable, often requiring sophisticated, skilled, and even specialty tissue culture techniques; (b) conventional gene transfer methods (e.g., calcium phosphate coprecipitation, retrovirus vectors, and electroporation) have been minimally effective for transfection of primary nerve cells, especially neurons (1–3); and (c) neural cell physiology often must be studied at the cellular level (4, 5), and therefore similar resolution is needed for transgenic techniques. Therefore, researchers have been exploring new gene transfer methods for nerve cell systems, making varying degrees of progress with herpes simplex virus, lipofectin, adenovirus, and particle bombardment methods.

In this chapter, we describe the Accell particle bombardment (gene gun) technology (Agracetus, Middleton, WI), which we have successfully applied to gene transfection of several nerve cell systems. Because the particle bombardment technique employs a physical means, it circumvents the need for specific cell membrane receptors or other components that mediate DNA uptake, resulting in gene transfer that is independent of the targeted cell

Methods in Neurosciences, Volume 21

types (6, 7). Using various rat brain tissue or cell systems, we effectively transfected fetal or adult brain cell explants prepared as freshly isolated tissue clumps, cell aggregates, single-cell suspensions, or as primary cultures. Neurons, glial cells, and purified oligodendrocytes were similarly transfected by this method. We also demonstrated that *ex vivo*-transfected fetal brain cell explants can be engrafted into adult brains for relatively long-term transgene expression *in vivo,* and that various promoter, reporter, functional, and candidate therapeutic genes can be effectively analyzed in these *ex vivo* gene transfer systems. Our laboratories are systematically evaluating further applications of the Accell method in basic research involving gene transfer to other nerve cell systems and gene therapy for brain diseases such as Parkinson's.

Accell Gene Transfer Technique

Particle Acceleration Mechanism

The Accell particle bombardment device developed by McCabe and Martinell (8, 9) was originally designed for plant gene transfer (10). More recently it has also been shown to be highly effective for gene transfer into a wide range of mammalian cell types, including those of the nervous system.

Within a small explosion chamber, a high-voltage electric discharge generates a strong burst of shock waves, which accelerate millions of DNA-coated gold particles to a supersonic velocity. Cell, tissue, or organ samples placed in the pathway are evenly bombarded, resulting in the penetration of the gold particles and DNA into the cells, effecting gene transfer (Fig. 1A). Gold particles are often chosen as the microprojectiles for gene delivery because gold is chemically inert, has no cytotoxic effects, and can penetrate deeper into intact tissue, due to its higher density and momentum on acceleration. The general design of the Accell instrument and its explosion chamber are shown in Figs. 1B and C (10a), respectively, and a hand-held device for *in vivo* gene transfer into selected somatic tissues is shown in Fig. 1D. Applications of other types of particle bombardment devices have been previously reviewed by Yang and Christou (11).

The Accell particle bombardment technique is highly versatile because several parameters can be fine-tuned to optimize DNA delivery for each tissue or cell type. The ballistic parameters include (a) a discharge voltage of 3 to 25 kV, which controls particle momentum and velocity, (b) gold particle size (0.7, 0.95, 1–3, 3–5, 5–9, or 9–15 μm in diameter), (c) bead loading density (about 0.5 particle per lymphocyte to five particles per fibroblast), (d) partial vacuum level (e.g., 250 mmHg), which reduces the shock wave impact on the cells, and (e) shape and form of the particles (e.g., pointed crystals, spheres, or clusters of aggregated beads). Optimal physical parameters can be selected on the basis of results of preliminary experiments. For nerve cell systems, the following conditions are highly effective: 5–7 kV, 0.95-μm gold particles, about one gold particle per cell, vacuum pressure of 250 mmHg, and spherical beads. Additional details of Accell transfection of brain or other cell types have been previously reported (1, 6, 7, 12, 13).

Molecular Biology Factors

As a physical means for gene transfer, the particle bombardment method delivers DNA directly into the nucleus or cytosol of target cells in a random fashion, circumventing the cell membrane receptors or structures that are biochemical or physical barriers to virus- or chemical-mediated gene transfer.

The method of precipitating DNA onto the surfaces of the gold particles is critical for optimal gene delivery (8–14). Our technique is to mix plasmid DNA, gold particles, spermidine or polyethylene glycol (PEG), and calcium salt in aqueous solution in sequence to precipitate the DNA onto the beads. The coprecipitates are then spun down, resuspended, and washed in 100% ethanol to remove excess salt. The ethanol suspension is gently sonicated to disperse aggregates, and is evenly loaded onto Mylar sheets. Because the DNA is coated onto the gold beads in a "dry," precipitated form, rather than in aqueous solution, it can intracellularly deliver high copy numbers of DNA into target tissue.

With these techniques, we found that submicrogram quantities of DNA (e.g., 0.32 μg of DNA per million cells per 35-mm dish) can be efficiently expressed in fetal rat brain cells (1). In comparison, tens or hundreds of micrograms of DNA were often required for other gene transfer methods in similar experiments (1, 15, 16). This differential is probably due to the unique combination provided by the Accell method of direct, instantaneous, and intracellular delivery of high-dosage DNA in precipitated form into the target cells.

The particle bombardment method can efficiently deliver large, plasmid, genomic DNA (~23 kb), and cosmid DNA (2). It remains to be seen if even larger DNA fragments, such as yeast artificial chromosomes, can also be precipitated and bombarded into mammalian cells.

The microenvironment of target cell cultures or tissue explants is an important factor for successful gene transfer. During bombardment a thin layer of aqueous medium should be applied to the tissue surface. For example, 20 to 30 μl of culture medium is commonly used on a 35-mm monolayer cell culture. More culture medium is added immediately after bombardment to facilitate cell recovery from wounding; membrane pores reseal within 10 min of bead entry (J. Decker and N. Yang, unpublished results, 1994). Similar

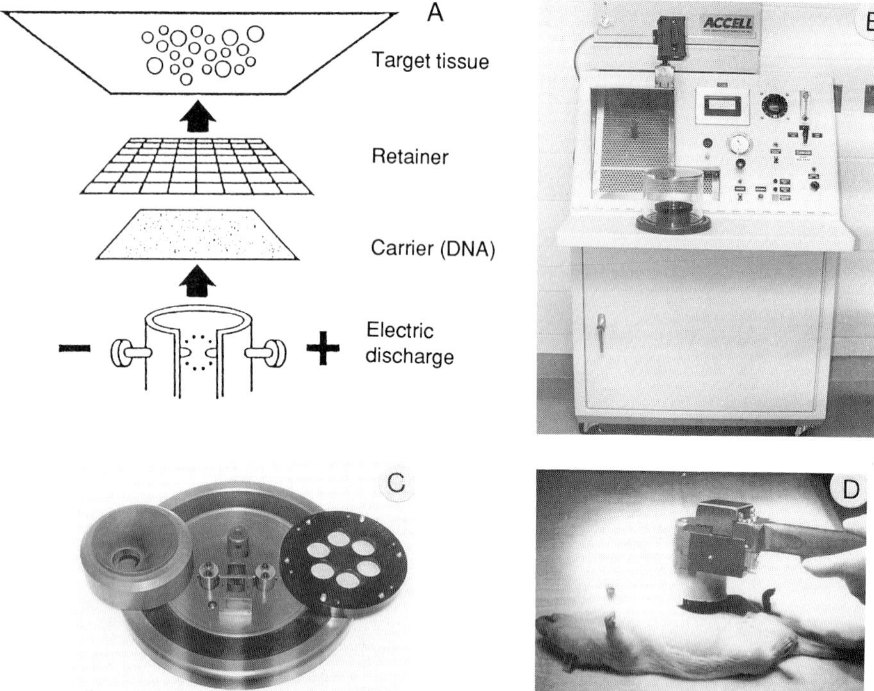

FIG. 1 Mechanism and design of the electric discharge-mediated particle bombardment device for gene transfer. (A) Diagram of the particle acceleration mechanism of the Accell instrument. (B) General design. (C) The electric discharge and explosion chamber. (D) The hand-held device for *in vivo* gene transfer. In (A) the motive force is generated in a spark discharge chamber containing two electrodes. A 10-μl water droplet is placed in between the electrodes, and a high-voltage capacitor is discharged through the water droplet, which vaporizes instantly, creating a shock wave. We have found that a polyvinyl chloride (PVC) pipe with an internal diameter of 13 mm is adequate for use at the spark discharge chamber. The electrodes are located opposite each other, project into the interior of the chamber approximately 5 mm below the top, and are protected at the tips with an arc-resistant alloy. The gap between the two electrodes can be adjusted by appropriately threading them into or out of the spark chamber. A spacer ring is placed above the spark chamber that, in a fixed apparatus for transformations of a single crop species, can be a vertical extension of the spark discharge chamber. However, a removable spacer ring allows the distance from the spark discharge to the carrier sheet to be varied so that the force of the shock wave can be adjusted. The motive force can also be adjusted by varying the voltage of the discharge. The carrier sheet on which the DNA-coated gold particles are precipitated in place on top of the spacer; the function of this sheet is to transfer the force of the shock wave from the spark discharge to the carrier particles. Located above the carrier sheet is a 100-mesh stainless steel screen that retains the sheet so that it does not proceed to the target tissue. The target tissue

measures are taken to provide minimal wounding and optimal transgene expression during bombardment of tissue explants or cell suspension samples (1, 13).

A major concern for any gene transfer technique is the viability of the treated cells. Although this process may seem destructive, we have shown that bombardment of many mammalian somatic cell cultures can confer high levels of transient gene expression and yet maintain high cell viability (1, 13). For example, 87 to 95% of bombarded fetal rat brain cells in primary cultures were viable (1). Our experience indicates that the particle bombardment system, when it is appropriately optimized, is an efficient tool for gene transfer.

Application to Central Nervous System Primary Cultures and Cell Explants

Ex Vivo Gene Transfer to Fetal and Adult Rat Brain Cells

Several cell transplantation techniques are being evaluated to treat human brain diseases such as Parkinson's disease. Transplantation of fetal brain or adrenal gland tissues into an adult host brain has been shown to exert a therapeutic effect on Parkinson's disease in animal models, and, more re-

---

can be placed on a water–agar plate in such a way that when the plate is inverted over the retaining screen, the tissue is in the direct path of the gold particles. The whole assembly is under a partial vacuum in order to minimize aerodynamic drag (10). In (C) the blast chamber consists of a PVC block milled to form a rectangular cavity divided into two chambers by a partial wall. In one of these chambers are two arc points spaced equidistant from the sides and rear wall. The points are set 0.5 mm apart and bridged by a 10-μl drop of water prior to each discharge. The spark chamber is covered by a wafer of PVC, which reflects the primary shock wave back into the chamber, avoiding energy loss. The cavity is partially obstructed by a partition that separates the spark chamber from the reflection chamber. The partition serves to prevent the primary shock wave from interacting directly with the carrier sheet. As secondary waves are formed by reflection from the chamber walls, their combined fronts distribute their force evenly over the carrier sheet, an 18-mm^2 piece of 0.5-mil metallized Mylar (Du Pont, Wilmington, DE). This sheet, which forms the roof of the reflection chamber, is accelerated upward until it encounters the retaining screen. The accelerated sheet is held by the retaining screen (100-mesh stainless steel) as the gold particles on its surface proceed to the target tissue. The energy for the arc is provided by a 25-kV, 2-μF capacitor charged from a 25-kV DC variable power supply. The capacitor is discharged through the arc gap by activating a solenoid-actuated double-pole double-throw switch. [Equipment, description, and design courtesy of D. McCabe (10a).]

cently, in human clinical studies (17,18). Genetic engineering may improve these donor cells by increasing their production of the deficient protein, tyrosine hydroxylase (TH). To explore this possibility, we have evaluated various gene transfer technqiues for brain cells.

Using primary cultures of fetal rat brain cells, we have compared the gene transfer efficiencies of four different DNA transfection methods: calcium phosphate coprecipitation, electroporation, lipofectin (DOTMA : DOPE = 1 : 1), and Accell particle bombardment. As shown in Fig. 2, the Accell method was over 100-fold more effective in transient gene expression than the three other tested methods (1). The high efficiency of the particle bombardment technique is not unique to fetal brain cells; neural cells derived from freshly excised adult brain tissues or from primary cultures of purified oligodendrocytes gave similar results (1, 19). These results, as well as our previous experience with a standard and a new lipofectin formulation (1, 20), lead us to suggest that particle bombardment is much more effective than most other DNA transfection methods for a variety of nerve cell systems.

Gene Transfer to Different Cell Types in Various Microenvironments

In fetal rat brain primary cultures, both neuron and glial cells can be effectively transfected by the Accell bombardment method. As seen in Fig. 3A,

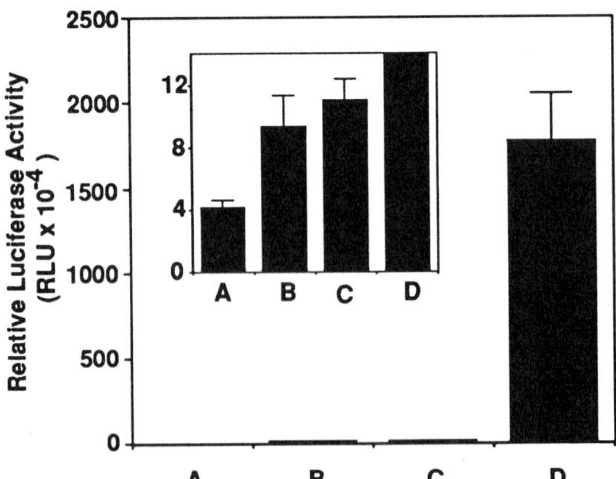

FIG. 2 Comparison of gene transfection methods in fetal rat brain cell cultures: (A) Calcium phosphate coprecipitation, (B) electroporation, (C) lipofection, and (D) particle bombardment. The same preparation of pCMVluc DNA was used for each transfection procedure, using four duplicate cell cultures. Luciferase activity was assayed 2 days after transfection. The error bars represent the standard error of the mean (1). Note: inset is a scaled up version of actual (A), (B), and (C) values.

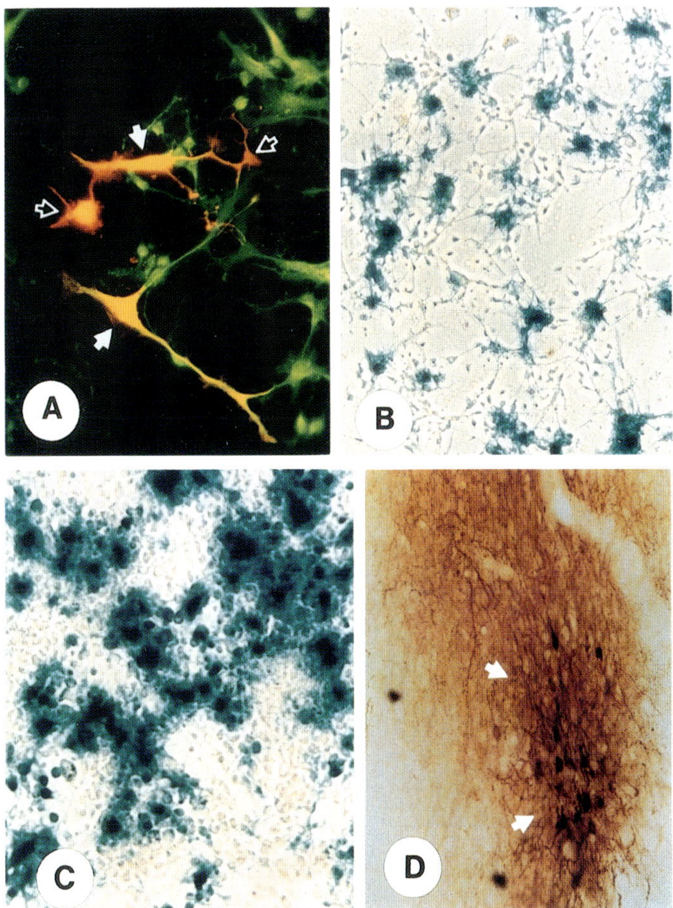

Fig. 3 Histological staining of transgenic β-galactosidase and tyrosine hydroxylase (TH) in fetal rat brain cells. (A) Double-immunofluorescence staining of fetal brain cells transfected with pCMVβ-Gal. (B) X-Gal staining of pCMVβ-Gal-transfected cells in culture derived from single-cell suspension. (C) X-Gal staining of tissue clumps bombarded with pCMVβ-Gal. (D) *In vivo* expression of pCMVTH in bombarded brain cells at 14 days posttransplantation. In (A) the cells were costained for β-Gal and neurofilament immunoreactivity. Photomicrograph was taken with an overlapping exposure under dual-excitation filters of an epifluorescence microscope. Cells in green fluorescence are neurofilament-immunoreactive cells (i.e., neurons). Cells in red fluorescence are immunoreactive to anti-β-Gal antibody, but not to anti-neurofilament antibody. These cells are β-Gal-expressing neurons, and are indicated by the closed arrow. Double staining of glial cells expressing β-Gal using anti-GFAP antibody, gave similar results (data not shown). Microscopic cell counting scored 1–2% of neuron and glial cells as double labeled for β-Gal expression. In (B) and (C), fetal cells in primary culture were formalin fixed, then stained with X-Gal for 10 to 30 min. In (D), arrows indicate the graft. In this experiment, cultured cells or brain sections were labeled by immunoperoxidase staining, using anti-TH antibody, and visualized by diaminobenzidine. Control sets of fetal brain cells were bombarded with pCMVβ-Gal and cultured *in vitro* or engrafted into adult host brains. Immunoperoxidase staining of these control tissues, using anti-TH antibody, showed no detectable immunoreactivity. Bars: (A) 50 μm; (B) 200 μm; (C) 140 μm; (D) 600 μm (1).

this was demonstrated by double-immunofluorescence labeling of the cell type-specific antigen and the transgenic β-galactosidase (β-Gal) antigen. With this double-labeling technique or with a histochemical staining assay of β-Gal activity, we have reported that approximately 1–2% of bombarded neurons and glial cells in primary brain cell cultures express high levels of pCMVβ-Gal transgene activities (Fig. 3B and C). A variety of tissue forms or microenvironments of brain cell samples can be similarly used for Accell-mediated gene transfer. These include primary tissue cultures prepared as single-cell suspensions (Fig. 3B) or as tissue clumps (Fig. 3C), and cell explants that are freshly excised from fetal or adult brain tissues before they are placed into primary culture or implanted into host animals. Thus, particle-mediated gene transfer would enable transgenic neuroscience research on a wide spectrum of biological systems.

One application to basic molecular genetic studies is a comparison of the relative strengths of various promoters in brain cells, using the bombardment method. Phosphoglycerate kinase (PGK) and cytomegalovirus (CMV) promoters exhibited the highest transgene activity among the tested mammalian cellular promoters and viral promoters, respectively (1). Also, protein expression levels of three different reporter transgenes [*Escherichia coli* β-galactosidase, firefly luciferase (Luc), and human growth hormone (hGH)] were determined in the fetal rat brain system, providing useful guidelines for future transgenic studies in nervous systems.

Unique Transgene Expression Pattern in Oligodendrocyte Culture

Transient gene expression in most mammalian cell cultures usually peaks during the first 2 days after transfection, followed by a rapid decline during the next few days, to a minimal level after 1 week. This pattern was observed for several cell culture systems we have studied (12, 13, 16), including fetal rat brain primary cultures (1). It was not, however, followed by purified rat oligodendrocytes bombarded in primary cell culture. Guo *et al.* (19; Z. Guo, S. Jiao, L. Cheng, N.-S. Yang, I. Duncan, and J. A. Wolff, unpublished results, 1994) observed that high levels of initial transgene expression, including those from pCMVluc and pCMVhGH reporter genes, were steadily maintained for 2–3 weeks following bombardment. These results provoke questions about the cellular physiology and control mechanisms for gene expression in oligodendrocytes, and possibly other nerve cell types as well. Transgene expression time course patterns may provide new means for analysis of gene expression behaviors in nerve cell systems, which should be investigated further in the future.

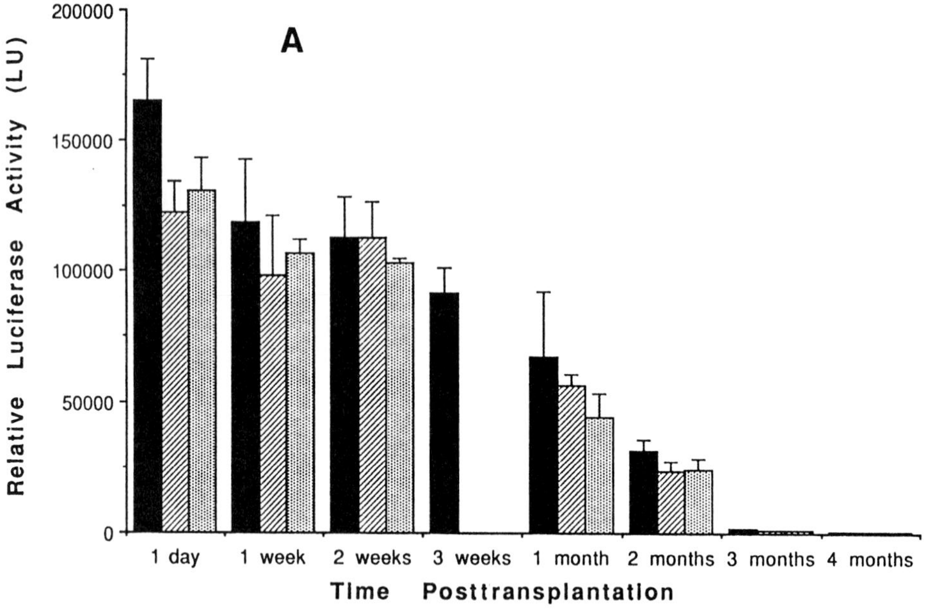

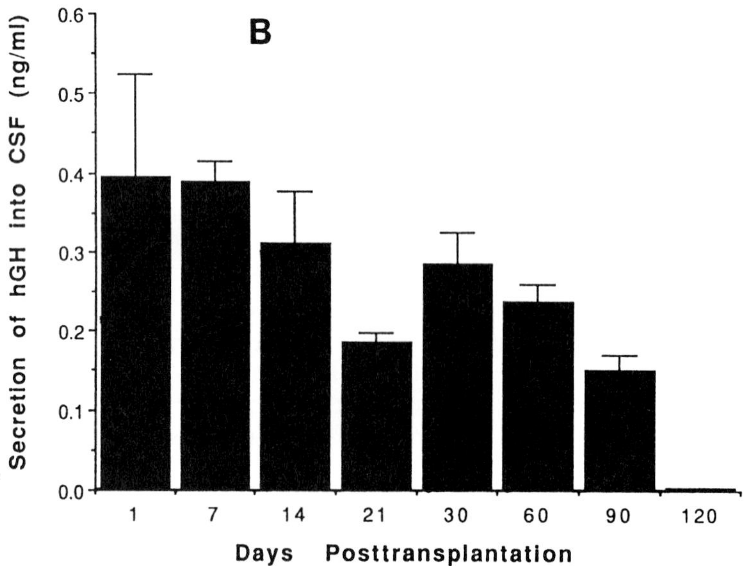

FIG. 4 *In vivo* transgene expression after transplantation of fetal brain tissues bombarded with (A) pCMVluc or (B) pCMVhGH genes. Black bars, tissue clumps; striped bars, tissue clumps embedded in collagen gel; stippled bars, single-cell suspension.

In Vivo Transgene Expression after Transplantation of Transfected Tissues

Tissue clumps and single cells in suspension can be conveniently obtained from freshly excised, fetal brain tissue explants. By using the Accell technique, they can be immediately bombarded for high-efficiency gene transfer and readily transplanted into caudate or cortex regions of adult host brains to investigate *in vivo* transgene expression (1). Significant levels of pCMVluc gene expression were detected *in vivo* in engrafted tissues at 2 months post-transplantation (Fig. 4A). Polymerase chain reaction (PCR) analysis of reporter gene sequence showed that transgenic DNA copies were present in transplanted cells.

An interesting observation on the secretion of transgenic proteins was obtained when a human growth hormone gene was transfected into fetal rat brain cells and immediately transplanted into adult host brains (Fig. 4B). Transgenic hGH protein was secreted into the extracellular space of brain tissue and a portion of it was transported into the cerebral spinal fluid (CSF) compartment of the host brain. Similar to the pattern of transgenic Luc activity, transgenic hGH expression in the CSF system was sustained for 2 to 3 months. These experiments demonstrate that transgenic studies of nervous systems can now be effectively investigated at the organ level as well as at the cellular and tissue levels, using the particle bombardment technique.

In Situ Gene Transfer to Adult Brain Tissue of Live Animals

By using a hand-held Accell device (Fig. 1D), a wide variety of mammalian somatic tissues has been shown to be susceptible to *in vivo* and *in situ* gene transfer to live animals, as discussed in Application to Mammalian Somatic

---

E15 donor cells were bombarded with test or control genes and immediately transplanted into host caudate regions. Between five and eight different animals were tested for each time point shown. Two control group animals transplanted with fetal brain tissues bombarded with pCMVβ-Gal DNA were included in each time point in grafting experiments. No luciferase activity was detected in any of the control samples. The error bars represent the standard error of the mean. Transgenic hGH proteins released into the cerebral spinal fluid (CSF) of adult brains were collected via the cisterna–magna puncture, and assayed with a commercial RIA kit. [(A) from Jiao *et al.* (1); (B) courtesy of S. Jiao, J. Sun, J. A. Wolff, and N.-S. Yang, unpublished results, 1994.]

Tissues in General, below. In a preliminary study of the efficacy of bombarding surgically exposed cortical tissues of adult rat brains, we found low but biochemically significant levels (e.g., $\sim 10^5$ relative light units/tissue sample) of transgenic pCMVluc activity (S. Jiao, J. Sun, J. Wolff, and N. Yang, unpublished data, 1994). Localized hemorrhaging and microscopic wounding of delicate cortical tissues drastically decreased transgene expression levels. This low-level expression can be used for basic research, such as for evaluating relative promoter strength *in vivo,* but is not sufficient for clinical applications. Future experiments are required to determine if surgical and bombardment techniques can be optimized to substantially improve *in vivo* gene expression in bombarded brain tissues.

Application to Brain Gene Therapy

To explore potential applications of the Accell method to gene therapy of human brain diseases, Jiao *et al.* (1) evaluated the transgenic expression of a tyrosine hydroxylase gene (*TH*), which corrects for the deficiency in Parkinson's disease, in rat brain cells. High-level expression of the CMVTH gene was detected in culture at the cellular level, at an efficiency similar to that obtained for the β-Gal reporter gene. *In vivo* expression of transgenic TH was also readily detected in fetal brain cell grafts bombarded with pCMVTH and transplanted into the caudate region of adult host brains (Fig. 3D).

Spencer *et al.* (21) and Freed *et al.* (22) reported that transplantation of mesencephalic tissues isolated from human fetal brains can result in significant reduction of symptoms in Parkinson's patients. In some of these cell therapy procedures, dopaminergic mesencephalic cells from four fetal brains were used to treat a single adult patient. We suggest that transfer of the *TH* gene into donor cells, combined with more effective transplantation procedures, may provide a more efficient treatment for Parkinsons' disease (1). Because dopamine-producing mesencephalic cells could be transfected *ex vivo* with high copy numbers of the *TH* gene to augment TH production, a greatly reduced amount of fetal cells would be required for each patient. In addition, even non-dopamine-producing cells, such as the much more abundant cortex tissues, could also be used as donor cells. Because the Accell technique takes only 1 to 2 min to complete gene transfer, and works efficiently on freshly excised tissues, it can be conveniently used with these brain surgery and tissue transplantation procedures.

In a related approach, Jiao *et al.* (23) reported that rat muscle cells, engineered with *TH* gene by lipofectin and transplanted into host brain, corrected the drug-induced Parkinson's symptom in rats. Because the Accell method is at least 10-fold more efficient in transfecting rat muscle cells than the lipofectin method (N. Yang, S. Jiao, and J. Wolff, unpublished results, 1994), its potential for brain gene therapy should be further explored.

Application to Mammalian Somatic Tissues in General

In Vivo and in Situ Gene Transfer

In addition to nerve cells, many different types of mammalian somatic tissues have been effectively transfected by particle bombardment techniques, including *in vivo* and *in vitro* systems. *In situ* bombardment of epidermis and liver tissues in rodents produced high levels of transient gene expression with minimal cell damage or inflammation of targeted tissues (12, 24). Cheng *et al.*(6) extended the *in vivo* transgene research to many rodent internal organs, including dermis, muscle, pancreas, kidney, spleen, and heart. In this study, relative strength, tissue preference, and induction of transgenic promoter activities were demonstrated for various viral and cellular promoters in five different tissues. Cheng and co-workers also compared marker gene expression in four different species (mouse, rat, rabbit, and rhesus monkey), demonstrating similar expression efficiencies among these animals. Because transgenic pCMVluc activity was sustained for over $1\frac{1}{2}$ years at greater than 40% of the peak level, dermal tissue, especially muscle cells in the panniculus carnosus layer, may be the best vehicle for long-term transgene expression.

Tang *et al.* (25) demonstrated that *in vivo* epidermis bombardment with the genes for an antigen is an effective genetic vaccination method for producing circulating antibodies against the expressed transgenic proteins. In similar studies, use of the Accell device produced both cytotoxic T lymphocyte and antibody responses against antigens or pathogens via genetic immunization (26, 27).

In vivo bombardment of skin or liver tissues in rats results in the release of transgenic secretory proteins, such as human growth hormone and human α anti-trypsin, into the circulatory system (J. Burkholder, L. Cheng, and N. Yang, unpublished results, 1994). Therefore this secretory effect may be used for physiological studies of transgenic proteins in serum.

Ex Vivo or in Vitro Bombardment

Because particle bombardment can transfer genes into freshly excised tissues, making them immediately available for transplantation, it is highly competitive with *ex vivo* gene transfer, the most common approach for gene therapy. Several laboratories (7, 12, 16, 28) have shown that mammary gland, liver, kidney, and skin explant tissues can be effectively transfected in organ culture via particle bombardment. In the mammary organoid system, the Accell method was 5- to 100-fold more effective than three other commonly used DNA transfer methods (16). Particle bombardment can be used on cell explants in many forms, such as tissue slices, cubes, clumps, small cell aggregates, or single cells. Suspensions of primary leukocytes—lymphocytes, macrophages, and splenocytes—were also transfected (13). New opportunities for gene therapy are hence created by the versatility of the particle bombardment technique.

A wide spectrum of mammalian cell lines in long-term culture were also transfected by the particle method, including those derived from epithelial, fibroblast, endothelial, and lymphocyte cells (12). Stable gene transfer into target cell chromosomes by the bombardment technique was observed at a frequency of $\sim 10^{-4}$, similar to that of other direct gene transfer methods (7, 12, 29).

Summary

Extensive progress in gene transfer, primary culture, and tissue transplantation technologies has provided new approaches for studying transgene expression and gene therapy. The particle bombardment method has been shown to be effective for gene delivery to a wide variety of mammalian somatic tissues, including *in vivo, ex vivo,* and *in vitro* systems. For gene transfer into several different central nervous system cell types, the Accell technique was shown to be more efficient than other direct gene transfer methods. High-efficiency *ex vivo* transgene expression can be similarly obtained with neuron, glial, or oligodendrocyte cells in primary cultures or cell explants. High cell viability and transient gene activity levels also facilitated the studies of *in vivo* transgene expression in host brains following transplantation of *ex vivo*-transfected nerve cells.

The use and efficacy of a variety of transgene constructions in rat brain systems, including those of several reporter, promoter, functional, or therapeutic genes, were systematically evaluated using particle bombardment technology. The techniques and results described in this chapter may provide useful tools for molecular genetic and cell biology research of nerve cell functions and gene expression. It is also our hope that the developing Accell gene transfer technology will provide means for future brain gene therapy.

Acknowledgment

We are deeply grateful to J. Decker for thorough editing of this manuscript.

References

1. S. Jiao, L. Cheng, J. A. Wolff, and N.-S. Yang, *Bio/Technology* **11,** 497 (1993).
2. N.-S. Yang, *CRC Crit. Rev. Biotechnol.* **12,** 335 (1992).
3. K. W. Culver, Z. Ram, S. Wallbridge, H. Ishii, E. H. Oldfield, and R. M. Blease, *Science* **256,** 550 (1992).
4. S. Popov, A. Brown, and M. Poo, *Science* **259,** 244 (1993).
5. P. M. Friden, L. R. Walus, P. Watson, S. R. Doctrow, J. W. Kozarich, C. Backman, H. Bergman, B. Hoffer, F. Bloom, and A.-C. Granholm, *Science* **259,** 373 (1993).
6. L. Cheng, P. R. Ziegelhoffer, and N.-S. Yang, *Proc. Natl. Acad. Sci. U.S.A.* **90,** 4455 (1993).
7. N.-S. Yang and P. R. Ziegelhoffer, *in* "Particle Bombardment Technology for Gene Transfer" (N.-S. Yang and P. Christou, eds.), pp. 117–114. Oxford Univ. Press, New York, 1994.
8. D. McCabe, W. Swain, B. Martinell, and P. Christou, *Bio/Technology* **6,** 923 (1988).
9. D. McCabe and B. Martinell, U.S. Pat. 5,149,655 (1992).
10. P. Christou, D. E. McCabe, B. Martinell, and W. F. Swain, *Trends Biotechnol.* **8,** 145 (1990).

10a. N.-S. Yang, J. K. Burkholder, L. Cheng, and P. R. Ziegelhoffer, "Gene Therapy: From Basic Research to Clinics." World Scientific Publishing, Singapore, 1993.

11. N.-S. Yang and P. Christou, eds., "Particle Bombardment Technology for Gene Transfer." Oxford Univ. Press, New York, 1994.
12. N.-S. Yang, J. Burkholder, B. Roberts, B. Martinell, and D. McCabe, *Proc. Natl. Acad. Sci. U.S.A.* **87,** 9568 (1990).
13. J. K. Burkholder, J. Decker, and N.-S. Yang, *J. Immunol. Methods* **165,** 149 (1993).
14. P. Christou, W. Swain, N.-S. Yang, and D. McCabe, *Proc. Natl. Acad. Sci. U.S.A.* **86,** 7500 (1989).
15. M. Krigler, *in* "Gene Transfer and Expression: A Laboratory Manual," p. 83. Stockton Press, New York, 1990.
16. T. A. Thompson, M. N. Gould, J. K. Burkholder, and N.-S. Yang, *In Vitro Cell Dev. Biol.* **29A,** 165 (1993).
17. A. Björklund, *Trends Neurosci.* **14,** 319 (1991).
18. A. Björklund, *Nature (London)* **362,** 414 (1993).
19. Z. Guo, S. Jiao, L. Cheng, N.-S. Yang, I. Duncan, and J. A. Wolff, *Soc. Neurosci. Abstr.* (in press).

20. S. Jiao, G. Ascadi, A. Jani, P. L. Felgner, and J. A. Wolff, *Exp. Neurol.* **115,** 400 (1992).
21. D. D. Spencer, R. J. Robbins, F. Naftolin, K. L. Marek, T. Vollmer, C. Leranth, R. H. Roth, L. H. Price, A. Gjedde, B. S. Bunney, K. J. Sass, J. D. Elsworth, E. L. Kier, R. Maruch, P. B. Hoffer, and D. E. Redmond, *N. Engl. J. Med.* **327,** 1541 (1992).
22. C. P. Freed, R. E. Breeze, N. L. Rosenberg, S. A. Schneck, E. Kriek, J.-X. Qi, T. Lone, Y.-B. Zhang, J. A. Snyder, T. H. Wells, L. O. Ramig, L. Thompson, J. C. Mazziota, S. C. Huang, S. T. Grafton, D. Brooks, G. Sawle, G. Schroter, and A. Ansari, *N. Engl. J. Med.* **327,** 1549 (1992).
23. S. Jiao, V. Gurevich, and J. A. Wolff, *Nature* (*London*) **362,** 450 (1993).
24. R. S. Williams, S. A. Johnston, M. Riedy, M. J. DeVit, S. G. McElligott, and J. C. Sanford, *Proc. Natl. Acad. Sci. U.S.A.* **88,** 2726 (1991).
25. D.-C. Tang, M. DeVit, and S. A. Johnston, *Nature* (*London*) **356,** 152 (1992).
26. J. Cohen, *Science* **259,** 1691 (1993).
27. J. Haynes, D. Fuller, and M. Eisenbraun, *in* "Particle Bombardment Technology for Gene Transfer" (N.-S. Yang and P. Christou, eds.), pp. 175–192. Oxford Univ. Press, New York, 1994.
28. A. V. Zelenin, A. A. Alimov, A. V. Titomirov, A. V. Kazansky, S. I. Gorodetsky, and V. A. Kolesnikov, *FEBS Lett.* **280,** 94 (1991).
29. S. Fitzpatrick-McElligott, *Bio/Technology* **10,** 1036 (1992).

Section XI

Viral Transfection of Intrinsic Cells within the Brain

[26] A Defective Herpes Simplex Virus Vector System for Genetic Intervention in the Adult Brain: Applications to Gene Therapy and Neuronal Physiology

Alfred I. Geller, Mathew J. During, and Rachael Neve

Introduction: Genetic Intervention in Brain

Genetic intervention in the brain is becoming an increasingly important strategy for answering questions pertaining to the molecular foundation of a wide range of brain functions, ranging from maintaining homeostasis to sensory information processing and cognitive functions. The genes encoding numerous molecules that are likely to be responsible for regulating neuronal physiology have been isolated and characterized. For example, cDNAs encoding proteins responsible for the generation of action potentials, for the synthesis and release of neurotransmitters, and for neurotransmitter receptors and components of the neuronal cytoskeleton have been isolated. cDNAs for signal transduction enzymes, transcription factors, and components of the neurotransmitter release machinery, which may play roles in altering the strengths of synaptic connections and thereby mediating changes in brain function as originally postulated by Hebb, have also been isolated. Much remains to be learned, however, about the roles played by these molecules in mediating alterations in neuronal physiology that lead to changes in complex behaviors. Genetic intervention in the brain can potentially produce precise information about brain functions by creating directed mutations in these cloned neuronal genes, and then introducing the mutated genes into their normal cellular milieu using gene transfer techniques.

Genetic intervention may also potentially be applied to many of the disorders that affect the brain. Some gene therapy strategies may use approaches that are specific to a disease. For example, expressing tyrosine hydroxylase in striatal neurons may be an approach to Parkinson's disease. Physical injury to an area of the nervous system might be treated by expressing neurotrophic factor(s) and/or their receptor(s) in specific groups of cells. Other gene therapy strategies might exploit the molecular pathways underlying normal neuronal function; a more detailed understanding of these pathways may lead to new insights into how defects in these pathways cause specific diseases. For example, a more detailed understanding of the mechanisms that modulate long-term changes in neurotransmitter release may suggest new approaches to diseases in which neurotransmitter release is altered, such as the epilepsies.

The brain, however, does not yield easily to genetic intervention. The postmitotic state of most neurons in the adult brain effectively blocks vectors, such as retroviruses, that are dependent on cell replication for stable maintenance in the cell. Moreover, the molecular determinants of specific behaviors and of neurological diseases may be confined to a precisely delineated type of cell at a precise time during a physiological event. Strategies for gene transfer into the brain, then, must utilize vectors that stably persist in postmitotic cells, and must be capable of altering the genetics and consequent physiology of a precisely defined class of neurons during a specific window in time.

Modern neuroscience research is moving rapidly in this direction. *In vivo* genetic intervention technology is being applied to an increasing number of neurobiological questions. The capability of retrovirus vectors to genetically label nerve cell progenitors and their progeny *in vivo* (1, 2) has been used to study the fates of single precursor cells in the mammalian brain. Immortalization of multiple types of neurons has been accomplished by using retrovirus vectors or transgenic mice to introduce oncogenes into these cells (3, 4). The potential of gene therapy to correct nervous system disorders first began to seem a reality when the shiverer phenotype was restored to wild-type by transgenic expression of a normal myelin basic protein gene (5) and when circadian behavioral rhythms in *Drosophila* per mutants were reestablished by gene transfer of a normal per gene (6, 7). Moreover, gene transcription regulatory elements that confer not only neuronal specificity, but also specificity for certain classes of neurons, are gradually being defined (8, 9). Thus, the promise of manipulating neuronal gene expression and hence neuronal function in a precise spatiotemporal fashion may be realized in the future.

Nevertheless, strategies for such manipulations of the adult mammalian nervous system have been hindered by the lack of a method to deliver genes directly into neurons. As a first step toward solving this problem, we have developed a defective herpes simplex virus type 1 (HSV-1) vector system that allows genes to be introduced directly into neurons, in culture, or in a defined region of the adult mammalian brain (10–13), thereby enabling a genetic analysis of the molecular events on which complex neuronal functions are based. The role of the protein expressed from the HSV-1 vector in neuronal physiology is assayed in electrophysiology, neurochemistry, protein biochemistry, immunohistochemistry, and behavioral studies.

Genetic intervention in neurons with HSV-1 vectors may support a precise analysis of the function of specific molecules in the brain. The resolution of the analysis is due to specific issues at each level of the experiment. First, the cellular changes are limited to those arising from changing the function of a specific protein. For example, expression of an unregulated adenylate cyclase in neurons reveals changes in both intracellular and transsynaptic pathways that result specifically from activation of the enzyme; in contrast, pharmacological agents that activate or inhibit adenylate cyclase often have pleiotropic effects that may confound the analysis. Second, genetic intervention results in a stable modification of the function of a protein, whereas pharmacological and electrophysiological interventions frequently act only transiently. Third, the class of neuron affected, and even the particular subcellular compartment within the neuron that is affected, may be regulated with molecular genetic tools.

Strategies for Manipulation of Neuronal Physiology by Genetic Intervention

Design of Recombinant Protein

Most proteins that neuroscientists wish to examine are endogenous to neurons. Therefore, if the goal is to perturb neuronal function by expressing a gene from an HSV-1 vector, the recombinant gene must be designed to have a dominant phenotype. Two types of dominant mutations are useful. Dominant positive mutations cause a protein that is normally regulated to function under all conditions (constitutive activity). For example, neuronal expression of the catalytic domain of adenylate cyclase will have a dominant effect on the cells because the wild-type adenylate cyclase is strictly regulated and is normally activated only in response to certain stimulii (14). In contrast, dominant negative mutations interfere with the function of the endogenous as well as the recombinant protein. For example, expression of a mutated ion channel subunit that can assemble into a channel but has altered voltage gating properties will result in the assembly of channels containing both mutated and normal channel subunits, thereby altering the voltage-gating properties of these specific ion channels in the neuron. A useful variation on the dominant negative mutation strategy involves stable inhibition of synthesis of a particular protein by expressing antisense RNA for the protein from an HSV-1 vector.

Cellular Sites and Molecular Targets

The specialized structure of neurons makes it possible to direct genetic intervention to functional compartments in the cell. Attractive molecular targets for perturbing presynaptic mechanisms include signal transduction enzymes, enzymes involved in neurotransmitter synthesis, and components of the secretory machinery. Specific perturbations of postsynaptic mechanisms might be caused by manipulating the activity of neurotransmitter receptors, ion channels, and signal transduction enzymes. More complex changes that affect the entire cell might be caused by altering neuronal gene regulation with genetically modified transcription factors. Recombinant proteins might be targeted to presynaptic or postsynaptic sites by fusion to sequences that contain axon- or dendrite-targeting signals. For example, a 10-amino acid domain at the amino terminus of the neuronal growth-associated protein GAP-43 can target another molecule to neuronal processes (15; R. Neve and A. I. Geller, unpublished data, 1994). A dendritic targeting signal is present in the adult form of microtubule-associated protein MAP2; clues to its location in the molecule are revealed by the absence of such a signal in the embryonic MAP2 (16). When the sequence encoding the signal is identified, it can be fused to specific coding sequences of neuronal proteins that the researcher wishes to direct to the dendrite. Also, sequences have been identified that can target a protein to the nucleus.

Alteration of Physiology in Adult Mammalian Brain in Vivo through Experimental Manipulation of Three Parameters of Defective HSV-1 Vectors

The design of an *in vivo* experiment with HSV-1 vectors is shaped by the three major variables that are vulnerable to experimental manipulation. These are, first, the location and number of the infected cells; second, the promoter directing transcription of the recombinant gene in the vector; and third, the identity of the recombinant gene itself.

The location and class of cells infected is determined by choice of the site of injection, the location and number of neurons that project to the injection site, the number of virus particles in the inoculum, and the extent of diffusion of the virus through the extracellular space before infection.

The promoter in the vector is the second variable subject to experimental control. pHSVlac contains a constitutive promoter, the HSV-1 *IE4/5* promoter, that functions in most cell types. We have used the human neurofilament L promoter (17) to restrict expression of recombinant gene from an HSV-1 vector to neurons. Expression may be further limited to a particular class of neurons; for example, the tyrosine hydroxylase promoter has been used to limit gene expression to catecholaminergic neurons (18). Thus, by placing a given gene under the control of a specific promoter, it should prove possible to restrict expression of the recombinant gene to neurons, or even to a specific type of neuron.

The recombinant gene is the third variable that is vulnerable to experimental manipulation. Virtually any gene may be inserted into an HSV-1 vector; for example, we have expressed the catalytic domain of the yeast adenylate cyclase, and have shown that neurons infected with this recombinant exhibit elevated intracellular cAMP levels and protein kinase A activity, resulting in a long-term increase in neurotransmitter release (14). Furthermore, if the gene is fused to subcellular targeting sequences, the expressed protein can be directed to a particular part of a neuron, as discussed above.

An example of an experiment that might potentially be performed following this experimental strategy is the following (see Fig. 1). In this case, consider an HSV-1 vector in which the yeast adenylate cyclase catalytic domain is expressed from the vasoactive intestinal polypeptide (VIP) promoter (19). Delivery of this vector to the occipital cortex would result in infection of cortical neurons and glia. The VIP promoter is transcriptionally active only in VIP neurons in the central nervous system (CNS), thereby potentially

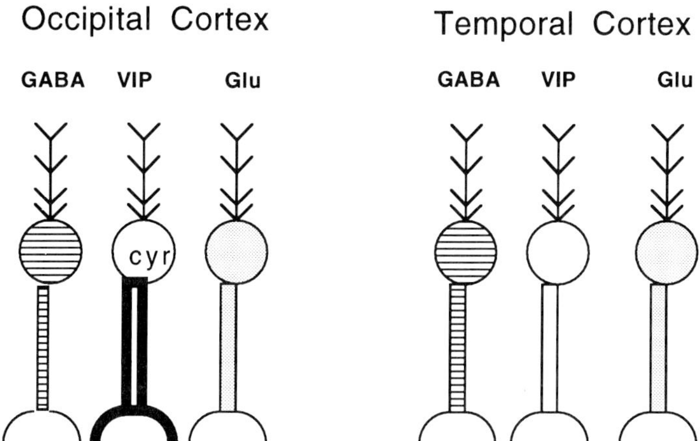

FIG. 1 A potential example of an experiment using HSV-1 vectors to alter the physiology of a specific type of neuron: increasing cAMP levels in VIP neurons in the occipital cortex. A defective HSV-1 vector is constructed that places the yeast adenylate cyclase catalytic domain under the control of the VIP promoter. Virus containing this vector is delivered by stereotactic injection into the occipital cortex, thereby infecting multiple cell types around the injection site. The VIP promoter may be active only in neurons that contain VIP, resulting in expression of the adenylate cyclase catalytic domain. The adenylate cyclase should direct an increase in cAMP levels. The physiological and behavioral consequences of activating the cAMP pathway in these VIP neurons can then be studied.

restricting expression of the adenylate cyclase to these neurons. The recombinant unregulated adenylated cyclase will raise cAMP levels in these VIP neurons, resulting in accumulation of cAMP selectively in occipital cortex VIP neurons. Specific neurons in the occipital cortex could be tested for altered biochemical or electrophysiological properties. Of note, possible behavioral consequence(s) of increasing cAMP in occipital cortex VIP neurons might be revealed by determining the performance of the animal in selected learning paradigms. In contrast, production of a transgenic animal with this construct would alter the function of VIP neurons throughout the nervous system, confounding the analysis.

We have begun testing this experimental strategy on a simple motor behavior in the substantia nigra. The catalytic domain of protein kinase C (PKC, rat β-II isoform) was expressed and found to potentiate neurotransmitter release from cultured neurons in an activity-dependent fashion (20). The PKC catalytic domain was placed under the control of the tyrosine hydroxylase promoter to limit expression to the catecholaminergic neurons of the substantia nigra compacta following delivery to the midbrain. This experimental protocol produced rats that demonstrated apomorphine-induced rotational behavior (21). These initial results suggest that the experimental strategy described in this section may be useful for analyzing specific brain functions.

Gene Therapy Approaches with HSV-1 Vectors

Parkinson's Disease

Parkinson's disease (PD) is a neurodegenerative disorder caused by the death of the substantia nigra compacta dopaminergic neurons, which project to the corpus striatum. Therapeutic strategies for PD have centered around restoring the lowered striatal dopamine levels; such strategies have included precursor loading of L-dopa, dopamine agonists (e.g., bromocryptine), and implantable dopamine delivery systems (both pump and polymeric strategies), with varying degrees of success. Typically, these treatments are effective initially but gradually lose their efficacy over a period of several years (23).

Tissue transplants (autologous adrenal chromaffin or fetal; 24, 25) have also been explored. Over the last several years, cell transplantation of genetically modified cells that produce either L-dopa or dopamine has been developed in animal models (26, 27). Although the effectiveness of cell transplantation is still under investigation, problems inherent to the approach include the following: first, L-dopa or dopamine must diffuse from the graft through the striatum, which is likely to be a more serious limitation in a large striatum (human); second, a graft is vulnerable to immune rejection; third, a graft secretes additional proteins and other molecules besides catecholamines, some of which may be beneficial whereas others may cause complications; and fourth, a graft disrupts local neuronal circuitry.

An alternative gene therapy approach to PD is to introduce the *TH* gene directly into neurons and glia in the striatum, using HSV-1 vectors. The potential advantages of this approach include the following: first, the production of L-dopa and dopamine is incorporated into the existing neuronal circuitry of the striatum and dopamine release should be regulated by these cells; second, graft rejection is not a potential complication; third, extensive diffusion of dopamine across large distances in the striatum is not required; fourth, neuronal circuitry is not physically disrupted. To test this approach we have constructed an HSV-1 vector that expresses the human TH type II (pHSVth). We have found that pHSVth expresses enzymatically active TH that directs the release of catecholamines from cultured striatal neurons. Furthermore, introduction of pHSVth into the striatum of the rat model of Parkinson's disease results in long-term behavioral recovery for up to 1 year, an increase in striatal dopamine levels, stable expression of TH as demonstrated by immunohistochemistry, and persistence of pHSVth DNA as detected by polymerase chain reaction (PCR) (28).

Gene Therapy Approaches with Neurotrophic Factors or Neurotrophic Factor Receptors

Nerve growth factor (NGF) is the prototype of the neurotrophin factor family, which includes brain-derived neurotrophic factor (BDNF) and neurotrophins 3, 4, and 5. Neurotrophic factors support the survival of specific types of neurons and direct the synthesis of specific proteins, including neurotransmitter systems, in selected neurons. Of particular note, NGF directs the maintenance of the cholinergic neurotransmitter system in specific types of neurons, notably the cholinergic forebrain neurons. Lack of NGF results in reductions in choline acetyltransferase activity and the size of the soma. Because delivery of NGF to the basal forebrain can reverse these alterations, NGF is used to treat patients with Alzheimer's disease, who consistently show a loss of functional basal forebrain cholinergic neurons.

HSV-1 vector-mediated delivery of neurotrophic factors and/or their receptors to the damaged nervous system has considerable therapeutic potential. Expression of NGF in the basal forebrain may prove useful in the treatment of Alzheimer's disease and we have found that expression of NGF can increase choline acetyltransferase activity in cultured basal forebrain neurons (28a). The neurons in the substantia nigra pars compacta that degenerate in Parkinson's disease require BDNF; consequently, expression of BDNF in the substantia nigra may have some potential therapeutic use in Parkinson's disease. Physical injury to the nervous system might be treated with expression of neurotrophic factors, and we have found that expression of NGF in the superior cervical ganglia can reverse specific effects of axotomy (29). Expression of neurotrophic receptors may be therapeutically useful and we have found that expression of the human NGF receptor $p75^{hNGFR}$ results in high-affinity NGF binding (30).

Diseases with Altered Neuronal Physiology

The strategy described above to alter the physiology of a specific type of neuron in a particular area of the brain (see example in Fig. 1) may be applicable to specific disease states. For example, epilepsies involve altered release of neurotransmitter(s) at specific site(s) in the brain. It has been hypothesized that some psychological disorders are caused by alterations in a specific neurotransmitter system such as the dopamine system. Advances in our knowledge of how specific types of neurons function to produce specific behaviors may result in new therapeutic approaches to disease states due to alterations in the function of these same neurons.

Defective HSV-1 Vector System for Gene Transfer into Neuronal Cells

Relevant Properties of HSV-1

Defective HSV-1 vectors have several attractive characteristics for genetic intervention in the brain (12); these features are based on specific properties of HSV-1. First, HSV-1 can infect quiescent cells, notably postmitotic neurons and glia in the adult mammalian brain. Second, HSV-1 has an unusually wide host range; HSV-1 can infect many different cell types such as fibroblasts, macrophages, glia, and neurons in many mammals, notably humans, nonhuman primates, and rodents (31). Third, an HSV-1 genome can be maintained in a latent state in neurons for the life of the cell (32). Fourth, in the latent state HSV-1 is remarkably quiescent; expression of viral genes is limited to a latency-associated transcript(s), HSV-1 DNA is not replicated, no progeny virus are produced, and electrophysiological properties of latently infected neurons are not changed (32).

When wild-type HSV-1 is injected into the brain, the lytic cycle results in the production of progeny virus and the infection spreads through the brain and rapidly kills the animal, often within several days. In contrast, intracerebral injection of temperature-sensitive (*ts*) mutants gives rise to a latent infection (33). These *ts* mutants contain a single base change in a gene essential for productive virus growth, resulting in a single amino acid substitution in the encoded protein. The mutant protein is functional at 31°C but not at the temperature of the brain, 37–39°C. Thus, the lytic cycle can proceed in tissue culture at 31°C, but not in the brain at 37°C. Thus, because these *ts* mutants do not grow in the brain, the infection is limited to cells around the injection site and to neurons that project to the injection site (33). We used these HSV-1 *ts* mutants (and subsequently deletion mutants in the same genes) to develop the defective HSV-1 vector system.

Experimental Procedure with HSV-1 Vectors

Initially, HSV-1 strain 17 *ts* K was used as the helper virus to package HSV-1 vectors into virus particles (10). This system was limited because *ts* mutants revert to wild-type HSV-1 at a finite frequency (33, 33a). In contrast, deletion mutants revert to wild type only at low frequencies. Subsequently, we developed a deletion mutant packaging system for defective HSV-1 vectors (34). A deletion mutant can grow in a cell line that contains the deleted gene in its genome and thereby complements the deletion mutant. To package vector DNA into HSV-1 particles using a deletion mutant as helper virus, the cell line harboring the deleted gene is transfected with vector DNA and then superinfected with deletion mutant virus.

We use the deletion mutant D30EBA as helper virus (35). Both D30EBA and *ts* K contain a mutation in the *IE3* gene in HSV-1 strain 17 and both mutants have the same phenotype; thus, switching from *ts* K to D30EBA should not alter the properties of the HSV-1 vector system. This deletion packaging system is a clear improvement over packaging using *ts* K as helper virus, establishes that defective HSV-1 vectors can be packaged using deletion mutants of HSV-1, and has supported experiments on neuronal physiology with HSV-1 vectors, both *in vitro* and *in vivo*. However, D30EBA, when grown on M64A cells, reverts to wild type at a frequency of approximately 1×10^{-5}. Consequently, this particular packaging system still has limitations and cannot support use in humans. Potential improvements (see below) to the deletion mutant packaging system, including a further reduction in the reversion frequency, will aid in experiments and may support use of HSV-1 vectors in humans.

Prototype Defective HSV-1 Vector, pHSVlac

The prototype HSV-1 vector, pHSVlac (10), contains three types of genetic elements (see Fig. 2).

1. A transcription unit that consists of the HSV-1 immediate-early 4/5 promoter, the intervening sequence immediately after the promoter, the *Escherichia coli lacZ* gene, and the simian virus 40 (SV40) early region polyadenylation site. This promoter is a constitutive promoter that functions in many cell types and the *lacZ* gene encodes a bacterial β-galactosidase,

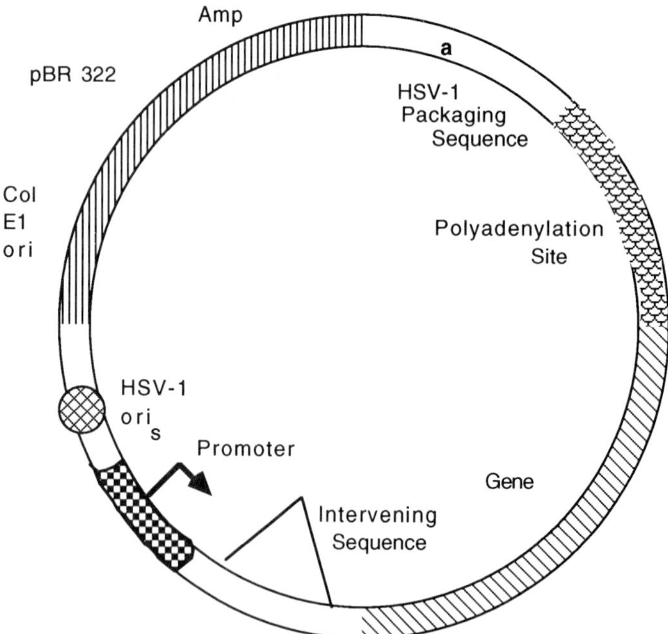

FIG. 2 The structure of a defective HSV-1 vector. A defective HSV-1 vector contains three kinds of genetic elements: (a) two HSV-1 packaging sequences required for packaging the vector into HSV-1 particles, the HSV-1 origin of DNA replication, ori_s, to support replication of vector DNA, and the HSV-1 **a** sequence, which contains the packaging site responsible for packaging vector DNA into HSV-1 particles; (b) the transcription unit, composed of a promoter, an intervening sequence, a gene, and a polyadenylation site; and (c) sequences from pBR322 required to propagate the vector in *E. coli*.

providing an assay for expression of this gene product. Thus, pHSVlac was useful for characterizing the properties of our system; however, the promoter and the *lacZ* gene can be replaced with other promoters and genes, respectively.

2. Two sequences from HSV-1 that are sufficient to package a vector into HSV-1 particles: (a) the HSV-1 **a** sequence, which contains the packaging site, and (b) HSV-1 ori_s, which supports replication of the vector DNA.
3. Bacterial sequences that allow growth of pHSVlac in *E. coli*.

Packaging Procedure Using the Deletion Mutant Packaging System

The packaging procedure (34) is diagrammed in Fig. 3. M64A cells are grown in Dulbecco's modified minimal essential medium containing 10% (v/v) fetal bovine serum at 37°C in the presence of 5% CO_2. M64A cells (1.5×10^5) are placed on a 60-mm plate. The following day, the cells are transfected by the calcium phosphate method, using a coprecipitate (0.5 ml) containing 9 μg of salmon sperm DNA and 1 μg of vector DNA. After a 4-hr incubation at 37°C, the transfected cells are treated with 15% (v/v) glycerol. Following an additional incubation at 37°C for 1 day, 8×10^6 plaque-forming units (PFU) of D30EBA is added to the plate. After 1 hr at room temperature, medium is added to a final volume of 5 ml, and 1 day later the virus is harvested. Virus is subsequently passaged three times; each passage is at a 1 : 2 dilution on M64A cells (34).

Gene Transfer by HSV-1 Vectors into Neurons and Glia

We established, in a detailed series of experiments using pHSVlac, that HSV-1 vectors can deliver a gene into mitotic and nonmitotic neural cell lines, human cells, cultured neurons and glia, and neurons and glia in the adult brain. Following infection with pHSVlac, expression of β-galactosidase was observed in many cultured neural cell lines (36), including N1E-115 mouse adrenergic neuroblastomas, NS-20Y mouse cholinergic neuroblastomas, PC-12 rat pheochromocytomas, AtT-20 mouse pituicytes, GH4 rat pituicytes, SK-N-BE(2) human neuroblastomas, Hs 630 human gliomas, and U1-Mel malignant human melanoma cells. Expression of β-galactosidase was also detected in several nonneuronal human cell lines, including GM2936B normal human fibroblasts, HEp-2 human laryngeal carcinoma, AT2052 ataxia telangiectasia fibroblasts, BS2548 Bloom's syndrome fibroblasts, FA2053 Fanconi's anemia fibroblasts, and XPV2359 xeroderma pigmentosum fibroblasts (37). In addition, expression was observed in two differentiated neuronal lines; N1E-115 cells treated with dibutyryl cAMP and PC-12 cells treated with NGF (36).

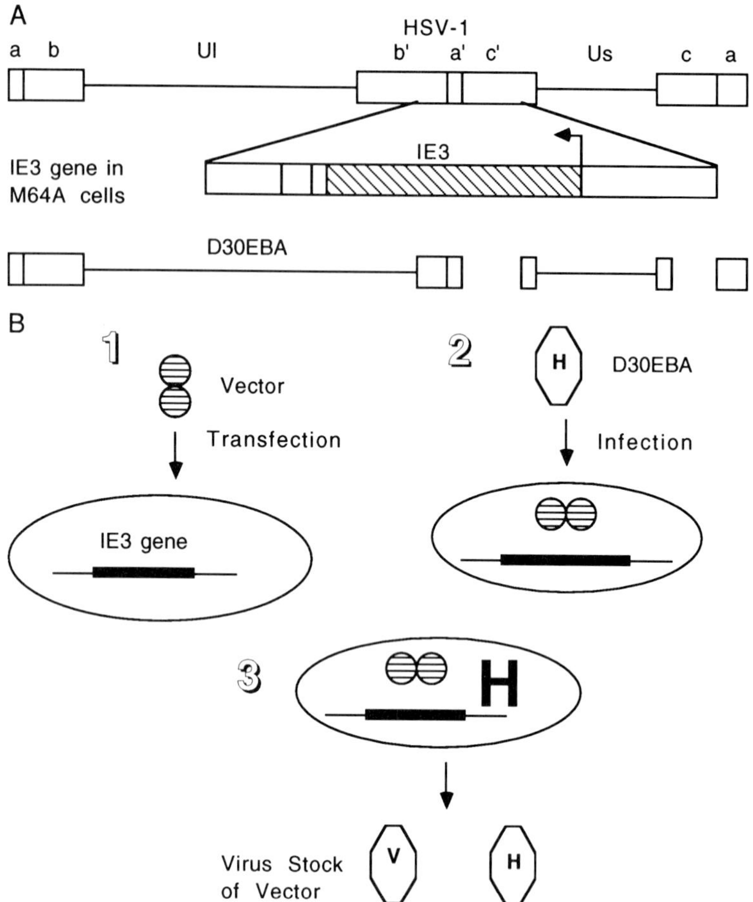

FIG. 3 The procedure for packaging a defective HSV-1 vector into virus particles. (A) *Top:* The structure of the HSV-1 genome: HSV-1 is a large, double-stranded DNA virus (150 kb) that contains approximately 75 genes. *Middle:* The portion of the genome containing the *IE3* gene, which is present in the M64A cell line. *Bottom:* The partial deletion of the *IE3* gene contained in D30EBA. (B) The procedure for packaging a vector into HSV-1 particles, using the deletion mutant packaging system. Step 1: Vector DNA is delivered by calcium phosphate DNA transfection into M64A cells. Step 2: The next day, these cells are infected with the helper virus, D30EBA. Step 3: The *IE3* gene in the cell line complements the *IE3* deletion mutant virus, resulting in a productive HSV-1 infection. The resulting virus stock is composed of identical HSV-1 particles that contain either the vector DNA (V) or the helper virus DNA (H).

Expression of β-galactosidase from pHSVlac was demonstrated in cultured cells from throughout the nervous system (10, 11). Peripheral neurons and glia derived from superior cervical ganglia and dorsal root ganglia were shown to express β-galactosidase, using X-Gal, 1 day after infection. Neuronal expression of β-galactosidase was also demonstrated in an immunofluorescent assay using a rabbit anti-*Escherichia coli* β-galactosidase antibody and a mouse anti-neurofilament antibody. Expression of β-galactosidase was demonstrated in cultured neurons from throughout the CNS, including spinal cord, cerebellum, thalamus, striatum, hippocampus, occipital cortex, temporal cortex, and frontal cortex. Expression of β-galactosidase was also detected in cells that did not contain neurofilament and that had glial morphology.

pHSVlac DNA was maintained in neurons and glia, and directed stable expression of β-galactosidase. Differentiated PC-12 cells, differentiated N1E-115 cells, and cultured neurons and glia from sensory ganglia, striatum, total neocortex, and hippocampus were infected with pHSVlac, and 2 weeks later expression of β-galactosidase was observed (10, 11, 36). pHSVlac DNA persisted in these cells for this period and was recovered following superinfection with HSV-1. pHSVlac stably persisted in an infected cell and was not horizontally transmitted to uninfected cells; the rate of horizontal transmission of pHSVlac was negligible as shown by the low titers of both the helper virus, *ts* K, and pHSVlac virus in the culture medium and by the maintenance of β-galactosidase-negative cells in these cultures. More recently, persistence of vector DNA in the adult rat brain has been demonstrated using PCR.

Following stereotactic injection of pHSVlac virus into the brain of adult rats, β-galactosidase was expressed in neurons and glia surrounding the injection site (hippocampus, occipital cortex, and superior colliculus), as well as in distant neurons whose axons project to the injection site (12, 13, 21, 22, 28). Expression was stably maintained for at least 1.5 months; pHSVlac escaped immune surveillance. Moreover, unlike wild-type HSV-1, pHSVlac did not spread throughout the brain, transfer of pHSVlac virus from one cell to another due to reactivation of persistent pHSVlac DNA did not occur.

Cell Type-Specific Promoter Restriction of Gene Expression from an HSV-1 Vector to a Specific Cell Type

pHSVlac contains the *IE4/5* promoter, which is transcriptionally active in many different cell types ranging from fibroblasts to glia and neurons. To limit expression to specific cell types, cell type-specific promoters have been inserted into HSV-1 vectors. Expression is then quantitated in multiple cell types, using the X-Gal assay, to determine cell type-specific expression. For example, the human neurofilament L promoter (pNflac) supports expression in PC-12 cells, but expression in fibroblasts is reduced approximately 50-

fold; similarly in cultured sympathetic or cortical cells expression is primarily observed in neurons rather than glia (17). The tyrosine hydroxylase promoter limits expression to catecholaminergic cells in culture or in the adult brain and deletions in the promoter can be used to study the regulation of this promoter (18). Furthermore, we have found that a neuron-specific enolase promoter restricts expression to neurons (S. Y. Bak, D. Hartley, R. L. Neve, and A. I. Geller, unpublished results, 1994). Thus, expression of a recombinant gene can be limited to a specific cell type by utilizing an appropriate promoter.

Limitations of Present System and Potential Solutions

Defective HSV-1 vectors clearly support genetic intervention in the brain; however, they are a developing, rather than a mature technology, and potential technological advances may improve the system in several areas. First, the current packaging system uses D30EBA, which carries a single deletion in the *IE3* gene, resulting in a reversion frequency to wild-type HSV-1 of approximately 10^{-5}. Use of a helper virus deleted in two or more essential genes should lower the reversion frequency below 10^{-10}. Second, an HSV-1 particle contains several proteins that have acute and temporary cytopathic effects; deleting these nonessential HSV-1 genes from the helper virus should allow an increase in the amount of vector used, especially with *in vivo* experiments in which multiple infection of cells proximal to the injection site, resulting in increased acute cytopathic effects, is likely to occur. Third, while cell type-specific promoters do confer cell type-specific expression on a recombinant gene, there is usually a low level of expression in inappropriate cell types. This inappropriate expression is likely due to either specific elements in the vector, particularly those proximal to the HSV-1 ori_s, or to specific genes in the helper virus. Thus, improvements in the vector and/or the helper virus may also enhance cell type-specific expression. In summary, if at least some of these improvements can indeed be made to the vector system, it is possible they will result in a defective HSV-1 vector system that can be used to perform human gene therapy.

Other Approaches to Direct Gene Transfer into Brain Cells

Many other approaches to direct gene transfer into neurons in the brain have been explored. Most have not yielded encouraging results, but two other approaches merit further study. Genes have been inserted into the HSV-1 genome and short-term expression from these vectors has been documented; however, it has not yet been possible to achieve stable expression *in vivo* with these kinds of HSV-1 vectors (38). Second, it has been shown that adenovirus vectors can express genes in selected neurons for at least 2 months (39). Because neurons are not the natural host for adenovirus, issues concerning the host range, stability of expression, and cytotoxic effects of this system remain to be resolved.

Alteration of Neuronal Physiology by Expression of Unregulated Adenylate Cyclase in Neurons

Signal transduction enzymes are particularly attractive targets for genetic manipulation of neuronal physiology because of the critical roles they are known to play in effecting both short-term and long-term changes in invertebrate neuronal function, as well as in effecting short-term changes in mammalian neuronal function. Many signal transduction enzymes are composed of a domain structure that lends itself to mutational analysis (see Fig. 4). Some enzymes involved in cyclic nucleotide metabolism contain such a domain structure: for example, the yeast adenylate cyclase (cyr) has distinct catalytic and regulatory domains (40). We hypothesized that expression of the catalytic domain of the yeast adenylate cyclase would result in a dominant positive unregulated activity in mammalian neurons, thereby increasing cAMP levels in the cell. We tested this hypothesis (14) and indeed found that expression of the cyr catalytic domain in neurons had specific effects on neuronal function: intracellular cAMP levels were greatly augmented, protein kinase A activity was elevated, phosphorylation of tyrosine hydroxylase by protein kinase A was stimulated, and basal neurotransmitter release was increased. These changes in neuronal physiology were stable for at least 1 week. The methods for these experiments, which are prototypic for studies involving infection of neurons with HSV-1 vectors expressing the catalytic domains of signal transduction enzymes, are presented below.

HSV-1 Vectors, Cell Culture, and Infections

The *lacZ* gene in pHSVlac was excised and replaced with the yeast adenylate cyclase catalytic domain (40) or with the pUC19 polylinker (pHSVpUC). The cDNA encoding the yeast adenylate cyclase catalytic domain was also fused to a sequence that encodes the 10-amino acid peptide Flag (41), for immunological detection using an anti-Flag antibody. [Flag has been fused to a wide range of proteins without noticeably affecting biological activity (41).] Vectors were packaged into HSV-1 particles as described above. Initially, we used the HSV-1 strain *ts* K as helper virus whereas later packaging procedures were performed with the deletion mutant packaging system (34). Virus stocks averaged 50% recombinant virus, at 2–6 $\times$ 10^6 infectious particles/ml. PC-12 cultures (2 $\times$ 10^5 cells/0.5 ml) grown in RPMI-1640 containing

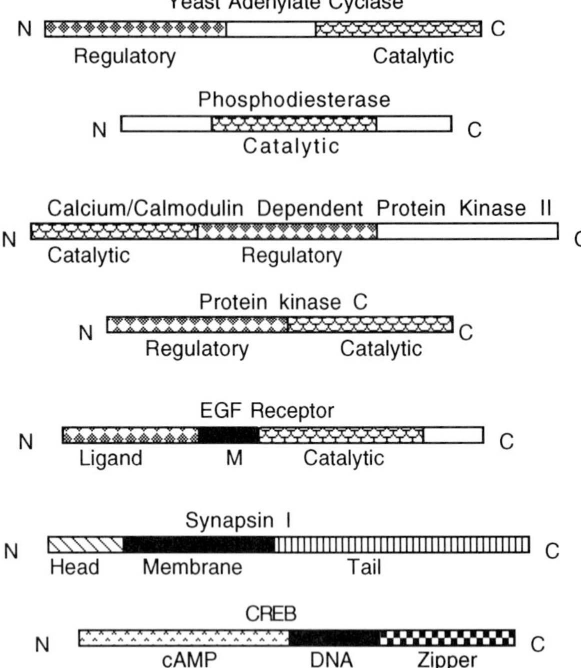

FIG. 4 Many components of signal transduction pathways contain a domain structure that is amenable to mutational analysis to derive unregulated proteins that are constitutively active. Regulatory domains (diamond segments) and catalytic domains (fish-scale segments) of five different signal transduction enzymes are shown. Components of the neurotransmitter release machinery, such as synapsin I, and transcription factors, such as CREB, also contain a domain structure that lends itself to mutational analysis.

10% (v/v) horse serum and 5% (v/v) fetal bovine serum were infected with virus stocks (7.5–12 μl), and assays were performed 1 day later. Cultures of dissociated superior cervical ganglia (10) were prepared using 4-day-old Sprague-Dawley rats and on days 5–6 the cultures were treated with the mitotic inhibitor cytosine arabinoside (40 μM). One to 3 weeks later, the cultures (2×10^5 cells/0.5 ml, 20% neurons) were infected with 7.5 μl of the virus stocks. Assays were performed on parallel sets of cultures that had been infected either 1 or 7 days earlier.

DNA and RNA Analysis

Total cellular DNA was isolated from infected cultures as described (11), digested with *Eco*RI, resolved on 0.7% (w/v) agarose gels, and transferred to a nylon membrane. The blot was hybridized with a probe for pBR sequences and for cyr; positive hybridization to the expected fragments indicated that the virus had been appropriately packaged. RNA was isolated 1 day after 2×10^7 CV1 fibroblast cells were infected with 1 ml of pHSVcyr or pHSVpUC. cyr cDNA was synthesized from the RNA and amplified using the polymerase chain reaction (PCR). In more recent experiments, reverse transcription (RT)-PCR (42) has been performed on primary neuronal cultures infected with HSV-1 vectors to confirm the presence of the recombinant RNA.

Neurotransmitter Release Assays

One day or 1 week after infection with HSV-1 vectors, cells were incubated (37°C, 15 min) in 1 ml (PC-12 cells) or 0.2 ml (neurons) of release buffer. The buffer was cooled (0°C, 5 min), and 1/10 vol each of 2 *M* $HClO_4$ and 1% (w/v) $Na_2S_2O_5$ was added. Release buffer consisted of 135 m*M* NaCl, 3 m*M* KCl, 1 m*M* $MgCl_2$, 1.2 m*M* $CaCl_2$, 2 m*M* $NaPO_4$, pH 7.4, and 10 m*M* glucose. Cells were lysed in 0.2 ml of ice-cold 4 *M* $HClO_3$ for 5 min and the lysates were buffered by addition of 100 μl of 1 *M* $NaPO_4$, pH 7.0, 80 μl of saturated NaOH, and 40 μl of $Na_2S_2O_5$. Catecholamines were separated by high-performance liquid chromatography and analyzed using a serial array of 16 electrode sensors (43; CEAS 55-0650; ESA, Inc.). Peaks were validated by comparison to standards (match criteria: retention time, ±2%; peak width, ±3 sec; peak ratio between sensors, >80%). The amount of catecholamines in each sample was quantitated on the basis of peak height (dominant sensor) relative to standards.Neurotransmitter release was measured over a 15-min period; therefore, this assay measured steady state changes in neurotransmitter release rather than changes in the initial rate of release.

Summary

We have developed and characterized a defective HSV-1 vector system that can support gene transfer into neurons and glia in culture or in the adult rat brain. Thus, HSV-1 vectors are likely to be useful both for studying neuronal physiology and brain functions as well as for performing gene therapy on neurological disorders. We have developed a strategy for studying neuronal physiology and brain functions by expressing the catalytic domains of signal transduction enzymes. Using this approach we have established that an unregulated adenylate cyclase causes a long-term increase in neurotransmitter release from cultured neurons. Initial results suggest that expressing these unregulated signal transduction enzymes from cell type-specific promoters in the adult brain can alter brain function and affect specific behavioral responses. A potential therapeutic approach to Parkinson's disease is to express the tyrosine hydroxylase gene in striatal cells. Expression of neurotrophic factors may be useful for treating specific neurodegenerative diseases. Only additional experiments can determine the potential of genetic intervention strategies to provide answers to basic questions about how the brain functions and to treat neurological disorders.

References

1. J. Price, D. Turner, and C. Cepko, *Proc. Natl. Acad. Sci. U.S.A.* **84,** 156–160 (1987).
2. J. R. Sanes, J. L. R. Rubenstein, and J. Nicolas, *EMBO J.* **5,** 3133–3142 (1986).
3. C. Cepko, *Trends Neurosci.* **11,** 6–8 (1988).
4. U. Lendahl and R. D. G. McKay, *Trends Neurosci.* **13,** 132–137 (1990).
5. C. Readhead, B. Popko, N. Takahashi, H. D. Shine, R. A. Saavedra, R. L. Sidman, and L. Hood, *Cell (Cambridge, Mass.)* **48,** 703–712 (1987).
6. T. A. Bargiello, F. R. Jackson, and M. W. Young, *Nature (London)* **312,** 752–754 (1984).
7. W. A. Zehring, D. A. Wheeler, P. Reddy, R. J. Konopka, C. P. Kyriacon, M. Rosbash, and J. C. Hall, *Cell (Cambridge, Mass.)* **39,** 369–376 (1984).
8. K. L. O'Malley, M. J. Anhalt, B. M. Martin, J. R. Kelsoe, S. L. Winfield, and E. I. Ginns, *Biochemistry* **26,** 6910–6914 (1987).
9. M. R. Montminy, R. H. Goodman, S. J. Horovitch, and J. F. Habener, *Proc. Natl. Acad. Sci. U.S.A.* **81,** 3370–3374 (1984).
10. A. I. Geller and X. O. Breakefield, *Science* **241,** 1667–1669 (1988).
11. A. I. Geller and A. Freese, *Proc. Natl. Acad. Sci. U.S.A.* **87,** 1149–1153 (1990).
12. A. Freese, A. I. Geller, and R. L. Neve, *Biochem. Pharmacol.* **40,** 2189–2199 (1990).
13. A. I. Geller, M. J. During, and R. L. Neve, *Trends Neurosci.* **14,** 428–432 (1991).
14. A. I. Geller, M. J. During, J. W. Haycock, A. Freese, and R. L. Neve, *Proc. Natl. Acad. Sci. U.S.A.* **90,** 7603–7607 (1993).
15. M. X. Zuber, S. M. Strittmatter, and M. C. Fishman, *Nature (London)* **341,** 345–348 (1989).
16. A. Papandrikopoulon, T. Doll, R. P. Tucker, C. C. Garner, and M. Matus, *Nature (London)* **340,** 650–652 (1989).
17. H. J. Federoff, A. I. Geller, and B. Lu, *Soc. Neurosci. Abstr.* **16,** 353 (1990).
18. Y. J. Oh, S. C. Wong, M. Moffat, D. Ullrey, A. I. Geller, and K. L. O'Malley, *Abstr. Soc. Neurosci.* **18,** 578.14 (1992).
19. S. Linder, T. Barkhem, A. Norberg, H. Perrson, M. Schalling, T. Hokfelt, and G. Magnusson, *Proc. Natl. Acad. Sci. U.S.A.* **84,** 605–609 (1987).
20. A. I. Geller, J. Bryan, O. Ashe, M. J. During, and R. L. Neve, *Abstr. Soc. Neurosci.* **17,** 240.11 (1991).
21. S. Song, P. Leone, Y. Wang, D. Hartley, J. Bryan, D. Ullrey, S. Y. Bak, K. Davis, K. L. O'Malley, R. L. Neve, A. I. Geller, and M. During, *Abstr. Soc. Neurosci.* **19,** 328.2 (1993).

22. P. Leone, M. Dragunow, K. Davis, D. Ullrey, K. L. O'Malley, R. L. Neve, A. I. Geller, and M. During, *Abstr. Soc. Neurosci.* **19,** 328.1 (1993). Deleted in proof.
23. M. D. Yahr and K. J. Bergmann, eds., "Parkinson's Disease." Raven Press, New York, 1987.
24. W. J. Freed, M. J. Perlow, F. Karoum, A. Seiger, L. Olson, B. J. Hoffer, and R. J. Wyatt, *Ann. Neurol.* **8,** 510–519 (1987).
25. O. Lindvall, E.-O. Backlund, L. Farde, G. Sedvall, R. Freedman, B. Hoffer, N. Nobin, A. Seiger, and L. Olson, *Ann. Neurol.* **22,** 457–468 (1987).
26. J. A. Wolff, L. J. Fisher, L. Xu, A. J. Hyder, P. J. Langinis, P. M. Iuvone, K. L. O'Malley, M. D. Rosenberg, S. Shimohama, T. Friedmann, and F. H. Gage, *Proc. Natl. Acad. Sci. U.S.A.* **86,** 9011–9014 (1989).
27. S. Jiao, V. Gurevich, and J. A. Wolff, *Nature* (*London*) **262,** 450–453 (1993).
28. M. J. During, A. I. Geller, A. Y. Deutch, and K. L. O'Malley, *Abstr. Soc. Neurosci.* **18,** 331.8 (1992).
28a. M. D. Geschwind, J. A. Kessler, A. I. Geller, and H. J. Federoff. Transfer of the nerve growth factor gene into cell lines and primary neuronal cultures using defective herpes simplex virus vectors. *Mol. Brain Res.* In press (1994).
29. H. J. Federoff, M. D. Geschwind, A. I. Geller, and J. A. Kessler, *Proc. Natl. Acad. Sci. U.S.A.* **89,** 1636–1640 (1992).
30. D. S. Battleman, A. I. Geller, and M. V. Chao, *J. Neurosci.* **13,** 941–951 (1993).
31. P.G. Spear and B. Roizman, *in* "DNA Tumor Viruses" (J. Tooze, ed.), pp. 615–746. Cold Spring Harbor Lab., Cold Spring Harbor, NY, 1981.
32. J. G. Stevens, *Curr. Top. Microbiol. Immunol.* **70,** 31–50 (1975).
33. K. Watson, J. G. Stevens, M. L. Cook, and J. H. Subak-Sharpe, *J. Gen. Virol.* **49,** 149–159 (1980).
33a. M. J. Davison, V. G. Preston, and D. J. McGeoch, Determination of the sequence alteration in the DNA of the herpes simplex virus type 1 temperature-sensitive mutant ts K. *J. Gen. Virol.* **65,** 859–863 (1984).
34. A. I. Geller, K. Keyomarski, J. Bryan, and A. B. Pardee, *Proc. Natl. Acad. Sci. U.S.A.* **87,** 8950–8954 (1990).
35. T. Patterson and R. D. Everett, *J. Gen. Virol.* **71,** 1775–1783 (1990).
36. A. I. Geller, *J. Neurosci. Methods* **36,** 91–103 (1991).
37. D. A. Boothman, A. I. Geller, and A. B. Pardee, *FEBS Lett.* **258,** 159–162 (1989).
38. A. T. Dobson, T. P. Margolis, F. Sedacrati, J. G. Stevens, and L. T. Feldman, *Neuron* **5,** 353–360 (1990).
39. G. L. G. La Salle, J. J. Robert, S. Berard, V. Ridoux, L. D. Stratford-Perricaudet, M. Perricaudet, and J. Mallet, *Science* **259,** 988–990 (1993).
40. T. Kataoka, D. Broek, and M. Wigler, *Cell* (*Cambridge, Mass.*) **43,** 493–505 (1985).
41. T. P. Hopp, K. S. Prickett, V. L. Price, R. J. Libby, C. J. March, D. P. Cerretti, D. L. Urdal, and P. J. Conlon, *BioTechniques* **6,** 1204–1210 (1988).
42. K. J. Ivins, K. A. Neve, D. J. Feller, S. A. Fidel, and R. L. Neve, *J. Neurochem.* **60,** 626–633 (1993).
43. W. R. Matson, P. G. Gamache, M. F. Beal, and E. D. Bird, *Life Sci.* **41,** 905–908 (1987).

[27] Expression of Neurotrophic Genes from Herpes Simplex Virus Type 1 Vectors: Modifying Neuronal Phenotype

Michael D. Geschwind, Bing Lu, and Howard J. Federoff

Introduction

Gene transfer into the mammalian nervous system promises to accelerate our understanding of complex neurophysiological processes and allow the delivery of therapeutic genes for inherited and acquired disorders affecting the nervous system. Development of an ideal gene transfer vector could be used to alter or change development, to modify the intact or diseased central nervous system (CNS), or to facilitate the generation of models for human disease. Such idealized vectors should be designed to cross the blood–brain barrier or to act in a targeted region, to be susceptible to regulation, and to express over an extended period of time. No single vector can fulfill all the criteria; however, herpes viral vectors transducing a gene driven by a regulatable promoter may have the greatest potential for being able to fulfill these criteria.

To date, herpes simplex virus (HSV)-based vectors are one of only three means of transferring genes into postmitotic cells such as neurons (1–4). HSV-1 is ideally suited as a vector for gene transfer for many reasons. It can infect a variety of cell types in many different organisms (5). Its large size (150 kb) suggests that HSV-1 vectors can be produced to carry relatively large genes. It can persist indefinitely in a latent state in neurons without affecting their electrophysiological properties (6), and HSV-1 genes are transcribed by cellular RNA polymerase II, suggesting that cellular promoters placed in the vector could be transcribed as well (7). It has a high level of expression (8), expression is often stable (9), and because it exists in an episomal state, there is little chance of insertional mutagenesis of host genes (9).

This chapter discusses methodologies used for one type of HSV-1 defective viral vector, the amplicon. This is a plasmid-based system of gene transfer that is effective for many cell types, including postmitotic neurons. The chapter presents methods for growing, titering, and applying defective HSV-1 vectors both *in vitro* and *in vivo*. These viral vectors are defective, nonreplicating HSV-1-derived viruses. The usefulness of these vectors for

Methods in Neurosciences, Volume 21

transducing genes to modify neuronal function is illustrated by vectors carrying neurotrophic factor genes. Specifically, the following areas are covered.

1. Amplicon-based viral vectors
2. Growing and maintaining the packaging cell line, the helper virus, and the amplicon virions
3. Specific details about packaging virus, including transfection of packaging cell line with the amplicon, passaging the virions, and troubleshooting
4. Analysis of the viral stock
5. Vector gene transduction *in vitro* and *in vivo*
6. Comparison of amplicon-based herpes vectors to other viral vectors for gene transfer in the nervous system
7. Potential developments of amplicon-based HSV vectors

Amplicon Vector System

Numerous articles review the life cycle and molecular biology of HSV (10–12) and thus this is not discussed here. Several observations have led to the development of the herpes amplicon. These include the definition of the *cis*-acting HSV sequences that are origins for viral DNA replication (ori) and sequences required for cleavage and packaging of DNA into virions (pac), identification of nonessential genes for virus propagation in tissue culture, and description of techniques designed for the genetic manipulation of the large genome of HSV-1 (13–20). The general principle of the amplicon system is as follows: the amplicon plasmid, which is replication defective, contains ori and pac sites, as well as the gene to be transduced. It is transfected into a cell, where it exists as an episome. These cells are then infected with a helper virus. All proteins needed for replication and packaging of the amplicon into virions are provided by the helper virus and complementing viral genes resident in the packaging cell line (see below).

The construction of the viral amplicon, design and insertion of the transcription unit into the amplicon, and the description of the packaging procedure has already been published (7, 21–23). Briefly, the components needed are (a) a helper HSV-1 virus deleted in at least one essential HSV gene, (b) a packaging cell line that complements the helper virus by containing the deleted essential HSV-1 gene(s) in its genome, and (c) the amplicon plasmid. The helper virus is replication defective, except when grown on the packaging cell line. The amplicon, which is transfected into the packaging cell line, consists of four main elements: (a) sequences for propagation in *Escherichia coli,* (b) an HSV 1 origin of replication (ori), necessary for replication of DNA, (c) an HSV-1 DNA packaging site (pac), needed for DNA to be packaged into virions, and (d) one or more transcription units.

Once the amplicon is transfected into the packaging cell line, the cells are then infected with helper virus. The HSV-1 genes present in the helper virus and packaging cell line allow for replication and packaging of a concatameric form of the amplicon DNA into virions. The resultant virus stock is a mixture of helper and vector virions that can then be used for gene transfer into neuronal and nonneuronal cells.

Packaging of Defective HSV-1 Viral Vectors

Care and Handling of Virus

Although the helper virus is replication defective, wild-type revertants resulting from recombination between the helper and the complementing cell

TABLE I Reagents Needed for Packaging Amplicon Vectors

Reagent	Description	Ref.[a]
Packaging cell line		
M64A	BHK TK(−)-derived cell line	1
E5	Vero-derived cell line	2,3
RR1	BHK TK(−)-derived cell line	4
Media		
For M64A cells (packaging)	DMEM, 10% FBS, penicillin (100 U/ml), and streptomycin (100 μg/ml)	
For M64A cells (maintaining)	DMEM, 10% FBS, penicillin (100 U/ml), streptomycin (100 μg/ml), and HAT	
For E5 cells	DMEM, 10% FBS, penicillin (100 U/ml), and streptomycin (100 μg/ml) and every 10 passages use G418 (400 μg/ml active) for maintaining cell selection	4
For RR1 cells	DMEM, 10% FBS, penicillin (100 U/ml), streptomycin (100 μg/ml), and G418.	4
Helper virus		
D30EBA	*IE3* deletion mutant	1
D120	*IE3* deletion mutant	2
14HΔ3	*IE3* deletion mutant and VP16 insertional mutation	4
Amplicon		5
Cup Sonicator (Heat Systems, Inc.)		

[a] Key to references: (1) see Paterson and Everett (24); (2) N. DeLuca, A. McCarthy, and P. Schaffer, *J. Virol.* **56**(2), 558 (1985); (3) N. DeLuca and P. Schaffer, *Nucleic Acids Res.* **15,** 4491 (1987); (4) see Johnson *et al.* (58); (5) see Geller and Breakefield (21) and Frenkel *et al.* (28).

line arise at various frequencies during production of the amplicon vectors (if wild-type virus occurs, at greater than 10^{-5}, make a new stock of helper virus). In addition to the possibility of wild-type virus, viruses transducing genes such as neurotrophins and receptors could also be potentially hazardous. Therefore, one should work under biological safety level 2 conditions and disinfect, with an iodine-containing solution, virtually all materials that come into contact with the virus, including surfaces.

Growing M64As and D30EBA

The reagents needed for packaging virus are shown in Table I. The details below on packaging are based on the use of the M64A packaging cell line and D30EBA helper virus. Other cell lines and helper viruses, such as those in Table I, can be used with some alterations in the protocol. The M64A cell line must be kept under hypoxanthine–aminopterin–thymidine (HAT) selection (24). Cells are maintained in Dulbecco's modified Eagle's medium (DMEM) with 10% (v/v) fetal bovine serum (FBS), penicillin (100 U/ml), and streptomycin (100 μg/ml) (P/S). We have found that M64A cells grow well in medium containing either low (1000 mg/ml) or high (4500 mg/ml) glucose. The protocol discussed below refers to M64A cells grown in low glucose. Some adjustments in the number of cells plated may be needed if using medium with high glucose.

Specifics about Packaging Procedure

The procedure for packaging virus takes 12 to 14 days if done continuously. This procedure is discussed in detail below and is outlined in Table II. We discuss the following protocols below.

1. Transfection of the packaging cell line
2. Determining transfection efficiency
3. Superinfection of transfected cells, passage 0 (P0)
4. Passaging the virus through three consecutive passages after superinfection

Transfection Procedure

For each virus to be packaged, we prepare 25–30 μg of sterile amplicon plasmid DNA in sterile water or DMEM, after two cycles of ethanol precipita-

TABLE II Outline for Passaging HSV-1 Defective Virus

Time	Procedure
Day 1	
−6 hr	Trypsinize and plate cells
0 hr	Transfect cells (transfect an extra *lacZ* plasmid)
5–6 hr	Add equal volume DMEM with 5% FCS
Day 2	1. X-Gal one β-galactosidase plate to determine transfection efficiency (see Transfection Procedure) 2. After confirming transfection, superinfect with helper virus for 1 hr (P0)
Day 3	Monitor cytopathicity
Day 4	Monitor cytopathicity. Assuming virus will be ready on day 5 (i.e., 100% cytopathic), plate cells for P1
Day 5	Harvest P0 virus (i.e., scrape cells, sonicate, spin down debris). Add undiluted to cells
Day 6	Monitor cytopathicity
Day 7	Monitor cytopathicity. Assuming virus will be ready on day 8, plate cells for P2 (100-mm plates)
Day 8	Harvest P1 virus. Add diluted 1 : 1 with fresh medium to cells
Day 9	Monitor cytopathicity
Day 10	Monitor cytopathicity. Assuming virus will be ready on day 11, plate cells for P3 (100-mm plates, twice the number of plates as for P2)
Day 11	Harvest P2 virus. Add diluted 1 : 1 with fresh medium to cells
Day 12	Monitor cytopathicity
Day 13	Monitor cytopathicity
Day 14	Harvest P3 virus. Aliquot, freeze, and titer

tion. Plate M64A cells in a 60-mm dish such that they are 70% confluent or higher, but not completely confluent. Leave at 37°C. Set up an extra plate that will be transfected in parallel with a plasmid containing a *lacZ* reporting gene and then treated with 5-bromo-4-chloro-3-indolyl-β-D-galactopyranoside (X-Gal) to determine transfection efficiency. Four to 6 hr postplating, gently wash the plates two times with 4 ml of serum-free medium (8 ml/100-mm dish). Leave in 2 ml of serum-free medium (5 ml/100-mm dish).

Add 40 μl of Lipofectin (GIBCO-Bethesda Research Laboratories, Gaithersburg, MD) per 60-mm plate, or 100 μl/100 mm plate, and rock gently to spread, and then let the plates sit 5 min at room temperature. After 5 min, add about 30 μg of the sterile-prepared plasmid vector DNA per 60-mm plate (about 70 μg/100-mm plate), rock gently to spread the DNA and return to 37°C. Approximately 6 hr after Lipofectin transfection, add 2 ml of DMEM–5% (v/v) FCS without HAT supplement (5 ml/100-mm plate). About 24 hr after transfection, perform histochemical staining for β-galactosidase on the dish transfected with the *lacZ* vector to determine transfection efficiency. Numerous published protocols are available (25). If transfection efficiency is greater than 0.5%, on the basis of X-Gal staining, continue with superinfection. After plating cells for transfection, all media used in viral packaging are without HAT supplement.

Detailed Passaging Procedure

In our laboratory, after the initial superinfection (passage 0 or P0), we carry out packaging for three consecutive passages (P1–P3). More or fewer passages can be done, depending on the desired ratio of vector particles to helper virus (see Analysis of Viral Stocks) (13). At any freezing step, the virus may be stored at −70°C until one is ready for the next step. The terms "day 1, day 2, ..., day 14" used in the packaging procedure assume the procedure is done continuously (see Table II).

On day 2 (the day after transfection), superinfect the transfected plates. Remove the medium from each plate, leaving about 0.5 ml behind, and add about 0.5–2 × 10^6 infectious particles (i.p.) of D30EBA virus. Ideally one should use virus at a multiplicity of infection (MOI) of between 0.1 and 1.0. Rock the plates every 15 min for a total of 1 hr at room temperature. After 1 hr add 5 ml of DMEM with 5% (v/v) FCS, 1% (v/v) P/S, and incubate at 34°C (26).

Over the next 2 to 3 days, on days 3–5, examine the cytopathicity of cells to determine whether they are ready to be harvested. Virus is ready to be harvested when all cells have a cytopathic effect (CPE). Cytopathicity is characterized by rounded cells (27). A plate should be harvested when basically all cells are rounded and just beginning to lift off the plate (100% CPE).

The harvesting procedures is as follows. Most HSV-1 will stay inside the cell between 23 and 34°C. At 37°C, the virus is released from the cell (P. Schaffer, personal communication, 1993). Therefore, before the cells are scraped, place the cells at 37°C for 1 to 2 hours to stimulate release of virus. Scrape the cells in the original medium, rotating the plate three to four times to ensure all areas are scraped. Collect the cell suspension in medium in a 50-ml polypropylene conical tube and quick-freeze in a dry ice–ethanol bath (virus can be left at −70°C at this step until M64A cells are ready for the next passage or, if the cells are ready, proceed with the harvesting). Thaw the virus at 34°C and sonicate for three 30-sec bursts, using a cup sonicator (setting 6–8; Heat Systems, Farmingdale, NY) cooled with circulating ice-cold water. Cool the virus on ice for at least 1 min between each burst. Spin down the cellular debris at 1200 rpm for 10 min. Remove the medium from the M64A plates for the next passage and add newly harvested viral supernatant (undiluted for P1, diluted 1 : 1 with medium for P2 and P3) and incubate at 34°C.

The next passage we refer to as P1, and it begins about day 5. Plate 3–4 × 10^6 cells/60-mm plate the day before use, on about day 4 (when 50%

or more of cells from P0 have CPE). The next day (day 5), harvest the virus from the cells and add virus from each P0 plate undiluted to 60-mm plates to begin P1.

Monitor cell cytopathicity over days 6–8, until 100% CPE is achieved. Harvest the virus in the same manner as for P0. One day before beginning P2 (i.e., about day 7), plate the same number of plates used for P1, but at 1×10^7 cells/100-mm plate.

On day 8, harvest the P1 virus and add supernatant (about 5 ml) to the 100-mm P2 plates. Dilute the virus 1 : 1 by adding 5 ml of DMEM, 5% (v/v) FCS, penicillin (100 U/ml), and streptomycin (100 μg/ml) to each plate for a total of approximately 10 ml/100-mm plate (one can also dilute the virus first and then add it to the plates). Incubate the cells at 34°C and monitor cytopathicity, over days 9–11, until 100% CPE is achieved. One day before beginning P3 (i.e., about day 10), plate 1×10^7 cells/100-mm plate (the number of plates will be double the number used for P2). When P2 reaches 100% CPE, probably on day 11, harvest the P2 virus. Dilute the 10 ml of viral supernatant from each P2 plate with 10 ml of medium and add 10 ml to each P3 plate.

Monitor cytopathicity over days 12–14, and harvest when 100% CPE is achieved. Aliquot, freeze, and titer virus.

Analysis of Viral Stocks

Virology

Adjusting Ratio of Amplicon Virus to Helper Virus

The HSV-1 amplicon vector method of gene transfer could be developed because of the observation that after serial undiluted passages of herpes viruses at high MOI in culture, defective interfering particles were generated. These defective viral particles still encapsulate a 150-kb genome; however, they consist of reiterations of small, repetitive DNA sequences as short as 3 kb (13). These defective particles can replicate only in the presence of wild-type virus. Because the defective particles contain many more origins of replication than in the wild-type HSV-1 they compete for the replication machinery encoded by the copropagating wild-type virus. This competition is the basis whereby passage at high MOIs promotes an increase in titer of the defective relative to the wild-type virus. On the basis of the molecular characterization of these reiterated pieces of DNA found within the defective particles, the minimum *cis* elements needed for DNA replication (ori) and packaging (pac) into virions were determined (13, 17, 18, 28). In the amplicon system, the amplicon vector is analogous to the defective particle and the mutated helper virus plus complementing cell line fulfills the role of the wild-type virus.

To ensure that the amplicon vector has not been rearranged during packaging, a Southern blot analysis can be performed on DNA extracted from stocks of virus. An example of such an analysis is shown in Fig. 1. As shown, the DNA extracted from separate viral stocks shows no evidence of rearrangement of its transcription unit; the fragment containing the transcription unit was the same size as in the original amplicon plasmid.

Titering Helper and Revertant Wild-Type Virus by Plaque Assay

In our laboratory, we have used several different methods for titering. The only difference between titering wild-type and helper virus is the cell line

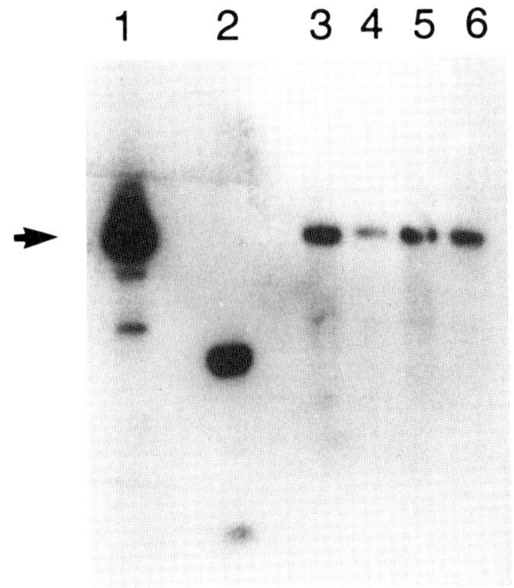

FIG. 1 Southern blot analysis of viral stocks. Determination of the integrity of amplicon transcription unit after third passage of virus-packaging procedure. DNA was phenol extracted from two separate viral stocks of the same amplicon in duplicate. This DNA, and DNA from the original amplicon plasmid, were cut with restriction enzymes to liberate the entire transcription unit, run on a gel, and hybridized with DNA that specifically recognizes the transcription unit. Lane 1, the amplicon plasmid transcription unit; lane 2, a 1-kb ladder; lanes 3 and 4, the P3 virus in duplicate; lanes 5 and 6, the same amplicon vector from a separate P3 viral stock in duplicate. The transcription unit is the same size in lanes 1 and 3–6. If the transcription unit in the amplicon had undergone recombination during the viral packaging procedure, it would be a different size than transcription unit cut from the original amplicon plasmid. The band hybridizing in the 1-kb ladder represents hybridization of the probe to a plasmid fragment of the standard.

used. For wild-type virus, we use the Vero (African Green monkey kidney) cell line and for helper virus we use the packaging cell line M64A or the E5 cell line (a Vero cell containing HSV-1 *IE3* gene; gift of N. DeLuca). We have used two different overlays, methylcellulose or low melting point (LMP) agarose, for titering (the latter is easier to make). The methods of making the overlays are discussed below, followed by methods for applying the overlay.

Making Methylcellulose

Methylcellulose is made by autoclaving 3.6 g of methylcellulose in 100 ml of distilled H_2O, shaking for 2 to 3 days at 4°C until all methylcellulose is dissolved. Add 100 ml of 2× DMEM without phenol red, containing 10% (v/v) FBS and 2× penicillin (200 U/ml) and 2× streptomycin (200 μg/ml) and shake for 10–20 min until homogeneous.

Making Low Melting Point Agarose

This recipe is from the laboratory of M. Horwitz (Albert Einstein College of Medicine, Bronx, NY). Make a 2% dilution of low melting point agarose in double-distilled water, autoclave, and store at room temperature. When ready to titer virus, melt the agarose in a microwave, and place in a beaker of water in a 45°C bath for a minimum of 10–15 min, to ensure the agarose is liquid. Place an aliquot of 2× medium (see above) in a 45°C bath (do not place the entire bottle of medium in the bath, as components may precipitate with repeated warming and cooling). Under a hood, mix the agarose and 2× DMEM medium (same medium as for methylcellulose) together at a ratio of 1 : 1 and place it in a beaker containing warm (37°C) water in the hood.

Plating Cells and Applying Overlay

Plate the cells in 60-mm dishes so that they will be just confluent the next day (for M64A cells this is about 1.6–2.0 × 10^5 cells). One laboratory uses 2.5 × 10^5 M64A cells/35-mm dish (R. Everett, personal communication, 1994) and another uses 10^6 Vero cells/35-mm dish (27). The next day, infect with at least 100 μl of serially diluted virus. Every 15 min for the next hour, rock the plates to ensure the inoculant is spread over the cells. Inoculation can be done at 37°C (26) or room temperature.

Remove the viral inoculant from the plates (optional). Gently add overlay, either methylcellulose or LMP agarose, warmed to 37°C, to each plate (5 ml/60-mm plate; 1.5–2.0 ml/35-mm plate) and incubate at 37°C.

Over the next 2 to 3 days examine the plates under a microscope for viral plaques. There are many different methods to facilitate visualization of plaques for counting, including dark-field illumination or by adding a stain such as neutral red diluted in phosphate-buffered saline (PBS); add enough to flood the plate and count the plaques within 3 hr (29). In addition to this method of titering, many authors have published other methods for titering HSV-1 (27, 30).

Biology: Titering Amplicon Vectors

Titering Viruses Containing Reporter Genes

It is relatively straightforward to titer a virus expressing a marker protein, such as β-galactosidase. The results of one experiment in which we determined the relationship between the number of viral particles added and the number of cells infected are shown in Fig. 2. Vero cells were plated at 1 ×

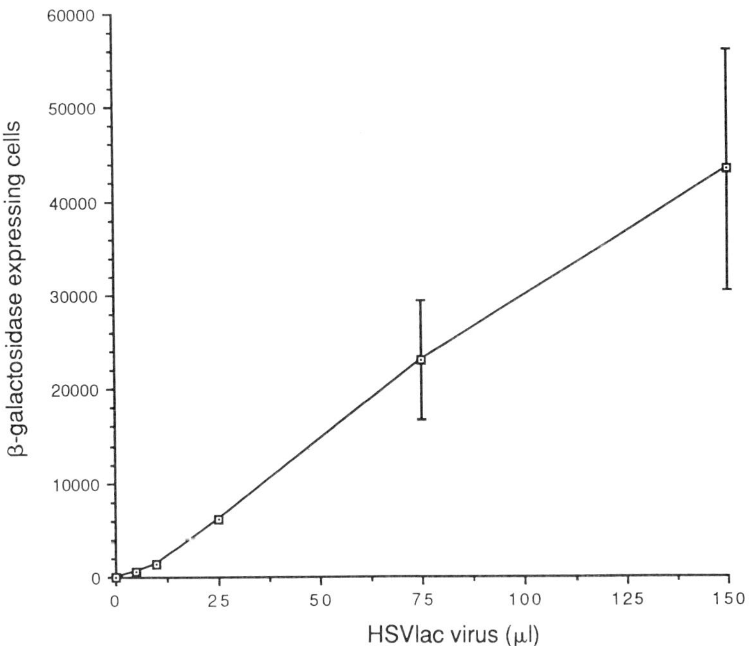

FIG. 2 Titering of HSVlac virus: the relationship between the volume of virus appleid and the number of cells expressing the β-galactosidase gene. Vero cells were plated (1×10^6 cells/35-mm dish) and infected in duplicate with increasing volumes, ranging from 0 to 150 μl of pHSVlac virus. Twenty-four hours after infection, cells were washed, fixed, and stained overnight with X-Gal. The next day blue cells were counted. There is a linear relationship between the volume of virus added and the number of blue cells. Bars represent standard error.

10^6 cells/35-mm dish and infected in duplicate with increasing volumes of HSVlac virus, ranging from 0 to 150 μl. Twenty-four hours after infection cells were stained with X-Gal and blue cells were counted. As seen in Fig. 2, there is a linear relationship between the volume of virus added and the number of blue cells.

Human growth hormone (hGH) is one of the frequently used reporter genes for detection of DNA transfection of mammalian cells (31, 32). Endogenous hGH is not detected in most mammalian cells, except where it is secreted by somatotrophs of the anterior pituitary. Because it is secreted and it is not found in most mammalian cells, hGH is very suitable to use as a reporter gene for HSV-mediated transduction of most mammalian cells. Levels of hGH can be monitored during an experiment using a commercially available kit (Nichols Institute Diagnostics, San Juan Capistrano, CA). In addition, hGH's very short half-life *in vivo* provides for a good correlation between serum hGH levels and gene expression (33, 34).

Molecular Biology

Titering by DNA Slot-Blot

Another method for quantitation of defective viral genomes, regardless of what gene it is expressing, is by slot-blot, as shown in Fig. 3. DNA, extracted from known volumes of viral stock, and also increasing amounts of amplicon plasmid DNA (1 ng to 800 ng) are bound to a nylon membrane and then probed with DNA that will hybridize to the amplicon DNA and not to the helper viral DNA. Using densitometry one can determine the amount of amplicon DNA per unit volume of virus stock. Since each defective virus contains concatamers of the ammplicon DNA up to 150 kb, one must correct for this number. This method gives the number of vector genomes per unit volume. Not all of these measured vector genomes will successfully transduce and express their heterologous genes as assayed by expression.

Troubleshooting

If viral titers are lower than expected, consider some of the following observations and make appropriate changes in technique.

HSV-1 viruses are sensitive to environmental conditions. Virus is stored by freezing in a dry ice–ethanol bath and then being placed at $-70°C$. We have found that repeated freeze-thaws may inactivate the virus. Therefore, after completing the final packaging step, aliquot the virus in volumes slightly larger than what will be used for experiments.

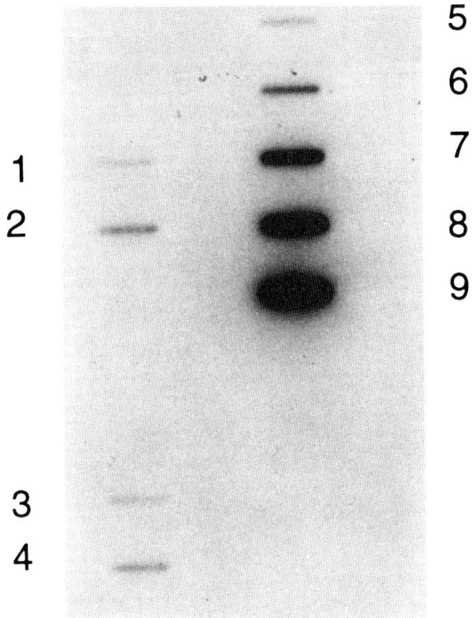

FIG. 3 Determining defective viral genomes by slot-blot. DNA was phenol extracted from 2 vol (lanes 1 and 3, 20 μl and lanes 2 and 4, 50 μl) of two different virus stocks (lanes 1 and 2, HSVlac; lanes 3 and 4, HSVgluR6) and run on the slot-blot along with a titration. Lanes 5–9 are a titration of defective viral DNA amplicons (1, 10, 50, 200, and 800 ng, respectively). Knowing the length of the DNA amplicon, one can estimate the number of amplicon units that can be concatamerized and packaged per virus. The length of the amplicon DNA is easily converted to a weight, giving a total weight of defective virus DNA per virus. Using the titration curve, one can determine the number of defective viruses per volume of viral stock.

As with many cell lines, we do not let stock M64A cells grow to high density. Cells plated at 5×10^5/100-mm dish can be left for 3 to 4 days without splitting. For viral passage 1 (P1), plate 3×10^6 cells/60-mm plate. For passage 2 (P2) and passage 3 (P3), plate 1×10^7 cells/100-mm plate and use the next day.

Viral Transduction

How to Apply Virus

Viral transduction of cell lines and primary cultures is relatively straightforward. We have found high levels of transduction simply by applying viral inoculant, at MOIs of about 1–3, to cells in medium. Prior to viral transduction, it is best to remove as much medium as possible to the extent that the cells will remain healthy. Depending on the conditions of the particular viral transduction, medium containing virus may be left on the cells or removed after a certain time period.

We have found expression of a reporter gene (β-galactosidase) by staining cells as soon as 3 hr after viral infection (cells were exposed to virus for 1 hr before rinsing; see Table III). For viral transduction of cells in culture, longer exposure to virus will allow greater absorption. As shown in Table III, increasing exposure of cells to the virus from 1 to 2 hr roughly doubles the number of cells infected. Lengthening the time of exposure of cells to virus from 2 to 4 hr increased the number of cells infected by about an additional 40%.

Use in Hippocampal Slice Cultures

We have shown, with others, that our amplicon-based HSV-1 vector can be efficiently applied to hippocampal slice cultures to express β-galactosidase or proteins that alter neuronal physiology (35). A complete review of this

TABLE III Expression of HSVlac Virus *in Vitro*[a]

Virus exposure time (hr)	Time after virus removal before staining (hr)	Total time before staining (hr)	Expressing cells (blue forming units/ml)
	2	3	0.80×10^6
	4.5	5.5	0.84×10^6
1	24	25	1.58×10^6
	2	4	1.17×10^6
	4.5	6.5	1.82×10^6
2	24	26	4.27×10^6
	2	6	1.82×10^6
	4.5	8.5	2.50×10^6
4	24	28	6.11×10^6

[a] NIH 3T3 cells ($2–4 \times 10^5$/well) were plated in a 24-well plate and 2 μl of virus was added for the times shown in column 1 before cells were washed and fresh medium added. Cells were left in the fresh medium for the times shown in column 2 until they were washed, fixed, and stained for β-galactosidase expression with X-Gal. Column 3 shows the total time the cells were allowed to express the construct before staining. The titer of expression (column 4) was determined by calculating the total number of blue cells per dish and dividing by the volume of virus added. The titers shown are averages of duplicate wells.

methodology has been described (36). In brief, organotypic slice cultures are established from 400-μm hippocampal slices from 10-day-old Sprague-Dawley rat pups and maintained for 3 to 4 weeks prior to viral transduction. Fifty to 250 nl of viral stock is microapplied at a flow rate of 50 nl/min with pulled glass micropipettes positioned with a manual micromanipulator (Narishige, Greenvale, NY) placed on a vibrationless table (Kinetic Systems, Spring Valley, NY). For identification of expression of a reporter gene such as β-galactosidase, cultures are generally maintained for an additional 24 hr and then stained with X-Gal.

Use in Vivo

Because of the small volume available for expansion in the brain, unlike most other organs, only microliter amounts of virus can be applied. We keep the virus at $-70°C$ on dry ice until the animal is ready for injection. We then thaw the virus to room temperature or 37°C. Some investigators inject as much as 10 μl of virus per site (37); however, we prefer to inject less (2–5 μl) over several minutes (3–5 min). Injections are done stereotaxically, using a Hamilton syringe with a 26S-gauge needle. One can also use a microapplicator (David Kopf, Inc., Tujunga, CA), which will facilitate a constant steady injection; however, we have not found this apparatus to be necessary. Withdraw the needle slowly so as to prevent viral reflux from the needle track. When finished, clean the syringe and needle with 95% ethanol to kill any remaining virus and then rinse thoroughly with sterile distilled water.

Altering Neuronal Physiology

A use of HSV-1 vectors with great potential for neurobiology is the transfer of genes into neurons to study the molecular basis of neuronal physiology (23; reviewed in Ref. 7). One approach would be to transfer dominantly acting mutated genes into a normal cellular environment. Such genetic intervention affords a means of altering physiology with precision not previously possible. With HSV-1 vectors, it is possible for several reasons: the cellular changes would be confined to those caused by changes in a single protein; the intervention would be relatively stable; it could be physically directed to specific location in the nervous system; and through the use of appropriate promoters its expression could be limited to certain cell types (7).

The amplicon vectors have been used to express several genes that can alter neuronal physiology. Expression of nerve growth factor (NGF) from our vector in an axotomized superior cervical ganglia (SCG) prevented some of the sequelae of axotomy (8) and in culture can support survival and neuronal phenotype in the absence of added growth factor (37a). We have also made a vector expressing brain-derived neurotrophic factor (BDNF) and shown that it can support survival of neurons normally requiring exogenous factor (38).

In collaboration with others, we produced a vector that transduces the gene encoding the high-affinity nerve growth factor (NGF) receptor, *trkA*, and thereby converts NGF-unresponsive neurons into NGF-responding cells (39, 40). Similar studies with an HSV vector that transduces the gene encoding the low-affinity NGF receptor have been described (41). In other studies, we have constructed a vector that expresses the GluR6 kainate receptor. This vector induced transsynaptic neuronal loss and epileptiform activity when introduced in hippocampal slice cultures (35). Other investigators have used the HSV-1 amplicon vector in the CNS to express the rat protein kinase C (PKC) catalytic domain, driven by the tyrosine hydroxylase promoter, in order to study the role of PKC in rat spatial navigation tasks and in the regulation of rat motor behavior (42, 43).

There are many other potential uses of HSV vectors. For example, these vectors might be used to study the role of neurotrophins in development. Using neural-specific promoters (see Neuronal Specificity, below) to express biologically active foreign genes may be advantageous for this purpose as well as for creating and/or ameliorating animal models of human neurological disease.

Promoter Mapping

One potential application of the amplicon vector system is its use to study promoter function and map *cis* elements *in vivo*. It should be stressed that this approach needs to be validated by comparing the same promoter constructs in amplicon vectors and in transgenic animals. There are several reasons to believe that the same promoter may function differently in the two different contexts.

First, in the vector the promoter will be adjacent to HSV ori and pac sequences that may alter promoter *trans*-activation. Second, the promoter will be in an episomal configuration in the vector, but will be integrated into a chromosome in the transgenic situation. Comparisons of promoter-containing constructs by transient or stable transfections *in vitro* and transgenic germ line transmission have suggested that the configuration of the promoter may influence its *trans*-activation properties (44). Third, vector particles deliver some DNA-associated proteins that are products of the HSV packaging process. These proteins could interact with cellular transcription factors and/or chromosomal proteins such that the transcriptional activity of the vector is transiently or chronically changed. Direct tests of this approach will determine the validity of the aforementioned concerns.

Neuronal Specificity

Because of the modular design of the amplicon, it is relatively straightforward to change the transcription unit in part or in its entirety. It may often be advantageous to use a promoter that is neuronal specific. Such a situation was mentioned previously for the study of neuronal physiology and may also apply in the case of gene therapy. Our group has produced a vector that provides neuronal-specific expression of β-galactosidase using the human neurofilament L (NFL) promoter (45). Another group has shown neuronal-specific expression *in vivo* of β-galactosidase and of the rat PKC BII catalytic domain, using the neuron-specific promoter for tyrosine hydroxylase (42, 43). Other investigators, using a recombinant-based HSV-1 vector (see below), have used the mammalian neuron-specific enolase promoter driving the β-galactosidase gene for expression in neuronal cell lines, primary neuronal culture, and in the CNS. β-Galactosidase-positive neurons were found 30 days following injection into the striatum (37).

Other Viral Vectors Systems

Retroviral Vectors

Retroviral vectors have been used to study the development of the nervous system, primarily by infecting fetal and neonatal mitotic neurons for cell lineage analysis (25, 46–48). As retroviruses cannot integrate into postmitotic cells, such as mature neurons, they are not suitable for gene delivery into the adult nervous system. In addition, retroviruses are difficult to concentrate because of their relative lability in comparison with other viruses (49), such as herpesviruses and adenoviruses. These last two points most likely account for the problems encountered with the use of retroviruses for *in vivo* viral transduction. Furthermore, a danger with the use of retroviruses is their ability to transform; because they integrate into the host genome, there is the possibility for insertional mutagenesis and activation of protooncogenes (50).

Adenoviral Vectors

Replication-defective adenoviral vectors have been used to transfer a reporter gene into neurons and glia of the adult mouse CNS by stereotaxic injection, resulting in expression of β-galactosidase for at least 8 weeks postinfection. However, the stability of expression decreased dramatically over this time period (1, 51). Davidson and co-workers (1) used the cytomegalovirus (CMV) promoter whereas Le Gal La Salle and colleagues (51) used the Rous sarcoma virus long terminal repeat (RSV LTR) promoter to drive the *lacZ* gene. It was not known whether the decline in reporter gene activity in the CNS was due to viral promoter repression, loss of transduced vector genomes, and/or potential cytotoxicity of the adenoviral vectors.

The biology and manipulation of adenovirus as a vector for gene transfer has been reviewed in detail elsewhere (52–54). Similar to HSV-1 vectors, adenovirus vectors also can transfer genes into a wide variety of mammalian cells (9, 54). Unlike retroviral vectors, gene expression from HSV-1 and adenovirus vectors does not require integration of the vector DNA into the host cell chromosome, making both suitable for *in vivo* gene delivery into highly differentiated nonproliferating cells, such as neurons.

The major advantages of adenoviral vectors over HSV-1 vectors are that they can be made without the use of helper virus (helper independent) (49, 54) and can be produced in high titer with routine cell culture and purification procedures (49). In addition, adenoviral recombinants are relatively easy to construct (54), unlike HSV-1 recombinant vectors, which require more difficult manipulation of the large genome (55). Although integration of adenovirus DNA into the target cell can occur, it is not an integral part of the life cycle and is relatively inefficient (49). The major limitation of adenoviral vector is the small size of foreign DNA (7.5 kb) it can accommodate (52–54) as compared with the HSV-1 vector. There is also the possibility that the helper-independent virus with an *E1* region deletion may still be capable of replication (49). If this is the case, there may be several safety concerns, particularly for use in gene therapy.

HSV-1 Recombinant Vectors

Several other HSV-1 vector systems have been developed (4, 37, 56; reviewed in Ref. 55). Recombinant vectors are the principal alternative to amplicon vectors. Recombinant vectors for gene transfer are also rendered replication defective by deleting one or more of their *IE* gene(s), which are essential for viral replication. The vectors utilize the full-length HSV-1 genome, which is modified by cloning heterologous transcription units into nonessential regions. The recombinant HSV-1 vectors have the advantage that they can be engineered without significantly perturbing the HSV genome. This nearly wild-type genome may be more efficient in establishing a latent infection in transduced neurons and perhaps other postmitotic cells. This approach also has some disadvantages, including complex manipulations to insert the desired DNA into its genome and then isolate such recombinants (57). In contrast, amplicon vectors are easily prepared because they are assembled from small plasmid DNA into which a foreign piece of DNA can be readily inserted without having to use homologous recombination (57). In addition, depending on the size of the foreign gene, multiple copies of the amplicon plasmid will be packaged per virion.

Safety and Other Issues Related to Vector Use

Several HSV genes have been demonstrated to cause cellular toxicity and/or damage in infected cells. The expression of HSV *IE* genes has been correlated with cytotoxicity (58) and may reflect their interaction with cellular transcription factors. The transcription of the *IE* gene set is strongly dependent on the HSV transcription factor VP16, a product of an HSV late gene. Thus, efforts to make packaging cell systems or recombinant viruses that are mutated in VP16 may well reduce cytotoxicity. Cytotoxicity appears to be less severe with amplicon than with recombinant vectors. This may reflect the fact that amplicon vectors do not contain *IE* genes although their copropagated helper virus does. Thus, amplicon stocks may contain fewer virions with *IE* genes than do recombinant vector stocks with comparable amounts of transducing particles. Other HSV genes, such as *UL41*, which encodes the virus host shutoff function (VHS), may also produce toxicity (58). Systematic testing of helper viruses with mutations in these genes could also lead to improvements that limit cellular toxicity.

Transduction with amplicon vectors of cells harboring a latent wild-type HSV genome could potentially produce activation of the latent virus. Moreover, such a scenario could also produce recombination between amplicon and latent HSV, leading to the generation of novel virus that may be replication competent and capable of transducing the heterologous gene. A similar scenario could occur in the reverse situation, in which a cell containing the amplicon vector is later infected with wild-type HSV-1. However, there are potential solutions to these problems. Agents such as acyclovir could be administered to recipients of amplicon vectors to prevent any latent or new HSV replication. Safer vectors can be designed in which the gene(s) of interest are controlled by induction with an exogenously administered biopharmaceutical. In addition, designing helper viruses containing multiple deletion mutations, such as in *IE* genes and the gene encoding VP16 (58), may help to reduce cytotoxicity and the frequency of recombination to wild-type HSV. A safer alternative would be the development of a helper-independent vector system. Owing to limitations in current technology, this remains to be developed.

Summary

It is clear that the amplicon-based HSV-1 vector system can be used to transfer genes into many different cell types, including postmitotic cells, such as neurons. Genes transferred can be used to express neuronal markers, neuronal tracers, or to alter neuronal physiology.

The amplicon-based system has several advantages over other currently used gene transfer systems. With a well-designed plasmid vector, it is easy to package genes into the vector. A size limit has not been established yet, but so far DNA fragments up to 15 kb have been transferred, and larger sizes are expected to be feasible. Large quantities of the viral vector can be made within about 2 weeks. Depending on the system, applying the virus is straightforward. Depending on the promoter and cell type infected, significant quantities of protein can be produced. Almost any cell type can be infected (11) and because HSV vectors transduce genes with high efficiency, only a small number of virions is needed to produce a biological effect (8, 35).

In its current form, the amplicon vector system is imperfect and there exists considerable margin for improvement before it can safely be used for gene therapy in the CNS; nevertheless, this system will continue to be extremely useful for gene transfer into the nervous system for modifying neuronal development and physiology as well as for modeling human disease.

Acknowledgments

We would like to thank Dr. Roger Everett for providing the M64A packaging cell line and the D30EBA helper virus, Dr. Neal DeLuca for providing the E5 packaging cell line, Dr. Priscilla Schaffer for helpful suggestions regarding viral passaging, and Dr. Ari Grunhaus for advice on titering virus using low melting point agarose.

References

1. B. Davidson, E. Allen, K. Kozarsky, K. Wilson, and B. Roessler, *Nature Genet.* **3,** 219 (1993).
2. Q. Huang, J.-P. Vonsattel, P. Schaffer, R. Martuza, X. Breakefield, and M. DiFiglia, *Exp. Neurol.* **115,** 303 (1992).

3. D. Fink, L. Sternberg, P. Weber, M. Mata, W. Goins, and J. Glorioso, *Hum. Gene Ther.* **3,** 11 (1992).
4. J. Wolfe, S. Deshmane, and N. Fraser, *Nature Genet.* **1,** 379 (1992).
5. P. Spear and B. Roizman, *in* "DNA Tumor Viruses" (J. Tooze, ed.), p. 615. Cold Spring Harbor Lab., Cold Spring Harbor, NY, 1981.
6. J. Fukuda, I. Kurata, A. Yamamoto, and K. Yamaguchi, *Brain Res.* **262,** 79 (1983).
7. A. Geller, M. During, and R. Neve, *Trends Neurosci.* **14,** 428 (1991).
8. H. J. Federoff, M. D. Geschwind, A. I. Geller, and J. A. Kessler, *Proc. Natl. Acad. Sci. U.S.A.* **89,** 1636 (1992).
9. R. Neve, *Trends Neurosci.* **16**(7), 251 (1993).
10. B. Roizman and A. Sears, *in* "Virology" (B. Fields and D. Knipe, eds.), 2nd ed., p. 1795. Raven Press, New York, 1990.
11. B. Roizman, *in* "Virology" (B. Fields and D. Knipe, eds.), 2nd ed., p. 1787. Raven Press, New York, 1990.
12. P. Schaffer, *in* "The Human Herpesviruses; An Interdisciplinary Perspective" (A. Nahmias, W. Dowdle, and R. Schinazi, eds.), p. 55. Elsevier/North-Holland, New York, 1981.
13. N. Frenkel, *in* "The Human Herpesviruses: An Interdisciplinary Prospective" (A. Nahmias, W. Dowdle, and R. Schinazi, eds.), p. 91. Elsevier/North-Holland, New York, 1981.
14. D. Vlazny and N. Frenkel, *Proc. Natl. Acad. Sci. U.S.A.* **78,** 742 (1981).
15. D. Vlazny, A. Kwong, and N. Frenkel, *Proc. Natl. Acad. Sci. U.S.A.* **79,** 1423 (1982).
16. R. Spaete and N. Frenkel, *Cell (Cambridge, Mass.)* **30,** 295 (1982).
17. N. Stow and E. McMonagle, *in* "Eucaryotic Viral Vectors" (Y. Gluzman, ed.), p. 199. Cold Spring Harbor Lab., Cold Spring Harbor, NY, 1982.
18. R. Spaete and N. Frenkel, *Proc. Natl. Acad. Sci. U.S.A.* **82,** 694 (1985).
19. P. Weber, M. Levine, and J. Glorioso, *Science* **236,** 576 (1987).
20. B. Roizman and F. Jenkins, *Science* **229,** 1208 (1985).
21. A. I. Geller and X. O. Breakefield, *Science* **241,** 1667 (1988).
22. A. I. Geller and H. J. Federoff, *Human Gene Transfer* **219,** 63 (1991).
23. A. Freese, A. Geller, and R. Neve, *Biochem. Pharmacol.* **40,** 2189 (1990).
24. T. Paterson and R. Everett, *J. Gen. Virol.* **71,** 1775 (1990).
25. J. Sanes, J. Rubenstein, and J. Nicholas, *EMBO J* **5,** 3133 (1986).
26. P. Schaffer, V. Carter, and M. Timbury, *J. Virol.* **27**(3), 490 (1978).
27. D. Latchman and L. Kemp, *Methods Mol. Biol.* **8,** 191 (1991).
28. N. Frenkel, R. Spaete, D. Vlazny, L. Deiss, and H. Locker, *in* "Eucaryotic Viral Vectors" (Y. Gluzman, ed.), p. 205. Cold Spring Harbor Lab., Cold Spring Harbor, NY, 1982.
29. G. Dreesman and M. Benyesh-Melnick, *J. Immunol.* **99**(6), 1104 (1967).
30. W. Russell, *Nature (London)* **195,** 1028 (1962).
31. R. Selden, K. Burke Howie, M. Rowe, H. Goodman, and D. Moore, *Mol. Cell. Biol.* **6,** 3173 (1986).
32. R. Selden, *in* "Current Protocols in Molecular Biology" (F. Ausubel, R. Brent, R. Kingston, D. Moore, J. Seidman, J. Smith, and K. Struhl, eds.), Ch. 9. Green Publishing Associates, New York, 1987.

33. J. Dhawan, L. Pan, G. Pavlath, M. Travis, A. Lanctot, and H. Blau, *Science* **254,** 1509 (1991).
34. E. Barr and J. Leiden, *Science* **254,** 1507 (1991).
35. P. Bergold, P. Cassaccia-Bonnefil, Z. Xiu-Liu, and H. Federoff, *Proc. Natl. Acad. Sci. U.S.A.* **90,** 6165 (1993).
36. P. Casaccia-Bonnefil, E. Benedikz, H. Shen, A. Stelzer, D. Edelstein, M. Geschwind, M. Brownlee, H. J. Federoff, and P. J. Bergold, *J. Neurosci. Methods* **50,** 341 (1993).
37. J. Andersen, D. Garber, C. Meaney, and X. Breakefield, *Hum. Gene Ther.* **3,** 487 (1992).
37a. M. D. Geschwind, J. A. Kessler, A. I. Geller, and H. J. Federoff, *Mol. Brain Res.* In press (1994).
38. M. Geschwind, J. Amat, and H. Federoff, *Soc. Neurosci. Abstr.* **19,** 255 (1993).
39. H. Xu, L. Parada, H. Federoff, and J. Kessler, *Dev. Biol.* (in press).
40. T. Van De Water, P. Lefebvre, W. Liu, H. Xu, J. Kessler, and H. Federoff, *Soc. Neurosci. Abstr.* **18,** 951 (1992).
41. D. S. Battleman, A. I. Geller, and M. V. Chao, *J. Neurosci.* **13**(3), 941 (1993).
42. P. Leone, M. Dragunow, K. Davis, D. Ullrey, K. O'Malley, R. Neve, A. Geller, and M. During, *Soc. Neurosci. Abstr.* **19,** 806 (1993).
43. S. Song, P. Leone, Y. Wang, D. Hartley, J. Bryan, D. Ullrey, S. Bak, K. Davis, J. Haycock, K. O'Malley, R. Neve, A. Geller, and M. During, *Soc. Neurosci. Abstr.* **19,** 806 (1993).
44. R. Kitsis and L. Leinwand, *Gene Expression* **2**(4), 313 (1992).
45. H. Federoff, A. Geller, and B. Lu, *Soc. Neurosci. Abstr.* **16,** 353 (1990).
46. C. Walsh and C. Cepko, *Science* **241,** 1342 (1988).
47. C. Walsh and C. Cepko, *Science* **255,** 434 (1992).
48. J. Price, D. Turner, and C. Cepko, *Proc. Natl. Acad. Sci. U.S.A.* **84,** 56 (1987).
49. R. Mulligan, *Science* **260,** 926 (1993).
50. T. Friedmann, *in* "Therapy for Genetic Disease" (T. Friedmann, ed.), p. 107. Oxford Univ. Press, New York, 1991.
51. G. Le Gal La Salle, J. Robert, S. Berrard, V. Ridous, L. Stratford-Perricaudet, M. Perricaudet, and J. Mallet, *Science* **259,** 988 (1993).
52. F. Graham and L. N. Prevec, *Methods Mol. Biol.* **7,** 109 (1991).
53. A. Grunhaus and M. Horwitz, *Semin. Virol.* **3,** 237 (1992).
54. K. Berkner, *Curr. Top. Microbiol. Immunol.* **158,** 39 (1992).
55. X. Breakefield and N. DeLuca, *New Biologist* **3,** 203 (1991).
56. A. Dobson, T. P. Margolis, F. Sedarati, J. Stevens, and L. T. Feldman, *Neuron* **5,** 353 (1990).
57. D. Latchman, *Methods Mol. Biol.* **8,** 175 (1991).
58. P. Johnson, A. Miyanohara, F. Levine, T. Cahill, and T. Friedman, *J. Virol.* **66,** 2952 (1992).

Section XII

Predicting the Future of Central Nervous System Delivery System Technologies

[28] Assessing Commercial Potential of Central Nervous System Delivery Approaches

John S. Swen, Thomas R. Flanagan,
and Thomas G. Wiggans

Introduction

Advances in identifying therapeutic agents and delivery systems have opened up new possibilities for treating neurological diseases. These innovations offer alternatives to existing therapeutic practices. However, developing these new technologies is costly. Consequently, an understanding of the commercial issues behind such technologies is important in predicting how they will develop.

Neuroscience researchers need funding to develop new technologies. As academic researchers increasingly look toward industrial sources for their funds, it is important to understand the methods that industrial sources will use to evaluate the potential fundworthiness of evolving technologies. This chapter describes an approach to assessing the commercial potential of central nervous system (CNS) delivery technology for selected chronic degenerative diseases.

Assessing Market Size and Value

A market analysis is a critical component in the decision to invest in a new technology. Market information related to CNS disorders can be obtained from publicly available sources such as *Pharma Projects,* annual reports, analyst's reports, Security and Exchange Commission (SEC) filings (particularly newly public companies), from the biotechnology press (e.g., *BioWorld Today*), and from industry overviews (e.g., Ernst and Young's annual review). A brief summary of the types of information that should be abstracted from such sources is offered below.

Market Size

Successfully treating CNS disorders represents one of the most significant medical, social, and commercial opportunities in health care. Diseases of

Methods in Neurosciences, Volume 21

the central nervous system affect approximately 12 million persons in the United States. The scope of various disorders ranges from over 3 million Alzheimer's patients, to fewer than 1000 dysautonomic patients. In fact, there are at least 25 CNS "orphan" diseases, those affecting fewer than 200,000 patients. This special "orphan" regulatory status indicates that new therapeutic approaches directed toward these targets are likely to be rapidly tested and, if effective, rapidly adopted into clinical practice. Taken together, market pressures and unmet clinical needs indicate that this field is ripe for rapid, clinically acceptable innovation. The diseases that affect the largest numbers of patients are shown in Table I and are drawn from a report from the National Brain Injury Research Foundation. The "orphan" diseases shown in Table II are reported by the National Information Center for Orphan Drugs and Rare Diseases.

Market Value

Most degenerative CNS conditions are characterized by a slow, progressive deterioration that results in prolonged periods of increasing incapacitation. The costs associated with increasing levels of medical care for these patients are enormous. Degenerative CNS diseases thus devastate not only the quality of life of affected individuals and their families but in addition require enormous personal and/or pbulic expenditures for secondary medical expenses. The total cost of CNS disease to the United States health care system is estimated to be over $400 billion (3), with costs directly attributable to the organic neurological disease contributing to only 25% of this expense. The

TABLE I Annual Cost of Specific Neurological Diseases of the Brain (Billions of Dollars)

Disease	Prevalence (U.S.)	Annual cost (U.S.)
Dementias	4,000,000–5,000,000	113.2
Head injury	1,000,000	48.3
Mental retardation	575,000	35.1
Spinal cord injury	175,000	22.6
Stroke	3,000,000	17.9
Other	~1,000,000	8.1
Multiple sclerosis	200,000–500,000	5.0
Cerebral palsy	600,000–750,000	1.2
Epilepsy	2,000,000	3.0
	10,000,000–14,000,000	254.4

TABLE II "Orphan" Diseases of Brain

Disease	Prevalence (U.S.)	Disease	Prevalence (U.S.)
ALS[a]	25,000	Leukodystrophies	>50,000
Blepharospasm	150,000	Muscular dystrophy	15,000
Brain tumor all types	1,000,000	Myasthenia gravis	100,000
Charcot-Marie-Tooth	125,000	Neurofbiromatosis	100,000
Creutzfeldt-Jakob	<1,000	Rett syndrome	~1,100
Dysautonomia	<1,000	Reye's syndrome	<500
Various dystonias	~1,000,000	Spasmodic torticollis	1 in 10,000
Gaucher's disease	20,000	Spina bifida	1 in 20,000
Guillain-Barré syndrome	2,000–4,000	Tay–Sachs	<100 per year
Huntington's disease	12,000–25,000	Tourette syndrome	~100,000
Joseph disease	<5,000	Tuberous sclerosis	~10,000

[a] Amyotrophic lateral sclerosis

total medical cost for degenerative CNS diseases is distributed across expenses that are difficult to assess fully. An appreciation of the total cost of a disease should include factors such as lost work, hospital and office visits, home care, lost work of spouse, and long-term care in addition to the costs of pharmaceuticals and hospitalization.

Identifying Key Issues for Analysis

Technical issues are evaluated by analysts who utilize primary research publications, research reviews, personal research contacts, presentations and interactions observed at professional meetings and opinions generated from other analysts. Researchers can develop an understanding of the potential commercial value of their technology by identifying public companies that operate in their field of interest, and then by requesting industry reports on those companies from investment advising houses.

Industry reports are available in four general forms: public service reports from federal agencies or otherwise funded by federal grants (such as reports from technology transfer offices and business schools), industry review articles that are published as advertising for industry analyst firms (such as articles that frequently appear in *Genetic Engineering News*), investment firms recommendations (such as Oppenheimer Reports), and major industry reports (as per Arthur D. Little, Inc., Decisions Resources, Inc.). This latter class of reports does not consist of publications per se; rather they consist of documents prepared for clients willing to purchase them. And they are expensive, costing $2000 to $4000 each. Copyright laws strictly apply to this type of material; however, purchased copies may be shared among readers. Examples of consulting firms that prepare major industry reports are shown in Table III. In addition, a company will often contract specific studies from such firms. It must be noted that analyst reports reflect what in their opinion is a reasonable statement of fact. Because such reports are forward looking they contain an essential element of uncertainty in the absence of knowledge of unexpected innovations in the field. Informed scientific responses to analyst reports can affect the response of the industry to those reports.

TABLE III Sources That Track Technical Progress within Selected Fields

Analysts, consultants, and contract research firms
Ernst & Young
Bose Allen
Drug and Market Development, Inc.
Investment bankers
Openheimer, Robertson Stevens, Morgan Stanley, First Boston, Paine Webber
Trade publications and special reports
Genetic Engineering News
Med Ad News
Pharma Projects, PJB Publications, Ltd.
Symposia and conferences; development firms
BioConferences International, Inc.
Biomarkets '93: Forecasts for Key High-Growth Markets, FIND/SVP
Biomedical Business International
Biotechnology Industry Organization, Biotechnology Meeting and Exhibition Keystone Symposia
The Pharmaceutical Division, Institute for International Research
International Business Communications USA Conferences, Inc.
Technology Transfer Conferences, Inc.
Newsletter publishers
Applied Genetic News, Business Communications Company, Inc.
BioWorld Today, The Daily Biotechnology Newspaper, Io Publishing, Inc.
DR Reports, Decisions Resources, Inc.
Prescription Pharmaceuticals and Biotechnology, F-D-C-Reports, Inc.
News from TMG, Technology Management Group
Health Care Delivery News, Business Communications Company, Inc.
Surveys from academic centers and economic development centers
Center for the Study of Drug Development, Tufts University
Strategic Developments in Biotechnology, Institute for Biotechnology Information, North Carolina Biotechnology Center
Databases maintained by government agencies and nonprofit foundations
National Brain Injury Research Foundation
National Information Center for Orphan Drugs and Rare Diseases, ODPHP National Health Information Center
National Parkinson Foundation
Parkinson's Disease Foundation

Investment bankers, whether in venture capital groups, investment brokerage houses, corporate organizations, or research teams, will assimilate information and identify both the barriers and the opportunities for innovation. Examlpes of areas in which scientific breakthroughs would improve efforts to deliver drugs into the CNS are presented below.

Addressing the Blood–Brain Barrier

Unlike most organ systems, the brain is separated from the blood by a protective cellular barrier. The blood–brain barrier (BBB), although essential in maintaining a defined biochemical environment within the brain, represents a significant obstacle to the effective delivery of neuropharmacological agents from the blood stream. Systemic delivery routes have been developed to address problems that affect the CNS globally, such as dispersed infections. Additional efforts have been directed toward systemic delivery of neurotransmitter precursors (i.e., L-dopa) and growth factors, but such efforts have required additional efforts to then control for systemic toxicities and adverse reactions. The problems with CNS delivery reduce to special needs of the intended target site, the intended duration, and the biochemical nature of the therapeutic product. Protein neurotrophic factors have been advanced as powerful agents for rescuing neurons that might otherwise die in neurodegenerative disease states. The limited ability of neuroactive proteins to cross the BBB efficiently has been viewed as severely limiting the clinical utility of such therapeutic proteins (2). Technologies that allow access of therapeutic proteins into the brain and/or allow chronic delivery of these and other therapeutic products into precisely defined target sites within the brain will offer significant advantages to the development of new CNS therapeutic strategies.

Interpreting Data from Studies with Animal Models of Human Diseases

Human neurological disease states are usually inadequately modeled by animal models; an animal model is typically created to duplicate some of the symptoms of a human disease state and therapeutic strategies are then developed to manage those symptoms in the absence of a means of directly treating the disease. Even in widely accepted animals models, such as the MPTP lesion for Parkinson's disease, no current therapy exists that is targeted to treat the disease itself. Developing acceptable animal models for complex, multifactorial degenerative processes, such as Alzheimer's disease, has proved correspondingly more difficult. It is therefore recognized that data from existing animal models must be interpreted with caution when predicting successful human therapy. Animal tests thus become largely tests for safety, rather than relevant tests for clinical efficacy. Innovations that lead to better animal models of human neurodegenerative disease will accelerate the development of therapeutic products; however, delivery systems that will allow clinical researchers to begin experimental treatments on carefully selected patient populations will advance this field of therapy most rapidly.

Developing General Therapies for Diseases of Unknown Etiology

An additional obstacle to developing effective treatments for neurological disorders is the complex nature of the diseases themselves. In parallel with earlier views that lumped all cancers and all schizophrenias into a class of disease for which single therapies were sought, there is a tendency to group neurodegenerative diseases with similar symptoms into corresponding single treatment groups. Disorders that manifest themselves by similar symptoms but that result from distinct, unidentified causes are not predicted to respond equally well to a single therapeutic treatment. The imperfectly known extent of neuronal populations that are involved in any major neurodegenerative disorder complicates efforts to manage the disease with therapies that rescue neuronal populations identified as at risk. Alzheimer's disease, for example, is known to involve disorders of at least basal forebrain, cortical, hippocampal, and locus coeruleus neurons. Additional neuronal populations may yet be identified that are also involved in the disease. Each distinct neuronal population is likely to require its own rescue therapy; consequently, an effective treatment for Alzheimer's may require a cocktail of therapeutic molecules targeted to all neuronal populations at risk. It is hoped that some measure of symptom management can be achieved even while we await an improved understanding of the etiology and the pathogenesis of the disease. Delivery approaches that are sufficiently flexible to allow rapid refinement in response to rapidly evolving clinical understanding will contribute to successful new therapies.

Establishing Intellectual Property Rights for Novel Therapeutics

When all indicators suggest that a promising therapeutic agent, a promising delivery approach, and a relevant means of assessing clinical success exist, where will the $100 to $400 million of funding come from to add this product to the clinical arsenal? This issue can be sorted out most rapidly when there is a clear indication of ownership for each component in the therapy. However, this will remain a major challenge in business development. If, for example, multiple factors are required to treat a disease, and the factors are owned by different companies and universities, it will be important to negotiate cross-licensing agreements prospectively, since there will remain considerable uncertainty over what works until the necessary, and costly, clinical studies have been performed. In the spirit of planning for success, it is almost universally true that individuals and institutions with their "own" potentially therapeutic neurotrophic factors will expect their invention to cure the disease single-handedly. This view may be correct, but it most certainly encourages such owners to ask for more than most codevelopers would be willing to give up in a joint effort to develop a clinical product. For this reason, new delivery approaches that also have secured access to key delivery products are predicted to have much greater commercial potential than either the delivery approach or the product alone.

Identifying Competitive Therapeutic, Economic, and Societal Advantages

Within the field of neurodegenerative diseases, academic, government, and corporate research laboratories have all contributed to components that are likely to appear in a multicomponent therapeutic product in the future. In addition to conventional, small molecule therapeutics, there has been an explosion of activity directed to identify potentially therapeutic neurotrophic factors. The range of activities in this field is summarized in Table IV.

In addition to discoveries of trophic factors, there has been explosive growth in strategies to deliver such products into the CNS (as indicated by the chapters within this volume). Competitions for delivery of therapeutic agents into the CNS will exist on many levels. A case study of therapies for Parkinson's disease illustrates how one might asseses the potential commercial success of a novel CNS delivery approach within this competitive arena.

Ranking Therapeutic Approaches

Parkinson's disease (PD) is a chronic, debilitating neurodegenerative disease neurobiologically characterized by an underlying progressive loss of a population of dopaminergic neurons within the brain and behaviorally characterized principally on the basis of motor disorders. In practice or in theory, it may be managed with four classes of treatment: palliative therapies, therapies focusing on reducing/halting progression of the disease, therapies focusing

TABLE IV Neurotrophic Factor Selectivity and Possible Indications

Disease	Factors
Alzheimer's	
Basal forebrain	NGF, BDNF, bFGF
Cortical neurons	BDNF, NT-3, NT-4/5
Hippocampal neurons	BDNF, NT-3, NT-4/5
Coeruleus noradrenergic neurons	NT-4, NT5
ALS	
Motor neurons	CNTF, BDNF, NT-4/5, IGF-1
Parkinson's	
Dopaminergic neurons	BDNF, GDNF, NT-4/5, TGF-α, EGF, IGF-1
Peripheral neuropathies	
Sensory neurons	NGF, BDNF, NT-3, NT4/5
Sympathetic neurons	NGF, bFGF
Parasympathetic neurons	CNTF
Huntington's disease	
Striatal interneurons	BDNF, NT-3, NT-4/5
Ischemic stroke	
Striatal, hippocampal, cortical neurons	TGF-β, IGF-1, bFGF
Acute brain injury	
All populations of brain neurons	TGF-β, IGF-1
Nervous system tumors	
Neuroblastoma, glioma cells	NGF, BDNF, NT-3, NT-4/5
Multiple sclerosis	
Oligodendrocytes	GMF-β, Heregulin
Acute brain–spinal cord injury	
Corticospinal neurons	??

on reversal of the disease, and therapies that prevent neuronal degeneration. In fact, this disease is managed poorly, and then only at the level of palliative therapy. The status of each therapy class is indicated below.

Palliative Therapies

The now classic pharmacological approach to treating Parkinson's disease is with L-dopa/carbidopa conjugates such as Sinemet. This therapy reduces tremor, bradykinesia,and rigidity but causes nausea and hypotension in the short term, and severe dyskinesia, often alternating with episodes of sudden unpredictable loss of mobility, in the long term (1). In addition, there is some evidence that L-dopa/carbidopa treatment may exacerbate striatal neuron death. Parkinson's disease patients remain responsive to this therapy for 2 to 5 years, whereupon more aggressive therapies incorporating dopamine agonists must be adopted. Direct costs for medication are low, but indirect costs for patient support are very high. Alternative means of introducing L-dopa into the target site affected by dopaminergic cell loss in PD patients may allow PD patients to enjoy the benefits of this therapy without the side effects (i.e., progressive loss of L-dopa responsiveness, and systemic toxicities and CNS psychotic responses). Even though systemic L-dopa therapy is inadequate, it represents the state of the art, and surpassing this therapy will be a critical objective of any commercially successful alternative.

An alternative palliative therapy consists of supplemental implants of L-dopa and/or dopamine-producing cells or genes for local L-dopa synthesis. The rationale for such therapies is based on the belief that the principal product that is missing as a result of lost dopaminergic cells can be locally produced and released into affected region of the brain. Clinical studies with both autologous adrenal cells and dopamine-producing cells have been reported with varying degrees of short-term success, and have been alternately cited as reasons for both going forward and for stopping this mode of therapy. The continued evaluation of the efficacy of cellular and genetic approaches, as with all PD therapeutic approaches, must be established in unambiguously safe clinical studies. To enable truly safe clinical studies, a means of fully terminating the cellular therapy once it has been initiated still needs to be developed. To date, cellular transplantatioan into the brains of patients with PD or PD-like disorders does at least appear to be more safe than efficacious.

Reducing/Halting Progression of Disease

No therapy yet exists that has been shown to reduce or halt the progression of PD. One growth factor, glial-derived neurotrophic factor (GDNF), has been shown to protect dopaminergic neurons *in vitro,* and thus holds some promise as a neuroprotective agent *in vivo*. GDNF is potentially active at low doses; however, it is a relatively large protein that, to be effective, must be introduced into areas of the brain that contain the neurites of neurons at risk in PD patients. Systemic delivery appears unlikely owing to the target requirement to precise nuclei within the brain (not all dopaminergic neurons are at risk in PD patients, and therefore the therapy would be most strategically targeted to specific dopaminergic cell types). It is presumed that this (or some yet unidentified similar) protein must be administered over an extended period of time, and it is further presumed that once this treatment has been initiated it should be continued. For this reason, the delivery device, if a device is used, should promise to provide a multiyear delivery cycle and should be rechargeable with minimal invasive manipulations. The cost of this therapy must compete with the aggregate costs of the current palliative therapy (direct when the therapy works and indirect costs after that therapy no longer is effective); thus, although potentially expensive, GDNF therapy has potential as a commercial product. This promise of commercial potential will drive efforts to evaluate its clinical efficacy.

Reversing Disease

Factors that underlie the progression of PD are a source of continued medical speculation. In the absence of this information, and in the absence of good animal models for PD, an empirically discovered therapy to halt the progression of PD is a challenging objective. Such an effort will require carefully monitoring PD patients who are willing to participate in experimental therapies at early stages of their diseases. For this reason, such therapeutics must be of both verified safety and complete reversibility with minimal trauma to the patient. Two approaches have been suggested by experimental studies: early neurotrophic factor treatments, or cellular replacement approaches.

The rationale for trophic factor treatment to reverse PD is based on the hope that any agent that can be shown to protect a PD patient from the progression of the disease might also be able to reverse some aspects of the disease process. The role of GDNF and related factors, either to effectively supplement hypothesized deficiencies in endogenous neurotrophic factor levels or to provide a protective effect from yet unidentified endogenous toxic agents, can be fully assessed only in clinical testing. Thus, the therapeutic practice that enables clinical delivery of GDNF is most likely also to enable experimental delivery of GDNF-like substances in efforts to reverse the progress of PD.

The rationale for cellular replacement therapy is based on the belief that selective dopaminergic cell loss is a process intrinsic to the afflicted cells, and that if equivalent cells from a different source are placed into the brain, these new cells will fully replace the functions of the lost cells. Clinical studies with fetal mesencephalic cells have been reported with varying degrees of short-term success, and disappointing results have been attribtued to difficulties in obtaining an appropriate cell type for these transplants. Efforts to create and genetically engineer neuronal stem cells have been initiated. Stem cells add the advantage that they can be expanded from a well-characterized and safe stock culture and can then be differentiated into a desired implantable cell population.

Preventing Neuronal Degeneration

The holy grail of PD therapeutics is to prevent the disease fully. One can hope that with the advent of projects with the scope of the Human Genome Project we may soon have the means of diagnosing degenerative disease predisposition in individuals at a stage early enough to allow them to take preventative measures. The success of a preventative therapy will be reflected by the certainty that indicators used to predict the disease do in fact predict the disease and then both the cost and the invasiveness of the preventative treatment. A therapy that is effective for treating the symptoms of, blocking the progression of, and/or reversing the damage done by PD might also offer a preventative effect from the onset of the disease. If a preventative therapy is discovered it is likely to have these properties because therapies directed at readily measurable symptoms will be among the first to be tested clinically. If preventative therapeutics exist that treat only the underlying cause and not the behavioral symptoms, they will be impossible to recognize in short-term clinical tests. Thus, symptom management therapeutics and appropriate delivery systems that can be safely applied to nearly normal "patients" will need to be developed to offer truly preventative treatments.

Approaches that provide the greatest symptomatic efficacy, the fewest side effects, and the lowest patient cost will come out on top. This is a complicated equation that must be carefully balanced for each disease type, stage, and extent. Balancing the equation will require consensus from a large number of stakeholders, including investors and stockholders who will fund commercial efforts (through venture capital placements and through publicly traded corporations), physicians who will have to make informed decisions on behalf of their patients, patients and their families who will have to assess their personal views toward novel therapeutic approaches, reimbursement agents who will have to recognize the value of costly therapies when weighed against even more costly medical expenses, and governmental bureaucracies who will have to establish guidelines for regulating new therapeutic products and practices.

Predicting Breakthroughs

Predicting who will produce the next breakthrough drug is extremely difficult. In assessing the competitive environment, however, it is useful to look for four primary ingredients of success: (a) ideas protected by intellectual property rights, (b) motivated and talented scientists, (c) capital sufficient for creative exploring, and (d) a managerial structure that can successfully negotiate in the entrepreneurial market place. These four ingredients are most frequently found within small, start-up companies who have committed themselves to bold discoveries. Researchers who have confidence in the commercial success of their ideas might consider initial discussions with highly energetic small companies; researchers who are looking for a long-term funding opportunity for early-stage research projects might consider first approaching cash-rich large companies.

In predicting the commercial potential of a novel CNS delivery approach, industrial decision makers will want to know who has used that approach and what the key thought leaders think of the approach. A delivery approach that passes the acid test of being adopted into a significant competitor's practice is a strong indicator of the potential of that technology. If ownership is initially disputed, this, too, is a good indicator of the value of the technology, for nothing is as difficult to track as the early lineage of a really good idea. The winner in the race to develop a new delivery technology will be the individual who recognizes and rapidly adopts the most good ideas, particularly if that winner can adopt those ideas while sustaining collegial relations with those from whom the idea has been adopted.

Funding is also a useful indicator in predicting who will be winning in the race to develop new technologies. Funding is both an indication of past successes and an opportunity to make new advances. Publicly traded corporations make their financial status available in their annual reports, and academic researchers who receive federal funds will be listed in a catalog of awarded grants that can be solicited from federal granting agencies through the Freedom of Information Act. Well-funded academic laboratories are generally well known among their colleagues; however, well-funded private research groups may be less obvious. The best strategy for becoming part of a winning team is first to secure one's intellectual property and second to become obvious through published reports and presentations at professional meetings.

Partnering is yet another powerful indicator of technologies that are on the path toward successful commercialization. Partnering activities are monitored and reported in technology newsletters (e.g., *BioWorld*). Licensing activity is a close parallel to partnering. Edited reports on recent licensing agreements can be obtained through specialty industry research services (e.g., Recombinant Capital). Such reports have a dual function; they will inform a researcher where ideas are being marketed and they will also provide some realistic guidelines for terms under which such ideas are successfully marketed. Realistic expectations are an important part of successful commercialization.

Additional Assessments

Trends in society will often determine the success or failure of new practices and new products. Religious beliefs lead some individuals to reject vaccinations or pharmaceutical treatments. Beyond moral issues, the principal public policy debate will be focused on the questions of how much we are willing to pay to treat diseases that primarily affect the aged, how we will measure cost/benefit for an aged population, and who will pay for this treatment. The public policy debate surrounding the treatment of neurological disease will be intense, and for good reason: the stakes are huge. With up to 12 million patients suffering from various neurological diseases, the cost implications of the outcome will be enormous, and the growing size of this population will only exacerbate the situation. Currently, of the $400 billion total cost of CNS disease, approximately $40 billion is spent for direct medical costs to treat patients with organic neurological disorders (3). This works out to about $6700 per patient, per year. The fact is, current treatment options, while unsatisfactory, are relatively inexpensive. If more expensive early-stage interventions alleviate a more costly later-stage therapy, or allow patients to continue contributing to society, these expensive therapies are sure to replace less expensive, less effective therapies.

New therapies, if they are widely adopted, will cost significantly more than is currently being spent. And one of the few principles that all participants in the health care debate agree on is the concept of universal access to effective therapies. There will almost certainly be a much larger, *insured* population following health care reform. In addition, following reform there will be much less cost shifting: one organization, whether it is local or national, will be responsible for caring for all patients. This will dramatically concentrate the purchase of health care. What this will mean is that pharmacoeconomic analysis will become absolutely critical to the success of a new therapeutic.

For neurological diseases, this will not be an easy argument to make. Neurological diseases are not uniform in progression and are often not easily diagnosed. Alzheimer's disease, for example, currently can be confirmed only on autopsy. Therefore there will be a tremendous debate about who will receive treatment, how much the treatment should cost, and when patients should receive treatment. However, the tremendous cost of debilitating CNS disease should provide substantial opportunities to develop therapies that result in substantial net savings in health care costs.

However, there is little doubt that any health care reform package should provide broad coverage for older Americans, and provide access to breakthrough treatments for neurological disease. Older Americans are extremely well organized, vote around health care issues, and support their lobbying organizations through contributions and letter-writing campaigns. The political clout of AARP was well demonstrated when they rolled back the catastrophic health insurance plan passed by the Congress in 1989. The reimbursement environment will be amenable to efficacious treatments for neurological disease, but only after the costs and benefits of these treatments have been carefully reviewed.

The correct product to win public support will consist of an affordable, safe, convenient, chronic acting, locally effective, and removable delivery system or delivery approach.

Conclusion

Advances in molecular neurobiology have provided potential breakthrough opportunities for therapies for neurodegenerative disease. Most developments have occurred in the area of neurotrophic factors, which affect various aspects of neuronal function, neurite growth, and cell division. The behavior of these molecules can be influenced by the test conditions used to evaluate them, such that their biological roles need to be assessed in *in vivo* studies. For this reason, it is critical that methods to deliver these protein agents into the brain be developed and refined. The principal problem that confronts their study and application is their limited ability to pass through the blood–brain barrier and their potential to produce systemic side effects when administered chronically. For this reason, strategies must be developed that will allow researchers, and later clinicians, to deliver protein agents chronically into well-defined regions of the brain. The effective delivery of these trophic factors could result in a major breakthrough in the treatment of previously unmanageable neurological diseases. These objectives are recognized by a venture capital community that has poured millions of dollars into start-up companies to attacking neurodegenerative diseases. Consequently, the discovery and delivery of growth factors have become, and will remain, major focuses of research and development.

References

1. D. Calne, Treatment of Parkinson's disease. *N. Engl. J. Med.* **329,** 1021 (1993).
2. P. Friden, Delivery of nerve growth factor across the blood–brain barrier. *Neurodegenerative Dis., Adv. Ther. Dev. IBC USA Conf.,* Lake Beuna Vista, FL, 1993.
3. R. J. Rubin and W. A. Gold, "The Cost of Disorders of the Brain." Natl. Found. Brain Res., 1992.

Index

Accell particle bombardment
  for delivery of DNA, into target cells, 429–430
  mechanism, 428–429
  neuron and glial cells, 432–433
  in situ gene transfer, to primate adult brain tissue, 435–436
  and *ex vivo* gene transfer, transplantation comparison, 438
  in vivo and *in situ* gene transfer, of mammalian somatic tissues, 437
Acetylcholine, ^{3}H-labeled
  delivery to brain parenchyma, using polyanhydride microsphere system, 179
  production, using genetically engineered fibroblasts, 336–337
Adenoviral vectors, and herpes simplex virus type 1 vectors, comparison, 478
Adenylate cyclase, expression, in neurons, 457
Adrenal chromaffin cells
  bovine, xenograft preparation procedure, 349–350
  and immobilization matrices, aggregation inhibition, 387–388
  increased survival rate, using nerve growth factor, 152–153
  isolation procedure, from adrenal medulla in nonhuman primates, 258–261
  macroencapsulation process, 393–394
    cytotoxicity assay, to confirm immunoisolation, 395–396
    in vitro evaluation, 394–395
  microencapsulation process, 388–389
    assays to determine catecholamine release, 397–398
    coseeding, 392–393
    cytotoxicity assay, to confirm immunoisolation, 395–396
    in vitro evaluation, 394–395
  for neuropeptide and catecholamine delivery, into brain, 348
  open microsurgical implantation procedure, into nonhuman primates, 268–270
  survival rates, effect of peripheral nerve on, 261–262
Adrenalectomies, in nonhuman primates
  adrenal chromaffin cells isolation procedure, 258–261
  retroperitoneal approach, 254–256
  transabdominal approach, 256–258
Adrenal medulla
  allografts
    and microsphere-delivered nerve growth factor, effect on tissue, 156–158, 163–165
    and midbrain periaqueductal gray
      assessing neuropeptide and catecholamine delivery, 361–366
      implantation into, 358–361
    nerve growth factor augmentation, in Parkinson's disease treatment, 152
    preparation procedure, 349
    in spinal subarachnoid space, reduction of pain via catecholamine delivery, 356
  and caudate nucleus transplantation
    pretransplant neurosurgical procedure, 273–274
    tissue preparation, 274–276
  and cortex, dissection objectives, 274–275
Albumin, serum, immunoexpression, as indicator of blood–brain barrier permeability, 27–28
Alginate, and microencapsulation procedure, in adrenal chromaffin cells, 389–392
Alzet osmotic pump, *see also* Osmotic minipumps
  for continuous infusion of drugs, into central nervous system, 201
  preimplantation procedure, 206–207
  stereotaxic implantation, 209–210
Alzheimer's disease
  developing general therapies for, 490
  and nerve growth factor, therapeutic usages, 150
Amino acids
  delivery into central nervous system, 190–191

estimating concentration levels in brain, using radiolabeled compounds, 197–198
γ-Aminobutyric acid, in central nervous system neurons, determining penetration of, 30
Amplicons
components, 463
and helper virus, adjusting ratios between, 468–469
vectors
titering procedure, 471–472
in vivo expression of promotor mapping, 476–477
Angiogenesis, localization techniques, [^{3}H]thymidine autoradiography, 21–23
Antibodies, *see* Ascites antibody; IgG_{2a} antibody
Anti-bromodeoxyuridine immunocytochemistry, and endothelial cells, visualization, 24
Anti-laminin immunocytochemistry, and angiogenesis, visualization, 24–25
Ascites antibody, preparation and purification, for transcytosis studies, 98–101
Astrocytes
culture preparation procedure, for implantation into brain, 296–299
differentiation from endogenous astrocytes, 302–303
growth factor secretion, and neuron survival in central nervous system, 305
implantation procedure, 294–295
functional effects on central nervous system, 303–304
verification, using immunohistochemical techniques, 300–301
implanted cells versus endogenous cells, differentiation procedure, 302–303
role in brain homeostasis, 294
Astrocytomas, treatment, using BCNU, 135
Astrogliosis, from epidermal growth factor-responsive stem cells, tests to determine, 288
Axons
degeneration, 7
regeneration
double-labeling technique, 16–17
studies in optic nerve, 12–13
studies in spinal cord, 13–16

BCNU, *see* 1,3-Bis(2-chloroethyl)-1-nitrosourea
Biodegradable polymeric implants
biocompatibility and elimination processes, 172–173
for delivery of anticancer drugs, 172–173
1,3-Bis(2-chloroethyl)-1-nitrosourea
controlled release into 9L gliosarcomas, efficacy studies, 142–147
and controlled release polymers, incorporation procedure, 140–141
and EVAc, release rate, 141–142
incorporation procedure
with ethylene–vinyl acetate copolymer, 140–141
with PCPP-SA, 141
and treatment of astrocytomas, 135
Blood–brain barrier
and angiogenesis, 20
and chemical homeostasis in brain, 35–37
effect of hypertonic solutions, permeability after infusion, 39–40
and horseradish peroxidase, determination of permeability, 27
intracranial delivery of amino acids and peptides, using osmotic minipumps, 187–188
and lipophilic drugs, 169
and metabolite exchange, in central nervous system, 52–53
and neurotransmitters, systemic delivery, 489
osmotic disruption
and carotid artery, importance of correct solute infusion rate, 59–63
and chemotherapy for brain tumors, 45
in dog, surgical procedure for, 56–58
effect of anesthetic agents on, 63
effects of drug delivery, 64
in rat, surgical procedure for, 54–56
and polypeptide growth factors, permeability limitations, 281
transcytosis studies, identification of peroxidase reaction, 103–104
transport mechanisms, 169
vascular permeability
effect of hypertonic solutions on, 39–40
molecular charge effects, 43
molecular size effects, 40–43
using radiolabeled neurotransmitters, 27–28
Blood–cerebrospinal fluid–brain barrier, injury to, neurotrophic mechanisms, 10
Bovine adrenal chromaffin cells
and catecholamine release, from microencapsulation process, 398–400
and spinal subarachnoid space
implantation procedure, 350–351

neuropeptide and catecholamine levels in, 351–352
xenograft preparation procedure, 349–350
Brain
caudate nucleus, transplantation of adrenal medulla tissue into, 272–276
chemical homeostasis in, role of blood–brain barrier, 35–37
interstitial fluid, role in drug distribution, 188
microinjection technique
coordination verification procedure, 216–217
guide cannula and stylet preparation, 217–220
insertion of guide cannula, 221–222
and nerve growth factor, intracerebral delivery, *in vivo* release from microspheres, 156
and OX-26–NGF conjugate delivery process, 77–78
parenchyma, cell injection, for Parkinson's disease studies, 229–233
ventricular section, microinjection procedure, 226–227
Brain–tumor barrier, and chemotherapy for brain tumors, 44

Camptothecin, polymeric delivery, efficacy as brain cancer treatment, 177–178
Cannulas, *see also* Stereotaxic implantation
and continuous infusion systems, 202–204
for microinjection procedures
insertion steps, into brain, 221–222
preparation, 217–220
for osmotic minipump placement in rat, procedural steps, 193–196
Catecholamines
assays to determine levels, in spinal subarachnoid space, 355
delivery into midbrain periaqueductal gray, assessing delivery success, 361–366
and microencapsulation process, in adrenal chromaffin cells, assays, 397–398
Caudate nucleus, and adrenal medulla tissue, autologous transplantation, 272–273
Cell lines
genetic manipulation production, 322
immortalized
cell labeling, advantages of retrovirus markers versus microspheres, 316–317
creation procedure, general guidelines, 309–310
differentiation, determining target cell population, 315–316
establishment procedure, 310–313
selection and characterization procedure, 313–315
stereotaxic transplantation procedure, 318–320
Central nervous system
angiogenesis in, temporal sequence, 25–26
astrocyte implantation effects, behavioral recovery, 303–304
continuous infusion systems, advantages over repeated injections, 201
drug delivery methods, assessing commercial potential, 485–489
fibrous scarring, effect of transforming growth factor β_1, 16
injury to
cellular response, 3
neurotrophic response, molecular hybridization and immunochemical techniques, 8–9
role of astrocytes, 294
microvasculature, 188
neurotrophic factor delivery, using genetically modified cells, 329
regeneration failure, 7
Cerebral blood vessel labeling, for receptor-mediated probe molecule detection, 105–106
Cerebral cortex, injury to, cellular and trophic responses, 10–11
Cerebrospinal fluid
formation in choroid plexus, procedure, 188–189
solute penetration into brain, limiting factors, 189
Chemotherapy agents
and blood–brain barrier, efficacy of osmotic opening, 43–46
and controlled release polymers, criteria for selecting, 137–138
modifications to cross blood–brain barrier, 37–38
Choline acetyltransferase assay, in genetically modified fibroblasts, to determine ChAT activity, 334
Cholinergic neurons
effects of peripheral OX-26–NGF, in intraocular septal grafts, 84–86
and nerve growth factor, effect on, 151
Choroid plexus, and blood–brain barrier formation, 35–36
Continuous infusion systems
infusion device, construction
cannula, 202–204
connection piece, 204–205

platform, 205
siliconization procedure, 206
infusion protocols, 208–209
stereotaxic surgery for, in rat, 209–210
Controlled release polymers
advantages, in drug delivery to central nervous system, 135–136
and chemotherapeutic agents, criteria for selecting, 137–138
criteria for selecting, importance of degradation ability, 136–137
Cortex, and adrenal medulla, dissection objectives, 274–275
Cytarabine
and DepoFoam, synthesis with, 119
half-life increases, in central nervous system, 130

Defective herpes simplex virus type 1, *see* Herpes simplex virus type 1, defective
DepoFoam
and cerebrospinal fluid, water-soluble molecule delivery, 118
encapsulation procedure
cytarabine, 119
interferon α, 120–121
methotrexate, 119
morphine sulfate, 119–120
DepoFoam-Encapsulated Ara-C, *see* DTC 101
DepoFoam-encapsulated methotrexate, intracisternal central nervous system pharmacokinetics, in rats, 124–127
Depression, catecholamine imbalance in, restoration with implanted chromaffin cells, 349
Dimethyl sulfoxide, and blood–brain barrier permeability, 53
Dopamine, *see also* Parkinson's disease
deafferentation of, effect of nigral grafts, 238–239
increased production, from adrenal medulla transplant to caudate nucleus, 272–273
Double-labeling technique, and axon regeneration, in central nervous system injury, 16–17
DTC 101
intralumbar central nervous system pharmacokinetics, in monkeys, 123–124
intraventricular central nervous system pharmacokinetics
in humans, 128–130
in rats, 122–123

Electron microscopy
microcapsules, wall structure examinations, 376–377
and vascular sprouts, 25
Endothelial cells, visualization of, using anti-bromodeoxyuridine immunochemistry, 24
Endothelium, nonfenestrated, role in blood–brain barrier, 93
Engineered cells, genetically, fibroblasts
acetylcholine production, neurotrophic delivery procedure, 336–340
preparation and grafting, for neurotransmitter delivery to brain, 341–344
production of nerve growth factor, 332–333
in vitro development and characterization, 331–332
Epidermal growth factor-responsive neural stem cells
cell differentiation procedure, 283–284
differentiation and survival rates, mouse cerebral cortex, 289–290
identification of donor cells
genetic tagging, 290–292
role of marked glial cells, 290–292
myelinating oligodendrocytes formation, 285–288
for neurodegenerative diseases, treatment for, 281–282
production and *in vitro* characterization, 283
in vitro formation, of mature oligodendrocytes, 285
Ethylene–vinyl acetate copolymer
advantages, in drug delivery across blood–brain barrier, 136–137
biocompatibility and toxicity studies, in rat brain, 142
fabrication and drug incorporation, 140–141
interstitial delivery of BCNU into central nervous system, 141–144
release rate of BCNU, *in vivo* determinations, 141–142, 145
EVAc, *see* Ethylene–vinyl acetate copolymer

Ferrotransferrin
and macromolecule delivery, across blood–brain barrier, 94
preparation and application, for transcytosis studies, 96
receptor-mediated endocytosis of, in cell, 95
transcytosis studies, peroxidase conjugation, 96–97

Ferrotransferrin–HRP conjugate, transendothelial transfer, across blood–brain barrier, 106
Fibroblasts, genetic modification
  choline acetyltransferase assay, to determine ChAT activity, 334
  lacZ transgene identification, 334–335
  nerve growth factor production, immunoassay to determine, 332–333
  for neurotransmitter delivery to brain
    immunohistochemical staining, 344–346
    preparation and grafting procedure, 341–343
    using *in vivo* microdialysis, 340–341
  neurotrophic factor delivery, for acetylcholine production, 336–340
  verification of transgene expression, 332
  in vitro development and characterization, 331–332
Fimbria–fornix lesions, and genetically engineered fibroblasts, implantation of, 337

GABA, *see* γ-Aminobutyric acid
β-Galactosidase, and immortalized cell lines, for cell labeling in, 316–317
GelFoam, and astrocyte implantation into brain, 299–300
Gene therapy, using neurotrophic factors, for treatment of Alzheimer's disease, 449–450
Genetic intervention
  in neurons, using HSV-1 vectors, 443–445
  recombinant protein design, 445
Gene transfer
  in fibroblasts, retroviral infection method, 331–332
  in neurons, using herpes simplex virus vectors, 462
  using Accell particle bombardment device, 428–431
Glia cells, *see also* Astrocytes; Oligodendrocytes
  and central nervous system regeneration failure, 7
  gene transfer into, using pHSVlac, 453–454
Glial-derived neurotrophic factor, effect on Parkinson's disease, reducing progression, 493–494
Glial fibrillary acidic protein, and astrocyte detection, in central nervous system, 4–5
Glial limitans
  and central nervous system, injury to, 5
  and reestablishment of blood–brain barrier, 304
Gliosarcomas, 9L
  and BCNU and controlled release polymers, pharmacokinetic studies, 141
  controlled release of BCNU, efficacy studies, 142–147
  and interstitial drug delivery studies, across blood–brain barrier, 139–140
Golgi complex, and OX-26–HRP conjugate, trafficking across blood–brain barrier, 111–115

Helper virus
  and amplicon virus, adjusting ratios between, 468–469
  titering, using plaque assay, 469–470
Hematoxylin–eosin stain, and immunoisolation devices, histological analysis, 409–410
Hemorrhage, acute, in central nervous system, from injury, 3
Herpes simplex virus type 1, defective
  IE gene expression, cytotoxicity, 479
  quantitation of defective viral genomes, slot-blot technique, 472
  wild-type, titering, using plaque assay, 469–470
Herpes simplex virus vectors
  advantages, for gene transfer into neurons, 450–452
  expression of β-galactosidase, 474–475
  gene therapy, for Parkinson's disease, 448–449
  and genetic intervention, in brain, 443–445
  gene transfer into neurons, 462, 475
  packaging, 464–465
  pHSVlac, gene transfer into neurons, 453
  recombinant, establishment of latent infection in postmitotic neurons, 479
  and *in vivo* alteration of adult mammalian brain, 446–447
Hippocampus, slice cultures, β-galactosidase expression, using amplicon-based herpes simplex virus type 1 vectors, 474–475
Histochemical imaging, *see* Horseradish peroxidase
Horseradish peroxidase
  conjugation
    ferrotransferrin, for transcytosis studies, 96–97
    IgG_{2a} antibody, procedure for, 102
    OX-26 antibody, procedure, 102
  and endothelial organelles, detection in, 107–109
  histochemical detection, as indicator of blood–brain barrier permeability, 27
HSV-1, *see* Herpes simplex virus type 1
Hydrogels, and immobilization matrices, 387

Hydrophilic drugs, and interstitial delivery into central nervous system, 138
4-Hydroxycyclophosphamide, and controlled release polymers, interstitial delivery into central nervous system, 138
6-Hydroxydopamine, and catecholamine neuron destruction, studies to mimick dopamine loss, 341–342
Hypercapnia, effect on blood–brain barrier, osmotic disruption, 63
Hypertonic solutions, and blood–brain barrier, osmotic disruption, 39–40
  in rat, 54–56

IgG_{2a} antibody, peroxidase conjugation, for transcytosis studies, 102
Immobilization matrix
  in adrenal chromaffin cells, aggregation inhibition, 387–388
  preparation procedure, 389–390
Immortalized cell lines
  cell labeling, advantages of retrovirus markers versus microspheres, 316–317
  creation procedure for, general guidelines, 309–310
  differentiation, determining target cell population, 315–316
  establishment procedure, 310–313
  selection and characterization, 313–315
  stereotaxic transplantation procedure, 318–320
Immunocytochemistry techniques
  anti-bromodeoxyuridine, and endothelial cells, visualization, 24
  anti-laminin, and angiogenesis, visualization, 24–25
  and genetically engineered fibroblasts, transgene identification in, 335
Immunohistochemical staining, for ferrotransferrin receptor detection, in rat brain, 102–103
Immunoisolation devices
  biological compatibility, with host tissue, 408–409
  histological analysis, using hematoxylin–eosin stain, 409–410
  and xenograft survival, membrane structure reproduction, 404
Implantable systems, polymer-based, advantages, as compared with systemically administered systems, 170
Infusate, and Azlet osmotic pumps, 207
Intercostal nerves, resection procedure for, 262
Interferon α, and DepoFoam, synthesis with, 120–121
Interstitial fluid, brain, role in drug distribution, 188
Intracerebroventricular delivery, of peptides, using graft, comparison with microinjection method, 190–191
Intracerebroventricular injection, microinjection, comparison with graft, 188–189
Intraocular septal transplants
  and cholinergic neurons, effects of peripheral OX-26–NGF, 84–86
  effects of peripheral OX-26–NGF, 84–86
  and OX-26–NGF conjugate, effect of doses, 80–82
Iron, role in cellular metabolism, 95
Iron–transferrin complex, and drug delivery, across blood–brain barrier, 72–73

Laminin, expression, using immunocytochemical localization, 24
Light microscopy, of microcapsules, cell localization in, 378

Macroencapsulation, methodologies, in adrenal chromaffin cells, 393–394
Magnetic resonance imaging, for target localization, in adrenal chromaffin cell transplantation, 264–265
Matrix, immobolization, *see* Immobolization matrix
Mesencephalon, and dopamine cell bodies, lesioning of, 227–229
Methotrexate
  and DepoFoam, synthesis with, 119
  dextran conjugates, delivery into brain, antitumor treatment, 175
  intracisternal injection, unencapsulated, comparison with encapsulated, 127
Microcapsules
  cellular preparation, 388–389
  cellular viability, MTT assay, 378–379, 381–384
  encapsulation procedure, 375
    advantages, compared with basic grafts, 371
    necessary materials, 372–375
Microdialysis, of genetically engineered fibroblasts, site-specific neurotransmitter delivery into brain, 340–341

Microinjection
biologically active substances
into brain
advantages, versus systemic delivery, 214–215
coordinate verification procedure, 216–217
diffusion limitations, 215
guide cannula and stylet preparation, 217–220
injection procedure, 222–226
into brain ventricles, injection procedure, 226–227
peptides, comparison with intracerebroventricular delivery method, 190–191
Microscopy, *see* Electron microscopy; Light microscopy
Microspheres
characteristics and release process, 159
and nerve growth factor, *in vitro* and *in vivo* release, 159159–162
preparation procedure, 154–155
in vitro dopamine delivery, for Parkinson's disease, 179
Midbrain periaqueductal gray, and adrenal medullary allografts
implantation procedure, 358–361
morphological analysis, to determine integration, 366
neuropeptide and catecholamine delivery, assessment, 361–366
Minipumps, osmotic, *see* Osmotic minipumps
Morphine sulfate, and DepoFoam, encapsulation procedure, 119–120
Morphological analysis
adrenal medullary allografts, in midbrain periaqueductal gray, 366
spinal subarachnoid–adrenal medullary graft relationship, 355–358
Multiple sclerosis, cell therapy applications for, 282

Nerve growth factor
and cholinergic neurons
degenerative prevention, 151
regeneration, 71–72
delivery across blood–brain barrier, 73
expression, using herpes simplex virus type 1 vectors, 475–476
HSV-1 mediated delivery, for choline acetyltransferase increase, 450
intracerebral delivery
determining *in vivo* release, 155–156, 162
using osmotic pump, advantages, 153
osmotic delivery methods, 153
and regeneration of septal cholinergic neurons, 336
verification of production, in genetically modified fibroblasts, 332–333
Neural stem cells, epidermal growth factor–responsive, *see* Epidermal growth factor–responsive neural stem cells
Neurodegenerative diseases, developing general therapies for, 490
Neurons
cholinergic, *see* Cholinergic neurons
death, pharmacological measures to prevent, 17
degeneration, effect of proteases on, 7–8
effect of chemotherapeutic drugs on, 44
effects of astrocytes on, 304
embryonic nigral, cellular interactions of, *in vitro* cultures, 2446–247
gene transfer into, using defective HSV-1 vector system, 450–452
nigral, clinical origins, 238–239
and osmotic pumps, for studies of neurotrophic factors, 211–212
physiology alterations, from unregulated adenylate cyclase, 457
septal cholinergic, role in cognitive deterioration, in Alzheimer's patients, 336
Neuropeptides
assays to determine levels, after bovine chromaffin cell implants, in spinal subarachnoid space, 352–354
delivery into midbrain periaqueductal gray, assessing delivery, 361–366
Neurotrophic factors, glial-derived, *see* Glial-derived neurotrophic factor
Nigral grafts, embryonic
cell suspension graft procedure, into brain, 240–242
clinical origins, 238–239
transplantation limitations, 240
strategies for improvement, 242–243
in vivo intracerebral, 248–249
Nondegradable polymer implants, for drug delivery into brain, 171–172
Nonfenestrated endothelium, role in blood–brain barrier, 93

Oligodendrocytes
mature, *in vitro* formation, from epidermal growth factor-responsive stem cells, 285
myelinating, *in vivo* formation, from epidermal growth factor-responsive stem cells, 285–288
transgene expression pattern, using Accell particle bombardment, 433–434
Oncogenes, *lacZ* identification assay, in genetically engineered fibroblasts, 334–335
Optic nerve, and axon regeneration studies, 12–13
Osmotic minipumps, *see* Alzet osmotic pumps
advantages, for *in vivo* studies, 191
and amino acids and peptides, intracranial delivery, 187–188
implantation, surgical procedure, 192–193
and nerve growth factor, intracerebral delivery into brain, 153
and neurons, for studies of trophic factors, 211–212
peptides, amino acids, and drugs infused with, 194–195
placement in rat
cannula insertion, verification procedure, 196–197
procedure for third ventricular cannulation, 193–194
OX-26, peroxidase conjugation, for transcytosis studies, 102
OX-26–NGF conjugate
antibody formation, immunoassays to determine, 87–89
biological activity, PC-12 assay to determine, 75–77
delivery into blood–brain barrier, 73
intraocular transplantation
blood–brain barrier formation, assay to confirm, 78–80
effect on cholinergic neurons, 80–82, 84–87
procedure, 73–74
visualization in brain vasculature, 77–78
production process, 74–75

Parkinson's disease, *see also* Dopamine
and adrenal medullary grafts, nerve growth factor augmentation, 152
attempts to prevent neuronal degeneration, 495
cell therapy applications for, 282
cellular replacement therapy, 494
effect of glial-derived neurotrophic factor, progression cessation, 493–494
effects of caudate nucleus transplanted with adrenal medulla tissue, 272–273
and embryonic nigral neurons, treatment using, 238–239
experiments using nonhuman primates, striatal grafting and cografting, 263–264
palliative therapy for, 492–493
treatment for, using transplantation of mesencephalic tissue, 436
and tyrosine hydroxylase, cell transplantation production, 431–432
in vitro dopamine release, using polyanhydride microsphere system, 179–180
PC-12 cells
intracerebral transplantation, into Parkinson's patients, 321
neurite outgrowth assay, to determine nerve growth factor biological activity, 75–77
and OX-26–NGF conjugate, determining biological activity, 75–77
PCPP-SA
advantages, in drug delivery across blood–brain barrier, 136–137
fabrication and drug incorporation, 140–141
neural biocompatibility, 142
release rate of BCNU, 145–147
Pentylenetetrazol, and blood–brain barrier permeability, 53
Peptides, estimating concentration levels in brain, using radiolabeled compounds, 197–198
Peripheral nerves
effect on survival of adrenal chromaffin cells, 261–262
intercostal nerve resection, for use with adrenal chromaffin cells, 262
sural nerve resection, for use with adrenal chromaffin cells, 263
Peripheral nervous system, angiogenesis in, temporal sequence, 25–26
Peroxidase immunohistochemistry, for trophic mechanisms, after central nervous system injury, 9
Phagocytes, role in blood–brain barrier, 93
Pheochromocytoma cells, *see* PC-12 cells
pHSVlac
expression of β-galactosidase, 455
for gene transfer into neurons and glia, 453–454
Polyanhydride microsphere system
and delivery of neurotransmitters, 178–180

and [^{3}H]acetylcholine, delivery to brain parenchyma, 179
Polyanhydrides, and anticancer agents, for treatment of brain cancer, 173–174
Poly[bis(*p*-carboxyphenoxy)]propane–sebacic acid copolymer, *see* PCPP-SA
Polymeric formulations, biodegradable
advantages, for systemic delivery of drugs, 153–154
intracerebral nerve growth factor delivery, preparation procedure, 154–155
and microspheres, *in vivo* release of nerve growth factor, 156–157
Polymer implants, nondegradable, for treatment of brain cancer, 171–172
Polymers, controlled release
advantages, in drug delivery to central nervous system, 135–136
and chemotherapeutic agent, criteria for selecting, 137–138
criteria for selecting, importance of degradation ability, 136–137
Polymer systems
for drug delivery, desirable characteristics, 170–171
drug release from, steps in, 171
Polypeptide growth factors, and blood–brain barrier, permeability limitations, 281
Primates, nonhuman
adrenalectomies in
retroperitoneal approach, 254–256
transabdominal approach, 256–258
experimental parkinsonian syndromes in, striatal grafting and cografting procedure, 263–264
open microsurgical implantation procedure, of adrenal chromaffin cells, 268–270
peripheral nerve harvesting in, 261–262
stereotaxic implantation procedure, of adrenal chromaffin cells, 264–267
Proteases, and neural degeneration, 7–8
Proteins, recombinant, design for genetic intervention in brain, 445

Recombinant proteins, design, for genetic intervention in brain, 445
Recombinant vectors, cytotoxicity, 479
Reporter genes, human growth hormone, for detection of DNA transfection, 472
Retroviral vectors
and central nervous system, studies via mitotic neurons infection, 477–478
and gene expression, comparison with adenovirus vectors, 478
Ribonuclease protection assay, for trophic mechanisms, in central nervous system injury, 8
Rostral mesencephalic tegmental cells, injection into cells, procedure, 233

Septohippocampal system
neurotransmitter delivery, into brain, *in vivo* microdialysis, 340–341
role in cognitive deterioration, in Alzheimer's patients, 336
Sink action, of solutes in cerebrospinal fluid, 189
Slot-blot technique, for quantitation of defective viral genomes, in defective herpes simplex virus type 1, 472
Spinal cord, and axon regeneration studies, 13–16
Spinal subarachnoid space
implantation of adrenal chromaffin cells
catecholamine levels after, 355
neuropeptide levels after, 352–354
procedure, 350–351
morphological analysis, to determine host–graft relationship, 355–357
Stereotaxic implantation
adrenal chromaffin cells, into nonhuman primates, 264–265
continuous infusion systems, in rat, 209–210
Stereotaxic transplantation, of immortalized cell lines, 318–320
Striatum, dopamine loss in, effect on Parkinson's patients, 341
Substantia nigra, and striatum, role in GABA delivery to brain, 341
Sural nerves, resection procedure, for use with adrenal chromaffin cells, 263
Systemic delivery, of biologically active substances, into brain, comparison with microinjection procedure, 214–215

Taxol, efficacy in brain tumor treatment, 175–176
[^{3}H]Thymidine autoradiography, and angiogenesis, visualization of, 21–23
Transabdominal approach, for adrenalectomies, in nonhuman primates, 256–258

Transcytosis
  ferrotransferrin
    peroxidase conjugation, 96–97
    preparation and application, 96
  receptor-mediated
    ferrotransferrin delivery across blood–brain barrier, 94
    and nerve growth factor, delivery across blood–brain barrier, 73
Transferrin
  and drug delivery, across blood–brain barrier, 72–73
  and iron transport, into central nervous system, 95
Transferrin receptors, effects on peripheral systems, 86–87
Transforming growth factor β_1, and fibrotic scarring in central nervous system, 16
Tyrosine hydroxylase
  expression in strial cells, 460
  and Parkinson's disease, 432
    infusion into neurons and glia, 449
  transgenic expression, for Parkinson's disease treatment, 436–437

Vascular sprouts, electron microscopic visualization of, 25
Vectors, *see also* Herpes simplex virus vectors; Retroviral vectors; Viral vectors
  recombinant, cytotoxicity, 479
Ventromesencephalon tissue
  cell suspension
    determining surviving dopaminergic neurons, 243–244
    preparation method, 242–243
  and vital stains, viability of cell suspension determinations, 245–246
  in vivo neural graft, 244–245
Viral vectors
  amplicon-based
    packaging, reagents needed for, 464–465
    passaging procedure, 467
    titering procedure, 471–472
  retroviral, and central nervous system, studies via mitotic neuron infection, 477–478
Vital stains, and ventromesencephalon tissue, viability of cell suspensions in, 245–246
VM, *see* Ventromesencephalon tissue

WGA–HRP conjugate, transcellular transfer, across blood–brain barrier, 111–114

Xenografts, encapsulated
  cell growth, nutrient flux measurements, 415–416
  implantation devices
    stereotaxic equipment, 417–419
    testing for sterility and endotoxins, 416–417
  measuring dosages from, 414–415
  survival rates, role of immunoisolation devices, 404–407
  validating safety of transplantable cell sources, 413–414